# REVIEW
## OF
## BASIC SCIENCE
## AND
## CLINICAL DENTISTRY

Volume II | Clinical Dentistry

Edited by

## JACK E. WELLS, D.D.S., M.S.D.

Dean, College of Dentistry,
University of Tennessee Center for the Health Sciences,
Memphis, Tennessee

## MARVIN WALLACE REED, D.D.S., M.S.

Professor and Chairman,
Department of Graduate Pedodontics,
School of Dentistry, University of Missouri,
Kansas City, Missouri

## VICTOR M. COURY, D.ED.

Professor and Chairman, Department of Behavioral Science,
University of Tennessee Center for the Health Sciences,
College of Dentistry, Memphis, Tennessee

With 25 Contributors

HARPER & ROW, PUBLISHERS
PHILADELPHIA

| Cambridge | | London |
| New York | | Mexico City |
| Hagerstown |  | São Paulo |
| San Francisco | | Sydney |

*1817*

# REVIEW OF BASIC SCIENCE AND CLINICAL DENTISTRY

Volume II | Clinical Dentistry

10

**Library of Congress Cataloging in Publication Data**

Main entry under title:
Review of basic science and clinical dentistry.
  Includes index.
  CONTENTS: v. 1 Basic science.—v. 2. Clinical dentistry.
  1. Dentistry.   2. Dentistry—Examinations, questions, etc.   3. American Association of Dental Examiners—Examinations.   I. Wells, Jack E.   II. Reed, Marvin W.   III. Coury, Victor M.
  RK51.R47      617.6′0076      79-27347
  ISBN 0-06-142657-1 (v. 1)
  ISBN 0-06-142658-X (v. 2)

The authors and publisher have exerted every effort to ensure that drug selection and dosage set forth in this text are in accord with current recommendations and practice at the time of publication. However, in view of ongoing research, changes in government regulations, and the constant flow of information relating to drug therapy and drug reactions, the reader is urged to check the package insert for each drug for any change in indications and dosage and for added warnings and precautions. This is particularly important when the recommended agent is a new and/or infrequently employed drug.

# CONTENTS

# CONTRIBUTORS

**Thomas G. Berry, D.D.S., M.A.**

*Chapter 5*

Associate Dean and Professor, Restorative Dentistry, School of Dentistry, University of Colorado, Denver, Colorado

**Diane M. Brown, Ed.D.**

*Chapter 1*

Assistant Professor and Assistant Chairman, Department of Behavioral Science, and Coordinator of Dental Biostatistics, College of Dentistry, The University of Tennessee Center for the Health Sciences, Memphis, Tennessee

**Victor M. Coury, D.Ed.**

*Chapter 1*

Professor and Chairman, Department of Behavioral Science, College of Dentistry, The University of Tennessee Center for the Health Sciences, Memphis, Tennessee

**Henry W. Fields, Jr., D.D.S., M.S., M.S.D.**

*Chapter 7*

Assistant Professor, Department of Pedodontics and Orthodontics, University of North Carolina, Chapel Hill, North Carolina

**Willard G. Fischer, D.D.S.**

*Chapter 12*

Associate Professor, Department of Diagnostic Services, School of Dental Medicine, University of Pittsburgh, Pittsburgh, Pennsylvania

**James F. Gardiner, D.D.S., M.P.H.**

*Chapter 4*

Associate Professor, Department of Community and Preventive Dentistry, School of Dentistry, Louisiana State University, New Orleans, Louisiana

**Bal K. Goyal, B.D.S., M.D.S.**

*Chapter 6*

Assistant Professor, Department of Restorative Dentistry, School of Dental Medicine, University of Pennsylvania, Philadelphia, Pennsylvania

**David F. Greer, D.M.D., M.S.D.**

*Chapter 13*

Associate Professor of Dentistry, Department of Dental Radiology, School of Dentistry, University of Alabama, Birmingham, Alabama

**James L. Gutmann, D.D.S.**

*Chapter 9*

Associate Professor and Chairman, Department of Endodontics, Baltimore College of Dental Surgery, Dental School, University of Maryland, Baltimore, Maryland

**James E. Hardigan, Ph.D.**

*Chapter 16*

Assistant to the Dean for Administration and Assistant Professor, School of Dentistry, Virginia Commonwealth University, Medical College of Virginia, Richmond, Virginia

**John H. Hembree, Jr., D.D.S.**

*Chapter 2*

Professor and Chairman, Department of Operative Dentistry, College of Dental Medicine, Medical University of South Carolina, Charleston, South Carolina

**Carole N. Hildebrand, D.D.S., M.Ed.**

*Chapter 10*

Associate Professor, Department of Periodontology, School of Dentistry, Temple University, Philadelphia, Pennsylvania

**Kenneth P. Hopkins, D.D.S.**

*Chapter 11*

Chief, Department of Dental Services, St. Jude Children's Research Hospital, Memphis, Tennessee, and Associate Professor, Department of Oral Pathology, College of Dentistry, The University of Tennessee Center for the Health Sciences, Memphis, Tennessee

**Benjamin J. Legett, Jr., D.D.S., M.P.H.**

*Chapter 4*

Associate Professor and Head, Department of Community and Preventive Dentistry, School of Dentistry, Louisiana State University, New Orleans, Louisiana

**Robert M. Little, D.D.S., M.S.D., Ph.D.**

*Chapter 8*

Associate Professor, Department of Orthodontics, School of Dentistry, University of Washington, Seattle, Washington

**J. Bernard Machen, D.D.S., M.S., Ph.D.**

*Chapter 7*

Associate Professor, Department of Pedodontics, School of Dentistry, University of North Carolina, Chapel Hill, North Carolina

**Lincoln R. Manson-Hing, D.M.D., M.S.**

*Chapter 13*

Professor and Chairman, Department of Dental Radiology, School of Dentistry, University of Alabama, Birmingham, Alabama

**F. Thomas McIver, D.D.S., M.S.**

*Chapter 7*

Associate Professor, Department of Pedodontics, Pedodontic Section Head, Division for Disorders of Development and Learning, School of Dentistry, University of North Carolina, Chapel Hill, North Carolina

**Clifford H. Miller, D.D.S.**

*Chapter 3*

Associate Dean and Clinical Coordinator, Department of Administration, Northwestern University Dental School, Chicago, Illinois

**Thomas J. Pallasch, D.D.S., M.S.**

*Chapter 15*

Associate Professor of Pharmacology and Periodontics, and Chairman, Pharmacology Section, School of Dentistry, University of Southern California, Los Angeles, California

**Marvin E. Revzin, D.D.S.**

*Chapter 14*

Dean and Professor of Oral and Maxillofacial Surgery, School of Dentistry, University of Missouri, Kansas City, Missouri

**Leslie M. Salkin, D.D.S., M.Ed.**

*Chapter 10*

Associate Professor, Department of Periodontology, School of Dentistry, Temple University, Philadelphia, Pennsylvania

**Terry R. Wallen, D.D.S., M.S.D.**

*Chapter 8*

Assistant Professor, Department of Orthodontics, School of Dentistry, University of Washington, Seattle, Washington

**Gerald S. Weintraub, D.D.S.**

*Chapter 6*

Associate Professor and Assistant Chairman, Department of Restorative Dentistry, and Director of Removable Prosthodontics, School of Dental Medicine, University of Pennsylvania, Philadelphia, Pennsylvania

**Joseph K. Wittemann, Ph.D.**

*Chapter 16*

Associate Professor, Department of Community Dentistry, and Director, Office of Educational Evaluation, Planning, and Research, Medical College of Virginia, Virginia Commonwealth University, Richmond, Virginia

# PREFACE

At present, over 50% of the licensing jurisdictions require candidates to pass Parts I and II of the National Board Examinations. The American Association of Dental Examiners assists by distributing an outline of the subject matter covered in the questions contributed by each of the 59 dental schools. Therefore, one can say that the National Board Examinations survey aspects of American dental school curricula.

Dental educators are interested in the knowledge and skills taught in other schools as well as in sharing their own most recent academic developments. Such faculty are generally dedicated and committed individuals who strive not only to impart the "common body of biologic knowledge," but also to develop in dental students the skills and attitudes needed to deliver excellent oral health care.

However, basic science educators feel a sense of frustration. Owing to a knowledge explosion in the basic sciences as related to dentistry during the past decade, members of faculty feel that they are proceeding faster than the students are assimilating the material. Their concern is that, with little time for review, students do not retain enough content. This situation leads to *memorization* as opposed to *comprehension*. Yet, the students themselves are aware that memorization is not the approach best suited for the problem-oriented examination questions.

Dental students like to compare performances with other dental students who take the Boards. Correspondingly, they are proud of their alma mater and want their schools to compare favorably with other schools.

The primary emphasis of this volume of *Review of Basic Science and Clinical Dentistry* is to present specific content areas covered by Part II of the National Board Examinations. Authors who are well-versed in the basic principles and current practices in dentistry have been selected to write on content areas as presented in the outline from the American Association of Dental Examiners. When a dental topic is covered in more than one test, the authors will identify this distribution of content. To illustrate, the chapter on Biomaterials will incorporate the related areas in Operative Dentistry and Prosthodontics. The chapter on

Community and Preventive Dentistry will deal with DAU-TEAM which is covered in Operative Dentistry, and with diet, nutrition, and preventive dentistry which are covered in Operative Dentistry, Pedodontics, and Periodontics. The chapter on Behavioral Sciences will discuss aspects of child and parent psychology, the handicapped child, recognition of fear, methods of management, and psychological aspects of temporomandibular joint dysfunction. Further, the authors have incorporated into each chapter representative questions similar to the National Board questions, which present difficult cases and complex problems.

The authors also stress the need for students to have a positive attitude, self-confidence, and mental readiness for the problem-solving questions. A student can study this volume from the viewpoint of comprehension instead of memorization—that is, by synthesizing the principles of the basic sciences. Students may still discover content which they have not covered when they take the National Board Examinations, but they should not rationalize their lack of knowledge by blaming the faculty. Instead, they should acknowledge that there are deficiencies in their storehouse of information and accept responsibility for remedying these deficiencies.

The editors hope that this volume will reinforce existing knowledge, upgrade the present level of education in dental students, and increase self-confidence and self-respect. It will prepare students to undertake the National Board, and Regional and State Licensing examinations.

A note to the practitioner: to justify legally one's position as an expert, a practicing dentist must maintain a practical knowledge of his or her profession relative to biologic dentistry. There have been remarkable developments in dentistry over the past ten years; diagnosis, treatment, and the approach to treatment are significantly different now. For those who may be required to take state board dental examinations for relicensing, this volume will be a friend. It will be equally valuable in assessing one's own knowledge in terms of both past and present norms.

JACK E. WELLS, D.D.S., M.S.D.
MARVIN WALLACE REED, D.D.S., M.S.
VICTOR M. COURY, D.Ed.

# REVIEW
# OF
# BASIC SCIENCE
# AND
# CLINICAL DENTISTRY

Volume II | Clinical Dentistry

# 1

# HOW TO PREPARE FOR AND TAKE THE NATIONAL BOARDS:

## SELF-ACTIVATION IS THE KEY TO SUCCESS

### Diane M. Brown  /  Victor M. Coury

Because adequate and effective dental service must take into account biologic needs, students must develop a working knowledge of oral–systemic relationships in both health and disease, of the biologic significance of preventive, restorative, and prosthetic services, and of the interdependence of the dental practitioner and physician in coping with the total health needs of the patient and community. Societal trends, which assist the dental educator in the identification of dental requirements, are making the following demands upon the practitioner: 1) the individual must demonstrate in practice a thorough understanding of the structures, functions, and diseases of the mouth; 2) the individual must be able to deliver dental treatment according to published criteria for acceptable dental procedures; and 3) the individual must be able to defend the dental treatment.

It is generally agreed that the dental graduate must be able to meet certain basic objectives. For example, the graduate must be able to

1. Develop a sound diagnosis and treatment plan
2. Perform acceptable restorative procedures
3. Detect, diagnose, and manage an oral cancer patient
4. Evaluate the safety in use of dental materials
5. Detect, diagnose, and treat periodontal problems
6. Manage a dental emergency
7. Adjust occlusion for oral harmony
8. Administer myofunctional therapy for temporomandibular joint (TMJ) disorders
9. Establish safeguards against mercury vaporization, radiation scatter, and transference of hepatitis
10. Utilize auxiliaries efficiently
11. Manage dental office personnel
12. Manage patients according to established principles of human behavior

The National Board Dental Examinations aid in the evaluation of these abilities by attempting to 1) survey and evaluate the curricula of dental schools, 2) offer each student the results as to the level of his or her basic knowledge of dentistry in comparison to the national population of dental students, and 3) assess the problem-solving abilities of students. The National Board Examinations, which cover the material taught in all 59 dental colleges, are divided into two sections, the second of which has seven tests.

PART II
Operative Dentistry
Pharmacology
Prosthodontics
Oral Surgery and Pain Control
Orthodontics and Pedodontics
Oral Pathology and Radiography
Endodontics and Periodontics

Students taking Part II should be aware that the examination on Operative Dentistry includes preventive dentistry, auxiliary utilization, TEAM, dental materials, disease control, and occlusion, as well as operative dentistry. The examination on Prosthodontics includes dental materials, occlusion, partial dentures, fixed bridges, and complete dentures.

A revision in National Board regulations allows a student who fails one or more examinations to take a reexamination in individual subjects only if the student's average score is 75 or higher. Students who earn average scores below 75 are required to repeat the entire part. For example, scores of 85, 75, 78, 60, 82, 76, and 70 on the seven parts of Part II indicate that the student passed five of the seven tests. The average of these seven tests, however, is 74; the student is therefore required to repeat the entire examination.

Presently, 28 of 53 licensing jurisdictions require a student to pass both Parts I and II to be a licensed dentist. All portions of Part I must be passed before a student may take Part II; there are no exceptions.

## CAN YOU PREPARE YOURSELF TO TAKE THE NATIONAL BOARD EXAMINATIONS?

Yes, you certainly can. Although this volume is not a complete dental education in itself, it is a high quality review.

To prepare for the tests you must motivate yourself and get into a frame of mind for learning. It has been demonstrated that studies initiated and pursued by an individual with a clear goal in mind are the most successful. Self-motivation is a key to success. This volume will give you the self-confidence you need to succeed.

This book will also give you the feel of the examinations. The content in this volume follows the content outline of the National Boards. The practice questions are problem-solving, multiple choice questions similar to those found in the National Boards. In answering them you will add to your knowledge by learning the correct answers. This will help you to remember much you thought you had forgotten.

There is no substitute for knowledge in the specific content areas; test-taking technique or guessing will not earn a passing score. This review will test your level of knowledge by assessing your areas of strength and weakness. Weak content areas can be explored further for new learning.

## WHAT IS THE BEST WAY TO PREPARE FOR THE NATIONAL BOARD EXAMINATIONS?

The best general rule for taking any examination is to "be prepared." This means having a thorough mastery of the material and having it so well organized that you can recall it in any form requested. It means being prepared for the kind of examination you are to take and for all possible questions. It means being rested and calm.

Some students prefer to review alone, while others prefer to study in groups. Small study groups of five or six students can be beneficial, since social learning tends to promote self-esteem and self-confidence. Groups should be a mixture of average and bright students in order for this to occur. Each student needs to discover that he or she is capable of selecting correct answers. Students should practice with diagnostic- and problem-type questions from this volume and from released National Boards. Each of the alternative answers should be discussed so that you understand *why* one answer is correct and others wrong.

Reprints of the most recently released National Boards are available through the American Student Dental Association (ASDA). These tests are distributed in cooperation with the American Dental Association (ADA) Commission on National Dental Examinations, and may be ordered from

ASDA
211 East Chicago Avenue
Chicago, IL 60611

Review sessions should be frequent in order to reinforce learning, but not too long in duration. If you continue to study after mental fatigue has set in, you will be unable to recall what you have studied. You will be working against yourself. The mind functions best when it has adequate rest.

### Types of Questions

You must be prepared for the types of questions included on the National Board Examinations. The Commission on National Dental Examinations has prepared a brief guide (4) to indicate the types and form of objective questions which are presently being used in the examinations.*

**COMPLETION.**   In one type of completion the problem or situation is posed in the stem of the item. The student, therefore, knows exactly what is being asked of him. The stem plus the correct answer makes a complete sentence.

1. The most frequent cause of failure of silver amalgam restorations is
    1. improper cavity preparation
    2. moisture contamination
    3. inferior alloy
    4. improper manipulation of the amalgam

In a second type of completion the stem may include several sentences, such as in a case study.

2. A tooth with a 3-month history of occasional severe pain began to ache steadily. The pain was worse when hot liquids were in the mouth. After extraction, the tooth was split open. The pulp chamber was completely filled with pus. A few remnants of pulp tissue were found in the apical end of the root canal. The condition described is
    1. acute partial pulpitis
    2. acute total pulpitis
    3. suppurative pulpitis
    4. strangulation of the pulp
    5. chronic total pulpitis

Another type of completion question has more than one correct answer.

* Examples are taken from National Board Dental Examinations: Guide for the Construction of Test Items. Chicago, Commission on National Dental Examinations, ADA, July, 1976.

3. The tension developed by a given muscle on its tendon is determined by
    a. the number of muscle fibers stimulated
    b. whether or not the stimulus is supermaximal for all fibers
    c. frequency of stimulation of each muscle fiber
    d. the wave form of the maximal stimulus
    e. the prestimulation length of the muscle fibers

    1. a
    2. a, b, and e
    3. a, c, and e
    4. b and d
    5. c and d

QUESTION. As in the completion question the problem is posed in the stem. In this case the stem is a complete thought in the form of a question. The choices may be nouns, adjectives, adverbs, phrases, clauses, or sentences, but all are the same in any given item.

4. Which of the following substances is believed to be essential, in the process of repair, for the chemical transformation of procollagen to collagen fibers?
    1. Vitamin A
    2. Vitamin C
    3. Thromboplastin
    4. Cortisone
    5. Prothrombin

Some questions will have more than one correct answer.

5. Which of the following cells or tissues have a good capacity for regeneration after injury or loss?
    a. Collagenous fibrous tissue
    b. Spinal cord
    c. Epithelium of mucous membranes
    d. Skeletal muscle
    e. Renal glomeruli
    f. Cardiac muscle

    1. a and b
    2. a, b, and c
    3. a and c
    4. a, c, e and f
    5. c, d, and e

CAUSE AND EFFECT. The sentences in these items consist of a statement and a reason for that statement. The student must decide if

1. Both statement and reason are correct and related.
2. Both statement and reason are correct and *not* related.
3. The statement is correct but the reason is *not*.
4. The statement is *not* correct, but the reason is an accurate statement.
5. *Neither* statement nor reason is correct.

6. Penicillinase will reduce blood levels of penicillin *because* this enzyme renders penicillin inactive by competitive inhibition.

7. Atropine is used as premedication in general anesthesia with cyclopropane *because* atropine will block reflex bradycardia.

8. Epinephrine is contraindicated in patients during cyclopropane anesthesia *because* under cyclopropane epinephrine may precipitate ventricular arrhythmia.

9. A patient who responds to aspirin with severe dyspnea should be given an immediate subcutaneous injection of epinephrine *because* epinephrine relaxes the bronchiolar spasm.

The six types of items discussed have been approved by the Commission for use in the National Board Examinations. True–false items are no longer used, and negative items are discouraged. Since the National Board Examinations are written according to test construction norms, there are few grammatical clues to the correct answer, such as the articles a, an, and the.

**Rest and Relaxation**

As stated previously, being prepared also means being rested and calm. It does not pay to go without food, sleep, and recreation to cram for an examination. The student who crams pushes himself beyond the point of efficiency. The learner is "wasting time in the sense of getting less return for the investment of energy" (2).

Research has shown that a good night's sleep is essential to consolidate memories (6). Scientists have known for a long time that rapid eye movement (REM) during sleep indicates periods of dream sleep which serves crucial needs, and it appears that memory is one of those needs. The evidence indicates that the student who stays up all night cramming for a test is only introducing information that really cannot be learned, because the effort involved in staying awake prevents it. The next day none of the information can be recalled, and it will be of no use in the future because it has not been fully incorporated in the student's mind. On the other hand, the student who gets a good night's sleep is consolidating the material and making it a part of his or her long-term memory.

It is wise to relax deliberately just before the examination. Do not try to do a last minute review. All you can do with last minute reviewing is to confuse yourself with details. Rather, spend the few minutes before the examination in small talk or in reading a newspaper.

**HOW TO TAKE THE NATIONAL BOARD DENTAL EXAMINATIONS**

The important point in taking any examination is to have a definite plan in mind. People who know what to do and how they are going to do it seldom get upset or panicky.

The first step in beginning the examination is to read all directions carefully so that you will be able to answer in exactly the way specified. Directions such as choose the "best" or "most closely related" indicate that all alternatives are plausible, but only one is correct.

Next divide the total number of questions in a section by the time allocated for them in order to judge how much time to spend on each question. Approximately 1 min per question is allocated. It is to the student's advantage to utilize the full 3½ hours in each session. A student who finished the test quickly in a session probably did not analyze the questions carefully.

Approach each question by identifying the stated problem in the stem. It is very important that the stem and alternatives/distractors be accepted exactly as written, because each word was selected for a purpose. The meaning of each word must be precise, as defined in dental textbooks.

The examination is a straightforward test of your basic knowledge; the test items and alternative answers are not intended to trick you. Answer each question from the general principle rather than from the exception. You may have learned to respond to the exceptions on test items from your past experiences; however, this procedure is not appropriate for a test of basic knowledge like the National Board Examinations.

The test score is the total number of correct answers. Therefore it is usually best to go through the examination first, answering all the questions of which you are sure. In surveying the test, you might use a T to code those questions which will require more time for answering; and a G to code those which may require guessing. Answer the "time" (T) questions the second time through the examination, and leave the "guessing" (G) questions until last.

Concentrate on one question at a time. This ability is sometimes called "bridge-player's mentality"; it simply means ignoring the preceding and following questions unless the question at hand is a diagnostic interpretation question. The fact that "guessing" and "time" questions tend to linger in your mind and further reduce your concentration for the question at hand, is another reason why these should be coded and dealt with after you've answered questions that are easier for you.

You will probably be tempted to change some answers. If some answers are changed, be sure the first markings are completely erased. If you are uncertain between two answers, however, leave the answer you set down originally. Research has shown that when you are guessing, your first guess, based on careful reading, is likely to be your best guess.

## HOW TO ATTACK OBJECTIVE QUESTIONS

You should determine a plan for dealing with those questions about which you are uncertain. Following are some comments on how to attack objective questions (5):

1. **Read everything that is written and use it.** For example, suppose there are seven questions about Mrs. Doe. Preceding the first question is a brief personal, medical, dental, and social history of Mrs. Doe. Between questions 4 and 5 is a progress note in large type which reads, "Mrs. Doe improves. Oxygen therapy is discontinued." The beginning of question 5 reads, "On the basis of the information provided about Mrs. Doe. . . ." In answering question 5, students should consider the information in Mrs. Doe's history that precedes the first question, the information given in the stems of the four preceding questions, and the information in the progress note immediately preceding question 5, plus, of course, whatever else is included in the stem of question 5. In a sense this use of cumulative information in a patient-centered test situation is analogous to a real patient's medical and dental histories, doctors' orders, and medical and dental progress notes.

2. **Do not read into items what is not there.** Focus on the question or problem as it is stated in the stem. All of the options of an item may be correct or best for some situation or patient, but only one option is correct or best in terms of the specific question or problem posed in the item's stem. If an item begins, "in general" or "as a rule," the focus is on that which is generally true, correct, or best, not that which is only rarely the case.

3. **Pay attention to words in the stems that are underlined or capitalized.** The deliberate accenting of certain words in stems is part of the design of the items.

4. **Select the best answer of those provided, even though there may be another answer just as good which is not included.** Some students become confused when they do not see their favorite answer to a particular problem. Good test construction avoids the obvious, that is, it excludes correct answers that are so common as to be cliches. In addition, the person prepared for professional life must understand not only the main or primary factors involved in a problem but also the subordinate and contributing ones.

5. **Try to select the correct answer directly; if you cannot, try to determine the answer by eliminating the distractors.** When distractors are well constructed, the indirect route to the correct answer

often requires more knowledge than the direct route, so the indirect method of selecting the correct answer to multiple choice test items is an acceptable practice.

6. **Do not add an "always," "all," or "every" which is not in the stem.** For example, "A great deal of bickering occurs among brothers and sisters." This is true. Some students will mark it false, however, because their mental item read, "A great deal of bickering occurs among *all* brothers and sisters." This is not the same question.

7. **Guard against omitting or dropping qualifying phrases such as "generally" or "to some extent."** One way to prevent dropping a qualifying phrase is to underline "generally," "not," "sometimes," "in part," etc.

8. **Do not change the question by adding or deleting a qualifying phrase.**

9. **Be alert to double negatives.** "No one is always incorrect" does not mean "someone is always correct."

10. **Do not change your answers.**

11. **There is no system in the listing of multiple choice answers.** Each statement must be answered on its own merit.

Guess intelligently since there is no penalty for guessing. If you can eliminate all but two alternatives, then it would be wise to flip a coin in order to obtain an unbiased choice between those two. If you knew the answer, there would be no choice to make; if you do not flip a coin, the chances are you will be snared by a word which surely introduces a bias. Flip the coin and give yourself a true 50–50 chance. If you are totally uninformed about the alternatives, randomly select one of the alternatives, making certain not to waste valuable time with such questions. You cannot pass the examination on guessing only, however. The probability of guessing 19 correct answers in a row, when given four choices, is 1 in 274,877,906,944 (Table 1–1).

A percentage of questions will fall into the category of the most difficult. When unable to answer these, do not be discouraged, but proceed with the test. No one is expected to get a perfect score. Your score will compare your performance with that of others taking the examinations.

## HOW ARE NATIONAL BOARD EXAMINATIONS GRADED?

One point is given for each right answer. There is no penalty for guessing, so be sure to answer every question. The examinations are graded on a curve. The national average raw score is always equated with a standard score of 85. For example, if the national average raw score on a test were 60

**Table 1-1. Probabilities for Guessing Successive Correct Answer from Four Choices**

| NO. OF CORRECT GUESSES | PROBABILITY* |
|---|---|
| 1 | $(1/4)^1 = 1/4$ |
| 2 | $(1/4)^2 = 1/16$ |
| 3 | $(1/4)^3 = 1/64$ |
| 4 | $(1/4)^4 = 1/256$ |
| 5 | $(1/4)^5 = 1/1,024$ |
| 6 | $(1/4)^6 = 1/4,096$ |
| 7 | $(1/4)^7 = 1/16,384$ |
| 8 | $(1/4)^8 = 1/65,536$ |
| 9 | $(1/4)^9 = 1/262,144$ |
| 10 | $(1/4)^{10} = 1/1,048,576$ |
| 11 | $(1/4)^{11} = 1/4,194,304$ |
| 12 | $(1/4)^{12} = 1/16,777,216$ |
| 13 | $(1/4)^{13} = 1/67,108,864$ |
| 14 | $(1/4)^{14} = 1/268,435,456$ |
| 15 | $(1/4)^{15} = 1/1,073,741,824$ |
| 16 | $(1/4)^{16} = 1/4,294,967,296$ |
| 17 | $(1/4)^{17} = 1/17,179,869,184$ |
| 18 | $(1/4)^{18} = 1/68,719,476,736$ |
| 19 | $(1/4)^{19} = 1/274,877,906,944$ |

* In general, the probability of guessing the correct answer from four choices $n$ times in succession is $(1/4)^n$.

points, *any student who answered 60 questions out of 100 correctly would receive a score of 85.* Without attempting to go into the statistics involved, two questions generally equal one standard point. In this example, when 60 right answers equal a score of 85, 40 right answers would equal a score of 75 [1].

## HOW MANY RIGHT ANSWERS DO YOU NEED TO PASS ANY ONE TEST?

This varies from year to year and from test to test. On Part II, if a test has 100 questions, *about 55 right answers are required for a passing grade,* except in pharmacology where about 40 right answers are required to pass [1].

You can see therefore why it is important to go straight through each test; you may know immediately if you have the minimum number correct.

## SOME PERSONAL REMINDERS

Glasses worn for corrected vision will probably be more comfortable than contact lenses when testing extends over several hours.

When brain cells are utilized to make discriminating judgments on each question, energy is consumed which results in a feeling of fatigue upon completion of each section. The students who does not experience some degree of fatigue after taking an examination probably did not answer the written questions but read the questions to fit preset answers. The chances are this student "blew" the test.

You should develop a disciplined diet control regimen which insures high protein intake for sustained energy release during the examinations. Adequate sleep is essential for maximum organization of ideas and recall of facts. A few minutes deep relaxation between exams will help allay synaptic fatigue. It is not advisable to take drugs since these may impede your performance.

Each candidate is responsible for protecting the integrity of his answers. If cheating is noted during the examination or evidence of cheating is disclosed by the computer during processing, candidates involved, whether they be copiers or those copied from, will be failed and there will be a minimum waiting period of one year before the candidate can re-apply [3].

It is sincerely hoped that this volume will help you in preparing for the National Board Dental Examinations. But remember, there is no substitute for knowledge.

## REFERENCES

1. American Student Dental Association: How to Prepare for the National Board. Chicago, 1976
2. Bugelski BR: The Psychology of Learning Applied to Teaching. Indianapolis, Bobbs-Merrill, 1964
3. Council of National Board of Dental Examiners, American Dental Association: National Board Dental Examinations Brochure. Chicago, 1976
4. Council of National Board of Dental Examiners, American Dental Association: National Board Dental Examinations: Guide for the Construction of Test Items. Chicago, July, 1976
5. Coury VM: Study Skills and How to Take Exams. Memphis, University of Tennessee College of Dentistry, 1973
6. Time: Sleep for Memory. New York, Time-Life Publications, August 23, 1976

## SUGGESTED READING

ARMSTRONG WH: Study is Hard Work, 2nd ed. New York, Harper, 1967
BENNETT ME: College and Life, 4th ed. New York, McGraw-Hill, 1952
HARRIS AJ: How to Increase Reading Ability, 4th ed. New York, Longmans, 1961
HERRICK MW: Reading for Speed and Better Grades. New York, Dell Publishing, 1963
KALISH RA: Making the Most of College: A Guide to Effective Study. Belmont, CA, Brooks-Cole, 1959
LAIRD DA, LAIRD EC: Techniques for Efficient Remembering. New York, McGraw-Hill, 1960
LEWIS N: How to Read Better and Faster, 3rd ed. New York, Crowell, 1958
LIBAW FL, MARTINSON WD: Success in College, 2nd ed. Glenview, IL, Scott, Foresman, 1967
MILES OS, BRACKEN DK, DOUGHERTY MA, KINDER RF: Tactics in Reading, II. Glenview, IL, Scott, Foresman, 1965
MILLER LL: Increasing Reading Efficiency, rev ed. New York, Holt, Rinehart, & Winston, 1964
MORGAN CT, DEESE J: How to Study. New York, McGraw-Hill, 1957
ORCHARD NE: Study Successfully: 18 Keys to Better Work. New York, McGraw-Hill, 1953
PAUK W: How to Study in College. Boston, Houghton Mifflin, 1962
PRESTON RC: Teaching Study Habits and Skills. New York, Holt, Rinehart, & Winston, 1959
ROBINSON FP: Effective Study, rev ed. New York, Harper, 1961
SMITH GL: Spelling by Principles: A Programmed Text. New York, Appleton-Century-Crofts, 1966

## ANSWER KEY

| | | | |
|---|---|---|---|
| 1. 1 | 4. 2 | 6. 3 | 8. 1 |
| 2. 3 | 5. 3 | 7. 1 | 9. 1 |
| 3. 3 | | | |

# 2
# BIOMATERIALS

### John H. Hembree, Jr.

## PROPERTIES OF MATERIALS

Two important questions must be asked about a material for use in the oral cavity: 1) what effect will the material have on its environment, and 2) what effect will the environment have on the material? The desirable qualities for materials used for restorations include indestructibility in mouth fluids, adaptability to the cavity walls, freedom from dimensional change upon setting, resistance to attrition, sustaining power against the forces of mastication, and anticarcinogenicity. To date, no material used in restorative dentistry fulfills all of these requirements.

The following terms must be understood before the dentist can select the restorative material with the desired mechanical properties. When a force is applied to a material, there is a resistance in the material to the external force. The force is distributed over an area, and the ratio of the force to the area is called the **stress:**

$$\text{Stress} = \frac{\text{Force}}{\text{Area}}$$

Several types of stress may result when a force is applied to a material; these various types are referred to as compressive, tensile, and shearing stress (Fig. 2–1).

The change in length, or deformation per unit length, when a material is subjected to a force is defined as **strain:**

$$\text{Strain} = \frac{\text{Deformation}}{\text{Length}}$$

A convenient means of visualizing the mechanical properties of a material is to apply various forces to it and to determine the corresponding values of stress and strain. When these values are plotted on a graph, the result is referred to as a **stress–strain curve** (Fig. 2–2). Such a curve may be obtained in compression, tension, or shear. Properties of various materials can then be compared by comparing their stress–strain curves.

The **elastic modulus** is equal to the ratio of the stress to the strain in the linear or elastic portion of the stress–strain curve:

$$\text{Elastic modulus} = \frac{\text{Stress}}{\text{Strain}}$$

**Proportional limit** and **yield strength** indicate the stress at which the material no longer functions as an elastic solid. Below these values the material recovers from the strain if the stress is removed, and above these values permanent deformation of the material occurs. The proportional limit is the stress on the stress–strain curve when it ceases to be linear; the yield strength is the stress at some arbitrary value of permanent strain and thus is always slightly higher than the proportional limit (Fig. 2–2). Materials are said to be elastic in their behavior below the proportional limit or yield strength and to function in a plastic manner above these stresses.

A material, when subjected to enough force, will eventually fracture or rupture. This point is known as the **ultimate strength** (Fig. 2–2).

The **percent of deformation** that a material can withstand before rupture is reported as the percent of elongation when the material is under tension or the percent of compression when it is under compressive stress. These are important properties in that they are measures of the ductility and malleability, respectively, of the material.

Resilience and toughness are two properties that involve the area under the stress–strain curve and thus the energy required to reach specified points on the curve. The energy necessary to fracture a material is a measure of its **toughness,** whereas the energy required to deform a material permanently is a criterion of its **resilience** (Fig. 2–3).

For dental purposes the surface **hardness** of a material is generally measured in terms of its resistance to indentation. Hardness has also been used as a measure of the ability of a material to withstand abrasion and attrition. In general the harder a material, the less likely it is to be abraded, although there are exceptions to this rule. The hardness of dental materials is reported by Knoop, Brinell, Vickers or Rockwell numbers, with the Knoop hardness numbers being the most commonly used. Brinell and Vickers numbers are used primarily

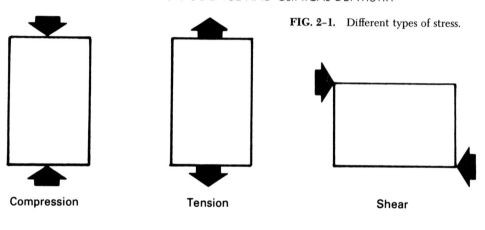

**FIG. 2-1.** Different types of stress.

Compression          Tension                    Shear

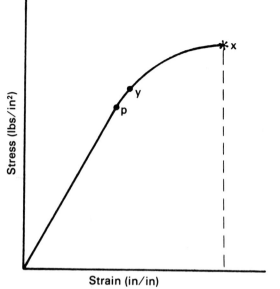

**FIG. 2-2.** Typical stress–strain curve indicating proportional limit (**p**), yield strength (**y**), ultimate strength (**x**).

for comparing casting alloys, and Rockwell numbers are used for composite resins.

### QUESTIONS

1. On a stress–strain curve, the area below the curve showing the energy required to fracture the material is known as
   1. resilience of the material
   2. toughness of the material
   3. the ultimate strength of the material
   4. hardness of the material

2. A measure of the malleability of a material is often expressed as
   1. the elastic modulus — *stiffness*
   2. toughness
   3. percent of compression
   4. percent of elongation

*ductility*

3. It can be said that a material behaves in certain ways above and below the proportional limit on a stress–strain curve. Which of the following is correct?
   1. Above the proportional limit a material functions in a plastic manner, while below the proportional limit it behaves as an elastic.
   2. Above the proportional limit a material functions in an elastic manner, while below the proportional limit it behaves as a plastic.
   3. Either 1 or 2 may be true.
   4. Neither 1 or 2 is correct.

## GYPSUM PRODUCTS AND INVESTMENTS

### Gypsum Products

The mineral gypsum, widely found in nature, is the dihydrate form of calcium sulfate ($CaSo_4 \bullet H_2O$). Gypsum has various applications in dentistry. It serves as a molding material in the construction of models and casts for dentures, is used to produce dies in which restorations are constructed, and acts as a binder for silica in casting investments (Fig. 2–4). The basic ingredient for plaster, dental stone and high-strength dental stone, and gypsum-bonded investments is a hemihydrate, or dehydrated form of the dihydrate form of calcium sulfate ($CaSO_4 \bullet 1/2H_2O$). The main differences among the basic powders lie with variations in the size, shape, and porosity of the particles produced by different methods of manufacture (Fig. 2–5). When water is mixed with the hemihydrate powders, they return to the dihydrate or gypsum form according to the following reaction:

Plaster     Water          Gypsum
$$(CaSO_4) \bullet H_2O + 3H_2O \rightarrow (CaSO_4 \bullet 2H_2O) + heat$$

It is in this reacted form that the dental gypsum products are used in their various applications. The mechanism of setting is due to the hemihydrate and dihydrate forms of calcium sulfate, with the dihydrate

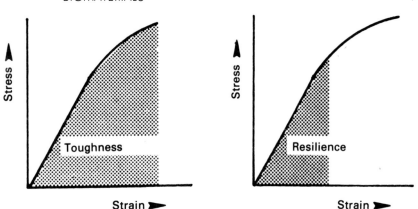

**FIG. 2-3.** Stress–strain curves. Shaded areas demonstrate toughness and resilience.

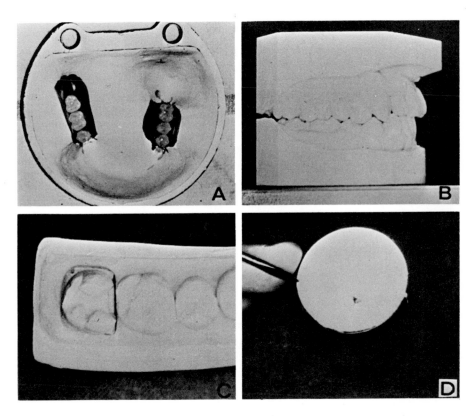

**FIG. 2-4.** Gypsum products. A. Denture mold. B. Cast. C. Die. D. Investment.

form being less soluble in water. During setting, growth and subsequent interlocking of gypsum crystals occur. The interlocking contributes to the strength and dimensional change of the gypsum. Manipulative procedures that influence the difference in solubility and the growth of the dihydrate crystals can influence the physical and mechanical properties of the gypsum mass.

Plaster, prepared by calcining in open kettles, is designated the $\beta$ form of calcium sulfate hemihydrate. Plaster is weaker than dental stone due to two contributing factors: 1) the porosity of the particles makes it necessary to use more water for a plaster mix, and 2) the irregular shapes of the particles prevent them from fitting together tightly.

Plaster products used in dentistry usually are made from commercial plaster modified to adjust setting time, expansion, or both. Impression plasters are modified by additions such as flavoring agents and/or starches, gums, and chemicals to give them desirable handling and physical properties. Model plasters are used for pouring primary impressions, study casts, and repair casts; for mounting interarch registration as-

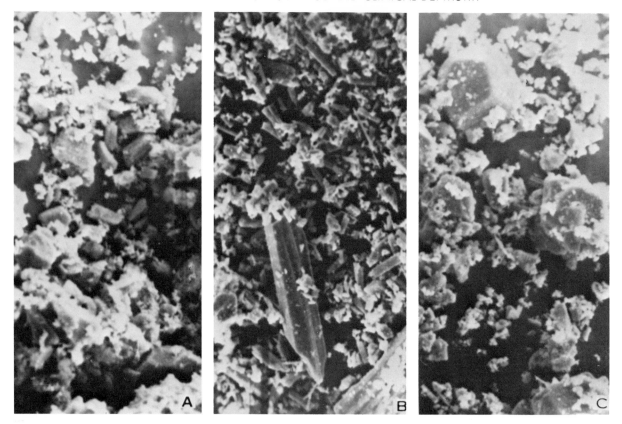

**FIG. 2-5.** Scanning electron photomicrographs showing particle shape of gypsum products. (× 500) A. Plaster. B. Stone. C. Improved stone.

semblies; for flasking dentures; and for a variety of other applications.

Dental stone, a dense, regularly shaped, relatively nonporous cuboidal crystal material, is manufactured by calcining gypsum under steam pressure in an autoclave. Dental stone (Hydrocal) has a crystal that is designated the α form of calcium sulfate hemihydrate. Because of their particle characteristics, the α hemihydrate stones require less gauging water and are about two and one-half times stronger than the β plaster. The α type stone is widely used in making casts and molds requiring a higher crushing strength and abrasion resistance, and as an ingredient for casting investments.

A still harder cast material than dental stone is produced by calcining gypsum by boiling it in a 30% solution of calcium chloride. The crystals of the hemihydrate resulting from this process are slightly larger and more dense than those of dental stone. This modified dental stone or high-strength stone originally was called Densite. Because of their increased strength and resistance to abrasion, the modified dental stones are especially suited for inlay, crown, and bridge casts and are often referred to as die stones.

A comparison of compressive strength for the gypsum products is shown in Table 2–1.

Deviation from the water:powder ratio recommended by the manufacturer affects setting time, strength, and setting expansion. Increasing the water:powder ratio produces a thinner mix that takes longer to set. A mix with a thinner consistency is weaker because excess water is used. When a gypsum product is mixed with a lower water:powder ratio, the mixed mass is thicker and more difficult to manipulate, but the set gypsum is stronger. Setting expansion is also influenced by the water:powder ratio; thicker mixes show increased expansion.

When a mixture of hemihydrate and water hardens, a measurable linear expansion takes place. This expansion may amount to as much as 0.5% with plaster. Dental stones also expand on setting, but the amount is less than that which occurs with plaster. Even though gypsum products develop a linear expansion during hardening, the true volume is the hemihydrate plus that of the water required for the conversion of the hemihydrate to the dihydrate.

Soaking or storing casts and dies in water, or exposing them to running water for prolonged periods should be avoided. Such treatment can lead to a mea-

**Table 2-1. Compressive Strengths of Dental Plaster and Stones**

| TYPE | CRYSTAL | W:RATIO (ML WATER TO 100 G POWDER) | COMPRESSIVE STRENGTH (POUNDS PER SQUARE INCH) 1 HR |
|---|---|---|---|
| Model plaster | $\beta$ | 40–50 | 1400–2000 |
| Dental stone | $\alpha$ | 30–40 | 3000–4000 |
| Dental stone, high strength | Modified $\alpha$ | 20 | 5000 |

**Table 2-2. Expansion Requirements of ADA Specification No. 2 for Casting Investments**

| CLASSIFICATION | SETTING (%) IN AIR | | SETTING (%) IN WATER | | THERMAL(%) TEMP. EXPANSION | | | COMBINED SETTING AND THERMAL | |
|---|---|---|---|---|---|---|---|---|---|
| | MINIMUM | MAXIMUM | MINIMUM | MAXIMUM | °C | MINIMUM | MAXIMUM | MINIMUM | MAXIMUM |
| Type I, inlay, thermal | 0.0 | 0.5 | | | 700 | 1.0 | 2.0 | 1.3 | 2.0 |
| Type II, inlay, hygroscopic | | | 1.2 | 2.2 | 500 | 0.0 | 0.6 | 1.3 | 2.7 |
| Type III, partial denture, thermal | 0.0 | 0.4 | | | 700 | 1.0 | 1.5 | 1.2 | 1.9 |

surable amount of crystals being dissolved from the surface of the cast.

## Casting Investments

Investments used with the wax pattern in forming molds for casting dental alloys of various types consist of a powder refractory, a binder, and modifiers. The refractory base is usually some crystalline form of silica. Usually quartz and cristobalite are used. Investments containing cristobalite expand earlier and exhibit greater expansions than those containing only quartz.

The usual binder for investments to cast gold alloys is an $\alpha$ calcium sulfate hemihydrate. Some of the investments used for casting cobalt–chromium alloys which solidify at low temperatures also have a gypsum binder. Investments for casting cobalt–chromium alloys which solidify at higher temperatures must have a binder other than gypsum. Organic and inorganic silicates and some phosphates are used to cast some high fusing golds, ceramic alloys, and gold substitute metals.

A number of modifiers are employed to prevent most of the shrinkage of gypsum when it is heated above 300°C. Among these modifiers are boric acid and sodium, and chlorides. Graphite, colloidal copper, and other substances are used to produce a nonoxidizing atmosphere in the mold.

The minimum and maximum limits for linear setting expansion and thermal expansion are set by the American Dental Association (ADA) Specification No. 2 for Casting Investments (Table 2–2). The setting ex-

pansion, hygroscopic expansion, and thermal expansion of the investments are the critical factors in accurate reproduction of the dimensions of the wax pattern because they must compensate for the casting shrinkage of the gold alloy.

Casting techniques for gold alloys are usually designated thermal expansion or hygroscopic expansion. Although the designation indicates the major expansion, all techniques involve both thermal expansion and hygroscopic expansion to some degree. The amount of thermal expansion depends primarily upon the composition of the investment and temperature but is also affected by such factors as water:powder ratio and rate or duration of heating. Hygroscopic expansion is dependent primarily upon composition of the investment, the time at which the investment is immersed in water, and the amount of water available during setting. It is also affected by such variables as water:powder ratio and restraining effects of the wax pattern.

QUESTIONS

4. Which of the following have a different chemical formula?
    a. Plaster
    b. Dental stone
    c. Hydrocal
    d. Phosphate-bonded investment
    e. Cristobalite

1. a, b, and c
2. b, c, and e
3. c and d
4. d and e

5. The refractory base in inlay casting investment powder is
   1. silica
   2. sodium chlorides
   3. calcium sulfate dihydrate
   4. calcium sulfate hemihydrate

6. The hardest type of dental stone available to the profession is manufactured by
   1. removing it directly from the earth
   2. calcining gypsum by boiling it in a 30% solution of calcium chloride
   3. calcining gypsum in open kettles
   4. calcining gypsum under steam pressure in an autoclave.

## DENTAL WAXES

Wax products can be broadly classified as pattern, processing, or impression waxes. Pattern waxes include inlay, casting, and baseplate waxes and are used to form models for a restoration or appliance. Processing waxes include boxing, utility, and sticky waxes and are used as auxiliary materials. Corrective and bite waxes are used as impression materials to record detail in the oral cavity (Fig. 2–6).

Waxes are made up of high-molecular-weight organic molecules. Dental waxes include both natural and synthetic waxes, gums, fats, fatty acids, oils, natural and synthetic resins, and pigments of various types.

The most common natural waxes used in the formulation of dental waxes are paraffin, beeswax, and carnauba wax. Synthetic waxes and resins were developed to solve problems with the use of natural products. Because the physical properties of the natural waxes vary, for example, manufacturers are faced with difficulties in formulation and cannot control properties from batch to batch. The synthetic waxes have a high degree of purity and dependable properties but do not possess properties equivalent to those of the natural waxes. Therefore synthetic waxes presently have limited use in dental formulations.

Some of the most important properties of wax are its melting range, thermal expansion, and mechanical properties such as flow and residual stress. Since waxes consist of similar types of molecules of different molecular weights, they have, not melting points, but melting ranges.

Waxes expand when subjected to a rise in temperature and contract as the temperature is decreased. Dental waxes and their components have the largest coefficient of thermal expansion of any material used in restorative dentistry. The coefficient of thermal expansion of inlay waxes is high enough that temperature changes in wax patterns after critical dimensional relationships have been established may be largely re-

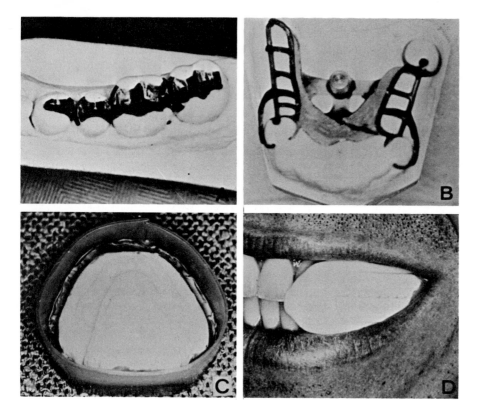

FIG. 2–6. Dental waxes. A. Inlay pattern wax. B. Casting wax pattern. C. Boxing wax. D. Bite wax.

sponsible for any inaccuracy of the finished restoration.

The elastic modulus, proportional limit, and compressive strength of dental wax are low compared to other materials. These properties, which are strongly dependent on the temperature, decrease as the temperature of the waxes increases. The mechanical properties of inlay wax are important in wax patterns of inlays and crowns as the wax is subjected to stresses during setting of the investment.

The flow of wax is most important when the wax is manipulated at a temperature below its melting range, when flow is actually a measure of plastic deformation. Flow greatly increases as the melting range of the wax is approached or as the pressure and the length of time the pressure is applied are increased.

Regardless of the method used to prepare a wax pattern, there is residual, or internal, stress in the completed pattern. It is developed when the wax is subjected to the stress that occurs during a carving procedure or during cooling under pressure. When released by the action of time and temperature, residual stress can result in a nonuniform dimensional change, or distortion. The higher the temperature of the wax at the time-that the pattern is adapted and shaped, the less likely it is that the wax patterns will be distorted. The manipulation of wax must be directed toward both minimizing the development of residual stress and keeping the stress that is developed from being released.

Since the release of residual stress and subsequent distortion is associated with storage time and temperature, greater distortion results at higher storage temperatures and during longer storage times. It has been suggested that, if inlay patterns must stand for longer than 30 min before being invested, they should be kept in a refrigerator. A refrigerated wax pattern should be allowed to warm to room temperature before being invested, however. The best way to minimize the warpage of inlay patterns is to invest the pattern immediately after it is completely shaped.

The principal waxes used for inlay patterns are paraffin, microcrystalline wax, ceresin, carnauba, candelilla, and beeswax; paraffin is the major component of inlay pattern wax. Factors that are very critical to a pattern wax are residue on burn-out, flow, and linear thermal expansion. When the burn-out oven is heated the wax should vaporize without leaving a residue which might prevent the reproduction of sharp detail in the casting. The wax should not flow during carving or upon removal from the model preparatory to the investing procedures and the wax should have a low coefficient of thermal expansion so that it will not change in dimension when it is removed from the mouth to room temperature.

The manufacturer has to blend the waxes very carefully to prepare an inlay pattern wax with optimum properties. The accuracy and ultimate usefulness of the resulting metal casting is dependent to a large degree on the accuracy and fine detail of the wax pattern.

QUESTIONS

7. What is the major constituent of an inlay pattern wax?
   1. Microcrystalline wax
   2. Ceresin
   3. Carnauba
   4. Beeswax
   5. Paraffin

8. If a wax pattern has been stored in a refrigerator, before the investment procedure the wax pattern should
   1. be allowed to return to room temperature
   2. have the margins reheated and readapted
   3. not be allowed to return to room temperature
   4. not be stored in a refrigerator under any circumstances.

9. The most important properties of dental wax are
   a. melting range
   b. thermal expansion
   c. mechanical properties
   d. flow
   e. residual stress
   1. a, b, and c
   2. b, d, and e
   3. a, d, and e
   4. All of the above
   5. None of the above

## METALS IN DENTISTRY

Metals play a major role in the restoration of teeth, both as fixed appliances and as removable appliances (Fig. 2–7). The metals used as restorative materials in the oral cavity must be noninjurious to both hard and soft tissues, inert and dimensionally stable, and strong enough to resist the forces of mastication and abrasion during use. Most metal alloys used in dentistry contain either high percentages of noble metals or utilize an inert oxide coating over a base metal in order to avoid long-term problems of corrosion and oxidation.

### Gold Casting Alloys

Gold alloys rather than pure gold are used as casting alloys in restorative dentistry, since alloying greatly increases the strength and hardness of gold without materially reducing its resistance to corrosion in the oral environment, providing that the gold and other precious metal content is kept above 75% by weight. The metals used with gold to produce suitable alloys include copper, silver, platinum, palladium, and zinc. Gold is the main constituent of all dental gold alloys. Its main contribution to the alloy is tarnish and corrosion

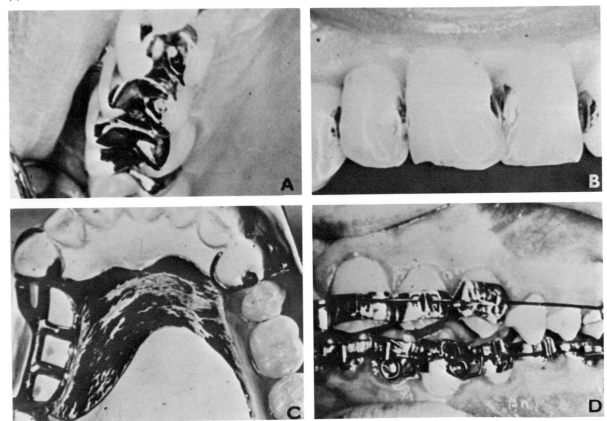

**FIG. 2–7.** Metals in dentistry. A. Cast gold inlays. B. Direct filling gold. C. Cobalt–chrome removable partial denture. D. Stainless steel orthodontic appliance.

resistance, although it also increases the strength of the alloy, its density, and its cost.

**OTHER METALS USED IN GOLD ALLOYS.** Copper, in combination with gold, platinum, or palladium, increases the hardness and strength of the alloy. Because the addition of copper tends to lower the tarnish and corrosion resistance, it must be limited in dental alloys to less than 15%. The addition of copper also tends to lower the melting point of the alloy and creates a narrow melting range.

Silver is added to the alloy to neutralize the pinkish color imparted by the copper. It also plays a small part in hardening heat treatments that can be applied to some alloys.

Platinum is added to some gold alloys to reduce the ductility and increase the strength and hardness. The platinum content of dental alloys must be kept below about 4%, because its presence raises the melting point of the alloy. Platinum also contributes to the age hardening, in conjunction with copper.

Palladium, because it is not as expensive as platinum, is sometimes used instead of platinum; its effect on the alloy's physical properties is similar. White golds used in dentistry contain palladium, as it is a very efficient whitening agent.

Zinc is sometimes present in alloys, because it tends to lower the melting point and also acts as an oxide scavenger.

**PROPERTIES OF GOLD ALLOYS.** Dental golds are classified by the American Dental Association according to their mechanical properties (Table 2–3).

All gold alloys can be softened by heating at 700°C for 10 min before quenching in water. For practical reasons this is generally accomplished after casting. When the button of gold becomes a dull red color, the investment is quenched in water to soften the appliance that has been cast.

Alloys containing approximately 15%–30% copper (Class III and IV alloys) harden after softening heat treatment if they are heated to 450°C and cooled uniformly to 250°C over a period of 15–30 min. Not only does the hardness increase, but also the proportional limit and modulus of elasticity. As would be expected, there is a corresponding drop in the ductility of the alloy.

**Table 2-3.  Composition and Physical Properties of Casting Golds**

| TYPE | USE | GOLD AND METALS OF THE PLATINUM GROUP (%) | VICKERS NUMBER (QUENCHED) | | MINIMUM % ELONGATION (QUENCHED) | FUSION. TEMP. (MINIMUM °C) |
|------|-----|------|------|------|------|------|
| | | | MINIMUM | MAXIMUM | | |
| I | Small inlays | 83 | 50 | 90 | 18 | 930 |
| II | inlays, 3/4 crowns | 78 | 90 | 120 | 12 | 900 |
| III | Crowns, bridges | 78 | 120 | 150 | 12 | 900 |
| IV | Partial dentures | 75 | 150 | | 10 | 870 |

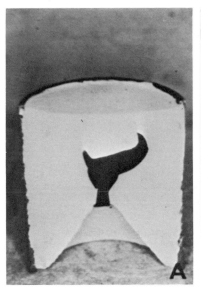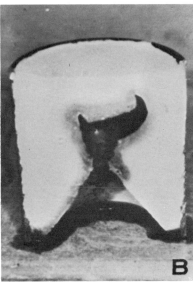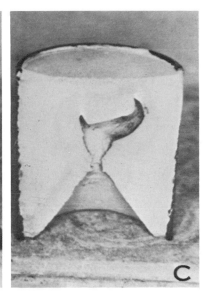

**FIG. 2-8.** Stages of wax elimination in cross section. A. Pattern prior to burn-out. B. During burn-out. C. Completed burn-out.

**CASTING.**    Since gold alloys must be cast, a pattern of the restoration is prepared in a suitable wax. To form a mold the wax pattern is then invested in a gypsum silica casting investment. The mold, which must be provided with an ingate or sprue to allow later ingress of the molten metal, is then heated so that the wax is completely eliminated (Fig. 2-8). The gold alloy is then melted and forced under pressure into the mold space where it solidifies. After removal of excess material, followed by adequate finishing and polishing, the restoration is ready for placement in the mouth.

When the molten gold alloy cools in the mold, it shrinks; this is known as the casting shrinkage. Since the wax pattern is an accurate reproduction of the appliance, the shrinkage of the gold alloy during solidification causes the casting to be too small unless the mold expands by the amount of shrinkage.

Porosity is quite common in commercial gold castings, but it is definitely to be avoided as much as possible in dental gold alloy castings to maintain the fine detail of the gold restoration. There are at least two causes for porosity. It may be caused by insufficient molten gold during solidification, for example, when too small a sprue is utilized, or it may be caused by gas inclusion. Some metals in the alloy dissolve oxygen while they are molten. When they solidify, the gas is precipitated in spherical porosities. Also, air may be trapped in the molten metal as it goes into the mold.

**ALTERNATE ALLOYS.**    Due to the increased cost of gold casting alloys, there has been an increased interest in less expensive alloy systems for the casting of inlays, crowns, and bridges. Alternate alloys are based on substantial amounts of palladium (22%–50% by weight) and silver (35%–66% by weight) in lieu of the more costly gold. Since sufficient data based on reliable long-term studies of fixed prostheses constructed from the palladium–silver alloys are not available, the clinical efficacy of these materials cannot be determined. The questions that must be answered concern the accuracy of fit of the cast appliances, the corrosion resistance in the oral environment, and the porcelain bond strength of high-palladium-content alloys.

## Wrought Gold Alloys

Gold alloys are also used in dentistry in the wrought form, usually as wires. These wrought materials often exhibit mechanical properties superior to those of similar cast alloys due to grain refinement and stored energy produced as a result of the cold working process. The only property that is not significantly altered by the cold working process is the modulus of elasticity. The wrought gold alloy wires have limited use in dentistry today due to the expense of the alloy. Generally gold wrought wires have been replaced by stainless steel wires and cast chrome alloys.

## Gold Solders

Gold solders are used for joining cast and/or wrought sections of a dental appliance which cannot be fabricated in one piece. Alloys used for solders are similar in composition to the casting gold alloys so that their color and mechanical properties will be comparable to the alloys being joined. To insure that the parts being soldered do not melt during assembly, gold solders must have a melting point of at least 50° C lower than the lowest melting point of the alloys being soldered. Thus the gold content of gold solders is usually about 8% less than the alloys on which they are used. Due to the lower gold content of the solder, the corrosion resistance of the joint may be decreased from the parts being joined.

## Direct Filling Golds

Gold may be used in its pure state for restorative dental purposes. It can be welded at room temperature by atomic attraction. The restoration is built up by incremental additions of gold, that is, each increment is welded or compacted to that already placed in the cavity. The compaction not only welds the pure gold, but the strain also hardens it, thus increasing both the strength and hardness of the finished restoration.

Pure gold is usually supplied to the dentist as cold worked foil, as mat gold which is prepared by electrical precipitation from solution, or as powdered gold formed by atomization or chemical precipitation. Since the presence of various gases on the surface of pure gold prevents it from being welded at room temperature, for ease of handling gold preparations are sometimes deliberately rendered noncohesive by the manufacturer. This is accomplished by allowing the gold to absorb ammonia gas onto its surface. Before use, both cohesive and noncohesive golds are given a degassing heat treatment at 340° C–370° C for 8–10 min by the dentist.

Gold foils possess adequate strength and hardness to give long-lasting restorations when properly inserted. Although pure gold has a Brinell hardness number of approximately 25, a well-inserted restoration will register a Brinell hardness number of 60 because of the strain which hardening induced in the material during placement.

## Chrome Alloys

Cobalt–chromium alloys have largely replaced gold alloys for the construction of metal partial denture frameworks. Their corrosion resistance in the oral environment is as good as that of the gold alloys because of the passivating effect of the chromium. The cobalt–chromium alloys are much less expensive and have only half the density of gold alloys.

The alloys are composed of approximately 70% cobalt and 30% chromium, although some of the cobalt can be replaced by nickel. Other elements, such as molybdenum, tungsten, manganese, and silicon, are added in small quantities to act as hardeners. Carbon is present in the alloy, but never above 0.5%. This small amount controls many of the properties of the material, since it can combine with all constituents to form hard, brittle carbides.

The melting point of cobalt–chromium alloys is in the range of 1250° C–1450° C. Thus the melting point is higher than that required to melt a gold casting alloy.

The proportional limit and ultimate strength of cobalt–chromium alloys are essentially similar to those of gold alloys in the hardened condition. The modulus of elasticity is approximately twice that of gold alloys. Thus, to obtain the same flexibility in a clasp arm, cobalt–chromium castings require only half the cross-sectional area of gold castings.

Cobalt–chromium alloys have been drawn into wires which have excellent properties for orthodontic wires. One wrought alloy, Elgiloy, differs from the casting alloys in that it contains some 16% iron as well as cobalt, chromium, and nickel. It is usually supplied to and used by the dentist in a cold worked form.

Recently a new nickel–chromium alloy has been marketed for use in fabricating fixed prostheses with particular emphasis on fused porcelain veneers. In general the nickel–chromium alloys show higher strength values than the gold alloys. The casting and handling techniques used on these alloys are quite different from those used on gold alloys. Careful attention to the technique differences is critical to obtain correct fit of the restoration.

## Stainless Steels

Stainless steels are used in dentistry in a number of situations, but the most common use is in the fabrication of orthodontic arch wires and retaining bands.

The addition of at least 12% chromium to a plain carbon steel makes the alloy resistant to corrosion because a tough, tenacious layer of chromium oxide

$(Cr_2O_3)$ known as the passivating film forms on the surface. This film, formed under oxidizing conditions, then protects the alloy from further oxidation and therefore makes it "stainless."

The most common stainless steels used in dentistry contain approximately 18% chromium and 8% nickel. The 18–8 stainless steels are also known as the austenitic type. Since these stainless steels can only be hardened and strengthened by cold working, and since many orthodontic appliances are assembled from several pieces of stainless steel by soldering or welding procedures which involve the use of heat, care must be taken not to overheat the material. When overheated, the stainless steel wires change in structure, becoming soft and losing their corrosion resistance.

Stainless steel wires and some wrought gold wires have essentially the same values for proportional limits and tensile strengths. The value of the modulus of elasticity of stainless steel is approximately twice that of the gold alloys, however, making stainless steels stiffer than gold alloys.

### QUESTIONS

10. To impart a hardening heat treatment to a dental gold alloy, the best method is to
    1. pickle the casting in a strong acid
    2. quench the hot casting in cold water
    3. bench cool from casting temperature to room temperature
    4. reheat the cooled casting to 450° C and cool uniformly to 250° C over a period of 15–30 min

11. According to the American Dental Association Specification for cast gold alloys,
    1. a decrease of the gold content is coupled with a decrease in the mechanical properties, except elongation, which increases
    2. a decrease of the gold content is coupled with an increase in the mechanical properties, except elongation, which decreases
    3. an increase of the gold content is coupled with an increase in the mechanical properties, except elongation, which decreases
    4. there is no correlation between the gold content of the gold alloys and their mechanical properties

12. If they are of the same composition, which is stronger, cast gold or gold wire?
    1. Cast gold is stronger as it can be heat treated.
    2. Wrought wire is weaker due to the stress relieving effect.
    3. Cast gold is weaker as it cannot be cold worked.
    4. Wrought wire is stronger due to the cold working effect.
    5. There is no difference in strength.

13. Although gold solders have a lower gold content than the parts being joined by the solder, the properties of the solder joint are essentially the same as the parts except
    1. yield strength
    2. elongation
    3. corrosion resistance
    4. ultimate tensile strength

14. The pure form of gold used in dentistry is known as
    1. class I casting gold
    2. cohesive gold
    3. noncohesive gold
    4. class IV casting gold

15. The carbon content of cobalt–chromium alloys is always below 0.5%, because the effect of carbon on the mechanical properties of these alloys is very strong. This statement consists of two parts, a statement and a reason. Which of the following best describes the statement and reason?
    1. Both statement and reason are correct and related.
    2. Both statement and reason are correct but unrelated.
    3. The statement is incorrect, but the reason is correct.
    4. The statement is correct, but the reason is incorrect.
    5. Both statement and reason are incorrect.

16. An orthodontic spring constructed from 18–8 stainless steel will exert twice as much force on a tooth as a comparable gold alloy wire, because the hardness value of stainless steel is twice that of gold alloy wire. This statement consists of two parts, a statement and a reason. Which of the following best describes both the statement and reason?
    1. Both statement and reason are correct and related.
    2. Both statement and reason are correct but unrelated.
    3. The statement is correct, but the reason is incorrect.
    4. The statement is incorrect, but the reason is correct.

## DENTAL AMALGAM

Amalgam accounts for 75% of all dental restorations. Amalgam alloy is commercially produced and marketed as small spherical or comminuted particles. The amalgam alloy is reacted with mercury in the dental office to produce dental amalgam.

Amalgam alloy is composed primarily of silver and tin with minor additions of copper, mercury, and sometimes zinc. Silver gives the composition adequate strength and prompt setting or hardening when it is mixed with mercury. High silver content tends to cause expansion in the dental amalgam. The presence of tin in small amounts aids in the amalgamation of the alloy with the mercury and also helps to keep the expansion within practical limits, but large quantities of tin reduce the strength of the amalgam, prolong the setting process, and reduce the corrosion resistance of the amalgam. Small amounts of copper improve the

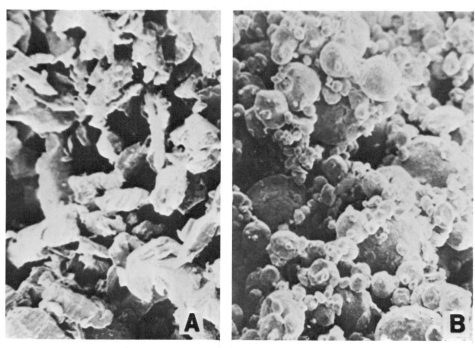

**FIG. 2-9.**    Amalgam alloys. A. Comminuted. B. Spherical. (300×)

**FIG. 2-10.**    Packaging of amalgam. A. Bulk powder. B. Tablets. C. Disposable capsules.

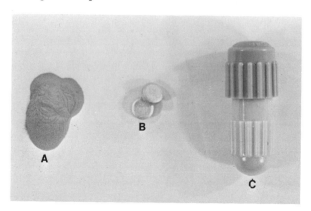

The shape of amalgam alloy particles may be one of two forms: 1) comminuted or lathe-cut and 2) spherical (Fig. 2–9). Amalgam alloy is available to the practicing dentist in bulk powder, tablets, and disposable capsules (Fig. 2–10), and the selection of the type of packaging is generally based on economy, accuracy, and convenience. The most expensive, but also the most convenient, package is the disposable capsule. In this type of packaging the mercury and alloy are separated by a thin membrane of plastic before use.

### Amalgamation

Amalgamation is the reaction that occurs between mercury and amalgam. The reaction is the following:

$$Mercury + silver–tin \rightarrow silver–tin\ phase \\ + silver–mercury + tin–mercury\ phase$$

The silver–tin phase is called $\gamma$ phase and is composed of the alloy particles before they have reacted with the mercury. The silver–mercury phase is called the $\gamma_1$ phase, and the tin–mercury phase is called the $\gamma_2$. Since amalgamation is a surface reaction, amalgam can be thought of as particles of $\gamma$ surrounded by a matrix of $\gamma_1$ and $\gamma_2$. The properties of amalgam are determined by the relative amount of each phase.

When mercury initially comes into contact with amalgam alloy, the $\gamma$ particles are wet by the mercury; then they begin to absorb it. The solution of mercury into the $\gamma$ particles leads to the formation on the surface

strength, hardness, and setting characteristics of the amalgam mass. Copper also tends to cause expansion in the dental amalgam.

Both zinc and zinc-free alloys are available to the dental profession. Zinc is primarily an aid in the manufacturing process, because a small amount of it helps to keep the alloy clean during manufacturing. The presence of 1% zinc in the amalgam alloy is responsible for an excessive delayed expansion in the amalgam mass, when the amalgam is contaminated with moisture from any source during the mixing and insertion process.

of $\gamma_1$ and $\gamma_2$ phases. The crystallization of the $\gamma_1$ and $\gamma_2$ phases and their subsequent growth causes amalgam to harden. At the same time this process occurs, voids that influence the mechanical properties of the hardened amalgam are formed.

## Properties

As amalgam hardens, dimensional changes occur that may cause the amalgam to expand or contract, depending on its manipulation. Either expansion or contraction, if excessive, is undesirable. The current ADA Specification for dental amalgam states that the dimensional change in 24 hours, either expansion or contraction, should be no more than $20\mu m/cm$.

The strength of amalgam is determined by the presence of the $\gamma$, $\gamma_1$, and $\gamma_2$ phases and by voids. The relative strengths of the phases are as follows: 1) the $\gamma$ phase is the strongest phase, 2) the silver–mercury ($\gamma_1$) phase is the second strongest, and 3) the tin–mercury phase ($\gamma_2$) and voids are the weakest. The manipulative techniques should be followed that result in sufficient formation of matrix ($\gamma_1$ and $\gamma_2$) to bond together the $\gamma$ particles and to reduce the presence of voids, the most important factor in reducing strength. Insufficient strength in amalgam may cause gross fracture or a marginal breakdown (Fig. 2–11). The rate at which an amalgam develops strength is an important clinical characteristic. If an amalgam restoration is subjected to pressure too soon after insertion, it may be sufficiently overloaded to be fractured clinically.

The flow of amalgam is a dimensional change that is a result of the viscoelastic properties of amalgam. Excessive flow under normal masticatory forces results in distorted cuspal portions of the restoration or in movement of the amalgam within the cavity.

Amalgam restorations will tarnish and corrode when exposed to conditions in the oral cavity. Of the phases present in amalgam, the $\gamma_2$ phase is the most susceptible to corrosion. Manipulation of amalgam to minimize the formulation of the $\gamma_2$ phase is therefore desirable.

## Manipulation

The clinical success of an amalgam restoration is highly dependent on the correct manipulation of the amalgam alloy. These manipulative factors include proportioning of mercury and alloy, mixing, condensation, and finishing.

**MERCURY : ALLOY RATIO.** The amount of mercury and alloy that is to be mixed is described as the mercury:alloy ratio. For example, a mercury:alloy ratio of 8:5 would indicate that eight parts of mercury are to be mixed with five parts of alloy by weight. The mercury:alloy ratio is a unique characteristic of each particular manufactured amalgam alloy; therefore the manufacturer's recommended mercury:alloy ratio should be followed. A 1:1 ratio is considered optimum

**FIG. 2–11.** Insufficient strength in amalgam can cause fracture or marginal breakdown. A. Fracture (**arrows**). B. Marginal breakdown (**arrows**).

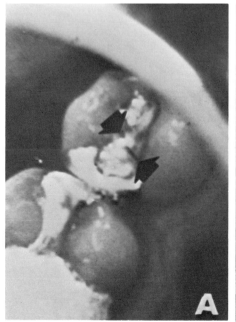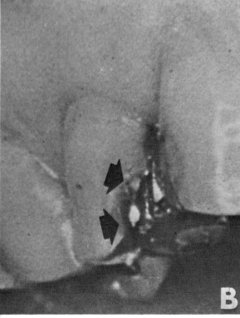

for many of the present day alloys. If excessive mercury remains in the amalgam (above 55%), it causes a high degree of expansion, a loss of strength, and a reduction in corrosion resistance.

TRITURATION. The principal purpose of mixing (trituration) is to coat the alloy particles with mercury. This process is generally accomplished by one of a variety of motor-driven amalgamators. These units contain a timing device which stops the motor after a desired interval of time. The alloy and mercury are placed, with a pestle, in a metallic or plastic capsule which is rotated eccentrically or with a reciprocating motion during trituration. The operating speed of different mechanical amalgamators varies. Not only must the mixing time be chosen with a particular unit, but also the proper capsule and pestle must be determined for the type of alloy to be triturated.

CONDENSATION. The objectives of condensation are to adapt the amalgam to prepared cavity walls and margins; to develop a uniform, compact mass with minimal voids; and to reduce excess mercury content. An increase in the final mercury content reflects the presence of excessive amounts of $\gamma_1$ and $\gamma_2$ phases, which decreases the strength of the amalgam. Selection of a condensing instrument and technique must be based on their effectiveness in removing excess mercury and in applying the pressure necessary for adaptation.

FINISHING. A properly condensed amalgam made from a modern alloy will be sufficiently hardened within a few minutes to permit carving with sharp instruments. Final finishing and polishing procedures should not be done for at least 24 hours after the initial carving of the amalgam. Clinical observations indicate that a well-finished and well-polished amalgam restoration retains its shiny metallic appearance for a longer period of time, is easier to keep clean, and undergoes less corrosion.

## High-Copper-Content Alloys

Recently several new alloys with high copper content have been introduced to the dental profession. These alloys appear to have superior and improved compressive strength, lower flow (creep) values, and the ability to reduce the $\gamma_2$ phase (Table 2–4). These advances are believed to lead to improved clinical performance. Three particle shapes are presently available in the high-copper-content alloys: spherical, spheroidal (a mixture of odd-shaped, rounded particles and spheres of varying sizes), and blends of fine-cut particles and spheres (Fig. 2–12). The inclusion of copper to replace a part of the tin component allows the copper to react with remaining free tin, thus reducing the amount of $\gamma_1$ in the final restoration.

QUESTIONS

17. Which of the following is the most accurate definition of the term amalgam? Amalgam is
    1. a metallic substance, supplied in the form of fillings, which is mixed with mercury
    2. a metallic substance composed of two or more metals which are mutually soluble in a molten state
    3. an alloy of two or more metals, one of which is mercury
    4. a metallic substance composed of silver, copper, tin, and zinc

18. The higher the mercury:alloy ratio in dental amalgam,
    1. the higher the strength
    2. the more matrix material will be formed
    3. the more of the $\gamma$ phase will be available
    4. the lower the creep value
    5. None of the above

19. Silver and copper in dental amalgam
    1. decrease expansion, flow, and compressive strength
    2. decrease expansion and compressive strength but increase the flow value
    3. increase expansion and compressive strength
    4. increase flow only
    5. increase expansion but decrease compressive strength

**Table 2–4. Comparison of Conventional Amalgam and High-Copper-Content Amalgam**

| ALLOY TYPE | COMPRESSIVE STRENGTH (POUNDS PER SQUARE INCH) | | | FLOW (%) |
| --- | --- | --- | --- | --- |
| | 1 HR | 24 HRS | 7 DAYS | 3–24 HRS |
| Conventional | | | | |
| Fine-Cut | 17,000 | 50,000 | 55,000 | 1.10 |
| Spherical | 16,000 | 49,000 | 50,000 | 1.40 |
| High-Copper | | | | |
| Blend | 33,000 | 64,000 | 65,000 | 0.25 |
| Spherical | 35,000 | 74,000 | 78,000 | 0.07 |
| Spheroidal | 33,000 | 68,000 | 74,000 | 0.26 |

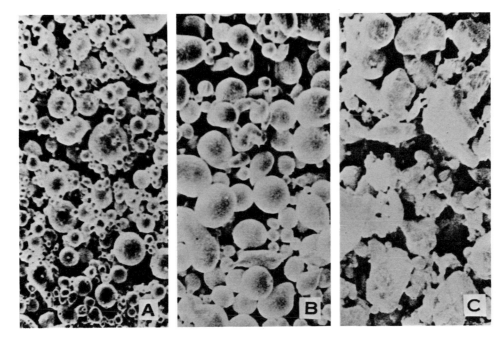

**FIG. 2-12.** Scanning electron photomicrograph showing particle shapes of high-copper-content amalgam alloys. (× 300) A. Spherical. B. Spheroidal. C. Blend.

20. The main achievement in developing the high-copper-content amalgam is the
    1. elimination of the $\gamma_1$ phase
    2. increase in the strength of dental amalgam
    3. decrease in the flow values of dental amalgam
    4. elimination of the $\gamma_2$ phase
    5. All of the above

## DENTAL CEMENTS AND CAVITY VARNISHES

Dental cements are used extensively in dentistry, because they have a low coefficient of thermal conductivity. When compared to other materials used in dentistry, the dental cements show low strength, high solubility and a lower resistance to conditions in the oral cavity. They are used as cementing agents for fixed cast restorations or orthodontic bands, as thermal insulators under metallic restorations, as temporary or permanent restorations, as root canal fillings, and for pulp capping.

### Zinc Phosphate Cement

The basic constituent of zinc phosphate powder is zinc oxide. The major modifier for the powder is magnesium oxide. The liquid is phosphoric acid, aluminum phosphate, and, in some cases, zinc phosphate. The metallic salts are added as buffers. The average water content of the liquid is approximately 33%.

When a zinc oxide powder is mixed with phosphoric acid, a solid substance is formed and a considerable amount of heat is liberated. The exact nature of the product of this reaction is not certain, but it is generally thought to be a tertiary zinc phosphate $Zn_3(PO_4)_2 \cdot 4H_2O$). Due to the presence of the phosphoric acid, the acidity of the zinc phosphate cement is quite high at the time it is inserted into the tooth. Three minutes after the start of the mixing, the pH is approximately 3.5. The pH then increases rapidly, approaching neutrality in 24–48 hours. The pH is lower and remains lower if thinner mixes of the cement are employed.

Zinc phosphate cement is used as a cementing medium for inlays and crowns, as a cementing medium for orthodontic bands, as an insulating base, and as a temporary restorative material. The consistency of the cement, which is different for each use, is related to the liquid:powder ratio. The more powder incorporated into the liquid, the thicker the mix. The temperature of the mixing slab also governs the viscosity of the mix by accelerating or retarding the setting reactions. Since the set is slower on a cooler mixing slab, more powder may be added during the mixing time. Generally speaking, the more powder added to the liquid the greater are its physical properties.

### Zinc Oxide–Eugenol Cements

Zinc oxide–eugenol cements are usually dispensed in the form of a powder and a liquid and are blended by the dentist just prior to use. They are used as a temporary filling material, temporary and permanent cementing media, insulating bases, root canal fillings, and soft tissue dressings. The wide range of uses is due to the sedative effect of eugenol on the pulp of the tooth. It should be noted that a zinc oxide–eugenol material should not be used under a resin.

The composition of a zinc oxide–eugenol cement powder is essentially zinc oxide, rosin, and zinc acetate. The rosin improves the consistency of the cement and promotes a smoother mix. Zinc acetate or zinc stearate, or both, usually are employed to accelerate the reaction between the zinc oxide and the eugenol.

The liquid is eugenol and cottonseed oil. The reaction which takes place when the liquid and powder are mixed is a chelation reaction, and the hardened cement can be envisioned as a matrix of zinc eugenolate binding particles of zinc oxide.

In an attempt to improve the zinc oxide–eugenol cements and create a cement with the properties desirable in a cementing medium, the zinc oxide–eugenol cements have been modified or reinforced. The addition of a polymer reinforcement and alumina, for example, increases the strength of the cement. Also, orthoethoxybenzoic acid (EBA) has been added to the eugenol liquid in an attempt to reduce the solubility of the cement; these cements are known as EBA cements.

## Polycarboxylate Cements

The polycarboxylate cements are powder–liquid systems utilized primarily as cementing media, although some manufacturers recommend them for an insulating base. The powder is similar in composition to that used with the zinc phosphate cement, that is, zinc oxide and some magnesium oxide. The liquid is an aqueous solution of polyacrylic acid and copolymers.

The newest of the dental cement systems, the polycarboxylate cement system is the only one for which there is evidence of adhesion to tooth structure. The adhesion of the polycarboxylate cement to tooth structure is due to the chelation of the calcium in the enamel apatite and dentin apatite by the carboxyl groups of the polyacrylic acid. It has also been suggested that some bonding may occur to the protein in the tooth. Since this cement demonstrates adhesion to tooth structure, a clean surface is necessary in order to provide intimate contact between the cement and the tooth.

Radioisotope studies have shown that the polycarboxylate cements and zinc phosphate cements have better sealing abilities than do the zinc oxide–eugenol cements (Fig. 2–13), which suggests that these two types of cements are less soluble than the zinc oxide–eugenol cements. Table 2–5 outlines the

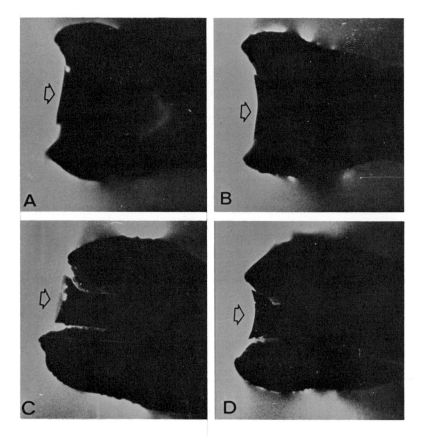

**FIG. 2-13.** Typical leakage patterns of cementing media at 1 year, indicating inlay (**arrows**) and leakage (**white lines**). A. Zinc phosphate cement. B. Polycarboxylate cement. C. Zinc oxide-eugenol cement. D. Reinforced zinc oxide–eugenol cement (EBA).

**Table 2-5. Solubility, Compressive Strength, and Film Thickness of Various Cementing Media**

| | WATER SOLUBILITY IN 24 HRS (%) | ACID SOLUBILITY IN 24 HRS (%) | COMPRESSIVE STRENGTH (POUNDS PER SQUARE INCH) | FILM THICKNESS ($\mu$m) |
|---|---|---|---|---|
| Zinc phosphate | 0.13 | 0.23 | 11,000 | 25 |
| Polycarboxylate | 0.12 | 0.41 | 7,800 | 30 |
| Zinc oxide–eugenol | 0.25 | 0.75 | 3,600 | 22 |
| Reinforced zinc oxide–eugenol (EBA) | 0.29 | 0.74 | 8,000 | 25 |

solubilities, compressive strengths, and film thickness of the major types of cementing media.

### Calcium Hydroxide Cements

The calcium hydroxide cements are the material of choice for capping a pulp that is exposed during a dental procedure, because calcium hydroxide tends to accelerate the formation of secondary dentin over the exposed pulp. This cement is often used as a base in deep cavities even if there is no obvious pulp exposure and is the material of choice to use as a base beneath the resin restorative materials.

Commercial preparations vary in composition. The formulas range from a very simple suspension of calcium hydroxide in distilled water to a preparation that contains six or seven components. The calcium hydroxide cements have a high pH in the range of 11.5–13.

### Cavity Varnishes and Liners

Cavity lining materials, used to coat the walls and floors of a prepared cavity, can be classified into two groups. A cavity varnish is principally a natural gum, such as copal, rosin, or a synthetic resin, dissolved in an organic solvent, such as acetone, chloroform, or ether. A cavity liner is a liquid in which calcium hydroxide and/or zinc oxide are suspended in the solutions of natural or synthetic resins.

A cavity varnish aids in reducing postoperative sensitivity when placed between metallic restorations, not because of its effective thermal insulation, but because of its tendency to minimize marginal leakage around restorations. The penetration of fluids is reduced around an amalgam restoration when a cavity varnish is used (Fig. 2–14).

The cavity varnishes have shown very little ability to prevent acid penetration through the dentinal tubules of a prepared cavity, but one of the subtle effects of the varnishes is the minimization of the discoloration of teeth caused by the penetration of metallic salts from an amalgam restoration. Cavity varnishes should not be employed under resin restorative materials, because the solvent may react with or soften the resin.

**FIG. 2-14.** Typical leakage patterns of amalgams, showing restoration (**arrows**) and leakage (**white line**). A. Amalgam with varnish. B. Amalgam without varnish.

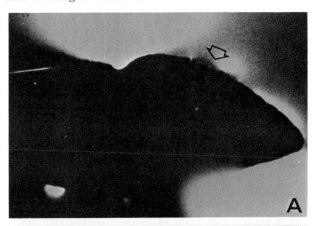

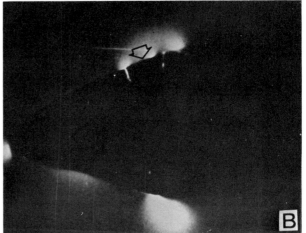

QUESTIONS

21. When compared to other materials, dental cements show
    a. less strength
    b. higher solubility
    c. lower resistance to conditions in the oral cavity
    1. a and b
    2. b and c
    3. a and c
    4. a, b, and c

22. In zinc phosphate cement liquid the buffering agents are zinc and
    1. magnesium
    2. bismuth
    3. aluminum
    4. silicon

23. The zinc oxide–eugenol cements are used as
    a. a temporary filling material
    b. an insulating base
    c. temporary and permanent cementing media
    d. a soft tissue pack
    e. a root canal sealer
    1. a, b, c, and d
    2. a, b, and c
    3. b, c, and d
    4. All of the above

24. The incorporation of orthoethoxybenzoic acid and synthetic resins into conventional zinc oxide–eugenol cements is said to
    a. increase strength
    b. reduce solubility
    c. reduce film thickness
    d. increase adhesiveness
    1. a and b
    2. b, c, and d
    3. a and d
    4. All of the above

25. Polyacrylic acid is the parent compound of the
    1. zinc oxide–eugenol cements
    2. zinc phosphate cements
    3. cyanoacrylate cements
    4. carboxylate cements

26. The most effective dental cement in stimulating growth of secondary dentin is one of the
    1. zinc phosphate cements
    2. calcium hydroxide cements
    3. zinc silicophosphate cements
    4. carboxylate cements

27. A solution of one or more resins from the natural gums, the synthetic resins, and rosin in an organic solvent is called a
    1. cavity varnish
    2. carboxylate cement
    3. liner
    4. cyanoacrylate cement

## ANTERIOR RESTORATIVE MATERIALS

Four types of materials have been developed for use as anterior restorative materials: 1) silicate, 2) unfilled acrylic resin, 3) composite resin, and more recently 4) a glass ionomer cement (Table 2–6).

### Silicate Cement

Silicates are supplied as a powder and a liquid. The powder is an acid-soluble glass, which has been prepared by fusing silica ($SiO_2$) and alumina ($Al_2O_3$) with a calcium fluoride flux. The liquid is a phosphoric acid solution in water, buffered by aluminum and zinc phosphate. The general setting reaction is as follows:

Alumina–silica glass containing fluorides + phosphoric acid + water → insoluble phosphate and fluoride matrix + unreacted glass covered with alumina–silica gel

The presence of the fluoride in the set matrix renders the silicates anticariogenic. The silicate cement reduces the enamel solubility of the tooth due to the fluoride uptake of the enamel.

Although a silicate is considered satisfactory for clinical use if it exhibits no more than 1% solubility in 24 hours, the fact that it disintegrates in oral fluids is a significant clinical problem. The larger the amount of matrix formed and the sooner the material is exposed to water after setting, the more disintegration occurs. The solubility value (Table 2–6) does not relate directly to clinical use, since it does not take into account the food debris and acids present in the mouth and the low resistance of the silicates to wear.

The mixing of silicates is critical. A satisfactory mixing temperature is from 70° F–75° F. Maintaining a cool slab allows the dentist some control over the setting time of the restoration and permits the addition of more powder to improve the properties of the final restoration. If the room temperature is higher than 75° F, the glass mixing slab can be cooled with water and dried just before mixing. The powder and liquid should be mixed by incorporating most of the powder first and then adding smaller amounts to adjust the consistency. The mixing should be done over a small area of the glass slab and each portion mixed to a smooth paste before the next portion is added. The total mixing time should be less than 1 min.

After the silicate has been placed in the prepared cavity, it should be held in place under compression with a matrix strip for about 4 min. When the strip is removed, the surface of the silicate should be coated with a layer of cavity varnish or a suitable lubricant to prevent dehydration of the surface. If a set silicate is allowed to dehydrate, the surface will crack and craze, rendering the restoration more susceptible to disintegration.

### Glass Ionomer Cement

Recently glass ionomer cements (Table 2–6) which, like the polycarboxylate cements, adhere to tooth structure have been developed. These cements are based on the hardening reaction between an aqueous solution of acrylic acid and a powdered calcium aluminosilicate glass. Setting results from the formation of a calcium polysalt gel matrix, which is subsequently reinforced by the aluminum salts. The cements are said

**Table 2-6. Properties of Anterior Restorative Materials**

| | SETTING TIME (MIN) | COMPRESSIVE STRENGTH (POUNDS PER SQUARE INCH) | SOLUBILITY IN 24 HRS (%) |
|---|---|---|---|
| Silicate cement | 4.5 | 30,000 | 0.6 |
| Glass ionomer cement | 4.5 | 21,000 | 0.3 |
| Unfilled resins | 4.0 | 10,000 | — |
| Composite resins | 2.5–4.0 | 35,000 | — |

to be, besides adhesive to enamel and dentin, aesthetic and anticariogenic.

### Unfilled Resins

Acrylic plastics with no reinforcing fillers have been used successfully to repair fractured anterior teeth. They are less susceptible to fracture by impact loads than the composites, but they do not have a high resistance to wear.

The materials are supplied as a powder and a liquid. The powder consists of a compound of high molecular weight called poly (methyl methacrylate), a catalyst such as benzoyl peroxide, and coloring and opacifying agents, which are usually metal oxides. The liquid is mainly methyl methacrylate but contains an inhibitor, hydroquinone, to lengthen shelf life and to prevent premature reaction of the liquid. The liquid also contains a reaction accelerator, which is usually an organic sulfinic acid compound.

The powder and liquid are mixed at a 3:1 ratio, and the accelerator from the liquid activates the catalyst from the powder, which in turn initiates the reaction of the methyl methacylate molecules with each other to from poly (methyl methacrylate) of a greater molecular weight than the original mixed parts. The reaction is inhibited by water and air and the mixture of powder and liquid should be protected from both during setting. The reaction is accelerated by increases in temperature.

The coefficient of thermal expansion is about seven times as great as that of tooth structure; as a result oral fluids have been shown to flow in and out of the marginal areas after a restoration, a process termed percolation, due to temperature changes in the mouth. This effect has been considered the principle cause of recurrent decay in unfilled resin restorations.

Because the insertion of acrylic restorations has been shown to cause pulpal responses, liners should be used under these restorations. Zinc oxide–eugenol cements and varnishes inhibit the setting reaction of the acrylic resins and should not be used beneath these materials.

### Composite Resins

The previous discussion of the anterior restorative materials has pointed out several drawbacks of silicate and unfilled acrylic resins. For example, high solubility of the silicates makes them vulnerable to disintegration in the oral environment; therefore, they must be considered a short-term restorative system. Since the silicates discolor and stain as dehydration occurs, their esthetic qualities also degrade with time. The unfilled acrylic resins are more resistant to solubility and have no problems with dehydration, but they become stained occasionally, undergo large dimensional change with temperature which results in percolation at margins, have little mechanical strength and stiffness, show low resistance to wear, and have problems with recurrent decay. Not surprisingly, continued attempts have been made to improve the qualities of direct anterior esthetic restorations. The composite restorative plastics incorporate recent advances in this area.

Most set composites consist of 50%–60%, by volume, inorganic particles that have been treated with special organometallic materials called coupling agents to provide a bond between the inorganic particles and the organic polymers. The majority of the composites have organic polymer systems based on bisphenol-A-glycidyl methacrylate (BIS–GMA). BIS–GMA is polymerized to a highly cross-linked polymer at room and mouth temperature by the addition of a peroxide catalyst and an organic accelerator. Polymerization also may be accomplished by ultraviolet light from a controlled concentrated source. These composite materials contain an ultraviolet absorber such as methylbenzoin ether.

The inorganic particles may be such materials as quartz, borosilicate glass, and a lithium aluminum silicate. The type of inorganic filler particles apparently controls the physical properties of the composites (Fig. 2–15).

The system is supplied to the dentist in a variety of forms: two pastes, a paste and a liquid, and a powder and a liquid.

The composites have about three and one-half to four times the compressive strength and three times the yield strength of the unfilled resins. The tensile strength of the composites is approximately twice that of unfilled resin. In addition the composites have improved resistance to abrasive wear, which is the result of the inorganic filler particles.

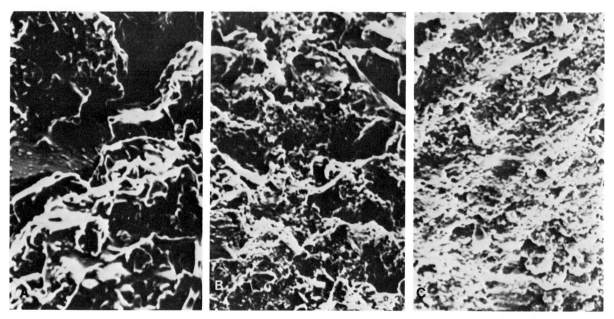

**FIG. 2-15.** Scanning electron photomicrographs on three different composites showing different filler particle size. (× 350)

A popular technique used with composites involves etching the enamel with etchants such as phosphoric acid to improve the tooth's retention of the restoration. Research has shown that the use of an unfilled BIS–GMA resin as an interface layer between the etched enamel and the composite is more effective in promoting retention than placing the composite directly on enamel. When unfilled BIS–GMA resins are bound to enamel, free-flowing liquids are produced which have the ability to wet the enamel surface and penetrate the micropores created by the etching. The thick, viscous consistency of the composite resins is not conducive to good wetting and penetration.

The use of an unfilled BIS–GMA resin in conjunction with the composite has also been shown to aid in minimizing the microleakage that occurs when the composite is used alone (Fig. 2–16). Marginal leakage is reduced significantly or eliminated in composite restorations where the cavosurface angle of the preparation and the enamel is etched and a layer of unfilled BIS–GMA resin in placed before and after the insertion of the composite restoration.

## QUESTIONS

28. A buffering agent for the phosphoric acid of silicate cement is
    1. $SiO_2$
    2. $AlPO_4$
    3. $Al_2O_3$
    4. $CaF_2$

29. When a silicate restoration dissolves in the oral fluids, the portion of the set restoration that disintegrates is the
    1. gel matrix
    2. $SiO_2$ particles
    3. $CaF_2$ flux
    4. $Zn_3 (PO_4)_2$ buffer

30. The only real advantage in properties the glass ionomer cement has over a silicate cement is that the glass ionomer cement has
    1. a shorter setting time
    2. greater compressive strength
    3. slightly less solubility
    4. less optical opacity

31. The initiator of the autopolymerizing resins is
    1. benzoyl peroxide
    2. hydroquinone
    3. methyl methacrylate
    4. p-toluene sulfinic acid

32. The activator (initiator) or the ultraviolet light activated BIS–GMA resins is
    1. a tertiary amine
    2. a peroxide
    3. a methyl ether
    4. hydroquinone

33. The common inorganic phase(s) used in the composites is/are
    a. BIS–GMA resin
    b. lithium aluminum silicate
    c. borosilicate
    d. poly (methyl methacrylate)
    e. quartz
    f. organic silane

1. a
2. b and c
3. a, d, and e
4. b, c, and e
5. f and e
6. a and f

## IMPRESSION MATERIALS

Impression materials can be classified as either inelastic or elastic. Inelastic impression materials such as plaster have very limited use today, however, so this discussion will be limited to the elastic type materials.

### Colloidal Sols

One of the popular types of elastic impression materials is essentially a colloid. Colloidal systems involve particles of a molecular size somewhere between the small particles of a true solution and the large ones present in a suspension. A colloidal solution may be referred to as a colloidal sol.

**REVERSIBLE HYDROCOLLOIDS.** Hydrocolloidal sols change into a gel when they are cooled. The temperature at which they change from the sol state to a semisolid material is known as the gelation temperature. Such a gel is reversible, since it can be changed back into a sol by raising the temperature above the liquefaction temperature. Thus the reversible hydrocolloids possess a property known as hysteresis, meaning that the temperature of gelation is lower than the liquefaction temperature. The change from the sol to the gel, and vice versa, is essentially a physical effect induced by a change in temperature.

The basic constituent of reversible hydrocolloid impression materials is agar (8%–15%), and the principal ingredient by weight is water (80%–85%). Small amounts of borax are added to increase the strength of the gel. Borax is a retarder for the setting of gypsum products, so potassium sulfate (2%) is generally added to commercial dental hydrocolloid impression materials as a hardener for the gypsum products.

Proper equipment is essential for the preparation and storage of hydrocolloid. Various types of conditioners are available. Specially designed syringes are used for injecting the fluid material in and around the prepared cavity, and special water-cooled trays are used for carrying the hydrocolloid into the mouth to form the impression.

The first step in preparing the material for use is to produce a fluid sol. The filled syringes and tubes are placed in boiling water for a minimum of 10 min. After liquefaction in boiling water, the material should be stored in the sol condition for a minimum of 20 min at 155°F. The material should be conditioned or tem-

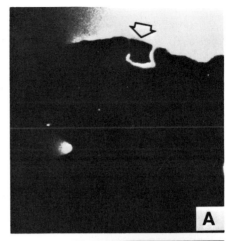

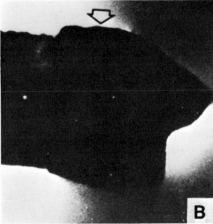

**FIG. 2-16.** Typical 1-year autoradiographs of restoration (**arrows**) with composite resins. A. Restoration with composite only, showing leakage (**white line**). B. Composite inserted following etching of enamel. A layer of unfilled resin was placed before and after insertion of composite.

pered for a minimum of 2 minutes at 115°F prior to inserting material into the mouth. The purpose of tempering the material is to increase the viscosity so that it will flow out of the tray, and to reduce the temperature enough so that the material will not be uncomfortable to the patient.

Gelation of the hydrocolloid material in the mouth is accomplished by circulating cool water in the tray at approximately 60°F–70°F, for not less than 5 min. Ice water cannot be used because it induces rapid gelation at the periphery of the material near the tray, and a distortion of the impression results.

The hydrocolloid gel is composed of fibrils of agar suspended in water. If water is lost the gel shrinks; this is known as syneresis. Likewise, if the gel takes up water the hydrocolloid swells and expands; this is called imbibition.

Because the gel is composed of a fibril network, it is important that the set impression be removed with a sudden application of force, which is less likely to distort or fracture the material than a force that is applied slowly. This fact holds true of any of the elastic impression materials.

There is no satisfactory method for storing a hydrocolloid impression. If storage is absolutely necessary, it should be for a minimum period at room temperature and 100% humidity. In view of the very real risk that the accuracy of a hydrocolloid impression may be lost during storage (Fig. 2–17), the importance of constructing the model immediately cannot be overemphasized.

ALGINATES (IRREVERSIBLE HYDROCOLLOIDS). The irreversible hydrocolloids, referred to as alginates, gel by means of a chemical reaction. Once the gel has formed it cannot be changed back into the sol condition by physical means.

Alginate impression materials usually consist of potassium alginate (12%), calcium sulfate (12%), trisodium phosphate (2%), and diatomaceous earth (74%). The major ingredient from the standpoint of the chemical reaction is the potassium alginate, which dissolves readily in water to form a viscous sol. The sol changes to a gel when the soluble alginate reacts with calcium sulfate to produce the gel structure of an insoluble calcium alginate. Since the reaction must take place in the mouth, it must be delayed until the impression material powder can be mixed with water, placed in the tray, and carried to the mouth. In order to delay this reaction and provide adequate working time, a third soluble salt, trisodium phosphate, is added to the solution to retard the reaction. Because the calcium sulfate reacts with the trisodium phosphate before reacting with the soluble alginate, the gelling reaction between the alginate and calcium sulfate is prevented as long as any trisodium phosphate is present.

The final structure of the gel then is a network of fibrils of calcium alginate holding the excess water and particles of the filler. The filler, which is usually diatomaceous earth, increases the strength and stiffness of the alginate gel and insures a firm surface.

The ideal gelation time usually specified by the manufacturer is approximately 3–4 min at a temperature of 70°F. A change in the temperature of the mixing water alters the gelation time of the material. The higher the water temperature, the shorter the gelation time, thus the cooler the water, the longer the gelation time. If gelation time is to be altered, the best method is to vary the temperature of the water used in making the mix.

The phenomena of syneresis and imbibition are also applicable to the alginate materials. Like the reversible hydrocolloids, the alginates are most stable when stored at room temperature in a humidor at 100% humidity. For most accurate results the model should be constructed immediately after the impression is obtained, however (Fig. 2–17).

FIG. 2-17. Comparison of the accuracy of various elastic impression materials. The data were collected from a series of models all poured from impressions made with each impression material. The discrepancy of fit was measured using a standard casting placed on each model.

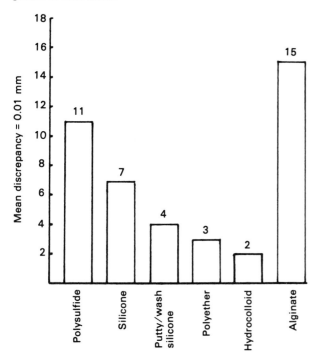

### Elastomers

In addition to the hydrocolloid gels, there are elastic impression materials which are synthetic rubbers known as elastomers. Three chemically distinct types of rubber bases are employed: polysulfide rubber, silicone rubber, and polyether rubber.

POLYSULFIDE RUBBER. The process of changing the rubber base product, called a liquid polymer, into the final rubberlike material is generally referred to as curing or vulcanization. The basic molecule of the polymer has a sulfide group attached to a terminal carbon atom. A compound containing such a group is called a mercaptan by the organic chemist. When the liquid polymer reacts with a certain chemical accelerator, usually lead peroxide in the presence of sulfur, or a hydroperoxide, the polymer grows or lengthens by a process known as polymerization; it therefore changes from a liquid to a solid. When the polysulfide base and the accelerator are properly proportioned and mixed together, the reaction occurs in 6–10 min, depending upon the product and the temperature.

Curing does not stop when the impression is removed from the mouth. The continued curing of the material after the impression has been made produces an increasing amount of shrinkage and distortion. Furthermore, some of the ingredients may volatilize, thus causing additional shrinkage. The stone die should be constructed within the 1st hour after removal of the impression from the mouth, particularly if polysulfide and some silicones have been employed (Fig. 2–18).

It is imperative that the tray be adjusted to provide a minimum thickness of impression material. The shorter the distance between the impression tray and the part to be duplicated, the more accurate the impression. In general the optimum thickness of material between the teeth and the sides of the tray is 2–3 mm. The best method to accomplish this is to construct a custom tray from a dental acrylic (Fig. 2–19).

**SILICONE RUBBER.** The silicone compound used for making dental impressions is a liquid, and consequently it must be combined with a powder to produce a paste that can be used to form a dental impression. The main powder or filler used for this purpose is silica of a fine particle size. The reactor used to polymerize the silicone is usually an organic tin compound known as tin octoate.

The silicone rubbers have several advantages: they are not as messy to handle as the polysulfide polymers,

they are esthetically more appealing, have a better odor and the equipment is easier to clean. The setting times of the silicone rubbers are much shorter than those of the polysulfide rubbers, although increased temperature and humidity shortens the setting times of both the silicones and the polysulfides.

As was the case with the polysulfides, maximum accuracy is obtained when a custom acrylic tray is employed. Some of the newer silicone impression products employ a putty/wash system whereby a custom tray is made in the patient's mouth with an extremely viscous, reinforced silicone putty material. There appears to be an increased accuracy with these materials (Fig. 2–17).

**POLYETHER RUBBER.** The newest of the elastomers, the polyether rubbers are supplied as two pastes. The elastomer contains the polyether polymer, a colloidal silica as a filler, and a plasticizer. The accelerator paste contains the alkyl-aromatic sulfonate in addition to filler and plasticizer. The working time of these materials is 2 min, and the setting time is 3–5 min, similar to that of the silicones.

The use of a custom tray does not appear to be a factor in obtaining maximum accuracy with polyether impression materials (Fig. 2–19), although research has shown that moisture may have an effect on their accuracy (Fig. 2–20). The polyethers appear to maintain their accuracy over a longer time period than the other elastomer impression materials, thus decreasing the demand for pouring the impression immediately.

**FIG. 2–18.** Comparison of the accuracy of elastomer impression materials over various time periods.

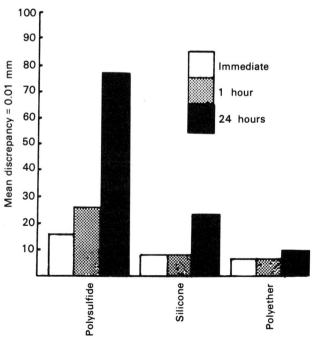

**FIG. 2–19.** Comparison of the accuracy of elastomer impression materials using a custom impression tray versus a stock impression tray.

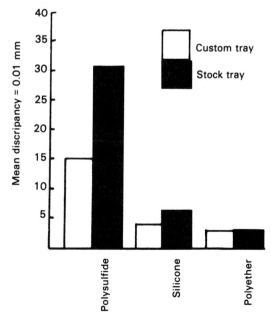

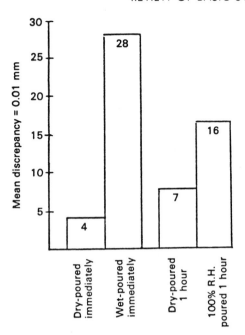

**FIG. 2-20.** Comparison of the accuracy of models made from polyether impression materials when subjected to moisture conditions. Models were poured when impression material was not subjected to a wet condition and when impression material was contaminated with 0.5 ml of water during polymerization. In addition, some impressions were poured 1 hr after polymerization and left in a dry environment and others were poured 1 hr after polymerization and left in 100% relative humidity.

The set material is quite stiff as shown by a high modulus of elasticity and percent strain in compression. The stiffness makes the impression difficult to remove from the mouth intact, as thin areas of the materials are easily torn.

### Impression Compounds

Impression compounds or tray compounds have limited use today in dentistry. In the construction of dentures they have been used to form a tray which can then be employed with other types of impression materials for reproducing the form of the mouth tissues. Because the formulas of impression compounds are trade secrets, any description of composition cannot be very specific. In general compounds are mixtures of waxes, thermoplastic resins, a filler, and a coloring agent.

The thermal conductivity of impression compounds is very low. Since the compound is softened by heat and should be uniformly soft when it is placed in the tray, adequate time must be allowed for the material to be heated throughout the mass. Whenever possible, compound should be softened by dry heat, although large amounts of compound are usually softened in a water bath. After being removed from the water bath, the compound is usually kneaded with the fingers in order to obtain uniform plasticity throughout the mass. Overworking, undue kneading of the compound, can incorporate water into the surface, and the flow after hardening will be increased. The flow of impression compound can be beneficial, but it can also be a source of distortion. After the compound has softened and while it is being pressed against the tissues, a continuous flow is desirable. Once the compound has cooled and solidified, however, flow should be at a minimum or the impression will be distorted when the compound is removed from the mouth.

Stress is induced while the impression is being obtained, and, although it can be minimized by proper handling, some stress is always present in the final impression. This stress may be released (as in dental waxes) once the impression has been removed from the mouth, so the safest procedure is to construct the cast as soon as possible after the impression has been removed from the mouth.

### Zinc Oxide-Eugenol Impression Pastes

Impression pastes are used as secondary impression materials in conjunction with materials like impression compound. The basic composition of these materials includes zinc oxide and eugenol. Plasticizers, fillers, and other additives are incorporated as necessary in order to provide the desired properties.

The reaction between zinc oxide and eugenol is complex and not completely understood. The reaction produces a type of compound referred to chemically as a chelate and involves a complex structural formula. The hardened mass may be visualized as particles of zinc oxide bound together with a matrix of zinc eugenolate, as is the case with zinc oxide–eugenol cements.

The composition of the individual pastes influences the setting time, and the type and amount of accelerator is the most important factor in the control of the setting time. Impression pastes set more rapidly in the oral environment than at room temperature, meaning that temperature and moisture accelerate their set.

QUESTIONS

34. Body and strength are given to the reversible hydrocolloid by
    1. potassium sulfate
    2. lead peroxide
    3. agar
    4. borax

35. The fact that the temperature of gelation of reversible hydrocolloid is lower than the temperature of liquefaction is known as
    1. syneresis
    2. gelling

3. hysteresis
4. polymerization

36. Calcium sulfate in the alginates is a
   1. retarder
   2. reactor
   3. Neither of the above
   4. Both 1 and 2

37. Warm water has which of the following effects on alginates?
   1. No effect
   2. Increase in the gelation time
   3. Decrease in the gelation time

38. The optimum thickness of polysulfide impression material is
   1. 0.5–1 cm
   2. 2–3 mm
   3. 6–8 mm
   4. 5–10 cm

39. The oxidizing agent(s) used in the polymerization of polysulfide impression materials is (are)
   a. lead octoate
   b. tin octoate
   c. hydroperoxide
   d. lead peroxide
   1. a and b
   2. c and d
   3. b
   4. c
   5. d

40. The advantages of the silicones over the mercaptans include
   a. longer working time
   b. better odor
   c. better esthetic characteristics
   d. easier to pour in stone
   1. a and b
   2. a and d
   3. b and c
   4. c and d

41. One of the problems with polyether impression materials is a
   1. low modulus of elasticity
   2. low coefficient of thermal conductivity
   3. dimensional instability in the presence of moisture
   4. consistency very similar to the reversible hydrocolloids

42. An impression compound impression should be poured in gypsum immediately to minimize inaccuracies related to
   1. dehydration
   2. stress relief
   3. syneresis
   4. further setting

43. An increase in temperature effects the setting time of the zinc oxide–eugenol impression pastes by

1. shortening the setting time
2. lengthening the setting time
3. An increase in temperature has no effect on the setting time.

## DENTURE BASE RESINS

Because of the complexity in chemistry and composition of resins, it is difficult to classify them. One classification system is based on their thermal behavior. If the resin is molded without a chemical change occurring, as when it is softened under heat and pressure and then cooled to form a solid, it is classified as thermoplastic. If a chemical reaction does take place during the molding process and the final product is chemically different from the original substance, the resin is classified as thermoset. The denture base resin is an example of a thermoplastic material, while the elastomer impression materials are thermoset resins.

Poly (methyl methacrylate) is the most common denture base resin. Although other types, such as polystyrene and vinyl copolymers have been marketed for the construction of denture bases, none have proved to be superior to poly (methyl methacrylate).

The dental resin is usually supplied in the form of a powder and liquid. The powder consists of polymer particles or beads which are very clear and transparent. In order to provide the proper color of the oral soft tissues or tooth structure, pigments are added to the polymer beads. The liquid is methyl methacrylate (monomer). A small amount of an inhibitor, such as hydroquinone, is present to help prevent premature polymerization of the monomer during storage. The monomer liquid and polymer beads are mixed together so that every polymer bead is wetted by the monomer. The mixed mass sets until it becomes doughy. At this stage the resin is molded into the shape of the denture or tooth. After molding, the monomer in the dough stage is polymerized and a solid polymer results.

The polymerization process occurs in three stages. The initiation or induction stage is when the molecules of the initiator become activated and transfer their energy to the molecules of the monomer. The result is a rapid propagation of the growth of the molecules, the stage where more of the polymerization occurs. Eventually the chain reactions cease; this is known as the termination stage.

There are two methods by which the polymerization or curing can occur. One is by heating; the other, by cold curing at room temperature. In both, a chemical, known as an initiator, is present in the polymer. Usually benzoyl peroxide is used. When the initiator is activated by some form of energy such as heat, it starts the polymerization, which takes place with extreme rapidity. This process is known as heat curing. (See also Unfilled Resins.)

The cold curing of the resin usually involves placing a second chemical, an amine activator, in the monomer. When the monomer is mixed with the polymer, the activator reacts with the initiator so that the initiator can begin the polymerization at room temperature. The reaction then proceeds without any need for heat.

The mold for the dental appliance is usually constructed in plaster or stone. The resin dough is inserted into this mold, which is closed tightly so that none of the dough can escape. If the heat polymerization method is used, the closed mold is usually placed in water, the temperature of which is gradually increased until the polymerization begins. This can be accomplished by placing the flasked mold in a water bath maintained at a temperature of approximately 165 °F for 4 hours, although most techniques involve increasing the water temperature to 212 °F for a shorter period of time.

The general effect of a temperature rise above 212 °F is to produce a porosity in the interior of a thick piece of resin. Although the rate of polymerization is extremely rapid, it is not instantaneous. If the temperature rises above the boiling point of the residual monomer, the monomer may boil, producing bubbles. This type of porosity is not present on the surface of a denture. The exothermic heat can be conducted away from the surface of the resin into the investing medium, and the temperature in this region is not likely to rise above the boiling point of the monomer.

Localized porosity positioned sporadically on the surface of or within the structure of a cured denture resin results from the monomer not being diffused homogeneously throughout the resin dough prior to curing. Porosity may occur throughout the denture if an acrylic resin of sticky consistency, not doughy, is used to pack the denture mold. A consistent porosity can also be caused if there is insufficient pressure on the denture resin in the denture mold during packing or insufficient denture resin was used to pack the mold.

If the cold cure polymerization method is used, the mold is kept closed at room temperature until the polymerization reaction has ceased.

The cold-cured resins are not used as often as other denture base materials or the heat-cured resins, although they are often used for the replacement of a denture tooth or the repair of a fractured denture. The cold-cured denture resins demonstrate less polymerization shrinkage, and the dimensional stability during usage is superior to that of a heat-cured resin; the surface of the denture is more porous, however.

### QUESTIONS

44. The principal difference between the heat-cured denture resins and the cold-cured denture resins is the

1. basic formulation
2. cold-cured resins contain an amine accelerator
3. cold-cured resins contain no initiator
4. heat-cured resins contain no initiator

45. The most generally accepted processing temperature for the heat-cured acrylics is
   1. 145 °F–155 °F
   2. 160 °F–170 °F
   3. 212 °F
   4. Any of the above

46. Inhibitors are added to the monomers of the denture base resins to
   1. activate the monomer
   2. increase shelf life
   3. speed up the reaction
   4. produce a softer polymer

47. Porosity will be seen in what area of a denture base when insufficient packing pressure is used?
   1. In the thickest portion of the denture
   2. At the periphery of the denture
   3. Consistently distributed throughout the denture
   4. At the junction of the teeth and denture base material

48. If a chemical activator rather than heat is used to generate free radicals from benzoyl peroxide in the initiation step, these polymers are known as
   1. condensation polymers
   2. self-curing polymers
   3. cross-linked polymers
   4. plasticized polymers

## DENTAL PORCELAIN

Porcelain has many uses in dentistry: denture teeth, jacket crowns, porcelain-fused-to-metal appliances, and inlays. Porcelain has an excellent cosmetic appearance, is kind to soft tissues, and resists wear.

Dental porcelain is composed of varying amounts of crystalline ingredients such as silica, feldspar, and alumina, in addition to other ingredients. The crystalline constituents are held together in glass, which is clear and has a liquidlike structure. The porcelain is manufactured by heating feldspar and other minerals together with materials called fluxes that form lower-fusing temperature glasses. These fluxes are oxides or carbonates of sodium potassium, lithium, and boron. The fused mass, called a frit, is quickly cooled to form the porcelain, which is then refired to add metal oxides that give the shades necessary to match natural tooth appearance.

Porcelains are classified according to their fusing temperature. The three fusing ranges generally recognized in dentistry for the porcelains are: low fusing (1600°–1950°F), medium fusing (2000°–2300°F), and high fusing (2360°–2500°F). The higher-fusing temperature porcelains contain more crystalline ingredients and usually have a more natural appearance.

Dental porcelains have several unique properties. They are brittle and cannot withstand tensile or bending stresses without breaking, but they are stronger in compression with strengths from two to three times those in tension. Care should be taken to design appliances to avoid tensile stresses.

The greatest use of dental porcelain in dentistry today is in the construction of porcelain-fused-to-metal appliances. Restorations of this type have the advantage over solid porcelain jacket crowns in that they are more resistant to fracture. These restorations are fabricated by firing a porcelain directly to a core made from a specially formulated metal alloy. Elements in the metal alloy that contribute to a satisfactory bond between the casting and porcelain are iron, tin, and gold because of the effectiveness of their oxides in penetrating the porcelain mass. The first layer of the porcelain, or the opaque layer, bonds to the oxide layer. Good wetting of the porcelain during the glass phase is essential to the bonding. It is also essential that the coefficient of thermal expansion of the metal and porcelain be matched so that the appliance does not crack on cooling. One of the major problems in firing dental porcelain is the high degree of shrinkage that occurs in firing.

QUESTIONS

49. If an alloy is to be fused to porcelain, it is essential that
   1. the compressive strength of the porcelain and alloy be the same
   2. the modulus of rupture of the porcelain and alloy be the same
   3. the coefficient of thermal expansion of the porcelain and alloy be the same

50. Porcelain is superior to plastic as a restorative material, because porcelain abrades more than plastic.
   1. Both statement and reason are true and related.
   2. Both statement and reason are true but not related.
   3. The statement is true, but the reason is not true.
   4. The statement is false, but the reason is true.

51. Porcelain-fused-to-metal restorations are superior to porcelain jacket crowns because a much better aesthetic result is obtainable.
   1. Both statement and reason are true and related.
   2. Both statement and reason are true but not related.
   3. The statement is true, but the reason is not true.
   4. The statement is false, but the reason is true.

52. Metallic oxides are included in the composition of dental porcelain to
   a. provide a refractory skeleton
   b. give color to the porcelain
   c. reduce the strength
   d. increase the strength

1. All of the above
2. b and d
3. a, b, and d
4. a, b, and c
5. None of the above

## MISCELLANEOUS BIOMATERIALS

### Pit and Fissure Sealants

Protection of enamel faults from dental caries remains a high priority in preventive dentistry. Although many questions remain unanswered, the pit and fissure sealants appear to be potential aids in these efforts against dental caries. The clinical procedure involved in sealant application is 1) prophylaxis of the teeth, 2) acid-etching of the enamel to promote resin bonding, and 3) resin placement.

Four types of resin materials have been utilized clinically: cyanoacrylates, polyurethanes, glass ionomer cement, and the BIS–GMA resins. Due to the hydrolysis of the cyanoacrylates in the oral environment, no commercial product of this type has been marketed. Only one polyurethane material has been on the market, but it has been withdrawn, due primarily to the fact that its bonds with enamel do not last for long time periods. Glass ionomer cement has been used as a pit and fissure sealant, but very limited clinical data are available. More data are available on the BIS–GMA resins, and they show the greatest potential as pit and fissure sealants. The formula is essentially the basic resin matrix in the composite restorative materials.

### Pins in Direct Restorations

When a tooth is so badly broken down that there is no longer any way of retaining a restoration by means of the remaining dental tissues, artificial aids for retention are necessary. Nonparallel pins may serve to retain restorative materials in such teeth, for example.

All pins used for the retention of direct restorations are similar in that they are rigid pieces of threaded or notched wires which are cemented, hammered, or screwed into holes made in the dentin of a tooth with a twist drill. The holes are drilled so that they are not parallel to one another, and the restorative material is placed around them and allowed to set.

Today there are basically three types of pins in common use: 1) the cemented pin, 2) the friction pin, and 3) the self-threading pin. In the cemented pin technique the pins are cemented into holes that are slightly larger than the pin, usually with a zinc phosphate cement or a cyanoacrylate cement. This technique does not depend on any intrinsic elasticity of the dentin for retention, and consequently it has been argued that this technique is the safest as far as the risk of fracturing the tooth structure is concerned and is the pin of choice when treating endodontically treated teeth.

The friction pin, or friction-locked pin, is placed into a hole that is slightly smaller than the pin. This pin is placed by driving it into the pin hole.

The third type of pin, the self-threading pin, is threaded into a hole that is smaller than the pin. This pin, like the friction pin, depends on the elasticity of the dentin for its retention.

A review of the literature concerning pins for direct restorations indicates that pins serve only to retain the restoration and that they tend to weaken, not reinforce, dental amalgam. Self-threading pins are consistently more efficient as retaining devices than either of the other pin types in common use today. The optimum length of a pin into a restorative material is 2 mm. In addition, the optimum depth of a self-threading pin into the dentin is 2–3 mm.

### QUESTIONS

53. Which of the following have been employed as a pit and fissure sealant?
    a. Cyanoacrylate
    b. Polyurethane
    c. BIS–GMA resin
    d. Poly (methyl methacrylate) resin
    1. a and b
    2. a, b, and c
    3. a and c
    4. All of the above

54. According to tests performed on pins in dentin, which pin has the greatest retention?
    1. Cemented pin
    2. Friction pin
    3. Self-threading pin

55. The pin of choice in endodontically treated teeth is the
    1. cemented pin
    2. friction pin
    3. self-threading pin

56. The optimum depth of self-threading pins for an amalgam restoration is
    1. 0.5 mm
    2. 2 mm
    3. 4 mm
    4. 5 mm

57. The pins designed to depend on the elasticity of the dentin for retention are the
    a. cemented pin
    b. friction pin
    c. self-threading pin
    1. a and b
    2. b and c
    3. a and c
    4. All of the above

## SUGGESTED READING

ANDREWS JT, HEMBREE JH: In vitro evaluation of marginal leakage of corrosion-resistant amalgam alloy. J Dent Child 42:367–370, 1975

ANDREWS JT, HEMBREE JH: In vivo evaluation of marginal leakage of four inlay cements. J Prosthet Dent 35:532–37, 1976

BARSH LI: Pin-retained amalgam restorations in restorative dentistry. J Gen Dent 19:24–27, 1971

COMBE EC (ed): Notes on Dental Materials, 2nd ed. Edinburgh, Churchill Livingston, 1975

Council on Dental Materials and Devices: Status report on silver amalgam. J Am Dent Assoc 91:618–21, 1975

CRAIG RG, O'BRIEN WJ, POWERS JM: Dental Materials, Properties, and Manipulation. St. Louis, CV Mosby, 1975

EAMES WB, MACNAMARA JF: Eight high-copper amalgam alloys and six conventional alloys compared. Oper Dent 1:98–107, 1976

EARNSHAW R, SMITH DC: The tensile and compressive strength of plaster and stone. Aust J Dent 11:415, 1966

GREENE EH, HARCOURT JK, LAUTENSCHLAGER EP: Materials Science in Dentistry. Baltimore, WB Saunders, 1973

Guide to Dental Materials and Devices, 6th ed. Chicago, American Dental Association, 1972

Guide to Dental Materials and Devices, 8th ed. Chicago, American Dental Association, 1976

HEMBREE JH: Comparative accuracy of elastomer impression materials. Tenn Dent J 54:164–167, 1974

HEMBREE JH: Comparison of compressive strengths of six dental amalgam alloys. Miss Dent J 31:18–19, 1975

HEMBREE JH: Comparative accuracy of impression materials used for indirect techniques. Tex Dent J 46:6–8, 1976

HEMBREE JH: Filler particles of composite restorative materials. Tenn Dent J 54:6–7, 1974

HEMBREE JH, ANDREWS JT: Accuracy of a polyether impression material. Ark Dent J 47:10–11, 1976

HEMBREE JH, ANDREWS JT: In situ evaluation of marginal leakage using an ultraviolet-light-activated resin system. J Am Dent Assoc 92:414–418, 1976

HEMBREE JH, ANDREWS JT: Microleakage of several acid-etch composite resin systems: a laboratory study. Oper Dent 1:91–97, 1976

HEMBREE JH, FINGAR W, DRAUGHN RA: Correlation of composite filler particle size and shape to compressive strength. SC Dent J 33:43–47, 1975

HEMBREE JH, HOWARD JL: In vitro evaluation of marginal leakage of four luting medias. Ark Dent J 46:13–16, 1975

HEMBREE JH, NUNEZ LJ: Effect of moisture on polyether impression materials. J Am Dent Assoc 89:1134–36, 1974

HOLTZ P, MCLEAN JW, SCED I et al: The bonding of glass ionomer cements to metal and tooth substrates. Br Dent J 142:41–47, 1977

HUGET EF, CIVJAN S: Status report on palladium-silver-based crown and bridge alloys. J Am Dent Assoc 89:383–385, 1974

KENT BE, LEWIS BG, WILSON AD: The properties of a glass ionomer cement. Br Dent J 135:322–326, 1973

MABIE CP: Petrographic study of the refractory performance of high-fusing dental alloy investments. I. High-fired phosphate bonded investments. J Dent Res 52:96–110, 1973

MABIE CP: Petrographic study of the refractory performance of high-fusing dental alloy investments. II. Silica bonded investments. J Dent Res 52:758–773, 1973

MAHLER DB: Hardness and flow properties of gypsum materials. J Prosthet Dent 1:188, 1951

MOFFA JP, HENKINS WA: Status report on base-metal crown and bridge alloys. J Am Dent Assoc 89:652–655, 1974

PEYTON FA, CRAIG RG: Restorative Dental Materials, 4th ed. St. Louis, CV Mosby, 1971

PHILLIPS RW: Elements of Dental Materials. Philadelphia, WB Saunders, 1971

PHILLIPS RW: Skinners Science of Dental Materials, 7th ed. Philadelphia, WB Saunders, 1973

SHORT GM, HEMBREE JH, MCKNIGHT JP: The bond strengths of resin systems to etched enamel. J Prosthet Dent 36:538–543, 1976

Status report on polyether impression materials. Council on Dental Materials and Devices. J Am Dent Assoc 95:126–129, 1977

WILSON AD, CRISP S, FERNER AJ: Reactions in glass-ionomer cements. IV. Effect of chelating comonomers on setting behavior. J Dent Res 55:489–495, 1976

## ANSWER KEY

| | | | |
|---|---|---|---|
| 1. 2 | 16. 3 | 30. 3 | 44. 2 |
| 2. 3 | 17. 4 | 31. 1 | 45. 2 |
| 3. 1 | 18. 2 | 32. 3 | 46. 2 |
| 4. 4 | 19. 3 | 33. 4 | 47. 3 |
| 5. 1 | 20. 4 | 34. 4 | 48. 2 |
| 6. 2 | 21. 4 | 35. 3 | 49. 3 |
| 7. 5 | 22. 3 | 36. 2 | 50. 3 |
| 8. 1 | 23. 4 | 37. 3 | 51. 3 |
| 9. 4 | 24. 1 | 38. 2 | 52. 2 |
| 10. 4 | 25. 4 | 39. 2 | 53. 2 |
| 11. 2 | 26. 2 | 40. 3 | 54. 3 |
| 12. 4 | 27. 1 | 41. 3 | 55. 1 |
| 13. 3 | 28. 2 | 42. 2 | 56. 2 |
| 14. 2 | 29. 1 | 43. 1 | 57. 2 |
| 15. 1 | | | |

# 3
# OPERATIVE DENTISTRY
## Clifford H. Miller

The subject of operative dentistry is allocated 100 questions on the National Board Dental Examinations, as are all other major subjects for examination. The content outline of operative dentistry incorporated in the National Board Dental Examinations encompasses five major topics: 8 questions are devoted to dental caries; 12 questions to examination, diagnosis, and treatment planning; 18 questions to general operative procedures; 27 questions to the preparation of cavities; and 35 questions to restorations of prepared cavities. The subject of dental materials is fairly heavily weighted in that section dealing with restorations of prepared cavities.

## DENTAL CARIES

### Disease Process

Four questions are devoted to the etiology of dental caries, and thus it is essential to be aware of the factors required to produce dental caries. Current theories concerning the etiology of dental caries require three components: 1) a susceptible individual, 2) a suitable substrate, and 3) a bacterial enzyme system. This has been demonstrated in the classic overlapping circles depicted in the work of Keyes. Dental caries is most commonly found in pits and fissures, followed by the proximal surfaces, and finally on the smooth surfaces of the facial and lingual sides of the teeth.

Dental plaque, the adherent material that is found on the surfaces of teeth that are not properly brushed and flossed, provides a suitable substrate for the initiation of dental caries. Dental plaque contains a variety of microorganisms including *Streptococcus mutans, Streptococcus sanguis, Streptococcus mitior, Streptococcus salivarius* and *Streptococcus milevi*. Fermentable carbohydrates are the chief offenders insofar as food is concerned in initiating dental caries. These fermentable carbohydrates are attacked by a bacterial enzyme system and, by a degradation process, are converted into acids which contribute to the decalcifi-

cation of the enamel, resulting in caries formation. *Streptococcus mutans* is the principal bacterial agent involved with the caries process. Dental caries is infectious and transmissible in nature.

QUESTIONS

1. Caries activity could well increase
   a. during pregnancy
   b. following radiation therapy in the head and neck region
   c. following a serious emotional problem
   d. following periodontal surgery
   1. a and b only
   2. b and c only
   3. a, c, and d only
   4. All of the above

2. The location of teeth in the arch and tooth morphology affect their caries susceptiblity. Those least susceptible to caries attack in the permanent dentition are
   1. maxillary cuspids
   2. mandibular incisors
   3. mandibular premolars
   4. maxillary incisors
   5. maxillary third molars

3. The principal bacterial agent involved in the caries process is
   1. *Lactobacillus acidophilus*
   2. *Streptococcus sanguis*
   3. *Streptococcus salivarius*
   4. *Streptococcus mutans*

4. Three factors required for the initiation of dental caries are
   1. polysaccharides, microorganisms, and enamel
   2. enamel lamella, lactobacilli, and polysaccharides
   3. susceptible tooth, suitable substrate, and a bacterial enzyme system
   4. bacterial plaque, suitable tooth, and polysaccharides

### Prevention

In simplified terms dental caries can be prevented in three ways: first, render the tooth less susceptible to the caries process; second, eliminate the suitable substrate or fermentable carbohydrate and adherent plaque; and third, attack the bacterial enzyme system.

The use of fluorides either topically or systemically has done a great deal to render the individual tooth less susceptible to dental caries. It is thought that the fluoride ion reacts with hydroxyapatite crystal by replacing the hydroxyl group to become a fluoroapatite crystal, which in theory renders the tooth more resistant to attack by caries. The critical pH for decalcification of a newly erupted tooth which has not been in contact with fluoride is approximately 5.2. In the presence of fluoride ion this critical pH is effectively lowered. It is generally agreed that fluoride taken systemically in the community drinking water is the most effective method of prevention and can reduce caries incidence up to 65%. One part per million (PPM) is considered ideal, since this appears to have the most beneficial effect on the teeth with no noticeable mottling. As the concentration of fluoride exceeds 2 PPM, the incidence of mottling greatly increases. Topical application of fluoride is considered an adjunctive method in preventing dental caries and is applied during routine recall visits using an acidulated phosphate fluoride.

Pit and fissure sealants are another means of rendering the tooth less susceptible to dental caries. Numerous brands of pit and fissure sealants are currently on the market and include cyanoacrylates, polyurethanes, and bisphenol-A-glycidyl methacrylates. The method of application is standard: isolating the teeth, drying them carefully, acid etching using 50% phosphoric acid for 1 min, and then flushing with water and drying. When the sealant is applied into the fissures and pits, every effort must be made to avoid the entrapment of air. Great caution should also be exercised to determine that no caries exist in the pits or fissures before the sealant is applied; many studies indicate that, unless applied properly, these sealants will leak and wash out in a fairly short period.

Emphasis is currently being directed towards proper patient education and home care instruction on how to keep the teeth in a plaque-free condition so that caries cannot be initiated. Proper brushing and flossing is required, as well as sensible dietary constraints. Finally, caries can be controlled or prevented by attacking the bacterial enzyme systems. Work is currently in progress to develop an effective vaccine or antienzymes to inhibit caries formation.

QUESTIONS

5. Fluorides affect the tooth structure in the following manner to make it more resistant to dental caries.
   a. Fluoride removes the organic component of the enamel matrix.
   b. Fluoride ions chemically react with the hydroxyapatite crystal and replace the hydroxyl ions.
   c. Fluoride ions react chemically with the calcium in the enamel.
   d. When topically applied, the fluoride ion only affects the outer layers of enamel.
   e. Fluoride ions react with the apatite crystal to make it more resistant to acid.
   1. a, b, and d
   2. b, d, and e
   3. c, d, and e
   4. a, c, and d
   5. All of the above

6. The optimum concentration of fluoride in the community drinking water is considered to be
   1. 0.5 PPM
   2. 0.75 PPM
   3. 1 PPM
   4. 2 PPM
   5. 4 PPM

7. Commonly used acid for etching teeth in conjunction with pit and fissure sealant is
   1. hydrochloric acid
   2. phosphoric acid
   3. acetic acid
   4. sulfuric acid

8. Bacterial plaque can be most effectively removed from the proximal surfaces of the teeth by using
   1. dental floss
   2. a tooth brush
   3. an interdental stimulator
   4. a water pick
   5. a periodontal aid
   6. All of the above

## EXAMINATION, DIAGNOSIS, AND TREATMENT PLANNING

### Dental Caries and Traumatic Injury

There are three basic ways of detecting caries: first, direct examination with a mirror and probe; second, bite-wing radiographs; and third, transillumination, using a fiberoptic light source.

Pit and fissure caries are not readily detected by radiograph, nor are smooth surface lesions on the facial or lingual surfaces of the anterior or posterior teeth. Proximal carious lesions are most readily detected by use of bite-wing radiographs. Transillumination is frequently effective for questionable lesions on the proximal surface of the anteriors. In detection of caries it is always wise to know the mode of spread of the carious lesion. In pit and fissure caries the spread is in the shape of a cone or pyramid with the tips of the cone at the outer surface of the enamel and the base at the dentoenamel junction. As the caries progresses into the dentin, it is again in the shape of a cone or pyramid with the base at the dentoenamel junction and the tip progressing along the lines of dentinal tubules towards the pulp.

Smooth surface caries present a different picture, although the progress of caries is again in the shape of a cone or pyramid. In this instance, however, the base of the cone is on the surface of the tooth with the tip at the dentoenamel junction. Again, as the caries spreads laterally along the dentoenamel junction, it can be depicted as a cone or pyramid with the base at the dentoenamel junction and tip following the dentinal tubules towards the pulp. Caries has always progressed further in the tooth than would appear radiographically.

Dental caries can be categorized as acute or chronic. Acute caries occurs in patients with high susceptibility. It progresses rapidly, usually with little if any staining, and can cause widespread destruction before cavitation is clinically evident.

Traumatic injury could be a fracture of the roots or crown, or a crack in the tooth itself. The cracked tooth syndrome is usually difficult to diagnose, but it can frequently be detected during cavity preparation when the tooth is dried or by means of topical stains. It exhibits vague symptoms such as occasional pain, sensitivity to heat or cold, discomfort on biting. A cracked tooth should always be suspected when other causes of pain and discomfort have been ruled out.

### QUESTIONS

9. Chronic dental caries differs from acute dental caries in that
    a. there is greater pigmentation of the lesion
    b. there is greater depth than width to the lesion
    c. the unsupported enamel is usually fractured away
    d. there is usually minimal sensitivity
    1. a and b
    2. a, b, and d
    3. b, c, and d
    4. a, c, and d
    5. All of the above

10. The radiographic appearance of a proximal carious lesion is
    1. larger than the actual lesion
    2. smaller than the actual lesion
    3. an accurate reproduction of the size of the lesion
    4. variable depending upon the exposure time and development process

11. Proximal caries typically progresses in a pattern characterized by a double cone or pyramid as it extends through the enamel and into the dentin. The apices of each cone are
    1. directed toward the pulp
    2. pointing in opposite directions
    3. touching each other at the dentoenamel junction
    4. directed toward the enamel surface

12. Bite-wing radiographs are a useful diagnostic tool for the detection of
    1. Class I carious lesions
    2. proximal surface caries
    3. caries on the facial surface
    4. caries on the lingual surface
    5. All of the above

13. The characteristic shape of smooth surface carious lesions in enamel relates to the
    1. striae of Retzius
    2. incremental lines of Owen
    3. direction of the enamel rods
    4. mamelons of the tooth
    5. direction of the Tomes fibers

### Odontogenic Pain

Patients may describe various types of sensitivity pre- or postoperatively. Frequently this pain or discomfort is associated with temperature changes or pressure related to occlusion. Hyperemia of the pulp can be brought about by pressure, chemical irritation, or thermal irritation, and if the trauma is not too great, is reversible in nature. The dental pulp has remarkable recuperative power but is handicapped by being in a confined chamber. Pulpal irritation has a cumulative effect and eventually can create an irreversible pulpitis that results in degeneration and necrosis. This is characterized by a more persistent pain which may be throbbing in nature, with or without swelling. It is generally aggravated by heat and tender to percussion.

Teeth may become sensitive to brushing in the cervical region. This is associated with exposure of the cementoenamel junction and cementum due to tissue recession.

### QUESTIONS

14. If, following placement of a metallic restoration, the tooth remains sensitive to heat, cold, and pressure after occlusal adjustment, the dentist should
    1. remove the restoration and place a sedative temporary restoration
    2. initiate endodontic therapy
    3. grind the opposing tooth to free it from any occlusal contact
    4. tell the patient to put up with the discomfort and it will eventually go away

15. A split tooth could well display which of the following characteristics?
    a. Not visible radiographically
    b. Sensitive to pressure
    c. Sensitive to temperature change
    d. Mild to moderate pain which comes and goes
    1. b and c only
    2. a and d only
    3. b, c, and d only
    4. All of the above

## Treatment Sequencing and Selection of Restorative Materials

Sequencing of treatment for full mouth dental care is generally the application of clinical judgment. Once the diagnosis has been finalized, pain or the threat of irreversible consequences must be eliminated. If there are teeth with pulpal involvement, they should be treated as a first priority. Those teeth that have deep carious lesions should be temporized. Once the threat of pulpal exposure is no longer a factor, the periodontal health and dental education of the patient must be considered. As patient cooperation develops and a home care regime is established, the routine restoration of the posterior and anterior dentition is accomplished. Upon completion of this stage, fixed prosthodontic appliances are cemented in the mouth; as a final stage any necessary removable prosthetic appliance is inserted.

In the selection of restorative materials a number of factors must be considered: the age of the patient, the caries susceptibility, the condition of the teeth as presented, any previous restorative work, the commitment of the patient to quality restorative procedures, the time which the patient has available to have the service rendered, the necessary aesthetic result, the occlusion and the masticatory stress which is to be placed on the dentition, and to some extent, the patient's financial situation. Amalgam would certainly be the material of choice for a teen-ager or young adult with moderate to severe caries susceptibility. The rationale for this selection is the time involved and physical response to the material. Amalgam restorations can be placed quickly, and the material itself is more resistant to caries because of its natural ability to seal margins and resist the recurrence of caries. Existing restorations can be modified conservatively with amalgam until the patient's home care is established and the caries susceptibility is controlled.

For those patients who have a very low caries susceptibility, who practice good preventive home care, and who are devoted to maintaining their teeth for the remainder of their lives, gold castings are the restoration of choice. The rationale for this is that the proximal contour and contact of a tooth can be more perfectly restored with gold castings than any other restorative material. Proper restoration of the mesiodistal dimension of the tooth, as well as the occlusal table and proximal contour, helps in the prevention of periodontal disease and maintains the correct occlusal relationships.

The selection of a restorative material may occasionally be determined by aesthetics, depending on the person's occupation or personality. In a situation such as this, masticatory forces and inherent strength of material are secondary to restoration of natural tooth color and form. For these instances porcelain jacket crowns, porcelain-fused-to-metal restorations, and even the composite resins may have priority in selection.

In the final analysis factors influencing the selection of materials are based on clinical judgment, common sense, and the ability to interact intelligently with the patient.

QUESTIONS

16. A proper treatment sequence would include the following in what order?
    a. Complete diagnosis and treatment plan
    b. Control of pain
    c. Prophylaxis and home care instruction
    d. Temporization of deep carious lesions
    e. Restorations placed

    1. a, b, c, d, and e
    2. b, d, a, c, and e
    3. c, b, a, d, and e
    4. b, c, d, a, and e

17. The restorative materials considered suitable for restoration of the distal of a canine involving the contact include
    a. direct filling gold
    b. amalgam
    c. gold casting
    d. composite resin
    e. filled acrylic resin using acid etching

    1. a and b
    2. a, b, and c
    3. b and d
    4. b, c, and d
    5. a, d, and e
    6. All of the above

## Postoperative Problems

Three questions are allocated to this topic and they are generally designed in the format of a differential diagnosis. In considering postoperative problems it is useful to place them into categories. The first category would be associated with the restoration or the treatment; the second, with the response of the dental pulp; and the third, with conditions involving the supporting tissues or periodontium.

Relative to the restorative treatment, a patient's postoperative symptoms might be associated with faulty occlusion, or improper contour and contact relationships. If a restoration were left in supraocclusion, the patient may well return complaining of discomfort on chewing and pain associated with pressure. This could create a hyperemic condition of the pulp with resultant sensitivity to cold or heat. Improper contact relationships or contours could cause the patient to complain of food impaction or, in the case of contour, of biting the cheek or tongue.

A frequent condition which occurs in relation to postoperative pulpal problems is hyperemia. This could be attributable to an inadequate base when the restoration has been placed in close proximity to the pulp or merely to the trauma associated with the restorative procedure. Occasionally a pulpal horn is violated in conjunction with the cavity preparation, and this should always be considered a possible cause for postoperative problems after deep restorations.

Postoperative problems associated with the periodontal supporting tissues are frequently in the nature of localized swelling or pain. This could be the result of a lateral abscess, or it could be the result of localized irritation due to the retention of something subgingivally. Impression material, alginate, a piece of rubber dam, a particle of amalgam, or temporary cement are all potential offenders.

### QUESTIONS

18. Pupal hyperemia results when some form of trauma causes an inflammation. The characteristics of hyperemia include
    a. pain of short duration
    b. no radiographic indication of pulp pathology
    c. increased sensitivity to cold temperature
    d. reversibility under usual conditions

    1. a, b, and c
    2. a, b, and d
    3. b, c, and d
    4. All of the above

19. Approximately 1 month following the placement of a large mesio-occluso-distal amalgam with deep proximal boxes, the patient experiences definite pain in the region of the tooth. The probable cause for the pain is

    1. moisture contamination of the amalgam causing delayed expansion
    2. an undetected exposure of a pulp horn
    3. supraocclusion
    4. gingival excess
    5. an open contact due to faulty matrix application

20. Pain following the placement of an amalgam restoration is most frequently related to
    1. heat
    2. cold
    3. occlusal pressure
    4. galvanic shock

## GENERAL OPERATIVE PROCEDURES

### Instruments and Equipment

The type of questions devoted to this topic has undergone some revision in recent years. Traditionally questions were asked relative to the formulation of instruments, and it is probably still a good idea to know what the numbers mean. For an 18–9–6 chisel, for example, the first number denotes the width of the blade in tenths of a millimeter, 18 meaning 1.8 mm wide. The second number denotes the length of the blade in millimeters, or 9 mm long; the third number denotes the angle of the blade to the shaft in degrees centigrade. Most of these questions have been removed from the examination, but occasionally one crops up; it is wise to be familiar with the formulation. The same holds true with the numbering system for burs. The single number digits (¼, ½, 2, 4, 6, 8) indicate round burs. The 30 series (33½, 34, 35, etc.) indicates inverted cones; the 50 series (56, 57, 58, etc.) indicates straight fissures; the 69, 70 series indicates tapered fissures; and the 500 series (556, 557) indicates cross cut straight fissure burs; and the 690 and 700 series (700, 701, 702) indicates cross cut tapered fissure burs.

Questions are asked regarding the effect on the pulp of heat generated by rotational instruments. Comparisons are ordinarily made between operating at ultra high speed and operating at a lower speed, between using carbide or steel burs and using diamond burs, and between working with or working without an air–water spray coolant. It should be relatively obvious that in all instances the least traumatic method of reducing tooth structures is with light pressure at ultra high speed and with an adequate air–water spray coolant. Describing all the instruments and equipment in dentistry which could serve as a source for questions is beyond the scope of this chapter, but most of these questions should be straightforward for anyone who has been involved in doing dental procedures.

### QUESTIONS

21. The rotational instrument which leaves the roughest surface on cut tooth structure is a
    1. medium grit diamond at low speed
    2. cross cut fissure bur at ultra speed
    3. cross cut fissure bur at low speed
    4. garnet disc at low speed
    5. medium grit diamond at ultra speed

22. The hazards of using air only as a coolant when cutting at ultra high speed are that it may
    a. cause dehydration
    b. supercool the tooth
    c. cause postoperative hypersensitivity
    d. result in the odontoblasts becoming disoriented and drawn into the dentinal tubules
    e. interfere with visibility

    1. a and b
    2. b, d, and e
    3. a, c, and d
    4. All of the above

23. The second number on those instruments having a three-number formula indicates the
    1. angle of the cutting edge in degrees centigrade
    2. length of the blade in tenths of a millimeter
    3. length of the blade in millimeters
    4. width of the blade in millimeters

## Relationship of Operative Dentistry to Other Disciplines

Three questions are devoted to this topic. Of course, operative dentistry is related to all of the disciplines of dentistry and is frequently considered the foundation of a general practice. In developing questions in this area, however, disciplines such as endodontics and periodontics, which have a more direct relationship to operative dentistry usually are selected.

Following endodontic treatment, it is always essential to place a permanent restoration, and an awareness of the result of the endodontic treatment must be taken into consideration. In selecting a restorative material when an endodontic procedure has been performed on an anterior tooth using lingual access, for example, it is essential that a restoration be placed that will seal the access preparation without darkening the tooth or causing it to lose translucency. If a metallic restoration is used, it is imperative that an opaque base be placed first. Amalgam would certainly not be the restorative material of choice. With today's products the material of choice would probably be one of the composite resins selected in a color to match the existing tooth.

Restoration of posterior teeth following endodontic treatment almost invariably involves protecting the weakened cusps, because the tooth becomes more brittle following an endodontic procedure. If amalgam is to be used, the cusp must be reduced 2–3 mm to provide adequate bulk for strength of the amalgam restoration. With gold restorations only 1–1.5 mm of tooth structure need to be removed, but care must be exercised in placing the bevels or chamfers on the working cusps in such a way that they will be out of the forces of occlusion.

The relationship of operative dentistry to periodontics involves the effect of operative restorative materials on the soft tissues, which generally applies to the gingival third. Silicates, composite resins, and amalgams tend to cause gingival tissue irritation because of their surface roughness or corrosion by-products. Gold foil properly polished and finished reacts very well with the soft tissue, as does fused porcelain that is properly glazed and polished. Proper maintenance of the contour and contact relationships in operative restorations is imperative to maintain periodontal health. Examination questions frequently relate to contact relationships, embrasure form, or marginal integrity as they affect the supporting tissues. It should be obvious that if the integrity of the tooth or contours are violated, an adverse reaction ensues.

### QUESTIONS

24. In order to maintain periodontal health the best position for the cavosurface margin is

a. in the gingival sulcus midway between the crest of the tissue and the epithelial attachment
b. at the epithelial attachment
c. at the free gingival crest
d. occlusal to the free gingival crest

1. a
2. a or c
3. b or c
4. c or d

25. An endodontically treated maxillary first permanent molar with a small carious lesion on the mesial and distal would be restored best by
1. a mesio-occluso-distal cast gold inlay
2. a mesio-occluso-distal amalgam
3. a mesio-occluso-distal cast gold onlay
4. a full crown
5. a ¾ crown

26. In restoring an endodontically treated maxillary central incisor with an abraded incisal edge and moderate composite resins on the mesial and distal, the treatment of choice would be
1. post-retained porcelain jacket crown
2. a pin ledge gold casting
3. composite resin using acid etch
4. post-retained porcelain–metal crown

## Control of the Operating Field

Controlling the operating field can involve isolating the area by using cotton rolls or a rubber dam. The three questions allocated for this topic almost invariably deal with the rubber dam, since when properly placed, it is the most effective method of control. Usually the extra heavy gauge material is recommended for a dam, since it provides better tissue retraction and improved protection for the patient and operator.

This topic can be considered from two standpoints: technique of placement and the manner in which the rubber dam controls the operating field. As far as technique of placement is concerned, one must be careful with the size of the holes, the spacing of the holes, and the position of the holes in relationship to the teeth. If the holes are punched too close together, there is a tendency for the dam to pull away from the necks of the teeth, causing leakage and also some tissue strangulation as a result of undue pressure on the papillae. Holes that are punched too far apart cause bunching of the rubber dam between the teeth, resulting in leakage and interfering with access and visibility. If the holes are not centered properly in the rubber dam, the rubber material could cover the patient's nose and impair breathing, or conversely, it could fail to cover the lips and allow moisture contamination.

The most likely questions associated with controlling the operating field relate to tissue retraction and accessibility for the gingival third lesion. The 212 clamp or retractor is used and must be stabilized with compound in order to prevent slippage or tissue laceration. The rubber dam must be carefully invaginated around the necks of the teeth in order to avoid leakage. For gingival third lesions that are well down on the cervical area of the tooth, the hole should be punched to the facial of normal tooth alignment to provide excess rubber and preclude the possibility of seepage.

### QUESTIONS

27. The rubber dam, in addition to maintaining a dry field, also serves to
    1. retract the cheeks and soft tissue
    2. protect the operator and assistant
    3. protect the patient
    4. improve accessibility
    5. save time
    6. All of the above

28. If the interdental papillae protrudes from beneath the rubber dam, the likely cause is
    1. failure to ligate each tooth
    2. too heavy gauge rubber dam material
    3. too light gauge rubber dam material
    4. punching the holes too close together
    5. punching the holes too far apart

29. When applying a rubber dam to control the operating field for a Class V restoration that is located at the cervical line, the dentist should
    a. place a ligature around each tooth to force down the papilla
    b. punch the hole for the involved tooth to the lingual of normal alignment
    c. use a 212 clamp for gingival retraction
    d. punch the hole for the involved tooth to the facial direction of normal alignment
    e. use a hatch clamp prior to placing the dam to retract tissue
    1. a
    2. b and c
    3. c and d
    4. b and e
    5. d and e

## Soft Tissue Management

In managing the soft tissues preparatory to making impressions for cast gold restorations, one should be aware of the various retraction cords and medicaments normally used for this purpose, as well as the electrosurgical techniques that are frequently employed. It is generally agreed that the use of a retraction cord containing an 8% racemic epinephrine solution is contraindicated because of untoward side-effects; there have been numerous cases reported of syncope and elevated blood pressure as a direct result of a high concentration of epinephrine in contact with tissues which may be bleeding.

Tissue can be retracted by means of pressure, using unimpregnated cord, or by a combination of pressure and chemicals. The chemical frequently used is an astringent such as alum. In all instances where tissue management is a factor, control of bleeding is a prerequisite to accurate impressions. If bleeding resumes when the cord is removed, the impression should not be taken, but rather the tissue repacked until such time as there is complete control of the tissues.

Electrosurgery has gained popularity in recent years and is widely advocated by many schools. It is important to be familiar with the different types of current used for electrosurgical procedures in order to prevent tissue necrosis with resultant recession or injury to the underlying alveolar bone. These types are commonly broken down into four categories: electrodesiccation, fulguration, electrocoagulation, and electrosection. The first two currents are dehydrating currents which are relatively destructive of tissues; their application is very limited for tissue management. A coagulating current is effective in controlling bleeding; however, it is not recommended for gingival retraction since it can result in excessive postoperative gingival recession. The most widely used current in dentistry is electrosection (acusection), since it can be controlled by the operator and is self-limiting in its destructiveness.

### QUESTIONS

30. The most widely utilized current for electrosurgery in dentistry is
    1. electrodesiccation
    2. fulguration
    3. electrocoagulation
    4. electrosection

31. Retraction cord containing racemic epinephrine has the potential hazard of
    1. localized vasoconstriction
    2. a caustic reaction on the tissues it contacts
    3. systemic vasoconstriction action
    4. a localized astringent action
    5. There are no hazards to its use.

32. The chemical tissue packs used for soft tissue management prior to impression taking are classified as
    a. caustics
    b. astringents
    c. anticoagulants
    d. vasoconstrictors
    e. vasodilators
    1. a and c
    2. b and d
    3. b and c
    4. c and e
    5. a and d

## Dental Auxilary Utilization (DAU) and Training in Expanded Auxiliary Management (TEAM)

Only two questions are allocated to this topic at present—not because it is unimportant, but because it is difficult to develop questions in this area. Since there is no universal agreement on TEAM and the manner in which it is taught, it is seldom that questions are asked relative to this topic.

DAU implies four-handed dentistry in a sit-down position, and frequently questions concern stool positions for the operator and assistant. For the operator, the stool should be positioned to provide support for the back as well as the legs. The feet should rest flat on the floor, and there should be adequate support for the upper legs. The dental assistant, whose stool generally has a ring around the base to serve as a foot support, is positioned approximately 4 in. higher than the operator. The purpose of this is to aid visibility and facilitate the assistant's responsibilities as they relate to retraction of the cheek, aspiration of fluids, and transfer of instruments. Frequently the position of the operator and the assistant are related to the hands of the clock. If the position of the patient's head is designated 12 o'clock, a right-handed operator working on the upper arch would ordinarily be in the 11 o'clock position, with the assistant in the 3 o'clock position.

### QUESTIONS

33. In positioning an assistant so that a right-handed operator is assured of visibility and access to the field of operation, it is generally agreed that the assistant sit at
   1. the right rear of the patient and the same height as the operator
   2. the left side of the patient and somewhat higher than the operator
   3. the left side of the patient and the same height as the operator
   4. any position that is comfortable for the assistant.

34. The dental assistant must be comfortably seated on a stool which supports the back and legs and permits the feet to
   1. hang freely
   2. rest on the floor
   3. rest on a platform or ring approximately 8 in. off the floor
   4. rest on a ring or platform approximately 4 in. off the floor

## Pulpal Responses

Pulpal responses can be divided into two categories: responses to the cutting procedures and responses to restorative materials.

It is generally agreed that the pulp responds favorably to virtually every physical or chemical irritation as long as there is a remaining dentin thickness of 2 mm. As one encroaches upon the pulp in a cutting procedure, the incidence of adverse pulpal response increases until a point of approximately 0.5 mm is reached, at which time virtually all cutting procedures create irritation and subsequent pulpal response. If the irritation is of a minor nature, this response, which is characterized by pulpal hyperemia and some sensitivity to heat and cold, is reversible. As the severity of the trauma increases, however, the tendency for irreversible changes in the pulp also increases. The sequence is generally acute pulpitis, chronic pulpitis, and pulpal necrosis. Heat and pressure are the two main physical factors which affect the dental pulp.

Virtually all restorative materials serve as pulpal irritants, some as the result of thermal conductivity and others, such as silicates, acrylics, and composite resins, as the result of chemical irritation. The use of bases and liners is advocated to insulate the pulp from these irritations. Chemical irritants appear to be more insidious in the manner in which they affect the dental pulp than are physical or thermal irritants. In the case of silicates, for example, the irritation is frequently of a subclinical nature until the pulp develops a chronic pulpitis and eventual necrosis. Often this occurs with no clinical symptoms whatsoever.

### QUESTIONS

35. An adverse pulpal reaction is most likely to occur when which of the following materials is placed directly into a deep cavity preparation?
   1. Silver amalgam
   2. Zinc oxide–eugenol
   3. Polycarboxylate cement
   4. Silicate cement
   5. Zinc phosphate cement
   6. Calcium hydroxide

36. Following the placement of an amalgam restoration, the patient may experience sensitivity as a result of
   1. cold
   2. sweets
   3. heat
   4. biting pressure
   5. galvanic shock

37. Following the placement of a gold onlay in a mandibular second bicuspid, the patient experiences hypersensitivity under chewing pressure only. This indicates
   1. chemical irritation caused by the cementing medium
   2. irritation resulting from the high thermal conductivity of the gold
   3. hyperemia of the pulp
   4. periodontal ligament involvement

38. When a patient experiences a throbbing pain in a specific tooth which is sensitive to pressure and when the pain is aggravated by heat and relieved by cold, the most likely diagnosis is
   1. suppurative pulpitis
   2. a radicular cyst
   3. a follicular cyst
   4. occlusal hyperfunction
   5. hyperemia

## PREPARATION OF CAVITIES

### Basic Principles, Instrumentation, and Nomenclature

Numerous questions are devoted to this fundamental topic, and generally the basic principles of cavity preparation and nomenclature are stressed more than the instrumentation. The reason for this is that there is no real standardization of instrumentation for cavity preparations.

STEPS IN CAVITY PREPARATION. The basic principles have been outlined in the classic steps of cavity preparation as listed by Black. The sequence of development of a cavity preparation is 1) outline form, 2) resistance and retention form, 3) convenience form, 4) remaining carious dentin removed, 5) enamel walls finished, and 6) cavity cleansing, or the toilet.

The outline form is the form of the area of the tooth which is included within the enamel margins of the finished cavity. This is determined by the operator's clinical judgment and frequently includes pits, fissures, and extensions into the embrasure forms on the proximal surface. This outline form is controlled by the extent that the enamel has been directly penetrated by caries, by the lateral spread of caries along the dentoenamel junction, and by those extensions which must be made along fissures and into embrasures in order to secure smooth margins for finishing.

Resistance and retention are generally considered together. Resistance form is that form designed into the cavity preparation so that the restoration can withstand the stresses being placed upon it by occlusion without being dislodged. This is most important in proximal occlusal cavities in the posterior regions. Resistance is created by flat pulpal walls, gingival seat, and the approach to parallelism of the opposing walls on the facial and lingual. Retention form is obviously that designed to hold the restoration in position and is generally accomplished by proximal retentive grooves placed at the expense of the axiofacial and axiolingual line angles.

Convenience form involves the modifications in the outline form which make it more convenient to place the restoration. This is most applicable in the proximal surface of anteriors and is frequently a major consideration in the placement of direct filling golds. The personal equation of the operator is a factor in the type of convenience form that is required.

Any remaining carious dentin is removed so as to conserve as much tooth structure as possible. In most situations the cavity preparation can be developed to an ideal depth and form with the required resistance, retention, and convenience established. In so doing, most, if not all, of the caries is removed. Any remaining caries can then be removed with a spoon excavator, and a base can be placed in the cavity. Occasionally, when a pulpal exposure with resultant endodontic treatment is anticipated, this procedure is performed first. This, again, becomes a judgmental factor for the operator.

Finishing and planing the enamel walls can be done with chisels or hatchets, fine grit diamond instruments, and, in positions of access, various grit disks or wheels. The purpose of finishing the enamel walls is to make the surface as smooth as possible for the interface between the tooth and restorative material; this enhances the fit and minimizes the degree of marginal leakage. The final step of cleansing or toilet of the cavity preparation is self-explanatory and involves removing all of the dust and debris so that the surface is clean.

TERMINOLOGY. Nomenclature on the examination can involve all of the terminology used in dentistry. The terms used are straightforward and simple, however. Concerning the relationship of the tooth to that segment of the face or mouth which they approximate, for example, the outer surfaces of the teeth that are covered by the cheeks or face are referred to as the facial surfaces. The tops of the teeth are referred to as the occlusal or incisal surfaces, depending on whether they are posterior or anterior. That surface approximating the tongue is referred to as the lingual surface. The proximal surfaces are divided into the anterior region, or mesial relating to the midline, and the posterior or distal.

The walls of the cavity preparation are similarly termed. Only the names of the internal walls of the cavity preparation sometimes present difficulty. On the occlusal surface that wall which approximates the pulp is termed the pulpal wall. On the proximal surface the wall which parallels the long axis of the tooth while still approximating the pulp is referred to as the axial wall. The line angles are determined by the walls which form the angle. For example, the three line angles on a proximal preparation are the facioaxial line angle, the gingivoaxial line angle, and the linguoaxial line angle. The fourth angle, the junction of the axial and pulpal walls, is termed the axiopulpal line angle.

CLASSIFICATION OF CAVITIES. There are five basic cavity classifications. Cavities in Class I are one surface cavities involving structural defects in the teeth, the pits, and the fissures. These are located in the occlusal surfaces of the posterior teeth, the occlusal two-thirds of the facial surfaces of the molars, and the lingual surfaces of the upper incisors, and occasionally in the lingual surfaces of the upper molars. Class II cavities are those which involve the proximal surfaces of the posterior teeth. Class III cavities involve the proximal surfaces of the incisors and cuspids, but do not include the incisal angle. Class IV cavities involve the proximal surfaces of the anterior teeth plus the incisal angle, and Class V cavities are smooth surface cavities in the gingival third of the facial and/or lingual surfaces of the teeth.

**INSTRUMENTATION.** The only likely examination questions in the area of instrumentation involve the specific function of major instruments. Hatchets and chisels are primarily utilized for planing enamel. Spoon excavators, as the name implies, are utilized for the removal of carious dentin. Margin trimmers are used for creating gingival bevels and cavosurface bevels, and angle formers are used to sharpen, define, or create retention form at line angles within the inner surface of the preparation.

## QUESTIONS

39. The reduction of cusps tends to decrease
    1. outline form
    2. resistance form
    3. retention form
    4. convenience form
    5. the width of the occlusal table

40. The form given to a cavity to resist displacement of the restoration in any direction is
    1. outline form
    2. retention form
    3. resistance form
    4. convenience form

41. Those instruments normally used for placing gingival bevels are
    a. safe side diamond disks
    b. margin trimmers
    c. angle formers
    d. tapered carbide burs
    e. fine tapered diamond stones
    1. a, b, and c
    2. a, b, and e
    3. b, c, and d
    4. b, d, and e
    5. All of the above

42. A line angle that can be found in a proximoocclusal cavity is the
    1. mesioaxial line angle
    2. faciolingual line angle
    3. gingivoaxial line angle
    4. facioocclusal line angle

43. The outline form of a cavity implies the shape of
    1. the cavity following removal of the caries
    2. the cavity after the resistance and retention form has been established
    3. the preparation as it relates to the surface of the tooth
    4. All of the above

44. That instrument which creates the roughest cut surface on a tooth is
    1. cross-cut fissure bur at ultra speed
    2. plane fissure bur at ultra speed
    3. cross-cut fissure bur at low speed
    4. plane fissure bur at low speed
    5. medium sandpaper disk at low speed

45. That form in Class III cavities which helps to insure the proper line of force for condensation of direct filling gold is
    1. outline form
    2. resistance form
    3. retention form
    4. convenience form

46. The retention form for a Class II amalgam preparation is achieved by:
    1. a flat gingival wall
    2. parallel facial and lingual walls
    3. facial and lingual grooves placed at the axial line angle
    4. walls converging in an occlusogingival direction
    5. All of the above

## Preparations

**AMALGAM.** Amalgam is probably the most widely used restorative material available in dentistry, and several questions are allocated to the topic of cavity preparations for amalgam. As one would expect, these range from the simplest Class I cavities to the most complex type of preparations involving pins for retention. Basic principles apply to every category of amalgam preparation, however.

Because amalgam is condensed into cavity preparations in a plastic state, all preparations to receive amalgam must have mechanical retention. Class I preparations pose no particular problem with retention because there are four surrounding walls to retain the material. In Class II preparations, however, proximal retentive grooves placed in the dentin at the axiofacial line angle and axiolingual line angle must be used to help retain the restoration. Proximal boxes are generally prepared with a slight divergence toward the gingival surface. Because the tensile strength of amalgam restorations is somewhat less than ideal, it is important that the cavosurface angles on all classifications of cavity preparations approach 90° to provide bulk at the cavosurface which will resist fracture. All unsupported enamel, however, must be removed.

In those areas where amalgam is placed under unusual occlusal stress, such as cuspal regions, sufficient bulk must be provided to lend the necessary strength. When tipping cusps, 2–3 mm of reduction are generally required. As the preparations become larger and more complex, it is frequently necessary to provide additional forms of mechanical retention so that the final restoration will not be dislodged. To this end, pins are frequently selected.

There are three basic types of pins: cemented pins, threaded pins, and friction lock pins. The friction lock pins have been shown to create a great deal of stress within the tooth, and thus the cemented pins or threaded pins appear to be the most generally accepted. Most research indicates that pins placed 2 mm within the dentin and extending into the preparation no more than 2 mm provide the desired retention. As to the number of pins, a general rule of thumb is one pin for each involved cusp. Cross pinning of cusps is frequently advocated, especially for endodontically treated teeth, to help the weakened cuspal areas resist fracture. It is generally agreed today that the use of pins enhances the retention of the amalgam but in no way adds to its inherent strength.

### QUESTIONS

47. Finish of the enamel margin at the gingival cavosurface on a cavity prepared for amalgam is
    1. not indicated because of the poor tensile strength of amalgam
    2. accomplished by creating a steep cavosurface bevel
    3. not required since no stress is placed on the restoration in this region
    4. accomplished by removing all unsupported enamel rods or prisms

48. Stainless steel pins are principally used in conjunction with amalgam restorations to enhance the
    1. retention
    2. strength
    3. resistance form
    4. All of the above
    5. Only 1 and 2

49. To provide maximum strength in an amalgam restoration, the cavosurface angles should
    a. approach a 75° angle with the outer surface
    b. approach a 90° angle with the outer surface
    c. be supported by sound dentin
    d. be located in areas free of occlusal stress
    1. a, c, and d
    2. a and c
    3. b, c, and d
    4. c and d

50. In tipping the cusps for a complex amalgam restoration, the cusps should be reduced
    1. 0.5–1 mm
    2. 1–1.5 mm
    3. 1.5–2 mm
    4. 2–3 mm
    5. 3–4 mm

51. When utilizing self-threading, friction–locked pins for the retention of amalgam, it is generally agreed that the pin should extend about equally into the dentin and alloy. The recommended depth is about
    1. 1 mm
    2. 2 mm
    3. 3 mm
    4. 4 mm

**CAST GOLD.** The principles involved in preparing a cavity for cast gold are similar to those involved in preparing a cavity for amalgam. The major difference is that in cast gold restorations there can be no undercuts within the preparation since a wax pattern must be fabricated from the tooth or die and the resultant casting placed without distortion. Therefore, for all cast gold restorations, the walls of the cavity must diverge slightly as they approach the occlusal. Too much divergence, however, results in a loss of frictional retention and a loose or sloppy fit. Dovetail locks are useful in improving retention in Class II restorations when using cast gold.

Since the nature of gold is conducive to burnishing, it is desirable in cast gold restorations to have acute cavosurface angles. These are created by means of margin trimmers, stones, or burs, so that the gold can be burnished and drawn out to a fine layer, which helps to improve the marginal integrity of the final restoration.

The advent of ultra high speed cutting instruments has significantly altered the traditional concept of cavity preparation for cast gold. More delicate reduction of the tooth is now possible, and veneers and pin ledges can be used to conserve tooth structure and maintain the tooth's aesthetic appearance in a manner never before possible. Finishing of margins is greatly expedited also through the use of the ultra high speed instrument. Delicate chamfers and contrabevels are now permitting an infinite variety of cavity preparations to restore lost or diseased tooth structure. The use of tapered pins or parallel pins has increased the retentive capability of castings so that occlusal and proximal boxes are no longer mandatory for retention.

### QUESTIONS

52. Posterior teeth that have been endodontically treated are better restored by a cast gold onlay because
    1. gold is more aesthetic than amalgam
    2. gold renders the tooth more resistant to recurrent caries
    3. maximum protection is afforded to the tooth
    4. gold is less likely to disturb the gutta-percha filled canals than condensation of amalgam

53. The gingival margin and occlusal cavosurface angles are beveled for a gold inlay preparation because this

a. protects the enamel at the margins
b. improves marginal adaptation
c. helps to evaluate the accuracy of the impression
d. improves the seal of the cavity
e. facilitates finishing
1. a, b, and d
2. a, c, and e
3. b, d, and e
4. b, c, and d
5. All of the above

54. Gold inlays have improved retention when
1. there is a large cement film thickness
2. the opposing walls diverge toward the occlusal
3. there is less surface area involved in the preparation
4. the axial length in the cavity preparation is increased

55. To help insure maximum gingival adaptation of a gold inlay restoration the dentist should
1. use a soft gold alloy
2. employ the direct wax pattern procedure to avoid inaccuracies in the die
3. employ the indirect wax pattern
4. utilize a gingival reverse bevel
5. establish a precise gingival cavosurface bevel

56. In the preparation of proximal cavities the gingival extension is influenced by
a. the need to create adequate retention for a cast gold restoration
b. the degree of gingival recession
c. the position of the contact area
d. the location and extent of caries
1. a and d
2. b and c
3. b, c, and d
4. a, c, and d
5. All of the above

**DIRECT FILLING GOLD.** The questions devoted to direct filling gold preparations are usually confined to the Class III and Class V restorations. The most widely accepted Class V preparation today is the Ferrier preparation, which is trapezoidal in form with a mesiodistal curved axial wall, flared mesial and distal walls, and parallel incisal and gingival walls. The retention form for this preparation is placed at the expense of the occlusoaxial line angle and the gingivoaxial line angle. Sharp line angles are produced and precise cavosurface finish angles are attempted. The shape is trapezoidal in order to extend to the limits of the lesion, whether it is the result of caries, abrasion, or erosion. This precise outline form facilitates finishing and helps to insure the removal of all excess gold.

Class III preparations can be approached from either the labial or lingual surface. A separator is advocated for the Ferrier or labial preparation and should be carefully stabilized with compound, but separation should not exceed 0.6 mm. The approach to the preparation is from the labioincisal surface with the labial outline form carefully approximating the contour of the adjacent tooth to maintain aesthetic appearance. No further extension is made into the labial embrasure than absolutely required for convenience form, and the contact is broken on both labial and lingual surfaces. The primary retention form is at the labioaxiogingival, linguoaxiogingival, and incisal point angles. The lingual approach preparation, or inconspicuous Class III, can be done frequently with no separation by cutting through the linguoincisal marginal ridge and extending gingivally to the extent of caries involvement. The labial wall is brought just past the contact and in a line that parallels the contour of the adjacent tooth. The principal retention form is again at the labioaxiogingival, linguoaxiogingival, and incisal point angle.

As much of the lingual wall is retained as possible in the gingival third to aid in the retention of the direct filling gold and also to facilitate condensation if gold foil is used. If powdered gold is the material of choice, generally the access is from the lingual surface, and the lingual wall is removed entirely so that the axial wall and the lingual wall are the same. Retention form is created by rounded depressions at the labioaxiogingival, linguogingival, and incisal point angle. When powdered gold is used, no cavosurface bevels are prepared; rather a butt joint is advocated.

QUESTIONS

57. Retention form is created in a Class V cavity prepared for direct filling gold at
1. the mesial and distal axial line angles
2. the occlusal and gingival axial line angles
3. the four point angles of the cavity
4. circumferentially around all four walls.

58. Retention form for a Class III cavity prepared from either the labial or lingual approach is placed in the
a. incisal point angle
b. linguoaxiogingival point angle
c. labioaxiogingival point angle
1. a and b
2. a and c
3. b and c
4. All of the above

**TOOTH-COLORED RESTORATIVE MATERIALS.** The questions devoted to this topic, encompass the porcelain inlay, acrylic resins, silicate cements, and the more popular bisphenol-A-glycidyl (BIS–GMA) composite resins. In an effort to update the examinations, most questions are associated with the composite resins. Preparations for tooth-colored restoratives, with the exception of those for porcelain inlays, are usually determined by the extent of caries. Since these restorative materials are plastic in nature, no particular convenience form is required during placement, nor are extensions beyond the limit of caries desirable because of the inherent weakness of the restorative material.

Since the use of acrylics or composites are not widely advocated in the posterior region, it would be unlikely that any questions on Class II cavity preparation would be submitted. The primary preparations for tooth-colored restorative materials are for Class III, Class IV, and Class V cavities. Access to the carious lesion is made from the lingual surface on Class III cavities, and the carious material is removed. No cavosurface bevels are advocated, and the retention form is placed as rounded undercuts at the expense of the incisal and gingival surfaces. The contact area need not be included unless it is absolutely essential for the finish of the restoration.

For Class V preparations the outline form, again, is governed by the position and the extent of the carious lesion. No extensions beyond the limits of caries involvement are required. The retention form is made by rounded undercuts at the expense of the incisal surface or occlusal and gingival surfaces. In the event that acid-etching techniques are used, cavosurface bevels are frequently recommended in order to provide a wider surface of exposed enamel to be etched.

Preparations for fused porcelain restorations are generally limited to Class III and Class V lesions. The outline form for these preparations must be similar in nature to that for a cast gold restoration, since there should be no undercuts. Parallelism is attempted throughout with a flat axial wall to provide bulk of porcelain material for strength. The cavosurface angles are not beveled, but merely planed to avoid any loose, unsupported enamel rods. All walls are gently rounded to avoid any sharp corners.

### QUESTIONS

59. Retention form for composite resin restorations is achieved by
    1. a chemical bond with the tooth
    2. adhesion to the enamel and dentin
    3. mechanical undercuts
    4. All of the above

60. The margins of a porcelain inlay are fragile and must be considered in the design of a Class V preparation. This is accomplished by
    1. preparing the walls with a labial convergence
    2. preparing the walls with a large labial divergence
    3. deepening the axial wall
    4. preparing the cavosurface angles to approximate 90°

61. The primary factor in developing the outline form for a composite resin restoration on the proximal surface of an anterior tooth is
    1. the position of the contact
    2. the relationship to the adjacent tooth
    3. the aesthetics required

4. the extent of caries involvement
5. extension for prevention

62. Retention form for composite resin restorations in Class III preparations is achieved by
    1. sharp, well-defined line angles
    2. parallel walls
    3. rounded undercuts at the incisal and gingival point angles
    4. sharp, acute point angles at the incisal, labioaxiogingival, and linguoaxiogingival

63. In Class V preparations to receive composite resin the extension is determined by the
    1. position of the gingival crest
    2. contour of the tooth
    3. caries susceptibility of the patient
    4. extent of caries involvement
    5. All of the above

**PORCELAIN-FUSED-TO-METAL RESTORATIONS.** The two questions devoted to this topic generally deal with the additional tooth reduction required to accommodate a porcelain-fused-to-metal restoration. Additional tooth structure must be removed in the area where porcelain is to be applied, since both the porcelain and the metal thickness must be accommodated. Failure to do this results in a bulky-looking, overcontoured restoration.

On anterior teeth the lingual surface would ordinarily be finished like any gold restoration with a chamfer finish line, while the labial surface should have a distinct shoulder for the bulk of porcelain and a cavosurface bevel to finish the gingival margin of gold. The lingual margin can terminate at the crest of the tissue, but the labial margin should extend sufficiently below the free margin to cover the metal line at the cavosurface angle. Also there is generally a little greater incisal reduction to insure that the desired incisal translucency can be created in the final restoration.

### QUESTIONS

63. Preparations for porcelain-bonded-to-metal restorations should have a
    1. shoulder all around the tooth
    2. shoulder on the lingual and proximal surfaces and a chamfer on the labial surface
    3. beveled shoulder on the labial surface and a chamfer on the lingual surface
    4. feather edge around the entire tooth to facilitate finishing

64. When compared to a porcelain jacket crown preparation, a tooth prepared for a porcelain-bonded-to-metal restoration has
    a. more tooth structure removed on the labial surface
    b. more tooth structure removed on the lingual surface

c. less tooth structure removed on the labial surface
d. less tooth structure removed on the lingual surface

1. a
2. b
3. c
4. d
5. a and d
6. b and c

## RESTORATIONS OF PREPARED CAVITIES

### Properties of Restorative Materials

The questions on this topic are generally developed by a materials scientist and can be based on any of the physical properties or working characteristics of those materials commonly used in dentistry. In order to cover this subject adequately an entire textbook would be required, so only samples of information can be included here to familiarize the reader with the type of information that could be covered in the questions allocated to this topic.

AMALGAM ALLOYS. Dental amalgam alloys are composed primarily of silver and tin with small amounts of copper and occasionally some zinc. The silver, which comprises about 70% of an amalgam alloy, improves strength and decreases flow. Tin, which makes up about 26%, reduces the expansion and also cuts down on the strength and hardness of the resultant alloy. In order to keep the alloy from being brittle 3%–5% copper is added. It has the effect of hardening and strengthening the alloy, as well as decreasing flow. This percentage of copper, which is present in all alloys, should not be confused with the current high-copper-content alloys which are on the market. In the so-called high-copper-content alloys copper is added to the conventional system as a separate eutectic particle.

Zinc is present only to the extent of about 1%. Like gold, it is used as a scavenger to deoxidize. In the presence of moisture, however, it creates an excessive amount of expansion. For this reason, in those situations where moisture cannot be eliminated from the field of operation, zinc-free alloys are recommended.

Most of the alloys are manufactured by placing amalgam ingots on a lathe or milling machine and sifting the resultant filings through screens to produce the various grades of particle sizes. Spherical alloy has gained popularity in recent years, and this is prepared through an atomization process.

DIRECT FILLING RESINS. Direct filling resins, and especially the composite resins, are very popular dental restoratives today. Since none of these forms a true adhesion to tooth structure, there have been a variety of methods employed to improve the marginal seal and retentive qualities of this restorative material.

The most popular and effective method currently used is the acid-etching technique wherein the enamel wall of a cavity preparation is etched with acid prior to the placement of the resin restoration. Citric acid or phosphoric acid are suitable materials for this purpose, and various concentrations have been recommended. It is generally agreed that a 50% phosphoric acid solution is a very workable solution for etching the enamel surface. The dentin and deeper layers of the preparation should be protected from the acid with either a cement base or a cavity varnish. The acid is allowed to contact the enamel surface for approximately 1 min; the preparation is then flushed with water to remove the excess acid and dried. Then the resin is applied.

The most popular of today's tooth-colored restoratives is the composite resin, a restorative material that contains an inorganic filler together with a resin matrix. Most of the present composite restorative materials make use of the BIS–GMA molecule because it is a good binder for reinforcing fillers, has a low polymerization shrinkage, and hardens rapidly in the oral environment. Fillers comprise the bulk of composite resins, and while they vary in concentration from product to product, they are usually present in the range of 70%–80%. Various forms of silica, quartz, and glass have been used as fillers in a variety of shapes ranging from powders and spheres to whiskers.

Another popular use of resin is as a pit and fissure sealant. This is a preventive procedure accomplished by applying resin to the developmental pits and fissures in newly erupted teeth, allowing the resin to polymerize and theoretically seal the areas against oral microorganisms. Both filled and unfilled resins have been utilized for this purpose. One of the more popular brands employs benzoin methyl ether as the initiator, which allows ultraviolet light to be utilized as an activator rather than a tertiary amine type of chemical.

Silicate cement is another tooth-colored restorative, but it is not widely utilized today. As a result, virtually all questions relating to silicate have been removed from the operative section of the National Board Examinations.

CASTING GOLD. Basic gold alloys are primarily gold, copper, and silver, with small amounts of platinum, palladium, and zinc. Platinum and palladium can be added in increased amounts to increase strength and hardness. Surface hardness and strength generally are in a direct relationship.

Casting gold alloys are usually classified according to type: I, II, III, and IV. Type I is the softest; Type IV, the hardest. Type I has the highest percentage of gold, and this percentage decreases through Types II, III, and finally IV. The gold imparts tarnish resistance to the alloy and contributes ductility. Copper in gold alloys increases strength and hardness; thus there is considerably more copper in a Type IV alloy than in a Type I. Silver has no appreciable effect in the gold alloy, although it can be used to replace the gold to a limited extent. It affects the color somewhat and can contribute to the ductility. Platinum is used to harden the alloy, and palladium is merely a replacement for platinum because it is less expensive. Zinc tends to be a scavenger and combines with oxide present to help improve the casting characteristics of the gold alloy; it also effectively reduces the melting point.

Gold should always be melted using the reducing zone of a torch. Never should the oxidizing zone be used, since the temperature is lower in the oxidizing zone and it also causes oxidation of the metal.

**DIRECT FILLING GOLD.** Direct filling gold can be divided into three different categories: 1) gold foil; 2) mat gold, which is an electrolytic precipitate; and 3) powdered gold. Direct filling golds are pure golds and as such have excellent tarnish and corrosion resistance. By virtue of its purity, increments of gold can be welded together in the oral cavity by means of condensation pressure.

Gold foil is fabricated by being rolled into very thin sheets and then pounded to the desired thickness. It is calibrated by the thickness of a 4-in. square sheet such that if a 4-in. square sheet of gold foil weighs 4 grains it is referred to as a number 4. Gold foil is generally processed into pellets, and pellets are categorized by their size. A 1/64th pellet is made from 1/64th of a number 4, 4-in. sheet of gold foil. A 1/32nd pellet is made from 1/32nd of a sheet of a number 4, 4-in. square, etc. Mat gold is prepared by an electrolytic precipitation and then sintered. It is supplied in small strips, frequently coated with gold foil to hold the particles together. Powdered gold can be prepared either by chemical precipitation or atomization; it is spherical in appearance and fabricated for the dentist in small pellets encased in gold foil.

All pure gold is naturally cohesive; however, it can be supplied in a noncohesive form through the use of surface contaminants. Ammonia is the most commonly used since it can easily be driven off by heat to return the gold to a cohesive state. In some instances it is desirable to use gold in a noncohesive condition, particularly for lining the walls of cavity preparations.

### QUESTIONS

66. A commonly used acid solution for etching enamel in conjunction with composite resin restorations is
   1. 50% phosphoric acid
   2. 50% sulfuric acid
   3. 75% phosphoric acid
   4. 50% silicophosphoric acid
   5. 75% hydrofluoric acid

67. Direct filling resins can be activated by
   a. tertiary amines
   b. benzoin methyl ether
   c. benzoyl peroxide
   d. hydroquinone
   1. a
   2. a and c
   3. a and b
   4. b and d
   5. All of the above

68. Tin is incorporated into an amalgam alloy for the purpose of
   1. increasing expansion and strength
   2. reducing expansion and hardness
   3. increasing strength
   4. acting as a scavenger

69. Most amalgam alloys are comprised of approximately what percentage of silver?
   1. 50%
   2. 70%
   3. 80%
   4. 90%

70. In melting gold preparatory to casting, the appropriate zone of the flame to use is
   1. the reducing zone since it is not as hot
   2. the oxidizing zone to remove oxides
   3. the reducing zone since it prevents oxidation and is a higher temperature than the oxidizing zone
   4. Either zone may be used, since with the current type of alloys both provide satisfactory results

71. Hardness and strength are increased in a gold alloy by the addition of
   a. zinc
   b. silver
   c. copper
   d. platinum
   1. a and c
   2. b and c
   3. b and d
   4. c and d
   5. d

72. Direct filling gold can be supplied in a noncohesive condition by
   1. alloying the metal with calcium
   2. employing a special sintering process
   3. applying surface contaminants
   4. None of the above

73. Gold foil, mat gold, and powdered gold differ from each other by the
   1. percentage of pure gold present
   2. degree of cohesiveness
   3. method of fabrication
   4. All of the above
   5. None of the above

## Manipulation and Finishing of Restorative Materials

Numerous questions are devoted to this broad range topic, which is broken down into a number of sub-headings. As one would expect, questions on dental materials appear in this segment of the examination also, although in a more direct correlation to actual operative procedures.

AMALGAM. Amalgam is prepared for restoring a tooth by mixing it with mercury. The percentage of mercury to alloy is measured by weight and is referred to as the mercury : alloy ratio. Most texts refer to the so-called conventional alloy as having a mercury : alloy ratio in the neighborhood of 8:5, meaning eight parts mercury to five parts alloy by weight. In recent years, however, the mercury content has been reduced to a minimal level. This change of philosophy was the result of the work of Eames, who advocated equal parts of mercury and alloy. The minimal amount of mercury that can be utilized varies somewhat with the different brands of alloy. In some instances 46% mercury is effective in maintaining plasticity, while in other brands 52% or 53% is required. The minimal mercury technique has gained favor since it produces higher 1-hour strength and sets more rapidly than the higher mercury levels.

Mechanical amalgamators are the method of choice for trituration of amalgam, and they should employ a capsule that is threaded to avoid leakage of mercury. With a minimum mercury mix it is no longer necessary to express excess mercury prior to condensation, and the alloy should be condensed into a cavity preparation quickly and thoroughly while the mix is still plastic. Depending upon the alloy used, 3–4min is the maximum length of time that any single mix will remain plastic. For large preparations multiple mixes should be utilized to maintain a plastic working mass.

In condensation an effort should be made to incorporate each new increment into that which has previously been condensed in order to prevent a layering effect. Small condensers with a lateral scrubbing action are useful for accomplishing this objective, as well as for insuring that the restoration adapts to the lateral walls. Every cavity preparation should be slightly overfilled so that the mercury-rich alloy is brought to the surface and removed prior to carving and finishing.

In carving the amalgam care should be exerted to remove all of the excess material so that no thin fins or spines of amalgam remain. While it is desirable to reproduce normal tooth form and anatomy, the carving should complement the cavity preparation to insure that the bulk of amalgam is adequate at the cavosurface.

Since amalgam is condensed into the prepared cavity in a plastic state, it must be confined in all cavities involving the proximal surfaces. This is accomplished by means of a matrix. The matrix, when properly applied, makes it possible to restore the proximal surface to its correct anatomic form and relationship to the adjacent tooth. In this manner the contact area is maintained. In order to accomplish this, the matrix should be contoured and wedged at the gingival surface and stabilized by means of a mechanical retainer and/or compound.

QUESTIONS

74. Silver amalgam should be condensed within 4 min following trituration because
   1. excess will be more easily removed
   2. the final set takes place within 5 min
   3. time studies indicate this is the most efficient working time
   4. beyond this time the residual mercury retention is markedly increased

75. A minimal mercury level for amalgam varies with the brand of alloy used but it falls within the range of
   1. 40%–50%
   2. 46%–53%
   3. 50%–55%
   4. 55%–60%

76. When an amalgam is prepared using the minimal mercury technique and compared with a high-mercury-content technique, it is found to
   a. have a high 1-hour strength
   b. set more rapidly
   c. require less pressure during condensation
   d. have greater plasticity and thereby better adaptability to cavity walls
   e. eliminate the need for a squeeze cloth
   1. a, b, and c
   2. a, b, and e
   3. b, c, and d
   4. b, c, and e
   5. d

77. The principal reasons for using a wedge in conjunction with a matrix preparatory to condensing a Class II amalgam are to
   a. retract the gingival tissue
   b. separate the teeth minimally to insure the creation of proper contact
   c. adapt the matrix band firmly against the tooth cervical to the gingival margin
   d. prevent seepage of fluids into the prepared cavity
   1. a, b, c, and d
   2. b and c
   3. a, b, and d
   4. b
   5. c

CAST GOLD. Cast gold restorations can be fabricated by either the direct or the indirect method. The direct approach involves directly adapting wax in the prepared tooth, then carving and finishing the wax pattern in the mouth. Indirect techniques employ impressions of the prepared tooth which have been made with any of the elastic impression materials, i.e., polysulphide rubbers, silicones, and reversible hydrocolloid. The impression is poured in a suitable die stone and mounted, with centric and protrusive records, on an articulator. In this manner the patterns are fabricated on accurate models outside of the mouth.

Sprues are affixed to the pattern in a manner which minimizes the turbulence of the molten gold and insures direct flow to the most inaccessible areas of the preparation. In order to accomplish this, the sprue is generally placed in the long axis of the preparation with a slight flare to the attachment. A variety of investment materials can be used, and the pattern is invested in an asbestos-lined ring. The purpose of the asbestos is to provide for the lateral setting and thermal expansion of the investment which compensates for the casting shrinkage of the gold. The pattern should extend within ¼ in. of the end of the ring to permit venting of gases during the casting procedure.

Proper attention to the investing technique must be employed, and the manufacturer's recommendations should be strictly followed. Gold, as it goes from the liquid to the solid state, shrinks anywhere from 1¼% to 1½%. This shrinkage must be compensated for by an expansion in the mold in order to insure accurate castings. This compensation can take place in three or four ways. If a hygroscopic technique is employed, some expansion of the wax pattern results from the controlled temperature in the hygroscopic bath. There is setting expansion and thermal expansion with all types of investments, although the hygroscopic setting expansion is greater than the setting expansion of other types of investments. Those investments that do not employ a hygroscopic setting expansion undergo a higher thermal expansion, however, so that the final result is a mold expanded in direct relationship to the casting shrinkage of the gold.

The finish and polish of the gold casting is accomplished on the die or in the mouth, using graded disks or stones; then the margins are burnished and finally polished with pumice, after which tin oxide or rouge is applied. The softer inlay golds are amenable to burnishing, and with properly prepared cavities possessing adequate cavosurface bevels, a well-fitting casting with good marginal integrity can be achieved. The principal advantage of gold as a restorative material is that a more accurate restoration of proximal contour and contact relationships, as well as occlusion, can be made.

### QUESTIONS

78. When carving a wax pattern, the occlusal surface should be
    1. left a little high so that the final restoration will be certain to have adequate occlusal contact
    2. carved to establish a proper occlusal contact relationship in centric as well as the excursive movements
    3. carved just out of occlusion to provide for the thickness of cement during the seating of the restoration
    4. carved according to the opposing arch relation when the mandible is in its most retruded position

79. One of the principal advantages of a cast gold restoration is its
    1. aesthetic qualities
    2. ability to inhibit recurrent caries
    3. pulp protection because of the thermal insulating qualities of the cementing medium
    4. ability to restore anatomic form

80. Asbestos is utilized to line a casting ring in order to
    1. help uniformly distribute the heat throughout the mold
    2. facilitate venting of the mold
    3. permit expansion of the mold
    4. All of the above

81. The main reason for placing a cavosurface bevel on an inlay preparation is to
    1. remove the undermined enamel
    2. facilitate marginal adaptation
    3. reduce marginal percolation
    4. improve the visibility for the operator
    5. increase the resistance form

**DIRECT FILLING GOLDS.** The questions devoted to this topic, are generally directed toward methods of condensing direct filling golds. One must remember that the size of the condenser point, the amount of force applied, and the direction of force are the three most important factors in the proper condensation and adaptation of the direct filling gold to the preparation.

In Class I and V preparations where there are four surrounding walls it is always essential that the condensation build-up be greater in the region of the walls; there should be a shallow, hollowed out area in the center of the preparation. This allows for the proper line of force to insure adaptation to the walls and cavosurface angles and to seal the margins. The last step of the build-up should be in the center to develop the contour and final form. In Class III preparations the force is generally in the long axis of the tooth when gold foil is used and in a facial–axial direction when powdered gold is utilized.

Care should always be exercised to fill the most inaccessible areas of the preparation first and logically and sequentially build the restoration to full form and contour as one proceeds. Failure to do this results in blocking out or creating an inaccessible area after condensation. Since the condenser point is stepped, a careful overlapping of each condensing blow actually wedges the gold into the line angles and point angles to insure proper adaptation and retention. Various techniques can be employed in condensation, ranging from hand pressure to hand malleting to mechanical malleting, using either a pneumatic or electromagnetic force to control the frequency and intensity of the condenser blow. All of these techniques have been demonstrated to be effective in the hands of a skilled operator.

Following placement of the direct filling gold, a final condensation, which is again a logical and sequential stepping of the condenser point over the surface of the restoration, is employed to insure that compaction is complete and that there are no voids or soft spots. This step also has a tendency to harden the surface of foil and facilitate the ultimate finish. If the foil restoration has not been grossly overbuilt in contour, but merely slightly overfilled, during the finishing process one merely has to burnish and remove the indentations created by the serrated condensing points and go through a graded polishing procedure to obtain either a satin finish or high polish, depending on the preference of the patient and/or operator.

### QUESTIONS

82. The amount of force which must be applied in order to compact direct filling gold adequately is influenced by the
    1. angle of the compacting instrument relative to the surface of the tooth
    2. depth and therefore the bulk of the restoration
    3. surface area of the condenser point
    4. annealing time

83. During condensation the surface hardness of a direct filling gold
    1. increases
    2. decreases
    3. remains the same
    4. increases or decreases in relation to the amount of force applied

**TOOTH-COLORED RESTORATIVE MATERIALS.** The composite resins can be purchased commercially in a variety of ways. Currently most manufacturers supply them in a two-base system, although they can be purchased in a powder–liquid combination or a paste–liquid combination. In all cases the manufacturer's directions should be strictly followed. It is generally recommended that plastic or wood instruments be used in mixing a composite resin. Metal instruments should be avoided because the fillers are highly abrasive and during mixing some metal can be incorporated into the mix, discoloring the final restoration.

The handling time for most composites is fairly short: It is important that a homogeneous mix be established and placement into the cavity preparation should be done quickly and efficiently. Composites can either be packed into the cavity using a plastic-tipped instrument or injected with any of the commercially available syringes. The advantage of injection is that there is a lower risk of incorporating air bubbles.

The contour of the restoration is created by means of a matrix strip, and this should be held in position until the polymerization takes place. After polymerization is complete, which generally takes in the range of 4–6 min, the matrix can be removed and polishing initiated. Because of the fillers, however, it is very difficult to finish composite resin restorations; most polishing techniques affect the softer matrix and leave exposed filler. This creates a rough surface which tends to accumulate debris. For this reason it is desirable whenever possible to maintain the surface which has been created by the matrix band.

The selection of the correct shade is an extremely important consideration for the aesthetic qualities of a tooth-colored restoration. Irrespective of whether a silicate, filled resin, or unfilled resin is to be used, the same principles for shade selection apply. The shade should be selected prior to placing a rubber dam, when both the tooth and shade guide are moist. Natural light is preferred, although the normal room lighting can be employed. A shade should not be selected under the bright operating light.

### QUESTIONS

84. Compared to unfilled resins, composite resins have
    1. greater compressive strength
    2. less solubility
    3. greater working time
    4. smoother finished surface
    5. greater color stability

85. Metal instruments are contraindicated for use with composite resin because the
    1. metal is abraded by the filler and discolors the restoration
    2. monomer reacts with the metal and forms corrosive products which affect the final shade
    3. polymer reacts with the metal to affect the shade
    4. metal inhibits the polymerization

86. The best surface finish on a composite resin restoration is created by
    1. the 12 fluted finishing burs
    2. fine silica grit disks
    3. lubricated cuttle disks
    4. the matrix band with no additional finish

87. One should select the shade for a composite resin utilizing a
    1. bright light
    2. dry shade guide
    3. dry tooth isolated by the rubber dam
    4. All of the above
    5. None of the above

**PORCELAIN-FUSED-TO-METAL RESTORATIONS.** In preparing a casting to receive porcelain in a porcelain-bonded-to-metal restoration, it is important to follow certain procedures. Whenever possible it is desirable to check the metal portion of the restoration for contact and occlusion in the mouth prior to the addition of porcelain, and any modification should be made at this time. The surfaces of the metal casting which will not receive porcelain should be finished to final contour and given a preliminary polish with stones and wheels.

Attention must be given to the cervical area gingival to the site for veneering. It should be thinned out and chamfered so that it will be covered by the gingival tissue when seated and there will be no excess contour. This enhances the aesthetic appearance and minimizes gingival irritation.

All of the interior angles of the surfaces to be veneered are rounded to avoid poor adaptation and lessen the potential for cleavage along the sharp angles as a result of shrinkage. The cavosurface angles at the porcelain–metal interface should approximate right angles to permit a bulk of porcelain and minimize a metal "halo" effect or porcelain fracture.

### QUESTION

88. When a metal casting is prepared to receive a porcelain veneer, the interior angles of the area to be veneered should
    1. have sharply defined undercuts to help retain the porcelain
    2. have rounded channels to enhance porcelain retention
    3. not have undercuts but sharply defined angles for uniform thickness
    4. have rounded interior angles to enhance adaptation

**CEMENT BASES AND LINERS.** The principal cements currently utilized either as bases or luting agents are zinc phosphate, zinc oxide–eugenol, the polycarboxylates, and calcium hydroxide. Zinc phosphates and polycarboxylates are primarily utilized as luting agents for the cementation of gold restorations. Polycarboxylates have come into prominence in recent years because they are believed to have some degree of adhesion to tooth structure.

In addition to being utilized as luting agents, cements are used for pulp protection. In those areas that are very near to the pulp or involve an actual pulpal exposure, calcium hydroxide is the base of choice since it acts as a mild irritant and stimulates the odontoblasts to form secondary dentin. When used in the case of a direct exposure, it is referred to as a direct pulp capping. An indirect pulp cap procedure is used in those situations where the operator leaves a small amount of residual caries or decalcified material, because complete removal would potentially result in a pulpal ex-

posure. Calcium hydroxide is placed over the remaining carious material to permit the pulp to respond by developing secondary dentin. The zinc oxide–eugenol cements tend to be among the least irritating and are frequently used as temporary restorations or thermoinsulating bases. Because of the eugenol content, they cannot be used as bases under resin restorations.

Cavity varnishes are very popular since they have been shown to improve the marginal seal of most restorations. Under amalgam restorations they also serve to reduce tooth discoloration.

### QUESTIONS

89. Calcium hydroxide is regarded as a good pulp capping agent because
    1. the pulp responds by forming secondary dentin
    2. it creates a better cavity seal than other materials
    3. its alkaline nature is nonirritating to the pulp
    4. it has a sedative effect on the pulp

90. Cavity varnish is desirable under amalgam restorations because it
    1. eliminates the possibility of galvanic shock
    2. improves the marginal seal of the restoration
    3. completely seals all the dentinal tubules
    4. is an effective thermal insulator
    5. All of the above

91. One of the best materials for pulpal sedation is
    1. cavity varnish
    2. zinc oxide–eugenol
    3. calcium hydroxide
    4. zinc phosphate
    5. polycarboxylate cement

92. A material which is contraindicated as a base under a resin restoration is
    1. carboxylate cement
    2. calcium hydroxide
    3. zinc oxide–eugenol
    4. zinc phosphate

**INTERIM RESTORATIONS.** The selection of a material as an interim restoration depends to a great extent on the type of preparation and the reason for the interim restoration. For an inlay or cast gold restoration, the interim dressing must be such that it can be removed without altering the marginal integrity of the preparation. Zinc phosphate cements are therefore contraindicated because of their hardness. Zinc oxide–eugenol, gutta-percha, or acrylic temporaries are the materials of choice. For caries control where no definitive preparation has been made and a long-term interim dressing is desired, zinc phosphate, polycarboxylate cement, or reinforced zinc oxide–eugenol can be used along with acrylic temporaries.

Whenever interim restorations are being placed, the effect on the pulp must be considered; for long-term procedures the mesiodistal dimension of the tooth, as well as the occlusal relationships, must be taken into consideration. The failure to do so can result in arch collapse or malocclusion as the result of the continued active eruption of a tooth that is out of contact with its antagonist.

QUESTIONS

93. The interim restoration of choice for placement between completion of the cavity preparation and the seating of the cast mesio-occluso–distal inlay restoration is
   1. zinc oxide–eugenol
   2. zinc phosphate
   3. polycarboxylate cement
   4. an acrylic onlay cemented with zinc oxide–eugenol

94. Interim restorations which will, of necessity, be in the mouth for longer periods of time must take into consideration
   1. pulp response
   2. occlusion
   3. contact and contour
   4. patient comfort
   5. 1 and 4
   6. All of the above

95. An interim dressing cement is condensed down into the pin holes of a pin ledge inlay preparation because failure to do this will result in a nonretentive temporary.
   1. Both the statement and reason are correct and related.
   2. Both the statement and reason are correct but not related.
   3. The statement is correct but the reason is not.
   4. The statement is not correct but the reason is an accurate statement.
   5. Neither statement nor reason is correct.

**OCCLUSION.** Entire texts have been written on this much discussed subject, and it would be impossible to review the topic in even the most superficial terms in one or two paragraphs. Only a few questions on the examination are devoted to occlusion and thus only a sampling of the type of material considered relevant will be included here.

A popular approach to occlusal reconstruction is based on the "functionally generated path." This is a static registration of the patient's dynamic occlusion and is achieved by having the patient open and move the jaw to the right or left and then contact the teeth. From this position the patient slides into a normal bite position on the back teeth of one side. The procedure is repeated for the opposite side.

Most cases which involve the restoration of the contacting occlusal surfaces of one or more teeth should be evaluated for potential occlusal correction. This is properly performed initially, prior to treatment, and as a final procedure following restoration.

QUESTIONS

96. Which of the following relates to the functionally generated path for occlusal registration?
   1. Centric relation
   2. Anatomic registration
   3. Vertical dimension
   4. Most retruded mandibular position
   5. Static registration of dynamic occlusion

97. Occlusal correction is
   1. only considered when patient presents with temporomandibular joint problem
   2. never essential if only one tooth is affected
   3. a terminal treatment performed only after all restorative work is complete
   4. performed as an initial and final procedure

## SUGGESTED READING

BASSET RW, INGRAHAM R, KOSER JR: An Atlas of Cast Gold Procedures. Los Angeles Department of Operative Dentistry, University of Southern California, School of Dentistry, 1964

BAUM L: Advanced Restorative Dentistry: Modern Materials and Techniques. Philadelphia, WB Saunders, 1973

BELL B, GRAINGER D: Basic Operative Dentistry. Philadelphia, Lea & Febiger, 1971

BLACKWELL RE: Black's Operative Dentistry, Vols I, II. South Milwaukee, Medico-Dental, 1955

COURTADE GL, TIMMERMANS JJ: Pins in Restorative Dentistry. St. Louis, CV Mosby, 1971

GILMORE HW, LUND T, BALES D, VERNETTI J: Operative Dentistry, 3rd ed. St. Louis, CV Mosby, 1977

GREENER E, HARCOURT J, LAUTENSCHLAGER E: Materials Science in Dentistry. Baltimore, Williams & Wilkins, 1972

INGRAHAM R, KOSER JR: An Atlas of Gold Foil and Rubber Dam Procedures. Los Angeles Department of Operative Dentistry, University of Southern California, School of Dentistry, 1961

ORINGER MJ: Electrosurgery in Dentistry. Philadelphia, WB Saunders, 1975

PHILLIPS RW: Skinner's Science of Dental Materials, 7th ed. Philadelphia, WB Saunders, 1973

SELTZER S, BENDER IB: The Dental Pulp. Philadelphia, JB Lippincott, 1965

STILES HM, LOESCH WJ, O'BRIEN TC: Microbial Aspects of Dental Caries, Vols I, II, III. Washington DC, Information Retrieval, 1976

## ANSWER KEY

| | | | |
|---|---|---|---|
| 1. 4 | 12. 2 | 23. 3 | 34. 4 |
| 2. 2 | 13. 3 | 24. 4 | 35. 4 |
| 3. 4 | 14. 1 | 25. 3 | 36. 1 |
| 4. 3 | 15. 4 | 26. 4 | 37. 4 |
| 5. 2 | 16. 2 | 27. 6 | 38. 1 |
| 6. 3 | 17. 2 | 28. 4 | 39. 3 |
| 7. 2 | 18. 4 | 29. 3 | 40. 2 |
| 8. 1 | 19. 2 | 30. 4 | 41. 4 |
| 9. 4 | 20. 2 | 31. 3 | 42. 3 |
| 10. 2 | 21. 2 | 32. 2 | 43. 3 |
| 11. 1 | 22. 3 | 33. 2 | 44. 1 |

**ANSWER KEY** (cont.)

| | | | | | | | |
|---|---|---|---|---|---|---|---|
| 45. 4 | 52. 3 | 59. 3 | 66. 1 | 73. 3 | 80. 3 | 86. 4 | 92. 3 |
| 46. 3 | 53. 5 | 60. 4 | 67. 3 | 74. 4 | 81. 2 | 87. 5 | 93. 4 |
| 47. 4 | 54. 4 | 61. 4 | 68. 2 | 75. 2 | 82. 3 | 88. 4 | 94. 6 |
| 48. 1 | 55. 5 | 62. 3 | 69. 2 | 76. 2 | 83. 1 | 89. 1 | 95. 5 |
| 49. 3 | 56. 4 | 63. 4 | 70. 3 | 77. 2 | 84. 1 | 90. 2 | 96. 5 |
| 50. 4 | 57. 2 | 64. 3 | 71. 4 | 78. 2 | 85. 1 | 91. 2 | 97. 4 |
| 51. 2 | 58. 4 | 65. 5 | 72. 3 | 79. 4 | | | |

# 4

# COMMUNITY AND PREVENTIVE DENTISTRY

## PART I
## DENTAL HEALTH ECOLOGY

**James F. Gardiner** / **Benjamin J. Legett, Jr.**

If ecology deals with the interdependence of people and institutions, then dental ecology may be defined as that branch of dentistry concerned with the relationships of dentists, patients, and the community. These relationships form a delivery system. Although dentistry is less often described today as a cottage industry than it was 10 years ago, the use of the more popular term dental delivery system requires explanation if it is to be used correctly. According to the *Oxford English Dictionary,* a system is "a set or assemblage of things connected or interdependent so as to form a complex unity." Dentistry is that. It *is* a set of things like dentists, offices, laboratories, professional organizations, training institutions, and patients. They *are* connected, and their relationships *are* complex. But is there unity—unity of purpose, for example?

Looking at this concept another way, a system can be defined as "sets of components that work together for the overall objective of the whole." (3) Systems are defined by purpose rather than by parts, e.g., health systems, not doctor systems. We get out onto thin ice when we apply that definition to the somewhat disorderly multidirectional elements involved in today's dental health. To see dentistry as system theorists intend is to see it as a set of interrelated components moving toward (or away from) a goal. Its manpower resources, facilities, regulatory agencies, suppliers, information components, and its market (patients) must all be included in the set.

The dental delivery system is primarily a social one; the ultimate exchange is between people. As a social system it is in a constant and dynamic relationship with the political, economic, technologic, and legal systems which constitute the supersystem in which it functions. To begin to think of dental delivery in terms of general system theory helps create a constant awareness that no single issue, event, or problem should be considered without regard for the consequences of its interaction with other elements of the system or with its environment.

Both dental and total health services have evolved rapidly in the United States, and they have done so without an imposed order or structure. Until recently health care operated as a somewhat closed system, protected from environmental input, resistant to change which was not initiated from within. But in recent years the users of the health system have, through union and political representatives and through consumer advocacy groups, become a force for change despite contradictory reports on health care. On the one hand, there is continuing evidence of near miraculous progress; on the other, there are constant expressions of discontent and allegations of unacceptable access, availability, continuity, cost, and quality.

## CHRONOLOGY OF MAJOR HEALTH LEGISLATION

Any analysis of the dental health ecologic system must include a review of events outside the dental delivery system which affect it. Since the early 1930s there have been a number of significant federal laws which have disturbed the system's equilibrium. Following the economic crash of 1929, there came loud calls for federal assistance. Both Presidents Hoover and

Roosevelt took action to provide relief, and public acceptance of government responsibility for relief grew.

In 1935 the *Social Security Act* was passed, establishing a system of old age benefits for retired workers, a federal–state system of unemployment insurance, and a grant-in-aid program to give financial assistance to specified categories of needy people. Although it did not have immediate universal acceptance, it firmly established the role of the federal government in matters of social welfare and gave many Americans an awareness that wages can and do stop for a number of reasons beyond the individual's control.

It is interesting that as early as 1939 a national compulsory health insurance proposal was made to Congress but did not pass. In 1946 the Hill–Burton Act provided federal matching funds for building health facilities. In 1960 the Kerr–Mills Amendment to the Social Security Act introduced the first large-scale program of medical care in which doctors could be paid directly for providing care to certain groups. This laid part of the foundation for the third party payment concept.

In 1965 and 1966 Medicare and Medicaid began. Medicare introduced a compulsory hospitalization insurance and a voluntary medical benefits package for the elderly. Now for the first time a public health benefits program was not based solely on need. Medicaid provided comprehensive care for certain categories of persons, including all recipients of federally aided public assistance, comparable groups of medically needy, and all children under 21 whose parents could not afford to pay their medical bills.

Also in 1965 regional medical programs were set up and awarded grants to plan and develop cooperative arrangements for action against heart disease, cancer, stroke, and related diseases. Then, in 1966, the concept of comprehensive health planning was introduced with PL 89–749. The Comprehensive Health Planning and Public Health Services Amendments were to link together all elements of health service delivery, enabling them to develop a cooperative, coordinated approach to the system goal of good health for every individual.

The most recent and perhaps the most far-reaching health legislation to come out of Washington is the National Health Planning and Resources Development Act of 1974 (PL 93–641). It consolidates prior comprehensive health planning, regional medical programs, Hill–Burton programs, and experimental health services delivery systems legislation in an attempt to equalize access to care and to stabilize, if not reduce, costs.

This legislative chronolgy makes the direction in which the system is headed apparent. There is a merger, a diffusion of the public and private systems. It is almost as if the health delivery system could say with the comic strip character, Pogo, "we have met the environment and it is us."

QUESTION

1. Passage of the Social Security Act in 1935 represents a turning point in the U.S. welfare system because it
   1. provided for emergency relief to the unemployed
   2. firmly established the role of the federal government in welfare matters
   3. assisted business by setting up job programs
   4. developed pension programs in all states for widows and orphans

## THE DENTAL DELIVERY SYSTEM

### Dentistry in Transition

Dentistry is in a period of transition characterized by 1) an increasing disillusionment among dentists, financiers, and patients; 2) an increasing awareness by forward-thinking consumers, politicians, and professional leaders of the need for greater responsiveness to public needs and demands; and 3) increased experimentation in new models of organizing, delivering, and funding dental health. Although there is still little agreement on how extensive change will or should be, we can predict that the process is likely to be evolutionary rather than revolutionary. The dental delivery system will probably remain pluralistic and retain the solo practice model for some time, even though the trend toward dental groups accelerates.

Two policies of the American Dental Association (ADA) suggest the nature of the present dental delivery system. The first states that dental care should be available to all, regardless of income. Care should be provided as rapidly as resources permit, using both private and community programs and should be based on the following priorities: disease prevention and control in children, and the elimination of pain and infection in adults. The second policy contends that dental care should be the concern first of the individual receiving it, then of that individual's family, community, state, and nation—in that order. This is the principle of subsidiarity, and it places the responsibility for the development and implementation of any program with the smallest social unit which has the willingness and the capacity to carry out that obligation. This responsibility should not be passed to higher levels except for the strongest reasons.

QUESTION

2. Dentistry's present transitional period is characterized by
   a. a greater awareness of the need for responsiveness to the public

b. increased disillusionment with the dental delivery system from within and without

c. increased experimentation with dental care organization, delivery, and financing

1. All of the above
2. a and b
3. b and c
4. a and c

## Scope of the System

If the professional intent is to provide quality care for all who need it, then who are the potential consumers? Who speaks for them? Where are they served? Who pays? How does the present system meet demand?

According to the ADA policy described previously, dentistry should be available to all. This includes the indigent, the million or more institutionalized, and the ambulatory, semiambulatory and bed-ridden. Dental care for these groups is often totally or partially subsidized by government, religious organizations, or private philanthropic sources. These people are spoken for collectively by the sponsors of the programs attempting to provide care.

The present delivery system is for the most part still directed toward the private, self-pay segment of the market. For a variety of reasons the solo private practices, which comprise most of the dental service delivery resources, do not adequately meet the needs of these special patients. There is a lack of consensus on whether dentists are adequately trained to treat them, on whether they find it economically unattractive, or on whether their practice settings are geared to special patient care. Regardless of the basis for discontent, the major force for change seems to be energized by a real or perceived lack of access to adequate care among persons or groups who feel isolated from the system physically, socially, or economically.

The forces for change are rooted in the growth process of American society and involve public attitudes and expectations, the character of its economic life, and the nature of the health sciences. For example, technologic advances in health care create continually higher levels of minimal care. Changes in dental care come about not because of automatic planned responses to dentistry's environment, but because of specific developments, problems, or crises.

Dentistry must understand that although the nature and extent of change may be influenced by its own actions and attitudes, the final decisions will be made outside the dental delivery system by representatives of the nation's 216 million population, representatives of its 100 million union members and spokesmen for its 40 million poor or otherwise handicapped. The final decisions will not be made by the 124,000 dentists or ADA leaders. No longer will changes in the dental delivery system be determined by the profession alone.

### QUESTIONS

3. Unlike the private, self-pay segment of the dental market, handicapped patients are generally spoken for by
   1. their families
   2. insurance companies
   3. the sponsors of care programs
   4. themselves

4. The best explanation of why dentistry as a profession may no longer make delivery policy decisions unilaterally lies in
   a. numerical ratios of dentists to union members
   b. increased consumer involvement in health policy
   c. federal legislation
   1. All of the above
   2. None of the above
   3. c

## Needs, Demand, and Resources

The dental system's capacity to respond to its environment, i.e., to impact favorably upon health, is dependent on the interplay and balance of two forces. These are need/demand on one side and the system's capacity—its resources—on the other. It is not wise in planning a dental system (be it a solo private practice or a large national program) to consider only the prevalence of dental disease or a dentist:population ratio, however, because not everyone who has dental disease will seek treatment.

**NEEDS.** Need should be examined in two ways. An absolute need includes all dental disease—total prevalence. Detectable need, on the other hand, is that portion of the absolute which is identifiable and quantifiable. The extent to which need is detected is influenced by the reliability and validity of the diagnostic methods employed. Obviously an oral examination using natural light and tongue depressors will not detect all of the caries in a given population, for example. Estimates of the resources required of a dental delivery system must take into consideration both absolute and detectable need and are vulnerable to discrepancies between them.

**DEMANDS.** Need is often confused with demand. But a person can be aware of a need and not demand (seek) care, or may be aware and want to receive care but not have the access or financial resources to receive it. Potential demand is the unqualified desire for dental care; this desire plus availability and access is defined as effective demand. These demands, of course, also affect resource requirements.

Demand can be measured in terms of number of visits, costs, or kinds of services sought. In terms of visits about half of the U.S. population sought dental care in 1976. Or, looking at costs, 6 billion dollars worth of dental demand was measured in 1974. In terms of the kinds of care demanded variations occur in different socioeconomic groups; higher levels of care correlate to higher levels of education and income.

A change in any demand perspective will be reflected by a change on the resource side of the system. More visits or dollars means more resources required. Higher and more sophisticated levels of care also call for increases in the resource capacity.

***Demand Determinants.*** There are three basic determinants of demand. First there are those which are automatic and increase demand independently of dentists' attitudes or actions. For example, population changes, urbanization, education, changes in occupational level, and changes in buying power all have a positive correlation with dental demand. The second determinant is professional stimulation of the market by means of awareness programs like the ADA's Public Education Program. Although the question has been raised as to whether dentistry's resources can stay in balance with an increased demand resultant from such efforts, dentistry's spokesmen contend that they can. Natural attrition of patients, increased numbers and productivity of dentists, and the effect of prevention programs all tend to counteract demand increases due to such professional stimulation. The third determinant of demand is a financial one. The postpayment and prepayment methods which are now a part of the delivery system make it easier for patients to pay for necessary dental care so that they are more likely to seek it.

Summarizing the net effect of demand determinants, it can be said that need far exceeds demand. The backlog of accumulated disease attests to this. There is also evidence that average Americans will seek more care in the future than they do today because of improvements in the average income and education levels. These predictable increases in demand will be further augmented by new developments in methods of financing dental care.

***Utilization.*** A utilization review of a dental system or program gives another perspective on demand in that it may include, in addition to a simple quantification of demand, descriptions of the patterns of use and abuse in the relationship between the resource and need/demand sides of a delivery program.

The Bureau of Health Manpower of the U.S. Public Health Service has published a complete listing of factors which are linked to utilization of the dental care system. This checklist may be useful in understanding the dynamics of dental care utilization. Some factors on the checklist are

Dental manpower shortage in localized areas
Lack of public knowledge about improved dental techniques

Social structure of a community
Community's desire/acceptance of dental programs
Beliefs of religious groups
Dentist/patient relationship
Dentists' supposed lack of humanistic concerns or supposed sexual/racial bias
Lack of confidence in dental expertise
Age and sex of patient; parental/family influence
Physical and mental health of patients
Socioeconomic status and educational level of patients
Individual awareness of dental needs
Fear of pain
Racial/ethnic background
Social taboos of individuals; preference for folk medicine
Previous personal experience with dental treatment
Concern for personal appearance
Scheduling problems of patients
Availability of transportation

QUESTIONS

5. The extent to which absolute need becomes detected need directly depends on the
    a. reliability of the diagnostic methods
    b. validity of the diagnostic methods
    c. cost factors
    d. demand factors
  1. a and b
  2. a and c
  3. b and c
  4. a, b, c, and d

6. A person does not seek treatment for bleeding gums because of a financial handicap. Such an example comes under the category of
  1. potential demand
  2. effective demand
  3. Both a and b
  4. Neither a nor b

7. Which of the following determinants of demand is an example of professional stimulation? A
  1. dental health education program
  2. population change
  3. change in public buying power
  4. prepayment program

8. Which of the following are reasons for the projected increase in demand for dental care?
  1. Better education of the public
  2. Population increases
  3. Increased incomes
  4. All of the above
  5. None of the above

## Resources

Keeping the system in balance is a planning goal of both consumers and providers (Fig. 4–1), and substantial experimentation has been done on the organization

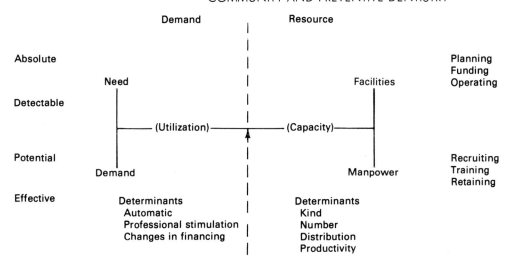

**FIG. 4-1.** Relationships of resources to demands in the dental delivery system. If there is an increased demand because of an automatic determinant, for example, the demand side can be lightened by reducing need, demand, or utilization; or resources can be increased in one or more ways. Manpower and/or facilities can be increased, or the productivity of existing resources can be increased by improving technology or the delivery system organization.

of dental care delivery. Two innovations which can greatly increase the dentists' productivity are Dental Auxiliary Utilization (DAU) and Training in Expanded Auxiliary Management (TEAM).

**MANPOWER.** There are about 124,000 dentists in the U.S.; the dentist:population ratio is 1:1710, but it is slowly decreasing. U.S. dentists are concentrated in New England, the mid-Atlantic, and the Pacific region, which includes Alaska and Hawaii. About 10% of the nation's active dentists are specialists, and more than half of these are in orthodontics and oral surgery. They are distributed this way:

| | |
|---|---|
| Orthodontics | 4667 |
| Oral surgery | 2937 |
| Pedodontics | 1256 |
| Periodontics | 1067 |
| Prosthodontics | 719 |
| Endodontics | 640 |
| Oral pathology | 68 |
| Public health | 83 |
| | 11,437 |

Nearly all practicing dentists employ some kind of auxiliary personnel. Because there is no across-the-board national or state certification, registry, or licensing required of all paradental personnel, it is difficult to estimate their total number. A reasonable guess would place the number of dental hygienists, dental assistants, and dental laboratory technicians at 180,000. The

dental hygiene training program capacity has doubled in the 1964–1974 period, laboratory technicians' training programs increased sevenfold in that period, and dental assistant/secretary/receptionist training opportunities have increased tenfold.

There are now 59 U.S. dental schools graduating approximately 5500 dentists a year—an increased output of slightly more than 40% since 1964. Minority and women enrollments are also up from less than 5% to near 10%. There is about a 40% increase in applicants for the period, about 14,000 for roughly 5,600 admissions. Since 1974, the number of applicants is decreasing, however. In an effort to retain those recruited and trained, most state university dental schools favor resident applicants.

Although the nation's overall dentist:population ratio may be adequate for the present, there is some doubt that it will be able to meet the anticipated future demand. A more serious problem centers upon an inequitable distribution. Regional differences range from a low of 1:1471 in the Pacific region to a high of 1:2624 in the East South Central area. Individual state ratios vary from 1:1302 in New York to 1:3425 in Mississippi.

Attempts to improve dental access by increasing the number of dentists seemed at first to be an obvious solution to the ratio problem. Further, it could be viewed as a long-range national strategy to give private enterprise and marketplace economics play. Although an oversupply in a free market may force redistribution, it takes time; more immediate solutions have been suggested in both governmental and professional proposals of the early and mid-1970s.

**REDISTRIBUTION PROGRAMS.** The ADA has authorized development of a health manpower policy planning model based on more localized supply and demand indices. Meanwhile, the Department of Health, Education, and Welfare (HEW) has implemented its own manpower distribution programs. One is the National Health Service Corps, which is a Public Health Service program begun in 1970 to bring health care to areas of the country where there are severe shortages of physicians or dentists (or physician extenders). As a member of the Corps, the dentist, for example, is a salaried officer of the Public Health Service working in a community which has agreed to underwrite or subsidize an office and ancillary personnel sufficient to practice efficient modern dentistry. The facility is equipped by the Corps, and the dentist's salary is paid by the Public Health Service until the practice is operating at a profit. Usually the subsidy continues for no more than 2 or 3 years. Part of any profits from the practice is returned to the U.S. Treasury during those 2 or 3 years and part to the community for additional upgrading of its health care. The community organization sponsoring the practice may terminate the relationship with the Corps sooner if it is mutually advantageous to do so.

While the dentist is on federal salary, the community collects fees for the dental services rendered in order to establish a firm economic basis for private practice. If the dentist chooses to remain in that community after the arrangement with the Corps ends, he or she is already established without the financial strain or risk usually attendant to setting up a practice.

Another less successful and more controversial attempt at changing distribution patterns is seen in the concept of reciprocity. That is, a dentist who is licensed in one state can practice in any other state which is a party to a reciprocity agreement with that state without reexamination.

The Health Education and Assistance Act of 1976 addresses manpower development and distribution through incentives such as capitation payments to schools for enlarging classes, for increasing enrollment from underserved areas, and for accenting primary care training programs. Through this legislation HEW intends to improve the numbers, kinds, and location of dental manpower. The legislation also provides economic incentives to dentists in the form of loan guarantees and educational loan repayment for practicing in critical shortage or underserved areas.

### QUESTIONS

9. The population of a one-dentist town is expected to increase by 75% in a 10-year period. What approaches are appropriate for planners in order to keep resources in balance with demand?
    a. Reduce the need through community fluoridation.
    b. Institute a school-based prevention program to reduce the need.
    c. Increase the dentist's productivity by adding auxiliary personnel and equipment.
    1. All of the above
    2. a and b
    3. c
    4. a and c

10. The mean ratio of dentists to U.S. population is closest to
    1. 1:500
    2. 1:1000
    3. 1:2000
    4. 1:4000

11. From the perspective of resources versus demand, the main problem in obtaining dental care is
    1. inequitable distribution of dentists
    2. shortage of general practice dentists
    3. inefficient delivery
    4. high cost

### Increased Productivity Mechanisms—DAU, TEAM

Major increases in a dentist's productivity can be brought about through the utilization of dental auxiliaries. Two trained aides can double production. Employing principles of sit-down, four-handed dentistry, i.e., good facility design, specified tasks, and preset instrument trays, not only increases productivity in a given time period but lengthens the time a dentist may remain productive because stress is reduced. Both Dental Auxiliary Utilization (DAU) and Training in Expanded Auxiliary Management (TEAM) concepts are approaches to the productivity issue.

Although TEAM is relatively new to the dental profession and represents a departure from traditional task and procedure delegations in the dental office, DAU is an old and well-proven aid to most dental practices.

DAU.    The concept of DAU implies somewhat more than having an assistant in the office to seat patients, perform light tasks, and clean up. DAU means the effective and efficient use of a well-trained auxiliary in the practice of four-handed dentistry. The hands of the auxiliary become, in effect, an extension of the hands of the dentist and free the dentist to perform the more complicated tasks and procedures. Four-handed dentistry involves scheduling patients so as to maximize the use of time by the dentist and assistant, standardization of operating procedures so that the assistant knows what is expected for any given procedure, the use of a standardized work setup (normally on prepared trays), efficient instrument transfer routines, and correct positioning of the patient in the dental chair.

In four-handed dentistry the patient is placed in a supine position with the head lower than the feet. Contoured dental chairs with thin backs most effectively support the patient while causing a minimum of interference to the dentist's knees and legs. The right-handed dentist would sit most often in approximately the 11 o'clock position (the patient's head is at 12 o'clock and feet are at 6 o'clock), with some variation allowed for working in different areas of the mouth. The dentist's feet should be on the floor, and the upper legs should be roughly parallel to the floor. Of course, the back should remain straight and should be gently supported by the seat back.

The assistant works opposite the dentist in approximately the 3 o'clock position and should be positioned higher than the dentist for better visual access. Because the assistant is positioned higher than the dentist, there should be a firm support which can be used as a footrest attached to the assistant's stool.

TEAM. A federally sponsored program to train dental students in the management of a dental team, TEAM uses expanded function auxiliaries (EFDAs) in some roles which have been traditionally reserved for dentists. Specifically the EFDA can perform most or all of the reversible procedures which the dentist wants to delegate.

The TEAM practice, whether located in a traditional one-dentist office or in a group setting, involves new roles for the dentist. The dentist must become an efficient and effective manager of the TEAM, and this requires skills in interpersonal communication, planning, and evaluation, as well as the determination to make the TEAM concept work. Not every dentist is psychologically suited to be a TEAM manager, for life is certainly different for the dentist in a TEAM practice. However, it is wrong to assume that the dentist in a TEAM practice is much busier and has little time to devote to dentistry. Actually the well-managed TEAM practice frees the dentist's time for those procedures which can only be performed by a highly trained dentist and therefore allows the dentist to do more of them. Many dentists avoid such procedures as endodontics or minor tooth movement, for example, because they know from past experience that these are time-consuming and cannot be conveniently fit into a crowded schedule. In a TEAM practice, however, they should be able to budget time for these procedures since an EFDA performs most of the routine reversible procedures.

Many dentists might express the opinion that managing an expanded practice is fine for the dentist who desires it, but that it's not for them. On the other hand, many dentists have objected to having EFDAs perform routine reversible procedures because they feel that these procedures are the prerogatives of the dental professional. "Why go to dental school to learn all these procedures if I'm simply going to let someone else do them in my practice?" Dentists with a knowledge of dental history will recall the same arguments voiced

with the same vehemence when dental hygienists and dental laboratories began to perform work traditionally done by the practitioner. Needless to say, both of these paraprofessional groups have contributed immensely to modern dentistry.

Although research conducted in the U.S. and abroad has demonstrated clearly that an EFDA can and does perform high quality work and under the supervision of a quality-conscious dentist will consistently perform to high standards, it should be remembered that it has never been and will never be compulsory to employ any paraprofessional. Any practitioner today can elect to use or not to use an assistant, hygienist, or commercial dental laboratory, and when state laws make the use of EFDAs possible the practitioner will have the same option regarding them. It is a reasonable assumption, however, that as third party payment removes financial barriers for many more potential patients and as some form of national health insurance is implemented, those practitioners who are willing to expand their practices and employ EFDAs will be providing a quality service to more persons.

QUESTIONS

12. You are planning your dental office. Which type of patient chair will be most convenient for your four-handed dental practice?
   1. Straight-backed, thin-backed
   2. Straight-backed, thick-backed
   3. Contoured, thin-backed
   4. Contoured, thick-backed

13. Your dental assistant consistently has difficulty visualizing the operating field and therefore is of minimal help to you during most procedures. What is the likely cause of the difficulty?
   1. The patient is too low.
   2. The patient is too high.
   3. The assistant is too low.
   4. The assistant is too high.
   5. You are out of position.

14. Where are the dentist's feet during any operative procedure when four-handed dentistry is being used?
   1. On the stool support rim
   2. On the floor
   3. On the dental chair base
   4. Wherever is convenient

15. Where are the assistant's feet during any operative procedure when four-handed dentistry is being used?
   1. On the stool support
   2. On the floor
   3. On the dental chair base
   4. Wherever is convenient

16. Which of the following is the major objective of TEAM programs?
   1. Training expanded function auxiliaries
   2. Changing state dental laws

(Continued)

3. Training dental students in expanded functions so that he can teach them in his practice
4. Training dental students in the management of an oral health team which uses EFDAs
5. Training auxiliaries to manage an oral health team which uses EFDAs

## Financing Mechanisms

The payment and financing of dental (health) care may be classified in a number of ways. One can consider the sources of funds, the timing of payment, the method of paying, or the one who pays. Regardless of how payment for medical care is classified, a basic point to remember is that the public must pay for care under any system of finance. The cost falls on families and individuals through taxes, higher prices, or lower take-home pay, even when the payment mechanism makes it appear that the bills are being sent elsewhere. The financing system can make a significant difference for high- and low-income families, but average tax-paying families all pay the same.

The present system for financing medical care in the U.S. is diverse—part self-pay, part government pay, and an increasing part third party payment through private insurance. Insurance is a method of sharing risk and often of spreading payments over an extended period. There has been a rapid growth in dental insurance in recent years; one out of seven families is now covered by some form of third party payment plan. By 1980 the ratio will probably be one in four. Dental prepayment, described by HEW simply as "a system for budgeting the cost of dental services in advance of their receipt," is a method of financing payment for all or part of the cost of dental care for persons covered by a plan (4). Usually a subscriber pays dues or premiums into a fund or to an insuring organization, and the money is subsequently used to cover the cost of dental services as the subscriber receives them.

Third party and prepayment arrangements can be made with a variety of organizational forms such as commercial insurance companies, health service corporations (such as Blue Cross), dental service corporations, and through group practices and clinics. Most of these arrangements are made with groups of patients rather than individuals.

Health service corporations are organizations which contract to provide a range of health care services. Dental service corporations are sponsored by the dental profession to administer dental care plans on a prepayment basis, for example, Delta Dental Plans. Both dental and health service corporations operate on a nonprofit basis.

Insurance companies differ from health service corporations in that they reimburse a subscriber for the cost of treatment, usually at a specified amount per service which may or may not cover the full cost. It should be noted that there is no contract between the dentist and the third party carrier. The arrangement in which the subscriber pays for the service and is then reimbursed by the insurance company is called indemnity benefit. In the service benefit plans the insurer pays the dentist to provide covered services and the patient is liable to the dentist only for any difference between the covered services and their costs.

### QUESTIONS

17. Regardless of whether health care is financed by self-pay, government subsidy, or other third party mechanism, the ultimate cost falls on
   1. only the taxpayers
   2. big business
   3. the middle class
   4. government
   5. the public at large

18. The insurance concept is essentially one of
   1. budgeting payments
   2. sharing risks
   3. subsidized financing
   4. capitation

## Practice Modalities

There is an accelerating pace to the changes occurring in equipment and facilities design for the dental practice; materials and work methods are continually undergoing improvements. Dentists can no longer expect that the physical aspects of practice or its staffing patterns will remain static for long periods if they are to keep up with anticipated demands. The trend toward larger and more complex group practices is indicated by several factors:

1. Increased demand from government subsidized programs necessitating greater productivity
2. The dentist's desire to use time more efficiently
3. Increased flexibility of dentists' time which accompanies utilization of expanded duty auxiliaries
4. Availability of grants for developing innovative primary health care groups in various settings

GROUP PRACTICE. Although solo private practice is still the dominant model for dental service delivery (about 60%), since 1950 there has been a noticeable increase in partnerships and salaried arrangements. The number of cost sharing arrangments for independent practitioners has changed sporadically, however. Hard data on group practices are difficult to come by, largely because of the lack of a universal definition of them and because the practice survey data collected by the ADA since 1950 do not have separate categories for "defined" groups.

In 1970 the Public Health Service undertook a survey which studied group dental practice as an organizational form, defining it as follows: "A group dental practice is a practice formally organized to provide dental care through the service of three or more dentists using office space, equipment and/or personnel jointly" (2). Even though the survey did not count two-dentist practices, 715 groups met the definition, which indicates a trend toward group practice.

OTHER ORGANIZATIONAL FORMS. Two organizational forms of dental service delivery deserve special attention in that they are major changes in the delivery system: health maintenance organizations (HMOs) and neighborhood health centers.

*Health Maintenance Organizations.* HMOs are health service delivery systems designed to provide comprehensive care to enrolled populations on a prepaid, capitation basis. They may either deliver or arrange for the delivery of health care. They are seen by some as alternatives to the present delivery models, as vehicles for medicare and medicaid, or ultimately as vehicles for the implementation of a national health insurance program. Since an HMO represents a big-business approach to the provision of health care, its success as a system depends on the relationship between the enrolled group of patients, the organization which provides the services, and its management.

HMOs differ from traditional prepaid group insurance in their more comprehensive service package, in the accent on preventive care and early intervention, and in the absence of third party financing. In an HMO the insurer is also the provider. The concept has unique economic incentives and other group model advantages built into it. Since payment is made in advance, it is to the physician's advantage to keep utilization of the system minimal, that is, to keep the patients well instead of intervening after they become sick or injured. For the first time in the U.S., the doctor, as part of the HMO, has a financial stake in the health of patients, and most persons feel this results in better quality control.

A further professional advantage is that with third party contract language removed, the doctor can more easily select the appropriate setting and timing of treatment. For example, the doctor would not be as inclined to hospitalize patients or keep them in the hospital solely because the insurance contract specifies a time period as a condition for reimbursement. Similarly, the doctor may not prefer to delay construction of a dental prosthesis until the end of a contract-specified waiting period.

There are two types of HMOs: the open panel and the closed panel. In the closed panel or group practice type physicians and dentists operate in the group's own facilities. The open panel or foundation type can involve a number of provider locations and facilities held together through formalized arrangements whereby enrollees can be served at any location or by any provider who is a part of the organization. Despite both legal and financial obstacles which have impeded development of HMOs, there are now over 200 covering more than 7 million people.

*Neighborhood Health Centers.* A natural strategy of the mid-1960s war on poverty was the movement toward "health rights" programs assisted originally by the U.S. Office of Economic Opportunity (OEO) and joined later by HEW. Their objectives were characterized as a positive pursuit of the healthright of individual families, neighborhoods and communities

"to assure that (health) services are made readily accessible to residents of concentrated poverty areas, are furnished in a manner more responsive to their needs and with their participation, and whenever possible are combined with . . . arrangements for providing employment, education, social or other assistance needed by the families and individuals served" (3).

The scarcity of physical facilities in which to conduct these programs, especially in poverty areas, led to a cooperative effort by OEO, HEW, the Department of Housing and Urban Development, the Office of Management and Budget, and sometimes private mortgage and insurance companies to obtain funds for neighborhood health centers. Most of them were free-standing but, to a lesser extent, hospital outpatient departments were used. The programs were developed with the active participation by neighborhood residents to assure maximum responsiveness.

Although there was an expressed desire for comprehensive services, it was not to be at the expense of personal care and the doctor/patient relationship. Neighborhood health center programs were characterized by special attention to prevention, early care, and outreach components to change the existing health behavior patterns of the poor. In contrast to families using HMOs, neighborhood health center families "register" rather than "enroll," which leaves them more freedom of choice in using or not using the center as their sole or primary source of care.

Because the care delivered by the neighborhood health center includes social work, outreach, education, and health supervision services, cost comparisons are difficult to make. Neighborhood health centers do not provide final answers for all questions on health care delivery systems, but they have provided planners with a better understanding of the systems' complexity.

QUESTION

19. The providers of care usually share in the responsibility for the financial success of an HMO. They theoretically do this by
   1. minimizing treatment
   2. reducing hospital admissions
   3. keeping patients well
   4. performing routine physical examinations

## Quality Assurance

ESSENTIALS OF GOOD MEDICAL CARE. The fundamental goal of the medical care system is to make good medical care available to the population, and there are four elements required to reach this goal: accessibility, quality, continuity, and efficiency.

Care, including facilities, equipment, drugs, and the practitioner's services, must be accessible where and when the individual needs it. Three criteria may be used to measure accessibility. Personal accessibility relates to an individual's point of entry into the system. Although it may vary from one person to another, it is primarily the physicians and dentists who deal with the patient in an ongoing relationship who can best serve as the entry point. Since comprehensiveness is another measure of accessibility, a good range of personnel, facilities, and services must be available at the system's entry point in order to make them accessible if or when they are needed. Quantitative adequacy, the third determinant of accessibility, means in simple terms that health services must be supplied in sufficient quality to meet the need for them, keeping supply in balance with demand.

The term quality is sometimes used as a synonym for good but is better defined as an optimum use of up-to-date knowledge and techniques to achieve the most desirable effect on the patient. Aspects of quality are professional competence, acceptability to patients, and conformity to minimum standards of care.

Continuity can be viewed from two perspectives. The patient wants to be treated as a whole person, and such person-centered care requires a continuing relationship with and coordination of care by a central contact, i.e., a primary provider. From the community standpoint it implies planning and coordination, and a minimum of aimless shuffling about in the system.

Efficiency involves the relationship between the quantity of resources used and the quantity of health effects produced. In addition to budgeting health care costs for patients, efficiency implies good compensation for providers. Efficient administration is the process of organizing the use of resources in an effective economical way.

Both the professional as an individual and the profession as a whole are responsible for the quality of health care provided. The dentist, for example, must be competent in diagnosis, treatment planning, and service delivery. The profession must cooperate with public agencies in activities such as aptitude testing, accrediting dental schools, licensure, and continuing education.

Although there is evidence that the quality of American dental care is high, it has never been documented. It was not until 1976 that currently quality assurance activities were studied with an eye to developing a model. The model is to be created by the professions and acceptable to them, while at the same time it is to address questions now being asked by an actively aware public. Such a model has yet to evolve. Dental prepayment has also increased interest in quality assurance, because as insurance companies and government continue to finance a larger segment of the dental care market, their insistence on high quality grows.

PROFESSIONAL STANDARDS REVIEW ORGANIZATIONS. In November of 1972 the Social Security Act was amended again under PL 92–603. The new law mandated the development and operation of a quality assurance system for health care delivery. It represents a federal effort to upgrade health care quality and control its costs. The law is being implemented through Professional Standards Review Organizations (PSROs) which review the quality and appropriateness of medical care provided to Medicare and Medicaid patients. The law requires that a PSRO must assure the public of quality care by the following methods:

1. establishing the necessity of treatment
2. establishing its consistency with regional professional standards
3. encouraging the use of less costly sites and modes of treatment
4. reviewing patient, doctor, and institutional profiles against regional norms of care.

PSROs are nonprofit professional associations representing physicians (dentists may have only an advisory role) which contract for the review of services in a designated area. (Much attention has been paid to regional differences in norms and standards.) PSRO review now covers only services in hospitals or long-term care facilities, but it is expected that ambulatory care will be included later. At the present time dentistry is only included when it is done in the institutional setting.

DENTAL PEER REVIEW. The general concept of peer review is especially needed in dentistry because the public is not able to evaluate dental care. Given that quality assurance programs will continue to develop in an attempt to meet the special needs of dentistry and given that they are needed as evidenced by the increased pressures for them, dentistry is now trying to determine the extent to which its existing peer review mechanisms can be combined with other measures such as PSRO for satisfactory quality assurance.

Dental peer review is a formalized system for resolving disagreements between dentists, patients, and third party carriers relating to the appropriateness or quality of care rendered. Unlike PSRO, peer review is voluntary. Its purpose is "to review matters concerning but not limited to the appropriateness of care, quality of treatment, and (acting in an advisory capacity) fees," and it is designed to function at the simplest level possible (1). At the local dental society level committees are composed of dentists having similar training and experience. Reviews are initiated by either the patient, the dentist, or the insurance company and are heard at the local level. Generally an attempt is made to mediate the dispute before referring it for full review. If a clinical examination is necessary, it may be done with permission of the patient and knowledge of the patient's dentist. All parties are notified of decisions and recommendations coming out of a review and have the right to appeal before final decisions are made. Reviewed cases may be continued in the courts but may be prejudiced by the Peer Review Committee findings.

## National Health Planning and Resources Development

Key words in the consumer perspective of health care beginning in the 1960s were quality, availability, and cost. Purchasers of health services sought to assure the highest level of health attainable for every person. In 1966 Comprehensive Health Planning and Public Health Services Amendments (PL 89–749) introduced the concept of linking together all elements involved in health services, thus enabling governmental, private health and related agencies, and interested groups to develop a cooperative and coordinated approach toward the good health goal. Besides establishing a comprehensive approach to health planning, this legislation gave access to the planning process to a wide range of persons, including consumers, opened the way for new relationships among health-related groups, and strengthened the decision-making process.

In 1974 problems in health care were no longer referred to as a crisis; however, large segments of the population were not yet receiving good care. Educational institutions were not producing the right kinds of health manpower, and a maldistribution persisted. Although substantial activity was underway to correct the problems, an orderly approach was necessary to achieve success in an economically feasible manner.

With that goal in mind PL 93–641, the National Health Planning and Resources Development Act of 1974, was passed. Its purpose was to assure equal access to quality health care at reasonable cost. Highlights of the law are as follows. It

1. establishes a National Council of Health Planning and Development
2. establishes the nation's ten highest health priorities
3. creates a network of Health Systems Agencies
4. calls for the designation of a specific state agency responsible for planning and regulatory functions (guided by State Coordinating Councils)

5. continues the Hill–Burton Program at the state level and requires that a state facilities plan be approved by the State Coordinating Council

The Health Systems Agencies (HSAs) are required to

1. gather and analyze suitable data
2. establish health systems plans (goals) and annual implementation plans (objectives and priorities)
3. provide technical and/or limited financial assistance to organizations seeking to implement provisions of the plans
4. coordinate activities with PSROs and other appropriate planning and regulatory entities
5. review and approve or disapprove applications for federal funds for health programs within the area
6. assist states in the performance of capital expenditures reviews
7. assist states in making findings as to the need for new institutional health services proposed for the area
8. assist states in reviewing existing institutional health services offered with respect to the appropriateness of such services
9. recommend annually to the states projects for the modernization, construction, and conversion of medical facilities in the area

HSAs are obviously more control oriented than the comprehensive planning agencies which preceded them. At the state level the law calls for designation of a State Health Planning and Development Agency to plan and implement governmental parts of the State Health Plan and of the HSAs. This agency assists in reviewing the state facilities plan and the capital expenditures of facilities receiving reimbursement under Section 1122 of the Social Security Act. By 1980 it must also administer a state certificate of need program, which mandates a review of the need for new health services. The existing Health Systems Agency network created by the National Health Planning and Resources Development Act may be viewed as a potential component of a national health insurance administrative or regulatory system.

That Congress will enact some form of national health insurance in the near future is hardly debatable. The only questions are when and what kind. There are three philosophical approaches to the issue. Some say it should be designed as a bona fide insurance scheme to protect individuals from catastrophic loss resulting from illness or accident. Others would design it as a redistributive mechanism that channels health care purchasing power from middle and upper income families to lower income groups and in so doing redistributes health services in the same manner. A third group sees it as a set of economic and administrative controls through which the public sector can reshape the organization of health care. Regardless of the form it takes, national health insurance planning must consider seven constants: 1) administration, 2) financing, 3) copayments, 4) benefit structure, 5) resources, 6) quality and evaluation, and 7) eligibility.

To date the numerous proposals can be classified into one of four categories. There are those that fall into the insurance group; the tax credit group; those administered mainly by public, government bodies; and those which represent a public and private administrative mixture.

### QUESTIONS

20. Which of the following is not in and of itself a criterion for evaluation of what constitutes good medical or dental care?
    1. Access
    2. Acceptability
    3. Quality
    4. Continuity
    5. Efficiency

21. The main reason for the increase in quality assurance mechanisms is
    1. the ADA code of ethics
    2. the competitive nature of the system
    3. increased third party purchases in the dental care market
    4. increased sophistication of the medical and dental technology

22. Which of the following is not a basic function assigned to PSRO by federal law or regulation?
    1. Establishing the necessity of treatment
    2. Establishing consistency with regional standards
    3. Encouraging the use of less costly sites and treatment modes
    4. Reviewing profiles against regional norms
    5. Establishing the reasonableness of fees

23. Dental Peer Review is intended to address disputes over
    a. fees
    b. appropriateness of care
    c. quality
    1. a
    2. b
    3. c
    4. a and c
    5. All of the Above

24. The main intent of the National Health Planning and Resources Development Act is to
    a. provide equity in access to care
    b. keep costs reasonable
    c. assure quality
    d. redistribute health resources
    1. a and c
    2. a and b
    3. a and d
    4. a, b, and c
    5. b

25. Which of the following is not one of the three most popular legislative approaches to national health insurance in the U.S.?
    1. To offer a bona fide insurance scheme protecting against financial disaster
    2. To redistribute the health care purchasing power more equitably
    3. To reorganize the delivery system
    4. To socialize medicine completely

# PART II
# PRINCIPLES OF DENTAL PUBLIC HEALTH

The specialty of dental public health, just as all the other public health disciplines, depends a great deal on the science of epidemiology. Epidemiology is concerned with gathering data in the community relative to disease, defects, disabilities, accidents, and health habits and conducting studies to elucidate causal relationships between these conditions and various risk factors associated with them.

## EPIDEMIOLOGY

Epidemiology is the study of the causes, occurrence, and distribution of diseases, defects, disabilities, or deaths in the community. This should be contrasted with disease etiology, wherein a disease cause is sought within the diseased entity. Epidemiologists examine the entire community as patient and therefore the causes of the diseases, disabilities, etc. are usually more general than those of disease etiology.

The word epidemiology formerly indicated a study of disease epidemics, especially infectious diseases. Today, except in the case of some lesser developed countries, infectious disease epidemics are relatively uncommon. The focus of epidemiology has therefore shifted to those diseases which have become more common in modern society. People seldom die from the infectious diseases which formerly ravaged the community; they live longer and therefore develop the diseases characteristic of old age, diseases which they might not have lived long enough to develop only a few decades ago. Specifically, epidemiologists have recently focused on the chronic diseases. By modern definition an epidemic is the occurrence of a disease, defect, or disability clearly in the excess of normal expectation. Thus it can be seen why cancer, stroke, heart attack, and dental caries have come under the intense study of epidemiologists.

26. As a science, epidemiology is concerned mainly with disease as it is manifested in
    1. individual patients
    2. selected populations
    3. the total community
    4. hospital cases

27. In modern epidemiology an epidemic is defined as
    1. an acute outbreak of infectious disease
    2. an acute outbreak of chronic diseases
    3. a chronically present disease
    4. an occurrence of a disease clearly in excess of normal expectation

## Rates—Incidence and Prevalence

Epidemiologists spend most of their working hours comparing populations—those who have the disease, defect, etc. of interest versus those who do not (the controls). Or, they compare a certain characteristic of one group which may predispose to disease (a risk factor) with that of another group. To do this, they employ rates. A rate can be defined as the number of cases of the disease, defect, etc. over the population at risk of getting that disease, defect, etc. expressed to some convenient multiple of 1000 as base.

$$\text{Rate} = \frac{\#\ \text{cases}}{\text{Population at risk}}\ (\times 1000)$$

The numerator is the number of cases; that's straightforward enough. The denominator is the number of persons who could have the disease in question. Why not the total population? It would not make sense to include males, prepubertal females, and postmenopausal females in the denominator of the puerperal fever rate, for example, since those persons cannot be affected by the disease. Thus epidemiologists speak of only the population at risk in the denominator.

Why should the fraction be expressed as some multiple of 1000? Consider the following rates. City A had a rate of disease X of 240/120,540 in 1976, and city B had a rate of disease X of 3,781/1,740,221 in 1976. Which city had the worse disease X experience? As presently expressed, there is no way to compare

the rates directly without performing the mathematics. If, however, both were expressed as a fraction with a base of, say, 10,000, you would have the following:

City A = 19.91/10,000
City B = 21.72/10,000

Now a direct comparison of cities A and B can be made concerning the occurrence of disease X.

The two rates most often encountered in epidemiology are incidence and prevalence. Incidence is the number of new cases of disease, defects, etc. arising among the population at risk during a given time period, usually one calendar year. The incidence rate is, of course, expressed as a fraction with a base of 1000 or a multiple thereof. Prevalence is the total number of disease, defect, etc. cases seen at the time of the study in the population at risk. Disease prevalence measures all new cases of disease which are extant at the time of examination plus any continuing cases of the disease. Thus disease prevalence depends not only on how often the disease occurs, but on how long the disease lasts. Generally a disease which occurs often but does not last long shows a higher incidence than prevalence rate. A disease which is long lasting shows a higher prevalence rate.

28. Which of the following is a properly expressed disease rate?
    1. Population at risk/cases of disease/100,000
    2. Total population/cases of disease/100,000
    3. Cases of disease/total population
    4. Cases of disease/total population/100,000
    5. Cases of disease/population at risk/100,000
    6. Cases of disease/number of cures/100,000
    7. Cases of disease/visits to doctor/100,000

29. City A had 54 cases of a certain disease last year while city B had 127. What, if anything, is missing to make a meaningful comparison of the disease experiences of the two cities?
    1. Nothing—city B's experience was worse than city A's
    2. The number of cases from a control city
    3. Total population of the two cities
    4. Populations at risk in the two cities
    5. Number of doctors in the two cities

30. An epidemiologist examines the population of a small town for both the incidence and prevalence rates of arteriosclerosis. Assume that all cases can be identified and that the cure rate is nil. Which rate is probably larger?
    1. Incidence
    2. Prevalence

31. An epidemiologist looks at the incidence and prevalence rates of upper respiratory infections. Assume that
(Continued)

all cases can be identified. Which rate is probably larger?

1. Incidence
2. Prevalence

## Indexes of Dental Disease

In dentistry incidence and prevalence rates are not as useful as they are in other medical areas because the two major dental diseases, dental caries and periodontal disease, are almost universal. If any two groups, say, freshmen and sophomore dental students, are compared, prevalence rates are likely to be in excess of 95% for these diseases. That is, almost everyone has or has had these two diseases. Therefore, incidence and prevalence rates do not distinguish well between two groups. Granting an almost universal prevalence to the dental diseases, dental epidemiologists have developed indexes of dental disease to measure the severity of the diseases among those persons who have it. An index can be generally defined as an indicator of disease severity measured on a scale with upper and lower limits. Groups can be distinguished by the average number of lesions.

INDEX OF PERMANENT DENTITION. The most common index of dental caries is the DMF (CER in some parts of Europe) which is an index of the permanent dentition. The D stands for a decayed tooth, M for a missing tooth, and F for a filled tooth. The rationale of this index is that dental caries is permanently observable in the mouth, that is, once an individual has it or has had it, an examiner will discover it either as an active lesion, a tooth which has been extracted, or a filling placed after caries removal. This index is most often based on 28 teeth. Third molars are usually excluded because of their frequency of extraction or impaction. The portion of the index that is most likely to give false scores is the M. The examiner may assume that a tooth is missing due to caries, whereas it may have been orthodontically extracted, it may have been lost due to an accident, or it may have been lost due to periodontal disease.

The DMF, sometimes written as DMFT, is an index of the entire tooth. If both D and F, or two separate lesions, on the same tooth cause a difficulty in scoring, the DMFS is often used; the S representing individual tooth surfaces.

### QUESTIONS

32. Why are incidence and prevalence rates less useful to dental epidemiologists than they are to medical epidemiologists? The dental diseases
    1. are almost universal
    2. occur infrequently
    3. are too difficult to measure
    4. are high in incidence but low in prevalence
    5. are low in incidence but high in prevalence

33. Which statement best describes the rationale of the DMF index?
    1. Adult teeth are easier to measure than deciduous teeth.
    2. Dental caries is permanently observable in the mouth.
    3. Dental caries is universally prevalent.
    4. Dental caries is best measured by scoring active lesions only.
    5. Dental caries is best measured by ignoring missing teeth.

34. A 12-year-old patient is scored using the DMF index. Data from this child revealed the following:

    2 missing permanent 1st molars
    4 missing 3rd molars
    3 filled permanent teeth
    4 active carious lesions on permanent teeth
    2 filled deciduous teeth
    2 missing deciduous teeth

    What is the DMF score for this patient?
    1. 6
    2. 9
    3. 13
    4. 15
    5. 19

INDEX OF DECIDUOUS TEETH. The index of deciduous teeth is the def (or df) index. Epidemiologists do not use an m for the deciduous teeth index because the deciduous teeth are naturally exfoliated and the use of an m would be a highly misleading indication of disease. The fact of exfoliation also leads to the paradox that a child with a def (or df) of 4 could actually have a better dental condition than a child with a score of 2. If the first child is 3 and has 20 deciduous teeth, that child's dental condition might be better than that of a child of 12 who has only 2 deciduous teeth left, both of which are decayed.

Like the D and F of the permanent tooth index, the d and the f indicate a decayed and filled tooth, respectively. Sometimes an e is used to indicate a tooth to be extracted. This is a judgmental call in which the examiner places a tooth otherwise to be called d into the e category to indicate severe caries. Often the "e" is just not used.

### QUESTIONS

35. A child of 8 is examined and found to have the following dental condition:

    2 filled permanent teeth
    4 missing permanent 2nd molars
    2 carious permanent teeth
    3 filled deciduous teeth
    2 missing deciduous teeth
    2 carious deciduous teeth

What is the df score for this child?

1. 3
2. 5
3. 7
4. 8
5. 11
6. 13

**PERIODONTAL DISEASE INDEXES.** Whereas most epidemiologists use the DMF, DMFS, or df indexes to measure dental caries, no single index is so widely used for periodontal disease that it can be considered standard. Periodontal disease indexes are termed reversible or irreversible depending on whether they are intended to measure reversible or irreversible gingival or periodontal conditions. One index commonly used for determining the oral hygiene status of a population of persons (an indirect indicator of periodontal disease) is the Oral Hygiene Index-Simplified or OHI-S. This index is a combined plaque and calculus index which is easily used in the community setting.

Generally periodontal disease is difficult to study epidemiologically because of the following:

1. Indexes are not standardized.
2. Two different disease processes can be involved; soft tissue and bone.
3. There is a reliance on x-rays for the irreversible diseases.
4. Periodontal disease is a disease of the elderly and it is difficult to know if tooth loss has been due to periodontal disease, to antecedent dental caries, or to other factors.

What then is found when dental epidemiologic methods are applied to most populations in the U.S. in the investigation of the two major dental diseases?

## Dental Caries

Dental caries is normally found to be a chronic disease which begins at a young age and progresses throughout life. Fewer than 5% of the total population can be expected to escape this disease, and the majority of the lucky few are likely to be those who have been born and raised in an area of optimum artificial or natural water fluoridation.

Extensive data on young children are lacking due to the difficulty of examining great numbers in this age group. However, available evidence indicates that dental caries begins shortly after tooth eruption. Most studies have shown that over 50% of preschool children have experienced some decay with as many as 20% experiencing severe decay. By age 6, when the first permanent teeth begin to erupt, approximately 80% of all children have decay in the deciduous teeth.

Permanent teeth begin to decay rapidly with the eruption of additional teeth. Although the process continues throughout life, incidence rates are higher at the ages of 6–20 than in later years. This is not due to any inherently gained resistance to decay but to a decrease in attackable surfaces as the disease progresses. By the time of the late teens and early twenties the prevalence of decay is almost universal.

These data are representative of the total population in the U.S. and do not reflect regional variations. There are regional variations, however, in relation to the natural and artificial presence of fluoride in potable waters.

QUESTIONS

36. Prevalence of dental decay in the adult population of the U.S. has been shown to be
    1. less than 50%
    2. 50%–75%
    3. 75%–95%
    4. 95+%
    5. 100%

37. Incidence rates of dental caries in the total population generally become smaller beyond the age of 20. Reduction in incidence rates of decay is primarily due to
    1. a reduction in attackable surfaces
    2. a natural resistance of mature teeth to decay
    3. a change in hormones in the older group
    4. a change in the constituents of plaque
    5. a change in the amount of measurable plaque
    6. better toothbrushing in the older group

38. When the first permanent teeth begin to erupt, the prevalence of dental decay in deciduous teeth is approximately
    1. 20%
    2. 50%
    3. 80%
    4. 95%
    5. 100%

## Periodontal Disease

Periodontal disease also affects nearly everyone, but its destructiveness, as measured by tooth loss, is confined mainly to the age group over 30. Periodontal disease can range from a mild gingivitis to the advanced states of a chronic, severe bone loss which results in tooth loss. Available data indicate that the milder forms of the disease do occur in youth and that gingivitis is common in adolescence. By the age of 45, people have commonly developed periodontal disease so severe that tooth extraction is required; eight of ten extractions performed on this age group are the result of periodontal disease. By age 50 half of the adult population is experiencing destructive periodontal disease, and by age 65 the percentage approaches 100.

39. Chronic destructive periodontal disease is a major problem in the population beyond the age of 30 in the U.S. By the age of 50 what percentage of the population can be expected to experience periodontal disease problems which involve bone loss?
   1. 10%
   2. 25%
   3. 50%
   4. 90%
   5. Nearly 100%

## Causative Factors of Dental Disease

Dental epidemiologists have carefully examined host, agent, and environmental factors which account for degrees of susceptibility to or severity of the dental diseases in individual patients or in populations. The interrelationships of these factors is complicated, and more research will be required before the causes of these diseases can be completely elucidated. However, both correlational and experimental studies have shown that a few factors can be clearly shown to be involved in the occurrence and severity of dental disease.

DENTAL CARIES.    Three factors are known to be the *sine qua non* of dental caries. These are as follows:

1. Host—a susceptible tooth
2. Agent—acid-producing bacteria
3. Environment—a suitable substrate, the dental plaque.

Host.    It is clear that there must be teeth for dental decay to occur, but few dentists would advocate prophylactic odontectomy. However, many host factors increase the susceptibility of the teeth to decay. The patient who snacks frequently, especially on sugary foods, increases the likelihood of decay. Poor positioning of the teeth in the arch may prevent adequate cleansing and result in decay. Personal habits such as failure to clean the teeth properly, a low socioeconomic status, and casual parental attitudes (especially the mother's) toward the child's oral hygiene can contribute to disease. The host factor which is most clearly helpful in the reduction of dental caries is the availability of fluoride, particularly during tooth development.

Agents.    Dental caries is clearly related to the presence of acid-producing bacteria in the environment of the teeth. Caries of the clinical crown seems to be mainly the result of *Streptococcus*, with the particular species depending upon the location of the plaque on the tooth. *Actinomyces* appears to be responsible for the majority of root caries. Root caries is normally associated with gingival recession, a common concomitant of the aging process.

Environment.    Dental plaque appears to be a common denominator for the initiation of most caries and periodontal disease lesions. The acid-producing bacteria colonize to operate efficiently in a substrate rich in sucrose. Particular strains of *Streptococcus* apparently split the sucrose molecule by means of an extracellular polymer, glucan or dextran, which also contributes to the adhesiveness of plaque. The fructose portion of the sucrose molecule apparently is used directly for energy by the bacteria, and its conversion into fructan or levan gives further nourishment to the substrate. The acid produced is lactic acid.

PERIODONTAL DISEASE.    The interrelationship of host, agent, and environmental factors in the production of periodontal disease has also been extensively studied. These factors in periodontal disease are as follows:

1. Host—teeth and supporting tissues
2. Agent—bacteria and mechanical irritants (calculus)
3. Environment—dental plaque

Host.    Studies of the factors which increase or decrease the susceptibility of the periodontium to periodontal disease indicate that the age of the host is most clearly related to this disease process. Periodontal disease increases in incidence and severity as a patient grows older. One other host factor that can contribute to an increased gingivitis is a rapid change in hormonal balance.

Agent.    The most important agent factors in periodontal disease are bacteria and calculus.

Environment.    Two factors can alter the environment in which periodontal disease is likely to occur: oral hygiene and nutrition. Both of these can be controlled by the host. Research data have shown consistent correlations of periodontal disease with poor oral hygiene, especially when coupled with poor nutrition.

40. Some host factors which can contribute to an increased incidence of dental caries in a patient are
      a. frequent snacking
      b. ingestion of optimum fluoride ion in potable water
      c. improper tooth alignment
      d. poor oral hygiene habits
      e. low socioeconomic status of the patient
   1. d
   2. a, b, and c
   3. a, c, and d
   4. a, c, d, and e
   5. All of the above

41. The primary culprit in caries of the clinical crown of the tooth appears to be

1. *Actinomyces viscosus*
2. *Streptococcus*
3. *Lactobacillus*
4. *Pneumococcus*

42. The primary culprit in caries of the root surface of the tooth appears to be
    1. *Actinomyces*
    2. *Streptococcus*
    3. *Lactobacillus*
    4. *Pneumococcus*

43. Acidogenic bacteria survive and produce acid best in a dental plaque rich in
    1. starch
    2. sucrose
    3. fructose
    4. galactose
    5. extracellular enzymes

44. A common factor in the diseases of caries and periodontal disease is
    1. dental plaque
    2. disturbed hormonal balance
    3. faulty restorations
    4. poor heredity (defective genes)
    5. lack of adequate professional care by the patient
    6. low socioeconomic status of the patient

## FLUORIDATION

The investigative epidemiology which led to the discovery and elucidation of the role of fluoride in the prevention of dental decay has been the greatest contribution of public health dentistry to the health of the nation.

Following a long period wherein a correlation between the characteristic enamel lesion called variously Colorado Brown Stain or mottled enamel and the relative absence of dental decay was noted but could not be accounted for, in the early 1930s the role of naturally occurring fluoride in potable water was discovered. Thereupon began one of the most thorough laboratory and clinical examinations of any environmental substance known to man. Fortunately, in order to study the effect of fluoride in drinking waters it is only necessary to match suitable cities, one with naturally occurring fluorides and one without them. Careful study consistently revealed no effect of fluoride on the human body, when available in optimum dosage, beyond the beneficial effects on teeth and bone.

In the 1940s clinical trials were begun to test the effect of drinking water artificially fluoridated to an optimum level. Once again the effects were nil except for a consistent reduction in the incidence of tooth decay in the range of 40%–60%. Such convincing evidence led public health and political officials to begin a movement toward optimum fluoride adjustment of city water supplies. Most major cities in the U.S. have enjoyed the benefit of this public health measure for over 20 years. A few states have mandated fluoridation for all municipal water supplies over a certain size, and the measure has been supported by every major reputable scientific and medical society and association in the U.S. Yet the job is far from complete in the U.S. and has hardly begun in most other countries of the world. Thus it is important for the dental student and the practitioner to know the basic facts of water fluoridation since, in those areas where the population still does not benefit from its use, the dentist is a major source of information to the public.

Fluoride is the 14th most commonly occurring substance in the environment. Because its presence in soils and waters is ubiquitous, it is impossible to plan a fluoride-free diet. At a fluoride concentration of approximately 1 part per million (1 PPM = 1 mg/liter) an optimum benefit accrues to the teeth with a minimal incidence of mottled enamel. At this level, which is adjusted in the range of 0.7–1 PPM depending on climatic variations among cities, mottling occurs in very few individuals and at a level usually detectable only by specialists. Although fluoride is taken in through water, food, and air, the primary source for most persons is water. Fluoride is rapidly absorbed by the body; 50% is stored in the bones and teeth, and 50% is excreted in the urine.

In teeth the primary protective mechanism seems to be an incorporation of the fluoride ion into the hydroxyapatite molecule of enamel. This apparently renders the enamel more resistant to acid dissolution but does not, in fact, make the enamel intrinsically harder. Most benefit is gained when the fluoride ion is available during enamel formation. Most naturally occurring, optimally fluoridated water occurs in the midwestern states.

QUESTIONS

45. Optimum water fluoridation concentration for most communities is
    1. 0.01 PPM
    2. 0.1 PPM
    3. 1 PPM
    4. 10 PPM
    5. 2 PPM

46. Fluoride ion concentration in city water supplies is varied from 0.7–1 PPM due to climatic conditions. Why?
    1. There is more naturally occurring fluoride in waters in colder climates.
    2. There is more naturally occurring fluoride in waters in warmer climates.
    3. People drink more water in colder climates.
    4. People drink more water in warmer climates.

47. Which of the following is the major modality of fluoride excretion in man?

*(Continued)*

1. Sweat
2. Urine
3. Feces
4. Expired air
5. Saliva

48. Which of the following statements best accounts for the effect of the fluoride ion on tooth enamel? It makes tooth enamel

   1. harder
   2. whiter
   3. more resistant to acid dissolution
   4. basic in pH
   5. more resistant to bacterial enzymes

49. When the fluoride ion is incorporated in the developing teeth in optimum amounts, what level of caries reduction can be expected for most persons in a community?

   1. 10%–20%
   2. 20%–40%
   3. 40%–60%

4. 60%–80%
5. 80%–100%

50. From your knowledge of the general location of most naturally occurring fluoridated waters, determine which of the following states is (are) likely to be home to Army inductees who show reduced DMF scores.

   a. Florida
   b. Massachusetts
   c. Colorado
   d. Oklahoma
   e. California

1. a
2. b
3. c
4. d
5. e
6. a and c
7. b and c
8. c and d
9. c and e

# PART III
# PREVENTIVE DENTISTRY

Disease prevention is a philosophy of dental practice which recognizes that disease is a continuum ranging from a prodromal state to a frank lesion or disability. As such, the preventive process can intervene in the process at any step along the way.

Primary prevention involves those measures which prevent the onset of the disease in question. Secondary prevention is recognizing the disease early in its progress and repairing damages while they are minimal. Tertiary prevention involves those measures taken after the disease process has done considerable damage. Primary prevention is prevention in the absolute sense, while secondary and tertiary prevention are relative terms because they must include those reparative and curative measures which arrest the disease process and prevent its spread and increased severity. Each procedure that a dentist performs makes a patient more or less susceptible to future diseases. If the procedure makes the patient less susceptible, then the procedure is preventive, regardless of how far along the disease was when intervention occurred.

Concepts of preventing dental disease have been espoused since the beginning of recorded history, although dentistry has become scientific in its approach to disease prevention only in the last few generations. Many concepts have proven sound; others have proven mere nostrums, ineffectual for the purposes for which they were advocated.

The most effective approach to the prevention of disease has always been that which involves the least patient effort. Hence, the public health measure of water fluoridation has always been the preferred first line of defense against dental caries. Yet, only approximately 50% of public drinking waters are fluoridated, and, of course, water fluoridation has little effect upon periodontal disease. Therefore those personal preventive measures which have been proven effective remain important for any person who desires to prevent or control both of the main dental diseases.

Research has demonstrated the importance of controlling dental plaque if dental diseases are to be controlled. Plaque is a clear, sticky gelatinous aggregation of bacterial colonies which adhere to the surface of teeth and to gingival tissue. Plaque is not a unidimensional or even a single entity. Certain types of plaque appear to be associated with initiation of dental caries, others with formation of calculus, and still others with certain inflammatory responses. Further research is required before the chemical and microbial variations in plaque can be more fully elucidated. It is known that plaque forms in phases. The first phase involves the deposition of a very thin mucoprotein coat, called the pellicle, on the tooth surface. In the second phase the pellicle serves as a nidus for the attachment of *Streptococcus* to the tooth surface. As the bacteria colonize and grow in the third phase they produce extracellular products which contribute to the adhesiveness of plaque. Maturation of plaque is often associated with mineralization; this process normally begins at the tooth surface and proceeds outward, ultimately producing dense calculus, an important etiologic agent in periodontal disease.

### QUESTIONS

51. Intervention in the disease process at a stage before the lesion occurs is
    1. primary prevention
    2. secondary prevention
    3. tertiary prevention
    4. preventive dentistry
    5. relative prevention

52. The first phase of plaque formation on the tooth surface is
    1. deposition of streptococci in the pellicle
    2. formation of a pellicle
    3. production of acids by the streptococci
    4. formation of materia alba

53. Mineralization of plaque usually proceeds from the
    1. tooth surface outwards
    2. center of plaque toward the tooth surface
    3. center of plaque toward the outer surface of the plaque
    4. sulcus of the tooth toward the occlusal surface of the tooth

54. The salivary mucoprotein which forms on the clean tooth surface soon after cleaning of the surface is termed
    1. bacterial colony
    2. materia alba
    3. plaque
    4. pellicle
    5. calculus

## Toothbrushing

Toothbrushing has been considered the mainstay in the fight against dental disease for many years. Most persons are perfectly willing to quote the figure of "three times a day" as a means to prevention, although few actually brush three times daily. In addition, when individuals do brush, they often do a poor job of it. Even when the brushing is thorough, it is practically impossible to remove all bacteria; after a thorough prophylaxis at the dental office, the pellicle soon reappears. Thorough toothbrushing is essential, however, because clinical gingival changes can occur in as little as 1 week without careful brushing.

Many techniques of brushing have been advanced as the "best" method of removing plaque. Generally any method that removes the plaque from the tooth surface and from the gingival sulcus (as demonstrated by disclosing solution), does not damage hard or soft tissue, and is relatively easy for the patient to perform should be satisfactory. Vigorous side-to-side brushing can result in abrasion of enamel and cementum, and this is one method to be avoided. The roll method, wherein the bristles of the brush are placed against the tooth as far gingivally as possible and the brush is rolled occlusally, is an effective method which is easy to learn. The Bass method, wherein the brush is pressed into the gingival sulcus at a 45° angle and moved back and forth in a short vibrating motion before being moved occlusally, is effective for patients with gingival inflammation or where gingival sulci are large. The method recommended ought to be individualized according to the patient's needs and abilities and the dentist's confidence in the recommended procedure. In recommending a toothbrush the dentist once again ought to consider the special needs of the individual patient, but for most patients a soft-bristled, straight-handled, small flat-headed brush is satisfactory. Synthetic bristles have the advantage of drying quicker than natural bristles.

Generally a thorough once-a-day cleaning of the teeth will prove sufficient in preventing disease and is certainly superior to a more casual three-times-a-day brushing. It should be emphasized, however, that a thorough cleaning involves the use of more than just a toothbrush.

### QUESTIONS

55. In the absence of proper oral health care, gingival inflammation of previously healthy tissue can occur in as little as
    1. 1 day
    2. 1 week
    3. 2 weeks
    4. 1 month

56. One toothbrushing method which is known to be potentially destructive of hard and soft tissue is
    1. side to side
    2. Bass
    3. roll
    4. up and down

57. When cleaning of the sulcus becomes particularly important, as in inflammation or pocket formation, a good toothbrushing method is
    1. side to side
    2. Bass
    3. roll
    4. up and down

## Flossing

Even the best toothbrushing method only cleanses those areas of the tooth which can be reached by the toothbrush. Other areas remain neglected, support a build-up of plaque and calculus, and become prime target areas for dental diseases. Although most patients readily accept the need for the toothbrush, they do not so readily accept the need for floss. It becomes incumbent upon the dental practitioner and the dental profession in general to do a better job of teaching the importance of flossing to clean the areas between the teeth. Floss is most useful in cleaning the interproximal areas of the teeth from the contact point down to the sulcus. Patients should be carefully guided in the proper use of floss since damage to soft tissue is a frequent sequelum of too vigorous use.

In general most practitioners recommend an unwaxed floss since the individual strands of unwaxed floss can flare out and cover a greater surface area. However, some patients have tight contact areas or rough contacts between fillings which can tear unwaxed floss; these patients should use waxed floss.

### QUESTIONS

58. Plaque lodged interproximally is best removed by
    1. a toothbrush
    2. mouthwash
    3. dental floss
    4. irrigation

59. Dental floss is useful in removing plaque from
    1. occlusal surfaces
    2. facial and lingual surfaces
    3. interproximal surfaces above contact point
    4. interproximal surfaces below contact point

## Dentifrices

Despite advertising claims to the contrary, there is little difference in the cleansing ability of commercial toothpastes—and for good reason. Government guidelines have severely restricted the range of abrasiveness, which is paramount in cleaning, permissible in toothpastes. Powder-type dentifrices are generally a little more abrasive than their paste counterparts and may be slightly more effective on stains. Toothpastes do differ in another important aspect, and that is whether or not they contain a fluoride compound which has been demonstrated effective in decay prevention. At least two such products, Crest and Colgate, are currently available and accepted by the Council on Dental Therapeutics of the American Dental Association.

Certain specialty toothpastes can be beneficial in the care of cemental pain associated with gingival recession (Thermodent or Sensodyne), and these can be recommended in the instance of individual need.

### QUESTIONS

60. The cleansing property of a toothpaste is primarily a function of its
    1. fluoride content
    2. physical form, paste or powder
    3. abrasiveness
    4. binding agents

61. In general there is only one distinction among toothpastes which is important for most dental patients. That is its
    1. abrasiveness
    2. color and taste
    3. possession of an effective fluoride compound
    4. possession of an antiplaque ingredient

## Mouthwashes

Despite aggressive claims by their manufacturers of effectiveness against germs, mouth odors, and other conditions, most mouthwashes have only a limited oral hygiene function. In general most dentists use them as a cover for blood and bad-tasting residues in the patient's mouth. Patients may use them in the home for a temporary flavoring of the mouth. It should be stressed, however, that the germicidal and therapeutic uses of mouthwash are questionable and that overuse can be unhealthy for most persons. A clean, fresh-tasting mouth is best accomplished by good oral hygiene measures.

### QUESTION

62. Which statement best describes the therapeutic usefulness of mouthwashes? Mouthwashes are
    1. very useful
    2. somewhat useful
    3. limited in usefulness
    4. positively dangerous to health

## ORAL IRRIGATORS

The use of oral irrigators has become widespread among patients, and it should be made clear that their usefulness is as an adjunct to a regular brushing and flossing regimen rather than as a replacement for them. They can be useful in removing debris from orthodontic appliances, from bridgework, and from areas where teeth are badly aligned. However, their ability to remove plaque has yet to be adequately demonstrated, and the patient who desires to use such a device should be cautioned as to this shortcoming.

### Topical Fluorides

The application of topical fluorides at the dental chairside remains an effective weapon against dental caries. Of the three types of solutions currently available—stannous fluoride (SnF), sodium fluoride (NaF), and acidulated phosphate fluoride (APF)—significant reduction in the incidence of tooth decay (20%–40%) can be expected with each. Careful weighing of the advantages and disadvantages of each product has led to the general recommendation of the acidulated phosphate fluoride solution in most cases. A prophylaxis should precede any of the three treatment regimens.

Sodium fluoride in a 2% solution is applied to teeth for approximately 3 min during the first visit. A second, third, and fourth application should be given at weekly intervals thereafter. A full series of treatments should be given at 3, 7, 11, and 13, ages which correspond to the eruption of major tooth groups which are then at full risk of decay. The solution is stable and accepted well by patients, but the treatment regimen does not correspond well to regular dental check-up schedules.

Stannous fluoride in an 8% solution is applied to isolated teeth for approximately a half-minute per tooth. Since this procedure should be done every 6 months, it fits well into most office recall systems. Stannous fluoride is unstable and disagreeable in taste, however, and it can cause discoloration of hypocalcified teeth and restorations. Acidulated phosphate fluoride in a 1.2% solution is applied in a regimen identical to that of stannous fluoride but has none of the attendant disadvantages.

Because of their convenience topical fluoride gels are currently more popular than solutions for chairside application, but two major disadvantages should be noted. First, it is impossible for the dentist to determine if all the teeth have been properly wetted by the gel since the gel is beneath a tray. Second, if the gel remains viscous, the solution may not flow well into interproximal areas. For these reasons flexible trays are preferred over rigid trays.

### QUESTIONS

63. Sodium fluoride solution for topical applications possesses fluoride in which concentration?
    1. 0.2%
    2. 1.2%
    3. 2%
    4. 8%
64. Stannous fluoride solution for topical applications possesses fluoride in which concentration?
    1. 0.2%
    2. 1.2%
    3. 2%
    4. 8%
65. Acidulated phosphate fluoride solution for topical application possesses fluoride in which concentration?
    1. 0.2%
    2. 1.2%
    3. 2.0%
    4. 8.0%
66. Which of the following topical fluoride preparations requires a treatment regimen which does not correspond to normal recall intervals?
    1. Sodium fluoride
    2. Stannous fluoride
    3. Acidulated phosphate fluoride
    4. Potassium fluoride

## Fluoride Supplements

Although water fluoridation is the most efficient and effective mode of supplying dietary fluoride to the community, a dietary fluoride supplement may be the only means of supplying the ion to patients in rural areas with no communal water supply and patients in cities or towns with no water fluoridation. It should be noted, however, that the regimen required (once a day for many years) means that only the most highly motivated parents will follow through with this procedure for their children. Too, the amount of supplemental fluoride given to a child must be adjusted according to the age of the child and the amount of fluoride in the water presently consumed by the family.

Generally most persons in areas with a fluoroidated water supply consume 2–4 mg fluoride per day, the largest proportion coming from water and a smaller amount from foods. Supplementation aims at attaining approximately similar levels.

One very convenient regimen for children above the age of 3 who do not drink fluoridated water involves chewing and swallowing one 2.2 mg sodium fluoride tablet daily (1 mg fluoride). Children under 2 should take one-fourth that amount; children from 2–3 one-half. Caution in prescription is indicated, and only 100 tablets should be dispensed at one time. In areas with limited natural fluoridation of water the dentist must be cognizant of the level of fluoride and carefully adjust the supplemental dosage according to the instructions accompanying the product of choice. Of course, the tablets should be stored in child-proof containers and should always be handled only by parents. If parents demonstrate an inclination to improper dispensing of the tablets (not enough, too many, skipping days, etc.), usage should be discontinued.

Fluoride supplementation is more effective in the prevention of decay than topical application but less effective than fluoridated water. Effects, as with fluoridated water, are more pronounced on smooth surfaces of teeth.

### QUESTIONS

67. Dietary fluoride supplementation has been shown to be an effective, if not efficient, method of decay prevention. What is the relationship of caries reduction levels seen with this method as compared to water fluoridation and topical application?
    1. Greater than water fluoridation and topical application
    2. Less than water fluoridation and topical application
    3. Greater than water fluoridation but less than topical application
    4. Less than water fluoridation but greater than topical application
68. Assume that your community lacks natural or artificial fluoridation of water. Dietary fluoride supplementation in general should be recommended for all

(Continued)

1. patients in your practice
2. persons in the community
3. highly motivated patients
4. children in your practice whose parents are highly motivated

69. Adjustment of dietary supplementation levels of fluoride should be a function of
   1. age and sex
   2. age and number of permanent teeth
   3. race and artificial fluoridation levels of water
   4. age and natural fluoridation levels of water
   5. sex and natural fluoridation levels of water

## REFERENCES

1. American Dental Association Council on Dental Care Programs: Peer Review Procedure Manual. Chicago, 1975
2. BROUSSEAU LS, HOGGARD, FM, Gribble JL: Group Practice in the United States, 1971. US Department of HEW, Publ No. (NIH) 72-189, Bethesda, 1972
3. US Congress: Economic Opportunity Act as Amended. 42, USC, 2809 Section, 272, (a), (4)
4. US Department of HEW: Prepaid Dental Care: A Glossary. Publ No. (NIH) 75–20, Bethesda, 1975

## SUGGESTED READING

ANDERSON OW: National Health Insurance: Implications for the Management of Hospitals. Chicago, American College of Hospital Administrators, 1974

AUSTIN DF, WERNER SB: Epidemiology for the Health Sciences. Springfield, IL, CC Thomas, 1974

BLUM JD, GERTMAN PM, RABINOW J: PSROs and The Law. Germantown, Aspen Systems, 1977

BROWN WE (ed): Oral Health, Dentistry, and the American Public. Norman, University of Oklahoma Press, 1974

BURTON LE, SMITH HH: Public Health and Community Medicine, 2nd ed. Baltimore, Williams & Wilkins, 1975

Chartbook of Federal Health Spending, 1969–74. Washington DC, National Planning Association, 1974

Congress and Health, An Introduction to the Legislative Process and Its Key Participants, 2nd ed. Washington DC, Barney Sellers, April, 1977

DUMMETT CO: Community Dentistry. Springfield, IL, CC Thomas, 1974

DUNNING JM: Principles of Dental Public Health, 2nd ed. Cambridge, Harvard University Press, 1970

EGDAHL RH, GERTMAN PM: Quality Assurance in Health Care. Germantown, Aspen Systems, 1976

ELZEY FF: A Programmed Introduction to Statistics. Belmont, Brooks/Cole, 1971

FRANKEL JM, BOFFA J: Prepaid Dental Care Technical Assistance Manual. Boston, Jerold Enterprises, 1974

FUCHS VR: Who Shall Live? Health, Economics, and Social Choice. New York, Basic Books, 1974

Health of the Disadvantaged Chart Book. US Department of HEW, Publ No. (HRA) 77–628, Hyattsville, 1977

Health Resources Statistics. US Department of HEW, Health Resources Administration, Rockville, National Center for Health Statistics, 1976

HIESTAND DL, OSTOW M: Health Manpower Information for Policy Guidance. Cambridge, Ballinger, 1976

JERGE CR, MARSHALL WE, SCHOEN MH, FRIEDMAN JW: Group Practice and the Future of Dental Care. Philadelphia, Lea & Febiger, 1974

LILIENFELD AA: Foundations of Epidemiology. New York, Oxford University Press, 1976

LINDSAY CM (ed): New Directions in Public Health Care, An Evaluation of Proposals for National Health Insurance. San Francisco, Institute for Contemporary Studies, 1976

MAURIZI AR: Public Policy and the Dental Care Market. Washington DC, American Enterprise Institute for Public Policy Research, 1975

MESKIN LH, LOUPE MJ, MICIK R: Workshop Proceedings on Current and Future Dental Roles in Primary Care. Division of Health Ecology, School of Dentistry, University of Minnesota Minneapolis, 1976

MOSS FE, HALAMANDARIS VJ: Too Old Too Sick Too Bad, Nursing Homes in America. Germantown, Aspen Systems, 1977

MYERS BA: A Guide to Medical Care Administration, Vol 1. Washington DC, American Public Health Association, 1973

National Health Insurance Resource Book, rev ed. Washington DC, US Government Printing Office, 1976

NEWBRUN E: Fluorides and Dental Caries. Springfield, IL, CC Thomas, 1975

Papers on the National Health Guidelines: Baselines for Setting Health Goals and Standards. Bethesda, US Department of HEW, Publ No (HRA) 76–640, 1976

Progress and Problems in Medical and Dental Education, A report of the Carnegie Council on Policy Studies in Higher Education. The Cargnegie Foundation for the Advancement of Teaching, San Francisco Jossey-Bass, 1976

SOMERS AR: Promoting Health, Consumer Education and National Policy. Germantown, Aspen Systems, 1976

SOMERS AR, SOMERS HM: Health and Health Care, Policies in Perspective. Germantown, Aspen Systems, 1977

SPENCE JT, UNDERWOOD BJ, DUNCAN CP: Elementary Statistics. New York, Appleton-Century-Crofts, 1968

ZOLA IK, MCKINLAY JB: Organizational Issues in the Delivery of Health Services. New York, PRODIST, 1974

## ANSWER KEY

| | | | |
|---|---|---|---|
| 1. 2 | 19. 3 | 36. 4 | 53. 1 |
| 2. 1 | 20. 2 | 37. 1 | 54. 4 |
| 3. 3 | 21. 3 | 38. 3 | 55. 2 |
| 4. 1 | 22. 5 | 39. 3 | 56. 1 |
| 5. 1 | 23. 5 | 40. 4 | 57. 2 |
| 6. 1 | 24. 2 | 41. 2 | 58. 3 |
| 7. 1 | 25. 4 | 42. 1 | 59. 4 |
| 8. 4 | 26. 3 | 43. 2 | 60. 3 |
| 9. 1 | 27. 4 | 44. 1 | 61. 3 |
| 10. 3 | 28. 5 | 45. 3 | 62. 3 |
| 11. 1 | 29. 4 | 46. 4 | 63. 3 |
| 12. 3 | 30. 2 | 47. 2 | 64. 4 |
| 13. 3 | 31. 1 | 48. 3 | 65. 2 |
| 14. 2 | 32. 1 | 49. 3 | 66. 1 |
| 15. 1 | 33. 2 | 50. 8 | 67. 4 |
| 16. 4 | 34. 2 | 51. 1 | 68. 4 |
| 17. 5 | 35. 2 | 52. 2 | 69. 4 |
| 18. 2 | | | |

# 5

# FIXED PROSTHODONTICS

## Thomas G. Berry

Fixed prosthodontics has been defined by Shillingburg et al (40) as "the art and science of restoring damaged teeth with cast metal or porcelain restorations and of replacing missing teeth with fixed or cemented prostheses." There are many stages involved in treatment with fixed prosthodontics.

## DIAGNOSIS AND TREATMENT PLANNING

Careful diagnosis and treatment planning are mandatory first steps in the treatment of any patient. To assure they are done in an intelligent and thorough manner information from many sources is required.

### Diagnostic Data

Mounted diagnostic casts provide information about tooth alignment, edentulous areas, and supraerupted and partially erupted teeth. The plane of occlusion can be determined from these casts, and the occlusal relationship of the two arches in centric and eccentric positions can be evaluated. These relationships can affect the whole sequence and scope of the treatment, because malocclusion may require occlusal equilibration and/or orthodontic movement of teeth, i.e., uprighting tipped molars. Additional teeth may be treated in an attempt to correct malalignment and malocclusion.

Radiographs reveal more than the presence of carious lesions. They disclose whether there is, or is likely to be, pulpal involvement from carious lesions or previous preparations. They reveal the bony architecture and the presence of infrabony pockets, as well as the number, size, and conformation of the roots of the teeth. Pathologic conditions such as tumors, periapical lesions, etc., otherwise undetectable, can be diagnosed through radiographs.

Knowledge of the patient's medical history helps the dentist to avoid complication from systemic or emotional conditions (allergies to drugs and materials, cardiovascular problems, mental illness). It may disclose

health considerations that directly affect the treatment plan.

Information about the patient's clinical condition should be carefully recorded in a chart to allow immediate access to the formation without the patient's presence. The chart should list the following:

1. carious lesions
2. missing teeth
3. periodontal pockets and their depth
4. existing restorations and their condition
5. mobility of the teeth
6. alignment and relationship of the teeth
7. oral hygiene

All of the information is designed to give an overview of the patient's general health, oral health, and attitude towards dental care. Without this overview the dentist is making "one tooth at a time" diagnostic and treatment planning decisions.

### Periodontal Considerations

The periodontal health of the patient must be evaluated prior to any treatment. Inflammation of soft tissue must be eliminated by removal of plaque and any factors that contribute to its formation (14). Some of the etiologic factors are

1. calculus
2. overhanging and/or rough restoration surfaces and margins
3. restorations with overclosed proximal embrasures
4. poorly designed pontics which prevent adequate access for cleaning

Bone loss, whether vertical or horizontal, must be halted, the causes eliminated, and the bony contours corrected before any fixed prostheses are done. If no attached gingiva surrounds the teeth involved, a gingival graft procedure is indicated. Otherwise, the gradual stripping away of the tissue and deepening of the pocket will continue. The level of bony support possessed by teeth chosen to serve as part of a fixed partial is important.

## Orthodontic Considerations

Stress is better borne when it is directed in the long axis of the tooth (12). There is little research to show how much tipping can be present before severe problems occur, however. The contours produced when a tipped tooth is crowned usually make it difficult for the patient to maintain good oral hygiene.

The degree of tipping can be determined from diagnostic casts, clinical observation, and radiographs. If the crown of an involved tooth has been altered by large restorations, the angulation of the tooth may be difficult to assess. Radiographs reveal the root inclinations and allow comparison to roots of other teeth.

The occlusal forces on rotated teeth may be transmitted primarily in the long axis of the teeth, but there are some special problems. Even if the teeth can be aligned during preparation, reduction of the axial surfaces of the tooth during preparation must be disproportional (3). Returning the tooth to a more desirable position via orthodontic treatment allows easier preparation and better control of contours, proximal contact, and occlusal relations (Fig. 5–1). Realignment also allows better proximal relationships and promotes better oral hygiene.

## Endodontic Considerations

Careful radiographic examination is necessary to reveal radiolucencies that might indicate nonvital teeth. The radiographs alone, however, do not indicate

problems developing with the health of the pulp. Teeth with large, deep restorations, discoloration, or a history of trauma should be tested for vitality. Lack of demonstrated vitality would indicate the need for endodontic therapy (24).

Endodontically treated teeth can serve well as abutments, but they do present two potential problems. The original damage to the tooth from caries and/or traumatic incident may have destroyed a significant amount of the clinical crown, and the access preparation for the endodontic therapy removes even more of the clinical crown. Added to this problem is the increased brittleness of the endodontically treated tooth. The result is a tooth that may not provide adequate strength to resist the stress that is placed upon it by occlusal forces (25). To create a more dependable foundation for a restoration, two procedures are available (21).

**POST AND CORE BUILD-UP.** The post and core is a cast metal post that extends into the prepared root canal of the tooth with a coronal portion that serves as an abutment for the retainer. Not only does it replace missing or fragile coronal tooth structure so a preparation can be made, it also extends into the root to prevent dislodgement and to decrease the possibility of fracture to the tooth or to the root. The size and depth of the post hole is determined by the root size and length. The post hole should extend approximately one-half to two-thirds the length of the root if possible (Fig. 5–2).

Commercially available in several sizes, they are sized in relation to the bur or reamer used to enlarge and shape the root canal. The use of the prefabricated

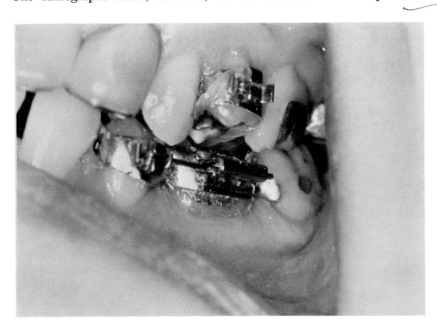

**FIG. 5–1.** Relatively simple orthodontic movement of malaligned teeth can produce a much more desirable relationship. Here a maxillary premolar in extreme buccoversion is being moved into a functional position.

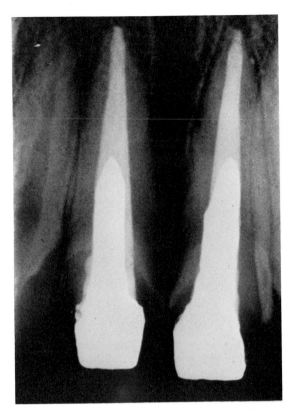

**FIG. 5-2.** A radiograph of two cemented post and core castings reveals the posts extending approximately one-half to two-thirds the length of the canals.

metal post and core is fast and relatively economical, but it is not indicated in situations involving teeth with narrow roots or roots with unusual configurations.

The post and core can also be custom-made by using wax or autocuring acrylic placed into the lubricated root canal to create the post portion. Additional wax or acrylic is used to form the coronal portion. The whole pattern is removed, invested, and cast. This method is adaptable to the many different shapes and sizes of root canals. Both types are cemented into place (Fig. 5–3).

**PIN-RETAINED BUILD-UP.** The pin-retained restoration is the second method of restoring an endodontically treated tooth. Pins may be placed into the remaining dentin to support a composite resin or amalgam core placed over them. After set, the material is shaped to serve as a preparation.

This approach offers no protection against fracture of the tooth as does the post and core. It may be difficult to find an adequate thickness of dentin into which to place the pins if the pulp chamber has been greatly enlarged to gain access for the endodontic therapy. A pin-retained restoration is primarily indicated in teeth

with small curving roots that would be difficult to prepare for a post and core.

QUESTIONS

1. A removable partial denture is indicated over a fixed one when
   1. the patient does not seem sufficiently motivated or capable of cleaning the fixed partial denture adequately
   2. supraerupted or submerged teeth have created an uneven plane of occlusion
   3. the proposed abutment teeth are malaligned
   4. there are missing teeth on both sides of the arch

2. What is (are) the benefit(s) to be derived from orthodontic uprighting of a molar prior to preparation?
   a. ease in aligning with other abutments
   b. occlusal forces directed in the long axis of the tooth
   c. improved prognosis for the health of the periodontium
   d. improved path of insertion and withdrawal
   1. a and c
   2. a, b, and c
   3. b and d
   4. b, c, and d
   5. All of the above

## ABUTMENT SELECTION

An abutment may be defined as the tooth over which the retainer or crown is placed. An abutment can support either a fixed or removable partial denture. Among the factors affecting the choice of teeth to serve as abutments are (34)

1. location of the tooth
2. alignment of the tooth
3. crown length
4. crown:root ratio, including the quality or condition of the bone
5. furcation involvement
6. the amount of the pericemental area
7. mobility
8. the aesthetic demands

### Crown : Root Ratio

The crown:root ratio refers to the occlusogingival length of the clinical crown contrasted to the length of root structure encased in bone. A ratio of 2:3 (crown:root ratio) is considered ideal. A ratio as low as 1:1 can be tolerated unless the span of the fixed partial denture is long or the occlusal stresses are severe (29).

### Ante's Law

Ante's law is not really a law but rather a rule of thumb which concerns the periodontal surface area. It

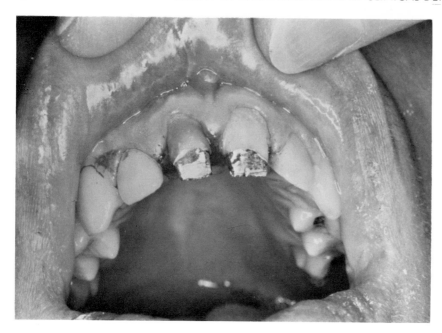

**FIG. 5–3.** Custom-made post and core castings are cemented into the prepared root canals of the tooth.

states that the pericemental area of the roots of the abutment teeth must equal or surpass the estimated original pericemental area of the roots of the tooth being replaced (20). The law is used to assure that the supporting structures are not overburdened by the increased load they have to accept when missing teeth are replaced.

## RETAINER SELECTION

The retainer is a crown, onlay, or inlay which fits into or over the tooth which is to be the abutment. It may be connected to other members of a fixed partial denture. There are several different types of retainers:

1. The inlay, designed to fit entirely within the tooth, does not cover or replace cusps. It is indicated only as a single tooth restoration in situations where the cusps are reasonably strong.
2. Like the inlay, the onlay gains retention by fitting within the tooth but it also overlays or covers one or more of the cusps. While primarily a single tooth restoration used in situations requiring protection of weakened cusps or realignment of the occlusal plane, the onlay can be used as a retainer for a fixed partial denture.
3. The three-quarter crown is an extracoronal retainer which completely covers all but one surface of the clinical crown, usually the facial surface. The three-quarter crown may serve as a single tooth retainer or as part of a fixed partial denture.
4. The full crown fits extracoronally, covering the en-

tire coronal portion of the tooth. It is indicated as a single restoration to protect and preserve severely involved teeth, to correct occlusal problems, and as a retainer for a fixed partial denture.
5. The jacket crown is a full crown made entirely of porcelain. It is a single tooth restoration which is indicated in situations where the aesthetic result is the prime concern.
6. The porcelain-fused-to-metal crown employs a porcelain veneer over a cast metal core, providing an aesthetic result. The porcelain-fused-to-metal crown can be used as a single crown or as part of a fixed partial denture.
7. There are several variations which are infrequently used—the pin ledge crown which relies almost entirely on pins for retention, the seven-eighth crown, and the acrylic-veneered crown.

The choice of retainer type is based upon the location of the tooth or teeth, aesthetic demands, crown length, amount of remaining tooth structure, whether single crown or part of fixed partial denture, and the length (span) of the fixed partial denture attached to the retainer.

QUESTIONS

3. Selection of an abutment tooth should be based upon
   a. the crown:root ratio
   b. whether the tooth has been endodontically treated
   c. the number and shape of the roots of the tooth
   d. the alignment of the tooth
1. a
2. a, b, and c
3. b, c, and d

4. a, c, and d
5. d

4. What factors generally determine the selection of the retainer type?
   a. Pulpal or axial extension of the decay
   b. Location of the carious lesion(s)
   c. Periodontal support of the abutment tooth
   d. Aesthetic demands
   1. a and b
   2. a, b, and c
   3. d
   4. b and d
   5. All of the above

5. All other factors being equal, the most retention is provided by the
   1. full crown preparation
   2. three-quarter crown preparation
   3. onlay
   4. inlay

6. The onlay gains most of its retention from
   1. the intracoronal portion
   2. the extracoronal portion
   3. proximal contact
   4. the cementing agent

7. Ante's law concerns the
   1. degree of tipping allowable in an abutment tooth
   2. amount of curvature acceptable in the plan of occlusion
   3. amount of increase in retentive factors with a full crown versus a three-quarter crown
   4. crown : root ratio
   5. None of the above

## PREPARATION OF THE ABUTMENT

There are three basic objectives of any preparation procedure. They are to 1) provide retentive features to support and hold the restoration in place, 2) remove any undercuts so the restoration can be seated onto or into the prepared tooth without distortion or significant stress, and 3) remove enough tooth structure to compensate for the required thickness of the restorative material. These three objectives must be met by all types of preparations.

Draw is a term meaning the preparation possesses no undercuts. Undercuts are areas that do not permit insertion and withdrawal of a wax pattern or casting without distortion or fracture. Undercuts may occur within a wall, between two or more walls, or between the abutment tooth and an unprepared adjacent tooth. Loss of a part of an old restoration or cement base or incorrect angulation of the bur or diamond stone can produce an undercut within a wall. When the undercut occurs between two or more walls, it is most often between opposing walls of different teeth involved in the

prosthesis. An undercut between the abutment tooth and an unprepared adjacent tooth occurs most frequently when a tooth is tipped or rotated so that the path of the wax pattern insertion and withdrawal is hindered by a surface of an adjacent tooth. No matter what the cause, all undercuts must be eliminated. If not, there can be no seating of an adequately fitting restoration.

The retention comes from frictional resistance to displacement created by the walls of the preparation. The amount of retention is a product of the degree of convergence (or divergence) of the opposing walls (the more nearly parallel the walls, the greater the retention) and of the length of those walls (33, 46). The retention can also be increased by grooves, pins, boxes, and other special means.

### Finish Lines

The finish lines on a three-quarter crown preparation may be any one of four types or a combination. They are 1) the knife edge finish line, 2) the chamfer finish line, 3) the shoulder finish line, and 4) the beveled shoulder finish line.

For a knife edge finish line the reduction of the tooth is decreased until it is very slight at the finish line in much the same way as a knife tapers to its edge. The finish line must be distinct. This type of finish line destroys the least amount of tooth structure but may be difficult to detect on the tooth in an impression, or later on the die. It provides the easiest fit and allows easy burnishing of the gold at the margins. It is indicated in situations where the anatomy of the tooth is constricted immediately cervical to the cervical line.

The chamfer finish line is somewhat like the knife edge margin except that the cut is made deeper into the tooth. This gives two advantages. It establishes a more readable finish line and provides more room for a bulk of gold. The chamfer finish line is indicated for the areas to be covered by a gold margin. It is slightly more difficult to establish the fit and to burnish the gold, however.

The axial reduction for a shoulder finish line is essentially even from the occlusal to the gingival finish line. The axial wall meets the finish line at a right angle to provide a shoulder or butt joint finish line. It is a very definite one which allows plenty of room for a thick, strong gold margin or for the bulk of a porcelain jacket crown (Fig. 5-4) or a porcelain-fused-to-metal crown. It has two important disadvantages. It is destructive of tooth structure to a greater extent than the other types and also demands a much more precise fit. If the restoration does not seat completely, the interface between the margin and the shoulder is open. Both the knife edge finish line and the chamfer finish line possess a "sliding fit" which allows the restoration to have rela-

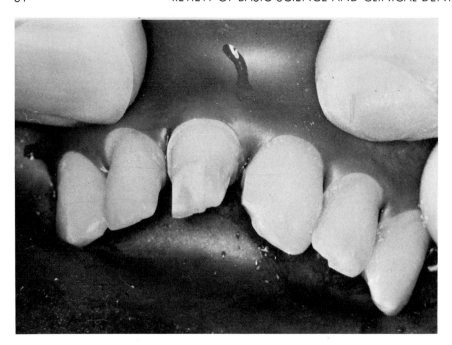

**FIG. 5-4.** Porcelain jacket preparation demonstrating a full shoulder finish line.

tively tight contact with the preparation wall before the restoration is even seated completely, but the shoulder finish line requires that the crown be completely seated before the crown walls contact the preparation tightly. The shoulder finish line is indicated only where bulk is required for strength or aesthetic results.

The beveled shoulder finish line is simply a modification of the shoulder finish line. After the shoulder is cut, a bevel is put on the shoulder to produce a fit like a knife edge finish line. This bevel is at approximately a 45° angle and should be about 0.5 mm long. This finish line is indicated whenever a shoulder has been prepared for any reason, as long as a metal margin will not adversely affect the final aesthetic results.

### Specific Preparations

The specific steps in preparation differ, however, according to several factors such as the amount of tooth structure to be replaced, restorative materials being used, and aesthetic considerations.

**INLAY PREPARATION.** The inlay restoration may replace one or both proximal surfaces as well as a portion of the occlusal surface. Occasionally the inlay may be used to replace an incisal edge or part of a facial surface.

The preparation is cut approximately 2 mm deep pulpally on its occlusal portion. The axial depth on each proximal surface is approximately 1 mm at the gingival margin. The buccal and lingual walls of the preparation diverge towards the occlusal at an angulation of 2°–5° (16), and the axial walls converge towards the occlusal at the same angulation. This convergence of the axial walls, combined with the divergence of all the other walls of the preparation, provides draw.

The proximal extensions to the buccal and lingual are carried slightly past the contact area. This extension allows proper smoothing of the finished lines of the preparation and adequate access for finishing the margins of the inlay.

The finish line of the preparation is beveled so that it can be covered with a thin layer of gold. Because gold is malleable and ductile, the thin layer can be burnished against the tooth structure to provide a better marginal seal (44). The bevel should be approximately 0.5–0.75 mm long and at an angle of 35°–45°. All of the finish lines of the preparation should end in a bevel (Fig. 5–5).

Because the inlay is a restoration which fits intracoronally, it does not protect the remaining tooth structure. It is indicated chiefly when satisfactory proximal contact is difficult to establish with amalgam or when other gold restorations should be opposed to prevent the potential galvanic shock if amalgam were used.

**ONLAY PREPARATION.** The onlay preparation fits both intracoronally and extracoronally. The intracoronal portion is prepared exactly as is the inlay. The extracoronal portion extends over lingual and/or buccal cusps to protect them against breakage because of occlusal stresses (Fig. 5–6). The amount of extension is determined by the degree of thinness and weakness in

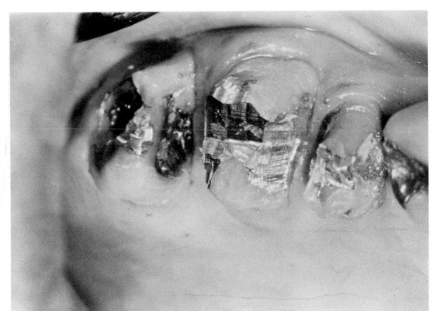

**FIG. 5-5.** The bevel is placed on all of the finish lines of the inlay preparation. A similar bevel is placed on the finish lines of the onlay preparation.

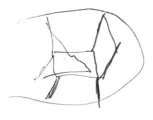

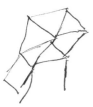

**FIG. 5-6.** Intracoronal and extracoronal features of the onlay preparation. Note how the preparation is designed to allow the casting to protect the cusps.

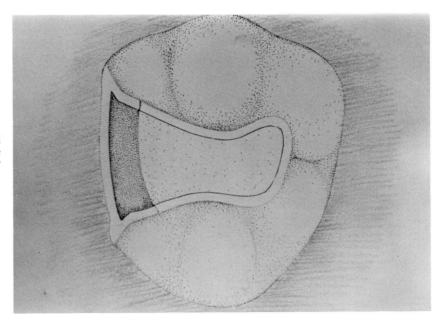

the cusps caused by caries or previous preparations. Nonworking cusps (maxillary buccal and mandibular lingual cusps) require less coverage than the working cusps simply because the stresses are less. Extensions over the buccal cusp may be modified somewhat to meet aesthetic demands (13a, 39).

The finish line on the onlay must be placed 0.5–1 mm beyond any area of occlusal contact to avoid distortion of the gold margin and subsequent leakage. The occlusal reduction over the cusp tip should equal 1.5–2 mm

on the working cusp (38). The nonworking cusp should be reduced approximately 1.5 mm near the central groove or fossae. The reduction may be gradually tapered towards the tip of the cusp to no more than 0.5 mm with a slight reverse bevel onto the buccal surface if there are aesthetic considerations. If not (as with the lingual cusps of mandibular molars), the nonworking cusps may be prepared just as the working cusps were prepared.

In summary, the onlay is a restoration which covers

one or both proximal surfaces, the entire occlusal surface, and the cusp tips for their protection. It is indicated in situations where cusps are poorly supported, where occlusal relationships need altering, or where proximal contact is difficult to establish.

**THREE-QUARTER CROWN.** As the name implies, the three-quarter crown covers three-quarters of the clinical crown of the tooth. It is primarily an extracoronal restoration, although parallel grooves cut into the proximal surfaces of the preparation help to retain it.

One axial wall, usually the facial surface, is left uncovered (Fig. 5–7). The appearance of the tooth therefore remains relatively unchanged. In some situations where appearance is not important (as with mandibular molars) and caries or existing restorations require the facial surface to be restored, the lingual surface is left uncovered.

The three-quarter crown is retained chiefly by two means: parallel or nearly parallel walls and retention grooves placed into the mesial and distal walls. The involved axial walls are converged towards the occlusal surface at a 2°–5° taper. The degree of taper varies, depending upon the length of the clinical crown. Short teeth demand less taper whereas teeth with very long clinical crowns allow more taper to assure draw is established (22).

The finish line is established about 1.5 mm supragingivally. This relationship of the finish line to the gingival tissue is less traumatic to the soft tissues (35, 43), allows easier cleaning by the patient, and is easier to capture in an impression. The presence of caries, an existing restoration, or decalcified enamel may require extension to the gingival crest or even beneath the gingiva, however. If the clinical crown is quite short,

extension into subgingival areas provides extra length of the wall for additional retention.

The occlusal reduction is much the same as that in the onlay preparation. It must allow a thickness of 1.5–2 mm of gold to prevent deformation of the casting. The reduction of the occlusal surface should be proportional to give an even reduction which provides adequate thickness of gold without overreducing any given area, increases the resistance of the casting to displacement lingually, and adds resistance to deformation. The latter benefit is due to the corrugated effect created.

Retention grooves are usually placed in the proximal surface. These grooves add to the retention against occlusal displacement. More importantly, they prevent displacement in a lingual direction. The grooves are placed in the buccal one-half of the proximal surface because the longer wall in this area allows for a longer groove. In addition, the resistance to a lingual or tipping force may be more effective if the grooves are in the buccal rather than the lingual one-half (39).

The axial walls of the grooves must be parallel or converging towards each other at an angle of 2°–5° (8). The buccal and lingual walls of each groove must diverge towards the occlusal surface. The grooves should be in the long axis of the tooth and extend gingivally to within 0.5–1 mm of the gingival finish line of the preparation. This assures that there will be a gold margin cervical to the gingival floor of the groove that can be burnished against the tooth. These grooves, which can be made with a tapered bur or stone, should be 0.5–1 mm deep into the axial wall at the gingival wall.

The location of the grooves varies somewhat according to the tooth. Anterior teeth require that the grooves be placed in the middle of the tooth buccolin-

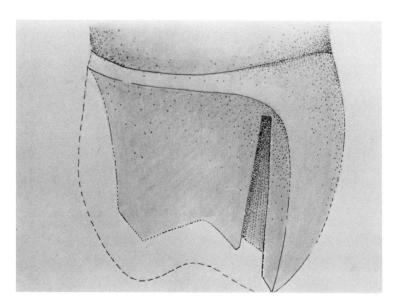

**FIG. 5–7.** The facial surface is usually the one left uncut on a three-quarter crown preparation.

gually in the incisal two-thirds of the teeth. As stated, in posterior teeth the grooves can be placed in the buccal one-half of the tooth just lingual to the buccal finish lines for optimum results.

**FULL CROWN.** The full crown preparation involves all of the surfaces of the tooth. The reduction of each surface is the same as that for the three-quarter crown. The facial reduction is essentially the same as the lingual reduction if a knife edge or chamfer finish line is to be used.

If the restoration is to be a porcelain jacket crown or a porcelain-fused-to-metal crown, a shoulder must be cut into the facial surface to a depth of 1.0 to 1.25 mm for a porcelain jacket crown or 1.5–1.75 mm for a porcelain-fused-to-metal crown. This reduction extends halfway into the proximal embrasure. Less reduction makes the thickness of the porcelain inadequate, resulting in a loss of some aesthetic quality or an overcontoured restoration. If the occlusal surface is to be covered with porcelain, a reduction of 2 mm is required to provide adequate space for the thickness of the metal plus porcelain. The full crown is indicated whenever there has been extensive damage to the tooth or when it is needed as a retainer for a fixed partial denture. The preparation is destructive of tooth structure, however, and should be used only when indicated.

### QUESTIONS

8. The walls of a full crown preparation should have
   1. a 2°–5° convergence towards the occlusal
   2. an 8°–10° convergence towards the occlusal
   3. a 5°–8° divergence towards the occlusal
   4. walls parallel to each other

9. Occlusal reduction for the three-quarter crown preparation should equal approximately
   1. the depth of all existing restorations
   2. 1.5–2 mm
   3. 0.75–1 mm
   4. 3–4 mm

10. The bevel is placed on the finish line of the inlay, onlay, and three-quarter crown primarily to
    1. provide ease of adaptation of the gold margin
    2. remove unsupported enamel rods
    3. provide increased strength to the gold margin
    4. produce a better defined finish line
    5. 2 and 4

11. Overcontoured crowns are most often the result of
    1. the need for added retention
    2. overbuilding by technicians
    3. insufficient tooth reduction
    4. periodontal considerations

12. How much labial tooth reduction is needed for a porcelain-fused-to-metal crown?
    1. 0.25–0.5 mm

   2. 0.5–1 mm
   3. 1–1.5 mm
   4. 1.5–1.75 mm
   5. 1.75–2 mm

13. The porcelain-metal crown requires what type of labial finish line on the preparation of anterior teeth?
    1. Knife edge
    2. Chamfer
    3. Shoulder
    4. Shoulder with a bevel
    5. The finish line type is not critical if the reduction is sufficient.

## TISSUE MANAGEMENT

The next step after preparation of the teeth is management of the soft tissue to facilitate impression making. If finish lines have been located supragingivally, tissue management is no problem. If, however, the finish lines are subgingival, the tissue must be temporarily displaced so that impression material can be injected into the area slightly apical to the finish lines of the preparation. There are two basic methods of displacing the soft tissue for impression making. They are chemomechanical and electrosurgical. If controlled, both can be done satisfactorily without undue damage to the soft tissue.

The chemomechanical means involves a cord impregnated with a chemical such as epinephrine or aluminum chloride. The cord is packed into the sulcus to displace the soft tissues physically from the areas of the finish lines. The chemical temporarily shrinks the tissue to a slight degree and also decreases bleeding. Epinephrine produces hemostasis, but it also can produce systemic reactions. It may be contraindicated therefore in patients with cardiovascular problems (7, 11).

A blunt, bladed instrument is used to pack the cord around the tooth into the gingival crevice (Fig. 5–8). While some pressure is necessary, it must be a controlled force to avoid tearing the gingival attachment. The size of cord chosen depends upon the location of the finish line and the size of the gingival sulcus. The area must be kept relatively dry to avoid diluting the chemical effect of the cord. Once in place, the cord is left for approximately 6 min. During this time, the area may be moist but not wet. After the proper time interval, the cord is removed and the area cleaned and checked for debris, blood, etc. The area must be dried completely prior to the impression making because moisture, blood, or debris interferes with the accuracy of the impression.

The electrosurgical method is suggested in certain circumstances by some authors (4, 27). A surgical tip is used with the instrument adjusted to a surgical current. The tip is carefully passed around the inside of the sulcus to remove the lining of the sulcus and thus in-

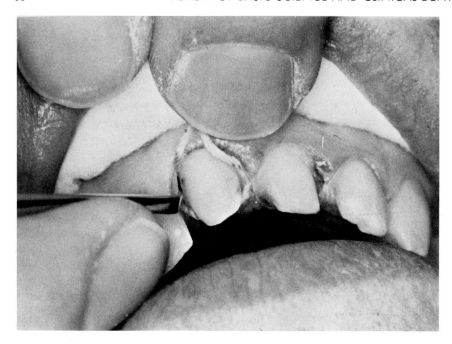

**FIG. 5-8.** An instrument with a blunt blade is used to place a chemically impregnated cord into the gingival sulcus to provide adequate tissue retraction prior to impression making.

crease the space between the tissue and the tooth. Handled carefully in select cases, the electrosurgical means provides good access for the impression material. Although this method does destroy some soft tissue, very thick and healthy gingival tissue returns to nearly its original height when it heals. Very thin soft tissue may not allow electrosurgical "retraction" without significant loss of tissue height, however.

QUESTIONS

14. Chemomechanical tissue retraction provides access primarily by
   1. displacing the gingival tissue laterally away from the tooth
   2. displacing the gingival tissue apically
   3. tearing the gingival attachment slightly
   4. removing the tissue on the inside of the sulcus
   5. chemically shrinking the gingival tissues

15. What is the chief contraindication for using epinephrine impregnated retraction cord?
   1. It is chemically irritating to the tissue, causing sloughing.
   2. It produces systemic reactions affecting the cardiovascular system.
   3. It produces inadequate retraction of the tissues.
   4. Its size makes it difficult to use where the gingival sulcus is shallow and the tissues firm.

## IMPRESSION MAKING

To be successful, an impression must reproduce

1. all finish line areas plus unprepared tooth structure slightly beyond them

2. the walls and occlusal surfaces without voids or bubbles, since even a very small void in a retentive groove can ruin the impression
3. the soft tissue area of the edentulous ridge
4. the occlusal and the axial surfaces of the other teeth to allow correct relationship of the casts

There are several types of impression materials available. Three types are accurate enough to be used to make impressions for fixed prosthodontics, and there is no clinically significant difference in their accuracy (6, 36). No matter what the material, it must

1. reproduce fine detail with absolute accuracy
2. be well tolerated by the tooth and soft tissues
3. be easy to handle
4. set, cure, or harden in the mouth in a reasonable time period
5. withdraw from undercuts without distortion
6. be dimensionally stable after removal from the mouth to allow adequate time for pouring the casts
7. have a shelf life long enough for the working characteristics to be dependable

### Types of Impression Materials

The three most commonly used types of impression materials are 1) polysulfide rubbers, 2) silicone rubbers, and 3) hydrocolloids. A polysulfide rubber consists of a base material of polysulfide polymer and an inert filler, lead peroxide plus sulfur and oil. These two materials are mixed to initiate the chemical reaction. Once initiated, the reaction continues until set is achieved. The material is used in an injection syringe in a less viscous form and in a medium or heavy-bodied form for use with an impression tray. The base material of a silicone rubber is a silicone polymer. Mixed with a reactor material of ethyl silicate and tin octoate, it follows a setting reaction similar to the polysulfide material. The material comes in a less viscous form for injection into the sulcus, and a heavier bodied form is used with the tray. The hydrocolloid is a distinctly different type of material. The reversible hydrocolloid, which has a base of agar, becomes a liquid when it is heated. Cooling the material reverses the process to return the material to a firm yet elastic state. No mixing is needed as the process is a physical rather than chemical change. Like the others, the material is supplied in a light consistency for injection and a heavier bodied form for use with the tray.

Other impression materials are used but not as frequently as the ones mentioned.

### Mixing the Material

The mixing of polysulfide rubber base and silicone rubber base materials is similar in many respects. Each requires the combination of a base material with a reactor material. The reactor may be in paste form, as it is for the polysulfide and some of the silicone rubber base materials, or it may be in liquid form, as it is for other silicone materials. The materials must be mixed in the correct proportions to assure that the working and setting times are sufficient and accuracy is not compromised. Once the reactor (or accelerator) material touches the base material, the chemical reaction starts.

Thorough mixing is a necessity, because inadequate mixing may alter the setting time or leave areas that never completely set. The base and reactor pastes are different colors; therefore a homogeneous mixture is one which exhibits no streaks. The mixing should be done on a firm mixing pad with a slightly flexible metal spatula.

There is no mixing needed with hydrocolloid. Instead the material is placed in a water bath which is brought to a boil. The tray material and injection material are left there a minimum of 10 min while the water is boiling to assure complete liquefaction before moving them to a conditioning bath at a temperature of 145°F–150°F. The hydrocolloid will remain fluid indefinitely at this temperature. The tray material is placed into a 115°F–118°F tempering bath for approximately 5 min prior to the actual impression making to cool it further. Cooling adds the necessary body to prevent it from running from the tray and also prevents it from burning the soft tissues of the patient's mouth. The injection material is used at 145°F to aid in its flow and because it is placed in such thin layers that it cools quickly.

### Impression Procedure

**INJECTION OF THE IMPRESSION MATERIAL.** The most critical part of the impression procedure is the placement of the material around the prepared tooth and into the gingival sulcus to capture all the details of the preparation and, most especially, the finish lines. To facilitate this, light-bodied material is placed into a syringe so the material may be injected into the sulcus and around the tooth (Fig. 5-9). This decreases the trapping of air and assures the impression material gets

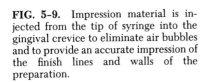

**FIG. 5-9.** Impression material is injected from the tip of syringe into the gingival crevice to eliminate air bubbles and to provide an accurate impression of the finish lines and walls of the preparation.

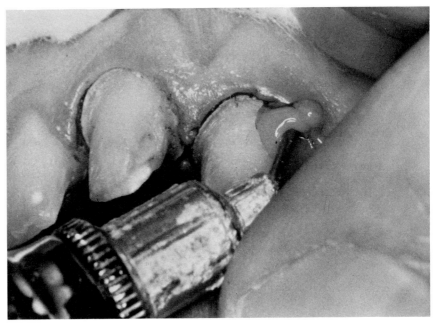

to all areas of preparation. The time allowed for injection depends upon the working time of the material. While the three materials differ in chemical make-up and the mechanism by which they set or solidify, the injection technique is basically the same.

**THE IMPRESSION TRAY.** The initial placement of the material is by injection, but the bulk of the material is used in a tray. Since the thickness of the material in a hydrocolloid impression is not critical, a stock metal tray can be used for hydrocolloid impressions. The tray has a rim which runs along its perimeter to hold the material in the tray. Cool water circulates through this rim to chill the material and solidify it.

Polysulfide and silicone rubber require a tray which fits more exactly because the thickness of the material in the impression does affect the accuracy. The optimum thickness of the material seems to be approximately 3 mm. To provide this thickness, a stock tray must be modified or a custom tray fabricated. The custom tray can be made from self-curing resin, leaving a space of 3 mm between the tray and the soft and hard tissues to be covered. To prevent the tray from being seated too far, three widely separated areas are left in contact with the teeth to serve as "stops."

The impression tray must be seated carefully until the stops in the tray signal complete seating. The careful seating is done by inserting the tray and seating it in the posterior region first and then slowly seating it in the anterior area. This procedure allows the air to escape ahead of the impression material as it flows forward.

**SET AND REMOVAL.** The tray is held firmly in place until the material is completely set or solidified. If the tray shifts prior to set or gelation, a distortion may occur. The setting time for the rubber base materials is approximately 8–10 min (136), but it can be varied by altering the proportions of reactor to base material and by the presence of moisture. Also affecting the setting is the shelf life of the materials.

Because of the variables mentioned, time alone should not be used as a determinant of whether either type of rubber base material has set. Set can be determined in other ways. The unused material on the mixing pad can be checked to see if it has set. Since it does not experience the same temperature and humidity that the material in the mouth does, it sets at a slightly slower rate. Another check is to press the accessible impression material in the mouth with a blunt instrument to see if it rebounds. If it has set, it will return, or rebound, to its original form as soon as the pressure is released.

The time required for gelation of the hydrocolloid material varies according to the water temperature as it circulates through the metal tray. When the water is

cool, 5–6 min is usually sufficient for the material to set. The material which has escaped beyond the rim of the tray can be tested with a blunt instrument for firmness.

No matter which type of material is used, the removal of the tray is important. The tray is freed all around its borders and then removed in one quick, controlled motion, if possible, because slow removal tends to place internal strains in the material which lead to distortion.

QUESTIONS

16. Why is a custom impression tray used for polysulfide rubber base materials?
   1. The material is too fluid to be retained in a stock tray.
   2. The material needs the additional support afforded by a custom tray.
   3. A custom fit tray controls the thickness of the impression tray.
   4. A custom fit tray is much easier to manipulate in the mouth.
   5. Both 3 and 4

17. The hydrocolloid tray material is placed into a 115°F–118°F tempering bath after boiling to
   1. make it less fluid so that it is easier to load and use
   2. allow the necessary chemical reaction to occur
   3. cool the material so that it will not burn the patient
   4. 1 and 2
   5. 1 and 3

18. To improve the accuracy of the rubber base impression
   a. impression material is injected into the sulcus area
   b. the area is kept free of moisture and debris
   c. a custom tray is used
   d. the loaded tray is seated first from the posterior and then seated forward
   e. the tray is removed slowly after the impression is completed
   1. a, b, d, and e
   2. b, c, d, and e
   3. a, c, and d
   4. a, b, c, and d
   5. All of the above

19. The chief disadvantage of hydrocolloid compared to the two rubber base impression materials is that it
   1. requires a stock tray
   2. is not as accurate
   3. requires a dry field free of blood, saliva, etc.
   4. is dimensionally unstable so it must be poured soon
   5. takes longer to "set" (solidify)

## TEMPORARY COVERAGE

After the impression has been made and before the patient is dismissed, it is important that the prepared tooth be provided protection and that the patient's comfort be assured while the final restoration is being fabricated. This is accomplished by means of a temporary restoration which has enough durability to serve during the interim period without fracturing or coming loose. The temporary must

1. protect the pulpal tissues from ingress of fluids and against thermal shock
2. restore the tooth to occlusal function so supraeruption does not occur and so the patient can chew
3. restore proximal contacts to protect the periodontal tissues and prevent drifting of the tooth
4. protect the preparation from possible injury
5. return the tooth to normal appearance if aesthetic concerns are important

Four types of material are commonly used for temporary restorations: 1) zinc oxide–eugenol cement, 2) soft metal crowns, 3) polycarbonate preformed crowns, and 4) autocuring acrylic resin. Zinc oxide-eugenol cement may be used for inlay preparations when the time interval will be brief. It is easy to use and soothing to the pulp, but it fractures easily and therefore is contraindicated for large preparations. Soft metal crowns (usually aluminum) can be used over three-quarter and full crown posterior preparations. Although the metal crowns come in various sizes, they are often difficult to adapt to the existing occlusion and proximal contacts. Some improvement in retention and marginal adaptation can be made by lining them with autocure acrylic and then adjusting them. Polycarbonate preformed crowns can be used for anterior preparations; they provide good aesthetic results. If the crown is modified with autocuring acrylic, good retention and

marginal adaptation, as well as proximal relationships, can be established. The external portion can be reduced to prevent overcontouring, especially in the marginal areas.

The most versatile material used is autocuring acrylic resin. It can be tailored to relationships required by the tooth, shaded to match the other teeth, and can be used for any type of preparation in any area of the mouth (Fig. 5–10). A matrix to confine and shape the acrylic is helpful. Such a matrix can be made by softening a sheet of celluloid with heat and then using a vacuum to conform it to a cast of the teeth before preparation. An impression of the unprepared teeth can also be used as a matrix. The celluloid matrix or impression is filled with acrylic in the doughy stage and then set over the teeth or preferably a cast of the prepared teeth. The matrix is removed when the acrylic reaches the rubbery stages so that the acrylic hardens off the teeth. After hardening, the acrylic is adjusted until the fit, contours, and relationships are satisfactory.

The acrylic should never be allowed to set on the tooth. There are several reasons why. The acrylic monomer is irritating to the pulp; therefore the length of time the acrylic is in contact with the cut tooth surface should be minimized. The setting reaction is exothermic, and the heat generated could be injurious to the pulp. The temporary restoration is likely to lock in place on the tooth when set, making it very difficult to remove for final contouring without damaging it or the prepared tooth. (Even if it possesses sufficient retention, the acrylic temporary does not have adequate marginal seal without cement.)

The metal, polycarbonate, and acrylic temporary

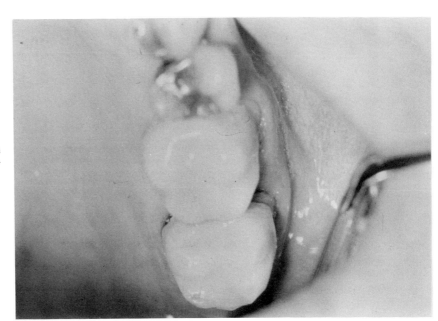

**FIG. 5-10.** Two temporary acrylic resin crowns which provide protection, function, comfort, and aesthetic results.

restorations need to be cemented in place, and the cement serves to seal the margins. The type of cement varies with the situation and the length of time the temporary coverage is to be in place. Usually a zinc oxide–eugenol cement or a similar type provides sufficient retention but can be removed cleanly and easily.

### QUESTIONS

20. A temporary crown should fulfill the same general requirements as the final restoration except for
    1. aesthetics
    2. occlusal contact
    3. durability
    4. marginal adaptation
    5. 1 and 2

21. Even if the retentive quality of the acrylic temporary crown is excellent, the crown should be cemented onto the tooth. In such a case, the cement would serve primarily to
    1. retain the restoration
    2. provide thermal insulation
    3. soothe the pulp
    4. prevent marginal leakage

## CREATION OF THE CAST AND DIES

### Pouring the Impression

Hydrocolloid is not stable enough dimensionally to remain in the room environment for very long. It exhibits syneresis or imbibition to a significant degree, depending upon the atmosphere (31a). If the impression cannot be poured quickly, it should be stored in a humidor or wrapped in a moist paper towel for a short period of time. Failure to protect the impression may result in a subtle distortion that is difficult to detect until the restorations are tried on the tooth.

The polysulfide and silicone rubber base materials are more stable than hydrocolloid. They not only survive some delay in pouring, they also profit from it. After removal from the mouth, the material gradually releases the strains incorporated during removal of the impression from around the undercuts in the mouth. A short delay of 30 min before pouring actually improves the accuracy (1).

Research has shown that the polysulfide and silicone rubber base impression cannot be left unpoured indefinitely. After 2 hours some measurable distortion does occur. By 6 hours the distortion may have reached a clinically significant level (2). Waiting until the next day or over a weekend to pour the impression is taking a real chance on the accuracy.

The casts and dies created from the impression must be exact reproductions of the mouth. A satisfactory working cast and dies must be as follows:

1. free of bubbles in any critical area, such as a finish line, groove or retentive area, or an occluding area
2. free of distortion
3. an accurate reproduction of the occlusal surfaces of the teeth so that the casts can be successfully articulated
4. an accurate reproduction of the axial contours of unprepared teeth to the extent that the restorations can imitate those contours
5. trimmed to allow access to the prepared teeth and their finish lines
6. designed to allow dies which can be easily removed and replaced for waxing

The correct pouring of the stone can achieve a good cast. The greatest potential problem is the entrapment of air in some critical area. The stone used should be one of the Class II densite stones, because the harder stone prevents abrasion during the laboratory procedures.

It is necessary to have a working die upon which the wax pattern can be perfected, and it must be possible to return the die to its original position on the cast to establish the necessary relationships. Two separate pours of the rubber base materials may be used, one as the cast for establishing relationships and the other to make a separate die for perfecting the fit and marginal integrity of the restoration.

If only one pour of the impression is used, as would be the limit with hydrocolloid, other means of forming dies that are removable and replaceable are needed. One method utilizes dowel pins and a double pour technique. A first pour is made in a hard stone, which can be mixed under vacuum to minimize the number of air bubbles. The mixture is then vibrated slowly into the impression. It should flow in a thin layer slowly along the sides of the impression and into the area of the preparation, because a thick, heavy layer of stone is more likely to entrap air. The impression is poured so that a base with a thickness of 5–6 mm is formed. A dowel pin with about 5 mm of serrations on one end to aid in retention is placed into the stone over the area of the preparation and supported until the stone hardens. The other end of the dowel pin, which is tapered, smooth, and flattened on one side, extends beyond the level of the first pour of stone.

Once the first pour has hardened, the area on the bottom of the stone surrounding the dowel pin is painted with a separating medium to prevent adherence by the second layer of stone. The other areas are left untreated. A hard stone in a contrasting color is selected, mixed, and poured over the first layer of stone. The second pour should be poured to a level 2–3 mm short of the tip of the dowel pin. This layer is allowed to harden.

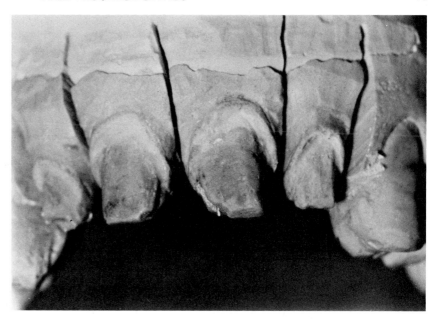

**FIG. 5-11.** Dies trimmed and sectioned to allow easy removal for waxing procedures. There should be a positive reseating when the dies are returned to their place.

After setting an hour or more, the cast is separated from the impression. Excess stone is cut away. The process to separate the dies is begun by using a thin saw blade to cut between the prepared tooth and the adjacent tooth (Fig. 5-11). These cuts should converge apically and extend to the junction of the first and second pour. After the cuts are made, a tap on the end of the dowel pin loosens the dowel pin, and the die can be removed easily. If the tap fails to loosen the die, there may be insufficient separating medium on the surface of the first pour, or the cuts may not converge apically so that the die is wedged in place.

The die is trimmed to allow easy access to the finish lines of the preparation. This trimming can be done with a round bur or a sharp-bladed knife. Care is needed to remove the stone apical to the finish lines without cutting or nicking the finish line itself.

### Mounting the Casts

It may be possible to fabricate the restoration without mounting the cast on an articulator in situations where there is no existing antagonist and the prepared tooth has adjacent teeth with desirable contours. In this situation, all the necessary relationships can be obtained from the cast itself. In most situations, however, it is necessary to mount the cast in correct relationship to the opposing arch on an articulator which allows close simulation of normal mandibular movements.

There are many different approaches to relating the casts to each other on an articulator. The complexity of the transfer records depends upon the complexity of the articulator itself.

**TRANSFER RECORDS.** The first record needed is a face-bow transfer. The face-bow is a device used to relate the maxillary cast to the condylar elements of the articulator in the same way the maxillary arch is related to the temporomandibular joints (24). Either an arbitrary position which approximates the location of the temporomandibular joint can be used, or the centers of rotations can be located and the information transferred to the articulator.

Wax or compound is placed over a rim referred to as a bite fork and an index of the maxillary arch is made. After the index is made, the bite fork is seated in the face-bow and the assembly is seated with the bite forked in the mouth. The ear pieces are guided into each ear and set as far medially and anteriorly as the patient can tolerate easily. This approximates the temporomandibular joints. The toggles surrounding the bite fork are tightened and the assembly removed. At this point the face-bow contains the following information:

1. the anteroposterior location of the cast to the condylar elements of the articulator
2. the mediolateral location of the cast to each condylar element of the articulator
3. the inferosuperior relationship of the maxillary cast to the condylar elements of the articulator
4. the approximate distance or width between the patient's condyles

This information is then programmed into the articulator.

The face-bow is set on the articulator and the maxillary cast seated in the indentations in the compound or wax on the bite fork. The cast is then luted to the upper portion of the articulator with a quick-set stone in approximately the same relationship to the condylar elements of the articulator as the patient's maxillary arch is to the patient's temporomandibular joint.

Then the mandibular cast is mounted to the maxillary cast. To establish a record of the relationship of the mandibular arch to the maxillary arch, a wax wafer is placed between the patient's teeth and the patient guided into closure in centric relationship. Centric relationship has been defined by Ramfjord and Ash (32) as "the most retruded position of the mandible from which opening and lateral movements can be performed comfortably." The wax wafer may be reinforced with metal foil and refined by adding warm drops of wax to three areas on the wafer. Each time the patient closes, he or she is guided into centric relationship. Materials other than wax, such as compound, can be used for the record.

The centric record is set against the maxillary arch and checked to assure the record is completely seated and stable. The articulator is then inverted and braced. The mandibular cast is set into the record and checked to assure the cast is completely seated and stable. Mounting stone is used then to lute the cast to the mounting ring on the lower portion of the articulator. The record is removed after the stone sets, and the occlusion is checked for correct mounting.

Eccentric movements can be recorded in several ways. If used with an arbitrary face-bow and other arbitrary settings, the lateral and protrusive records may consist of a reinforced wax horseshoe which records the relationship of the mandibular teeth to the maxillary

when the patient slides the jaw to the left several millimeters and closes into the wax horseshoe. This procedure is repeated for the other lateral movement and for protrusive movement.

If a fully adjustable articulator is used, the records must be much more precise. Pantographic tracings may be used to determine the exact centers of rotation and all movements from those points. This information is then programmed into the articulator settings.

**SETTING THE ARTICULATOR.** The articulator now must be set to reproduce the eccentric movements. The condylar guides are set at $0°$ and the side shift controls at their most open position so that the settings can be adjusted according to the wax wafers or rims. The right excursive record is completely seated on the teeth of the maxillary cast. Closing the articulator seats the mandibular teeth into the record. The left guide is set by rotating it downward until the superior wall of the guide touches the condylar element. The side shift is then set by rotating the side shift guide laterally until it touches the medial surface on the condylar element. The holding screw is then tightened.

The whole process for setting the right condylar guide is simply a reversal of the process for the left, this time using the left excursive record. The settings established can be written in the patient's record for future reference.

At this time the dentist has an accurate reproduction of the patient's teeth mounted on an articulator (Fig. 5–12) which is programmed to duplicate the relationships between the arches. It also reproduces the relationship of the arches to the temporomandibular joint.

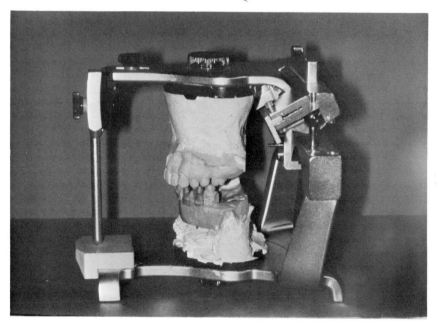

**FIG. 5–12.** Casts mounted on an adjustable articulator allow simulation of the patient's jaw movements as well as reproduction of centric relationship.

The casts are mounted and ready for fabrication of the restoration.

QUESTIONS

22. The advantage of the double pour technique for creation of the cast and dies is that it
    1. assures greater accuracy because of the second pour
    2. provides a second cast for checking occlusal relationships
    3. provides a removable die to facilitate waxing
    4. makes mounting on the articulator easier
    5. creates back-up dies in case the first pour is inaccurate

23. The face-bow registration gives a record of the
    1. relationship of the maxillary arch to the temporomandibular joint
    2. relationship between the maxillary and mandibular arches
    3. relationship of the mandibular arch to the temporomandibular joint
    4. condylar inclinations and the immediate side shift present
    5. None of the above

24. Centric relationship is defined as the
    1. most retruded position of the mandible from which opening and lateral movements can be made comfortably
    2. position in which the greatest amount of intercuspation of the teeth occurs
    3. position in which the supporting or centric cusp strikes the marginal ridge of the opposing teeth
    4. position in which the supporting or centric cusp strikes the fossa of the opposing teeth
    5. None of the above

25. Usually the biggest potential problem in pouring an impression is
    1. mixing the stone accurately
    2. entrapment of an air bubble
    3. achieving the proper thickness of the stone layer
    4. placement of the die pins
    5. None of the above

## LABORATORY PRESCRIPTION WRITING

If a laboratory technician is to make the restoration, the dentist must supply the technician with correctly mounted casts with accurate dies and a laboratory prescription. The dentist should trim the dies before they are sent to the technician in order to make the location of the finish lines clear.

The technician cannot legally fabricate restorations without proper authorization by prescription from the dentist anymore than the pharmacist can dispense drugs without a physician's prescription. The dentist should send with each mounted set of casts and dies a copy of the laboratory prescription and retain an office copy for the patient's records.

The laboratory prescription should contain the following information:

1. the patient's name
2. the tooth or teeth involved
3. the type of retainer(s) to be made
4. shade selected
5. pontic type or mold selected
6. pontic ridge relationship desired
7. special instructions such as staining, etc.
8. date or time desired

The technician must have the above information in order to fabricate restorations tailored to the individual patient.

QUESTIONS

26. Why does the dental technician need a written laboratory prescription before fabricating a restoration?
    a. It is legally required.
    b. The technician needs it to know the shade for the porcelain.
    c. The technician needs it to know the location of the finish lines on the preparations.
    d. The technician needs to know specific instructions about pontic design.

    1. a
    2. c and d
    3. a, b, and d
    4. a and b
    5. All of the above

27. Why should the dentist trim the dies before they are sent to a dental technician?
    1. The dentist should have better manual dexterity.
    2. The dentist should have a better knowledge of the location of the finish line.
    3. The dentist has the proper cutting instruments.
    4. The technician is not trained to recognize finish lines.

## THE WAX PATTERN

### Waxing Technique

The technique for making cast restorations is referred to as the "lost wax" technique. A wax pattern is produced on the die that possesses all the contours, contacts, and fit desired in the final product. A mold of investment stone is formed around the pattern, allowed to harden, and heated. The heat eliminates the wax to create a mold into which molten gold can be cast.

The first step involves coating the die with several coats of a lubricant to prevent the wax from sticking to the die. Excess lubricant is removed from the die by blotting or blowing away with an air syringe before wax is added.

The wax used may vary in color, hardness, and the way it is packaged. However, to be satisfactory the wax must

1. flow easily and retain its smoothness without chipping
2. undergo carving and shaping without chipping or distorting
3. be rigid and reasonably stable when cooled
4. be a color which contrasts with the die stone before used

Melted wax is allowed to flow in small amounts into all the confined areas, such as retentive grooves, first to assure good adaptation of the wax. When additional wax is placed, remelting the edges of the wax placed first helps the new wax blend with it and prevents voids or lines from forming on the interior portion of the pattern.

An alternate method of adding wax is to dip the lubricated die into a container of molten wax. This dipping can be repeated until sufficient bulk is added to begin carving and refining. After the wax has sufficient bulk, the pattern is removed from the die to assure it can be removed without fracturing. Before the wax is replaced, the die should be lubricated once more to prevent sticking. Wax is added until the correct contours and relationships are established, and any excess wax is removed. The pattern must reproduce the form of the original tooth except where improvements can be made.

## Relationships

Occlusal relationships can be established by adding an excess of wax to the occlusal surface and closing the articulator while the wax is still soft enough that the opposing teeth can indent the wax. The fossae and grooves are recorded in the wax by the opposing teeth. The excess is carved away and the indentations are blended together. The pattern is rechecked by closing the articulator again and then removing or adding wax as indicated.

The other method involves adding small increments of wax to build the areas into the proper occlusal relationships. While possibly a slower method, it tends to produce the relationship more exactly.

Ideally the occlusion should fall into one of two occlusal schemes, classified by where the working (functional) cusp meets the occlusal surface of its antagonist. The first occlusal scheme is the cusp–fossa. In this scheme the functional cusp of one tooth makes contact with the fossa of the opposing tooth. It is a tooth-to-tooth relationship which directs the forces along the long axis of the tooth. It is a difficult scheme to establish unless most of all of the teeth in both arches are involved. The second scheme is the cusp–marginal ridge relationship. This type is found most often in the natural dentition. It can be used even when dealing with a single restoration. The functional cusps fit against the opposing marginal ridges and the occlusal fossae. It is a tooth-to-two-tooth arrangement.

Either scheme may require modification to meet the needs or limitations of the situation. There are several principles which should remain consistent, however. The occlusal relationship must first create a stable relationship. It must direct forces in the long axis of the tooth as nearly as possible. There must be no prematurities in centric relationship or in excursive movements. Finally the occlusal relationship must create canine disclusion in eccentric movements or establish group function if the canine disclusion is not possible.

Proximal contacts are also important. The proximal surface must contact the adjacent tooth in such a manner and form that teeth are stabilized, underlying periodontal tissues are protected against food impaction and injury, and embrasures are open enough to prevent crowding and interdental tissues and to permit access for cleaning.

To accomplish all this the contact areas have several characteristics in common. No matter which teeth are involved, the contact area begins at the middle of the occlusal (incisal) one-third of the proximal surface and extends gingivally to include one-half of the middle one-third of the proximal surface. It is located more to the buccal than to the lingual surface, except in the case of the relationship between the maxillary first and second molars. Most importantly, it is a contact *area*, not just a contact point.

The contact areas are constructed so that four embrasures or open areas are formed around the contact area. They are a result of the contours of the proximal surfaces which are primarily convex occlusally, gingivally, buccally, and lingually. The embrasures are

1. the occlusal embrasure, which is the space between the teeth extending occlusally from the contact area to the marginal ridges
2. the facial embrasure, which is the space between the teeth facial to the contact area
3. the lingual embrasure, which is the space between the teeth lingual to the contact area. The lingual embrasure is usually larger than the facial embrasure.
4. the gingival embrasure, which is located between the teeth gingival to the contact area. This space provides room for the interdental papillae.

The embrasure form and location must be considered when the contact areas are established.

## Contours

The basic contours of the facial and lingual surfaces are gently rounded. The height of contour (area of greatest convexity) is in the middle of the gingival one-third on the facial surface. The surface is rounded from the top of the facial cusp through the height of contour to curve back inward at the cervical line. The lingual height of contour occurs at the junction of the middle and gingival one-thirds of the tooth in the maxillary arch. On mandibular teeth, the lingual height of contour is located about the middle one-third of the lingual surface.

The height of contour does not represent much of a bulge. The diameter of the tooth is only 1–1.5 mm greater through the height of contour than at the cementoenamel junction. Excessive contours invite food impaction, difficulty in cleaning, plaque accumulation, and periodontal problems (30, 45).

## Checking the Pattern

The marginal area must cover all of the prepared tooth structure and be adapted tightly at the finish line. The margins should extend to, but not past, the finish lines and be tightly adapted. They should be smooth and blended with the rest of the pattern. Burnishing with a warm (not hot) instrument helps to thin, adapt, and smooth the margin.

The finished pattern should be examined to assure the general contours are correct and the margins are well adapted (Fig. 5–13), and it should be remembered that poor margins are easier to identify if the die has been properly trimmed. The margins should be viewed from a gingival direction to detect open margins, that is, margins in which the wax is not tightly adapted to the finish line of the preparation. Overextension, in which the wax is extended beyond the finish line of the preparation, is another common discrepancy. If the wax extends into an undercut on the unprepared surface, it may fracture or distort when removed. If the pattern is not extended to the finish line, it is too short. It is advantageous to have the margins on a wax pattern slightly thick for casting purposes, but a thick margin on a completed restoration collects plaque because of its contours. The margin of a wax pattern should not be paper thin but should have only enough bulk to allow casting and finishing procedures. Although roughness or ripples can be eliminated by grinding, removal may also involve undesirable changes in the contours of the restoration; therefore the pattern must be checked for roughness also.

The pattern can be smoothed by wiping it with a piece of very smooth cloth, nylon hose, or a wet cotton roll. It is important that the pattern be very smooth to avoid extensive finishing of the casting.

### QUESTIONS

28. The technique for making cast restorations is referred to as the

    1. lost wax technique
    2. molten gold technique
    3. inlay investment technique
    4. G.V. Black technique
    5. centrifugal casting technique

29. Why should the wax pattern be invested soon after it is completed? (*Continued*)

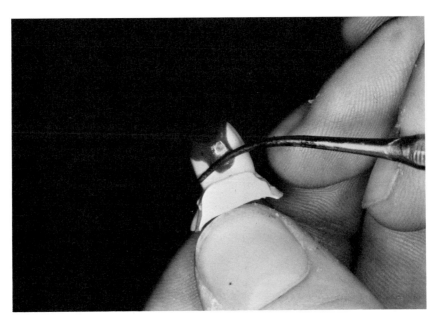

**FIG. 5–13.** The wax patterns should be checked to assure the marginal adaptation is correct.

1. The wax becomes brittle and subject to fracture.
2. The wax has "memory" and begins to distort.
3. The wax exhibits shrinkage after carving.
4. It is not critical how soon the pattern is invested.

30. The height of contour on the facial surface of posterior teeth is located
    1. in the gingival one-third of the tooth
    2. in the middle one-third of the tooth
    3. at the junction of the middle one-third and occlusal one-third
    4. at the junction of the middle one-third and the gingival one-third
    5. It varies considerably according to the tooth.

31. The margins of the wax pattern should be
    1. extended beyond the preparation finish lines to allow finishing
    2. left thick to allow finishing
    3. extended to the finish lines but no farther
    4. 1 and 2
    5. 2 and 3

## INVESTING AND CASTING

After completion of the wax pattern, there are several steps remaining to convert the pattern into a metal casting. The steps are 1) investment of the pattern, 2) burnout of the pattern, and 3) casting of molten metal into the mold.

### Investment Material

Investing the pattern is the first in a series of critical steps in converting the wax pattern into a cast restoration. The investment material must completely adapt to the wax pattern to assure the mold created is a perfect representation of the pattern, the entrapment of air bubbles can ruin the mold and result in a miscast. The material must have sufficient strength to withstand the heat of burn-out and the casting process without chipping or cracking and must provide the correct amount of expansion to offset the shrinkage of the gold alloy during solidification.

Various investment materials have been formulated. The investment materials used for Types I, II, and III gold alloys fall into two categories or classes: those that rely on thermal expansion and those that rely on hygroscopic expansion. Expansion is necessary to compensate for the approximately 1.5% shrinkage of gold during cooling and solidification (15, 31b).

Expansion occurs in two ways. It occurs during the setting reaction as a result of normal crystal growth. When the investment is placed in a 100°F water bath, the crystallization process has enough water to continue to completion and the amount of expansion is increased. Expansion which occurs in the presence of water is referred to as hygroscopic expansion. Thermal expansion is accomplished by the normal expansion that occurs from heating. (Refer to Chapter 2, "Dental Amalgams" section, for the composition of the matrix material.)

### Spruing

To assure that the pattern is located correctly inside the inlay ring before investment, it is attached to the crucible former at one end of the inlay ring by means of a small diameter rod made of wax, plastic, or metal. This rod serves a twofold purpose. It attaches the wax pattern to the crucible former, stabilizing the pattern during the investing process, and creates the inlet or passageway through the investment to the mold formed by the wax pattern so the gold can enter.

Various size sprues are used. Usually a number 8 or number 10 sprue is used on a large pattern and a number 12 sprue on a small pattern. The sprue itself should be no longer than 6–7 mm to prevent the gold from cooling before reaching all areas of the pattern, but it must be long enough to assure the top portion of the pattern extends to within 5–6 mm of the top of the inlay ring but no farther. Wax and plastic sprues are melted at the same time as the pattern itself, but metal sprues must be detached from the pattern after the investment ring has been heated enough to soften or eliminate the wax.

The sprue should be attached to the pattern at an area of bulk so the molten gold enters at an area that allows easy flow and prevents premature cooling (26). The sprue also must be attached at an angle which allows the gold to enter without making an abrupt turn to reach some area of the pattern. If the sprue is attached at right angles to the surface of the pattern, for example, the incoming metal will hit the wall of the mold and bounce, and the resulting turbulence can produce porosity in the casting.

### Investing

After the sprue has been attached, the pattern is removed from the die carefully. The sprue is set into the crucible former so that the internal surface of the pattern (the surface that contacts the tooth) is facing upward at a slight angle to decrease the chances of trapping an air bubble. The sprue is firmly attached to the crucible former with a drop of wax.

An asbestos liner is placed dry into the inlay ring and adapted to the walls of the ring. The asbestos serves as a cushion inside the ring to allow expansion of the investment and allows easier removal of the investment and the restoration after casting is completed. The asbestos must have very slight overlapping and extend to within about 3 mm of the end of the ring. Excessive overlapping of the ends of the asbestos strip can lead to excessive expansion.

The asbestos is wet before the investment material is poured into the ring.

Investment of the pattern can be accomplished by one of two methods. The pattern can be hand-invested or vacuum-invested. Either method works for the experienced technician.

If the procedure of choice is investing by hand, the pattern is painted with a debubblizing solution that lowers the surface tension. The investment material is then mixed, and a small brush is used to place a thin layer of the material on the pattern. The ring is then placed over the pattern onto the crucible former. The remaining investment is vibrated slowly into the ring until it is full. Entrapment of air must be avoided.

Vacuum investing requires more elaborate equipment but it has several advantages. It provides a denser investment and a slightly denser casting; there is less likelihood of trapping air against a critical portion of the pattern; and it is easier for the inexperienced person to use.

After the pattern is attached to the crucible form and the ring is in place, the investment is mixed under a vacuum of 25–30 lb pressure. The investment is then slowly vibrated around the pattern under vacuum until the ring is filled. The vacuum greatly decreases the chances of bubbles of air being trapped against the pattern.

After the ring is filled, it is set into the water bath at 100°F temperature for hygroscopic expansion. After the investment has set for 30 min, it can be removed. If hygroscopic expansion is not desired, the ring is not placed into the water bath.

## Burn-Out

Once the investment has set, it may be stored indefinitely. Some authorities suggest returning the invested pattern to a humidor for a few hours or soaking it in water for several minutes before burn-out if the invested pattern has been stored for many hours or days. This helps to prevent fracturing of the investment.

For burn-out the investment ring is set into an oven at room temperature, and the temperature is slowly raised to the proper level. If hygroscopic expansion has been used, the temperature should be raised to 900°F. If only thermal expansion is to be used, a temperature of 1200°F is required to provide adequate expansion. The burn-out temperature is designed to accomplish three things. It must 1) eliminate the wax pattern and its residue, 2) expand the investment to compensate for the shrinkage of the gold, and 3) prevent the premature solidification of the gold.

The investment should be left in the oven for a minimum of 1 hour.

## Casting

A gas–air torch can be used to melt the gold. There are four zones in a correctly adjusted flame (Fig. 5–14). The zones as they occur from the area closest to the torch outward are

1. the mixing of precombustion zone next to the end of the torch. It is a cool, colorless zone.
2. the combustion zone where some combustion takes place. It is greenish blue in color.
3. the reducing zone. It possesses the highest tem-

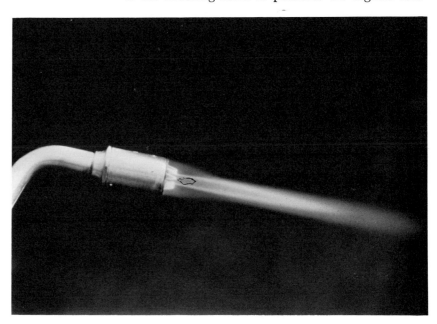

**FIG. 5-14.** A correctly adjusted gas–air torch showing the four zones of the flame.

perature and prevents the formation of oxides in the casting. The zone is dim blue in color.
4. the oxidizing zone. It is not used in heating the gold.

The crucible in which the gold is heated should be covered with a strip of asbestos adapted to the crucible. It protects the crucible and helps prevent contamination of the gold.

The reducing zone is used to melt the gold until it forms one round ball. When the crucible is tapped slightly, the gold should shimmer and have a shiny, mirrorlike appearance. Flux can be sprinkled onto the gold to add fluidity and decrease oxide formation.

The investment ring is removed from the oven and placed into the cradle of the casting arm. Then the casting arm is grasped and the holding pin is dropped. After making sure that the gold surface is shimmering and clean, the technician releases the casting arm. The centrifugal force throws the gold into the investment ring, completely filling the mold within the first quarter turn. The continued spinning holds the molten gold in place until it solidifies. No more than 30 sec. should elapse between the time the ring is removed and the gold is cast, because additional delay allows excessive cooling of the ring and contraction of the investment mold.

After 1 min the inlay ring is placed into cool water. This process is referred to as quenching. It anneals the gold to provide better working qualities. Placing the hot investment into cool water also helps to break up the investment material for removal of the casting.

After cleaning, the casting is placed into a pickling agent. Oxides and other impurities are removed by heating the pickling solution to a boil. The casting is removed from the solution and rinsed. It is ready for finishing.

### QUESTIONS

32. It is necessary that the investment expands to compensate for the shrinkage of gold during casting. The component in the investment material responsible is
    1. gypsum
    2. potassium oxide
    3. quartz
    4. potassium sulfate
    5. None of the above

33. Hygroscopic expansion of the investment material occurs because of
    1. 900°F heat in the oven
    2. the water present when the investment is mixed
    3. the 100°F water bath which increases the setting expansion by releasing a gaseous component
    4. the 100°F water bath which allows the crystallization process to go to completion

34. The pattern should be sprued
    1. in an area of bulk
    2. in a thin area to assure complete casting of the area
    3. near a margin to assure complete casting of the margin
    4. with a small sprue to minimize obliterating the anatomy carving

35. What purpose does the asbestos liner placed inside the inlay ring serve?
    1. It soaks up any excess moisture from the investment material.
    2. It helps to concentrate the heat from the oven in the center of the inlay ring.
    3. It allows room for the thermal expansion.
    4. It aids in removing the investment from the ring after casting.
    5. Both 3 and 4

36. At what temperature and for how long should the investment be heated when the hygroscopic technique is used?
    1. 900°F for 1 hour
    2. 1200°F for 30 min
    3. 1200°F for 1 hour
    4. 900°F for 30 min
    5. 900°F for 1-1/3 hour

37. The investment ring is heated to high temperatures to
    a. eliminate the wax pattern completely
    b. expand the investment mold to compensate for gold shrinkage
    c. prevent premature cooling of the molten gold
    d. eliminate contaminating gases formed by the melted wax
    1. a and c
    2. a, b, and c
    3. b, c, and d
    4. a, b, and d

## FINISHING AND POLISHING

No matter how well the wax pattern was finished, the surface of the casting is never smooth enough without some finishing. Finishing and polishing follow a logical sequence. First come the coarse finishing agents, followed by the medium, then the fine, and finally the polishing agents.

The sprue is removed by a separating disk. The gross roughness can be smoothed with a green stone or a finishing disk until normal contours are returned. The internal surfaces of the casting should be examined for holes, bubbles, or roughness. Much adjustment to the inside of the casting destroys retention and stability and should be avoided, however.

The axial surface is finished with disks used in order of decreasing abrasiveness. The occlusal surface is best smoothed by green stones followed by white stones. The axial and occlusal surfaces can be further smoothed using rubber points and disks. Grooves can be refined with finishing burs or small round burs.

Polishing should not be attempted until the final contours have been made and the surface smoothed. If finishing and contouring have been well done, the polishing will be quickly accomplished. The first step in polishing is the use of Tripoli or Williams Compound on a rag wheel or a soft bristle brush. This medium grit polishing compound removes scratches from the surface. The casting is then cleaned and a new rag wheel or soft bristle brush is used to apply jeweler's rouge, which produces a high luster.

Pressure and the speed of the rotary instruments must be diminished when nearing the finish line to avoid excessive thinning or shortening the margins of the casting. Rotary instruments should be turning from gold towards die rather than vice-versa to avoid catching and bending or breaking a margin.

Polishing is done for two purposes, the most important being to produce the smoothest possible surface because a smooth surface reduces plaque retention. The other is to produce a surface that looks and feels cleaner so the patient will be encouraged in home care efforts.

The occlusal surface can be left with either a high shine or air-blasted to dull the shine. A dull finish is helpful when checking the occlusal relationships. Marking ribbon and paper more readily produce marks on the dull surface than on a polished one. Prematurities may show as shiny burnish marks on the gold surface.

## TRY-IN OF THE RESTORATION

Although the crown has been fabricated upon a die considered accurate and related to the opposing and adjacent teeth on a good cast, it must not be presumed that the casting will fit and relate with complete accuracy in the mouth. Try-in of the restoration enables the dentist to determine if the restoration is suitable for cementation. The areas evaluated are 1) the marginal integrity, 2) the proximal contacts, 3) the occlusal relationships, 4) retention and stability, and 5) general contours.

Gold margins cannot be adapted completely to the preparation wall. There is a minimum opening of 15–20 $\mu$m. Even so, tight adaptation is essential to minimize marginal leakage. The tip of the explorer should not slip under the edge of the margin or catch against it. The margin may be improved by thinning and/or burnishing.

The proximal surface should touch the adjacent tooth with a firm, tight contact but without any pressure. The contact area should be located slightly buccal to the midline and slightly gingival to the marginal ridge. The gingival embrasure must be generous enough to assure no crowding of the papillae occurs.

The seated crown should strike its antagonist simultaneously with the rest of the teeth. If canine disclusion is present, the posterior teeth will not occlude in eccentric movements. If group function is present, the occlusion on the tooth in eccentric movements should be equal to that on the other teeth.

The occlusion can be evaluated in several ways. The occlusal relationships of the other teeth can be observed with the restoration in and with it out. Any variation would indicate prematurities. Marking ribbon or paper can be used, but the marks made by closing on ribbon or paper can be misleading; the dentist must interpret them to determine if they are heavier than those on the surrounding teeth. If so, the areas marked are reduced. Thin strips of wax, softened to eliminate any hindrance to closure by the patient, can be used instead of marking ribbon or paper. The heaviest contacts will pierce the wax while the lighter contacts will not. These areas are interpreted to determine exactly where to reduce the contacts. The patient can be asked if, the restoration feels like it strikes prematurely. Any complaint of extra pressure on the restoration by the patient must be considered because of the sensitivity of the patient's proprioceptor fibers in the periodontal membrane.

A little force such as a gentle tap, finger pressure, or a gentle prying action with an instrument should be sufficient to dislodge a well-fitted casting. If excessive pressure is required to seat and unseat it, the inside of the casting should be examined for burnished marks indicating areas that are binding. These areas should be relieved to allow the casting to be seated and removed with reasonable force. The uncemented casting must not exhibit any rocking or twisting motion when pressure is placed first on one corner and then on an opposite corner.

The crown should possess the same general contours as the teeth to either side and be a mirror image of its counterpart on the other side of the mouth. The height of convexity should be correctly located and not excessive. The axial surfaces should be rounded with the proximal surfaces flat or slightly concave gingival to the contact area. The occlusal surface should have well-defined, but not deep, anatomy. All surfaces should be rounded without sharp edges.

The final contouring, smoothing, and finishing are done. The crown is ready for cementation.

38. The proximal contact of the restoration should be located:
    a. in the midline of the tooth buccolingually
    b. at the marginal ridge
    c. in the middle of the occlusal one-third of the proximal surface
    d. buccal to the midline of the tooth
    e. in the middle one-third of the tooth occlusogingivally
    1. c and d
    2. a and d
    3. d and e
    4. b and d
    5. a and c

39. Premature occlusion can be detected by
    a. marking with a ribbon
    b. checking with thin wax for indentations
    c. visual observation
    d. patient's subjective symptoms
    1. a and b
    2. b
    3. a, b, and d
    4. All of the above

## FIXED PARTIAL DENTURES

The fixed partial denture or bridge is a fixed restoration which replaces one or more missing teeth (Fig. 5–15). Retention comes from the cemented retainers on the abutment teeth. The parts of a fixed partial denture are the following:

1. The retainer is the restoration cemented to one of the teeth involved. The retainer is connected to and provides support for the parts of the partial denture replacing the missing teeth.
2. The abutment is the tooth which supports the fixed partial denture and over which the retainer is cemented.
3. The pier is any tooth situated between the abutments at each end of the fixed partial denture which also provides support for denture.
4. The pontic is the replacement for the missing tooth.
5. The connector is the part that ties the pontic to the retainer. The connector may be a rigid (a cast or soldered) connector, or it may be a nonrigid connector.

### Preparation Considerations

The extra stress on the abutment retainer requires that it possess enough strength to prevent distortion of the retainer and that the preparation provides good retention. Inlays and even onlays are not generally considered to have adequate strength and retention to serve as retainers.

While each preparation must meet the general requirements of all preparations, the fact that a preparation is part of a fixed partial denture adds other considerations. Each preparation must be aligned with the other preparations. The path of insertion and withdrawal of the retainers must be common to each preparation unless a nonrigid connector is used. The design of

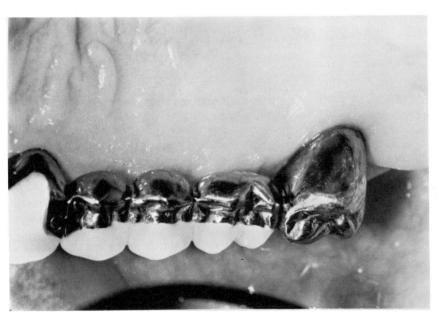

**FIG. 5–15.** A fixed partial denture. The anterior retainer on the canine and the posterior retainer on the molar support three pontics.

the pontic and its relationships to the other parts of the fixed partial denture are critical.

## Pontics

Pontics are made either of cast metal or a combination of cast metal and porcelain or acrylic resin. The choice depends upon cost, ease of fabrication, aesthetic considerations, and the functional requirements. All the combinations mentioned are acceptable, although cast metal has superior strength. All three are well tolerated by the soft tissues if the pontic design and surface texture are correct.

**REQUIREMENTS OF THE PONTIC DESIGN.** The most important element in the success of the pontic is its design. The design must assure that the gingival portion has the minimal contact with the ridge that is compatible with aesthetic considerations. This applies to the faciolingual and mesiodistal dimensions and the amount of ridge overlap. The occlusal relationships are like those established on any tooth; the pontic should have basically normal dimensions faciolingually. The pontic fills the space mesiodistally, and its proximal contours simulate those of a nature tooth.

In summary, the occlusal one-third or one-half of the pontic has normal dimensions (if space permits mesiodistally), normal occlusal and proximal relations, and normal appearance. The gingival one-half to two-thirds varies somewhat, depending upon the aesthetic demands. It has minimum soft tissue contact.

**PONTIC–RIDGE RELATIONSHIP.** It is imperative that the pontic be designed to facilitate cleaning. The patient will have limited access to the gingival and interproximal embrasure areas of the pontic because the connector on either side of the pontic prevents the passing of floss through the contacts into the gingival embrasure areas.

There are three basic designs for the gingival surface of the pontic. One does not approximate the ridge at all. It has a gingival surface which is convex faciolingually and mesiodistally. The gingival portion is a minimum of 3 mm off the ridge. This clearance and the convex surface provide easy access for cleaning. A variation has a shape that is concave mesiodistally (19), which allows easy cleaning and has the advantage of greater thickness of the connector for greater strength. Both of these designs are limited to areas of no aesthetic concerns.

The second type of pontic design is the ridge lap pontic design. It is used in areas where the aesthetic results are of prime importance. The ridge lap design attempts a compromise between good aesthetic results and good oral hygiene. With this design, the pontic

lightly touches the tissue, but there is no pressure and no contact with movable tissue. It contacts or approximates the tissue only on the facial portion of the ridge. Lingual to the height of the ridge, the pontic pulls away from the tissue in a convex shape. The shape mesiodistally is convex, while on the facial portion the gingival surface is straight or slightly concave. The degree of concavity is dependent upon the shape of the ridge and the degree of overlap. The pontic overlaps the facial portion no more than is required by the aesthetic need to match the length of the adjacent teeth. The less the need, the less the amount of overlap and the greater the ease of cleaning.

The third design, which is to be avoided, is the "saddle" design. In this design the gingival portion overlaps the facial *and* the lingual surfaces. The appearance is good, but the concave gingival surface created is very difficult to clean. Tissue irritation and inflammation are the inevitable consequences.

**PONTIC TYPES.** There are several types of pontics available, all using different combinations of designs and materials. They are

1. all cast metal
2. cast metal core with veneered porcelain. Connector areas and usually the occlusal surface are metal.
3. cast metal with a porcelain facing. The occlusal surface is metal, which provides the strength.
4. cast metal with an acrylic resin facing. The rest of the surfaces are metal.

Several types of porcelain facings are available. They require a metal backing for support, occlusion, and connection to the retainers. They are designed to produce good aesthetic results and/or to place a glazed porcelain surface next to the soft tissues. Because of its extremely smooth surface glazed porcelain has been traditionally considered the material of choice to place next to the soft tissues, even though research has shown that the design of the pontic influences tissue health more than the material being used (5, 18, 42).

The types of commercially available facings are 1) sanitary pontic, 2) flatback facing, 3) Trupontic, 4) pin facing, 5) long pin pontic, and 6) porcelain denture teeth.

The sanitary pontic is designed for the mandibular posterior regions only. Its purpose is to place porcelain next to the ridge. The porcelain portion is attached to the occlusal portion (which is composed of cast gold for strength) to provide the areas for the connector.

The flatback facing is composed of a facial portion of porcelain and a cast metal backing to withstand the occlusal forces proximal surfaces for the connectors. It is designed for the anterior regions.

The Trupontic is designed primarily for the maxil-

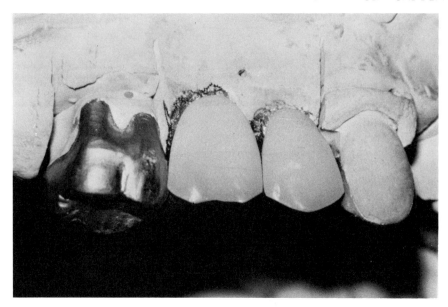

**FIG. 5-16.** The trupontic replaces the facial and gingival surfaces while relying upon a cast metal occlusal and lingual surface for strength and a surface for soldering.

lary posterior region. It places a bulk of porcelain next to the ridge and comprises the facial surface except for a small lip of gold overlaying the tip of the buccal cusp (Fig. 5-16). The aesthetic results are good.

The pin facing is designed much like a flatback facing, its primary purpose being aesthetics. The long pin pontic is similar in design and purpose to the Trupontic.

Porcelain denture teeth can be adapted as the veneer over a cast gold portion to satisfy aesthetic need.

The sanitary pontic, flatback facing, and the Trupontic are attached to the cast portion of the pontic by a metal lug which fits into a slot in the porcelain portion. The porcelain is cemented to the gold portion of the pontic before the prosthesis is cemented in place.

The pin pontic and the reverse pin pontic are retained by the use of pins. The long pin pontic has pins which fit into pinholes in the metal backing. The reverse pin pontic has pinholes drilled into the porcelain. Pins are cast as part of the metal to fit into the pinholes.

If the retainers are porcelain fused to metal, the best aesthetic and, possibly, functional result may come from a pontic of the same material. The match is better aesthetically because the porcelain is processed from the same batch of material. The metal core can be cast with one of the retainers to eliminate one solder joint.

**FABRICATION OF THE PONTIC.** If a porcelain facing is used, the first step is to adapt the facing to the ridge. The sequence is

1. selection of the shade and mold for the porcelain facing
2. establishment of the mesiodistal width

3. adaptation of the gingival portion to the soft tissues and establishment of the correct occlusogingival dimension
4. contouring of the linguogingival surface
5. contouring of the mesiogingival and distogingival embrasures
6. final contouring of the faciogingival surface
7. smoothing and blending of contours and surfaces
8. placement of bevels around the facing

The adaptation to the ridge contours is achieved by marking the cast with dark pencil lead. The pontic is placed against the marked area with slight pressure so the lead is transferred to the gingival surface of the pontic. The marked area is ground with a stone, returned to the ridge, and marked again. The marked area is ground until the gingival portion of the pontic is adapted to the contours and the occlusogingival dimension of the pontic is correct.

The facing must be aligned so that 1) its faciolingual alignment is the same as the retainers; 2) it is aligned with the same mesiodistal slant as the retainers; and 3) it has approximately the same occlusogingival length as the retainers. There must be clearance between the porcelain facing and the opposing cusps in both centric occlusion and excursive movements.

The gold on the occlusal surface must be a minimum thickness of 1.5–2 mm over most of the pontic, although it may thin out towards the facial cusp tip when the porcelain covers the facial surface. The gold–porcelain margin should not be placed in an area of occlusal function. Failure to provide proper thickness of gold may allow the gold to flex, which would loosen or fracture the porcelain facing.

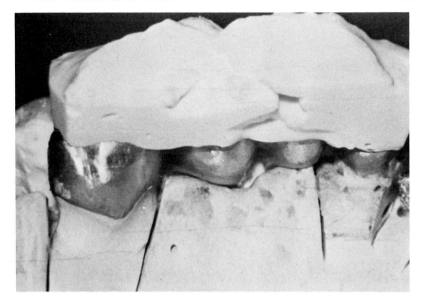

**FIG. 5-17.** Stone matrix which relates the castings to each other to allow removal for investing and casting.

After the facing has been adapted, a matrix of stone or tray resin is made to fit the facial surface (Fig. 5–17). It stabilizes the facing while the occlusal and lingual portions of the pontic are waxed and later adjusted after casting. The occlusal and lingual portions are waxed with the same objectives as were the crowns which serve as retainers (See section on The Wax Pattern). The attachment lug or pins are waxed into place and the casting made around them. If pinholes are made in the cast metal, the pinholes are preserved by insertion of substitute pins. The pattern is invested and cast in the usual manner. The substitute pins are removed by pulling or reaming them out.

The sprue is removed and the casting is adjusted and smoothed in the usual manner. The stone or resin matrix originally used in the waxing process serves to position the pontic during the adjustment period.

### QUESTIONS

40. What can be done to minimize the soft tissue irritation that is likely under a pontic?
    a. Place a highly polished surface or glazed porcelain next to the ridge.
    b. Design the pontic with minimum tissue contact.
    c. Design the pontic with convex gingival surfaces.
    d. Design the pontic with wide embrasures.

    1. a and b
    2. a
    3. b and d
    4. b, c, and d
    5. All of the above

41. The major advantage(s) of a Trupontic is (are) that it
    a. places porcelain next to the ridge
    b. is processed, not cemented, to the metal backing

    c. provides a facial surface of porcelain for aesthetics
    d. can be placed into occlusal function

    1. a and c
    2. a and d
    3. b
    4. a
    5. b and d
    6. c

42. For best results, the occlusion on a pontic should be
    1. eliminated by adjusting to remove occlusal contact
    2. confined to only the buccal portion of the pontic
    3. confined to only the lingual portion of the pontic
    4. essentially the same as on the other teeth
    5. confined to only the area next to strongest abutment

43. What is likely to produce fracture in an anterior porcelain pontic facing?
    1. Great vertical overlap of the teeth
    2. Great horizontal overlap
    3. Detrimental chewing habits
    4. Incorrect selection of facing type
    5. Incorrect design of cast backing

44. If the retainers have a porcelain veneer, the best aesthetic results from the pontic will probably result from:
    1. using a porcelain flatback facing
    2. using a porcelain Trupontic
    3. using an acrylic Trupontic
    4. processing a porcelain-fused-to-metal pontic

### Connectors

There are two types of connectors used with a fixed partial denture. The most commonly used connector is the solder joint. Soldering is the joining together of two metal parts by the use of another metal (the solder). The solder is fused to each of the metal components to join all the components into one solid piece. The other type is the non-rigid or broken stress connector, which involves a precision or semiprecision method of attachment.

**GOLD SOLDER JOINTS.** The solder used in fixed prosthodontics must possess 1) resistance to corrosion and tarnish; 2) strength equal to the casting alloys used; 3) the ability to flow freely, to wet metal surfaces, and to adhere to them; 4) resistance to pitting, usually due to burning out or vaporization of the base metals in the solder, which decreases strength; and 5) at least a 100°F lower fusing temperature than the alloys being soldered (37).

The solders for fixed prosthodontics can be classified in terms of fineness, which is the number of parts of gold per thousand found in solder alloy. The higher the fineness of the solder, the higher the melting range and the greater the resistance to corrosion. Lower fineness indicates a solder with a lower melting point, one more likely to corrode and to have poor flow characteristics. A solder of 580 fineness is the minimum which should be used.

There are several other elements necessary for successful soldering. The surfaces to be soldered must be free of debris, oxides, sulfides, polishing compounds, and other contaminants for the solder to wet the surfaces, flow, and adhere to the metal retainers. The blow torch must allow fine adjustment to produce a flame with a well-defined reducing zone. There must be adequate access or airways so heat from the flame reaches all areas surrounding the solder joint area. The investment and casting should be preheated because the solder needs a high temperature to spread evenly throughout the whole assembly.

**Relating the Castings.** Soldering transforms the individual castings into one solid unit, so the castings must be correctly related. Incorrectly related castings will prevent the fixed partial denture from seating. There are several approaches to correctly relating the units of the fixed partial denture. If the original cast has not been sectioned, it may be possible to place the retainers on the dies and then relate the pontic to them. If the cast has been sectioned, the relationship must be verified in the patient's mouth.

Whether in the mouth or on the cast, the castings can be luted together with an autocuring resin (such as DuraLay) or related by creating a matrix or index while the castings are in place. The use of autocure resin affords the simplest and fastest method. A brush is wet with the liquid and dipped into the powder; the wet bead is then spread over the solder joint area. This is continued until the individual units are securely locked together with the cured resin. The whole assembly is transferred to the mouth to assure that the units can be completely seated without any rock. Any discrepancy indicates the alignment is incorrect, so the casting must be separated by breaking loose the acrylic.

An index can be made either on the cast or in the mouth. The castings are seated with the pontic stabilized with wax or the plaster matrix. A mix of quick-set plaster is placed onto a suitable surface (such as a wet tongue blade) and then placed plaster side against the castings and vibrated gently. The vibrating motion helps the plaster to adapt to the surfaces for a more accurate and stable index. The plaster should extend 4–5 mm beyond the occlusal surface. The plaster should be trimmed so 1–2 mm of the margins of each crown is showing. The index is cleaned of any debris because debris may prevent the castings from seating completely, thus altering the relationships.

The castings are reseated and checked for complete seating and adequate space. There must be some space between the castings; if they are touching, there will be no room for the solder to flow into the proximal surfaces. In addition, expansion during the soldering process would cause the castings to press against each other and fracture the investment. On the other hand, excessive space makes the flow of the solder from one casting to the other difficult. Even if the flow does occur, the shrinkage of the solder as it cools may pull the castings towards each other and thus out of alignment. The correct amount of space to leave is equal to the thickness of a sheet of paper, approximately 0.005 in.

**Investing the Castings.** If the castings are correctly aligned and the interproximal space is correct, the castings are ready for investing. It is helpful to flow wax around the embrasure areas if the plaster matrix or the DuraLay does not cover them. The wax covering the embrasure areas can be eliminated prior to the soldering process so access for the heat is available. This will improve the likelihood of the solder flowing into the desired area.

Soldering investment is mixed and then very gently vibrated into the inverted casting assembly. All the interior of the castings must be filled, and the investment must extend over the margins of the castings to protect and stablize them. The investment should be poured to the depth of 1 in. to provide strength and should be allowed to sit for about 1 hour to reach adequate strength.

Any wax used to limit the areas covered by investment can be quickly eliminated by rinsing with hot water. DuraLay will be eliminated by the blowtorch. Any debris should be gently blown away.

Soldering requires an even heat throughout the investment assembly. The investment block itself must be strong enough to withstand stress yet be small enough that the whole assembly can be kept at the proper temperature. To meet these two objectives it is recommended that the investment be

1. approximately 1 in. thick
2. extended ¼ in. beyond the widest casting
3. extended ⅛–¼ in. beyond the retainer on each end of the fixed partial denture

Flux can be added to the warm castings in the areas where the solder is to flow. Antiflux can be placed on the other areas to help confine the flow.

*The Soldering Process.* The investment block is preheated in an oven, over a flame, or with a blowtorch until the whole assembly is nearing soldering temperature. If an oven is used, the temperature should reach about 1500°F. If a burner flame is used, the investment block should be set over a wire screen over the flame and heated for 10 min.

A sharply refined reducing zone is used only after the investment block is sufficiently preheated. The flame is played across the investment assembly until all areas quickly turn a dull, dark red when the flame is held on them. The burner under the investment block should be left on during this time to aid in the heating. Attempts to place the solder before sufficient preheating has been done may cause the solder to ball up and refuse to flow. Overheating of specific areas of the castings is also likely to occur.

The amount of solder used depends upon the size of the solder joint needed. Usually a piece 2–3 mm long is sufficient and permits controlled handling. The solder is placed in the occlusolingual embrasures, and the flame is applied from the facial side. The heat of the investment and castings, as well as the flame itself, melts the solder. The solder flows towards the greatest heat, which is the flame. The space around the soldering area, which was preserved with wax to prevent investment from covering the area, provides access for the heat so that it can draw solder gingivally to complete the joint. As soon as the solder flows, the torch should be moved away to prevent overheating.

The investment assembly should air-cool for approximately 5 min. More rapid cooling may result in thermal stresses and distortion. The investment assembly is then quenched in cool water. Cooling too long or slowly may result in excessive crystallization and grain growth weakening the solder joint. Quenching after 5 min minimizes distortion and allows the gold and solder to undergo an ordering heat treatment, increasing hardness and strength while reducing elongation. The fixed partial denture can be removed easily from the investment after quenching.

A good solder joint covers the same area generally occupied by the contact area, has no pits or voids, is smooth and rounded on its surfaces, and does not impinge upon or approximate too closely to a margin (Fig. 5–18). If these criteria are met by the solder joint or joints, the fixed partial denture is checked to see that it can be seated completely without any rock when pressure is applied. The presence of a rock, incomplete seating, or a tendency of one retainer to come slightly unseated after being seated would indicate an inaccurate relationship. A solder joint must be severed and the retainers realigned.

**NONRIGID CONNECTORS.** Nonrigid connectors may be either a precision or a nonprecision type. The pre-

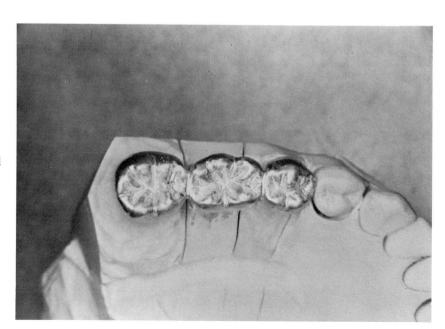

**FIG. 5–18.** A correctly soldered fixed partial denture.

cision type is prefabricated and is incorporated into the wax pattern to become part of the casting. After the pattern is waxed, a large box is cut into its proximal surface. The key and keyway are seated with the help of a surveyor so they are parallel to the path of insertion of the distal retainer. The keyway is blended into the rest of the pattern. The key is withdrawn and the keyway and pattern are cast. After casting, the key is replaced and the pontic is attached to it. The pontic and key are then cast as one unit. After casting, the mesial retainer with the keyway is seated first. The distal retainer and pontic are seated with the key fitting into the keyway on the mesial retainer.

Another type of nonrigid connector is the semiprecision one. It is created by carving a keyway on the distal surface of the mesial retainer and then fashioning a corresponding key on the mesial surface of the pontic. The keyway is T shaped to provide retention against distal displacement. The semiprecision attachment operates on the same principle as a precision one but the fit is not precise. There is less stress on the mesial abutment but not as much support for the pontic.

The broken stress or nonrigid connector has one very great advantage. It is not necessary that all of the preparations be aligned to draw. Tipped or poorly aligned teeth can be used as abutments for fixed partial dentures. Discrepancies in the line of draw between abutments is compensated for by the alignment of the keyway. If the keyway can be aligned with the line of draw of the other teeth, the fixed partial denture can be placed. Its disadvantage is that the nonrigid connector does not offer the same support for the restoration that a solid connector does. Even the precision attachment has some movement of the key in the keyway, which means a loss of support by the teeth. Nonrigid connectors are indicated when circumstances dictate nonparallel abutment preparations. It also may be used to avoid having to parallel all the abutment teeth for very long span fixed partial dentures.

## QUESTIONS

45. Gold solders are classified in terms of their fineness. The lowest fineness gold solder that should be used is
    1. 725 fineness
    2. 650 fineness
    3. 580 fineness
    4. 500 fineness
    5. Fineness is not a critical factor.
46. To complete the soldering procedure successfully, which of the following are necessary?
    a. Clean surfaces
    b. Preheated castings and investment
    c. Near contact between the surfaces to be soldered
    d. A finely adjusted oxidizing flame
    e. A finely adjusted reducing flame
    1. a, b, and e
    2. b, c, and d

3. a, b, c, and e
4. a, c, and e
5. a and e
6. c and e

47. The resistance to breakage of the solder joint by occlusal forces is mostly determined by the
    1. buccolingual width of the joint
    2. fineness of the solder used
    3. type of retainer involved
    4. occlusogingival thickness of the joint
    5. None of the above
48. What is the chief indication for the use of a nonrigid connector?
    1. The load on the anterior abutment should be decreased.
    2. The abutments cannot be aligned without significant tooth reduction.
    3. The occlusal load on the posterior abutment should be decreased.
    4. Some physiologic tooth movement by each abutment is necessary.
49. The keyway for a nonrigid connector is usually placed in the
    1. most mesial abutment
    2. abutment with the porcelain veneered retainer
    3. abutment with the all metal retainer
    4. most distal abutment
    5. Either abutment can be used.

## TRY-IN OF THE FIXED PARTIAL DENTURE

After determining that the fixed partial denture has no rock and can be seated completely, the dentist evaluates it for marginal integrity, proximal contact, contours, and function. Inadequate proximal contact can be improved by adding solder, and large pits or voids that do not perforate the casting can be filled with solder. However, repair of defective or deficient margins or holes completely through the casting is technically difficult, not usually successful, and often a waste of time. After the occlusal relationships are perfected, the fixed partial denture is ready for placement.

## PORCELAIN

Porcelain is used in fixed restorative dentistry for aesthetic reasons. If it constitutes the entire restoration, it is referred to as a jacket crown. Porcelain may be veneered over a ceramic metal to combine the fit and strength of metal with the aesthetic effects of porcelain.

### Characteristics of Porcelain

Porcelain is primarily a noncrystalline glass composed of silicon and oxygen ($SiO_4$ tetrahedra). Dental porcelain must possess 1) a low fusing temperature, 2) high viscosity, and 3) resistance to devitrification. These properties can be achieved by adding other oxides to the basic structure.

The fusing temperature can be lowered by the addition of glass modifiers such as potassium oxide, sodium oxide, and calcium oxide to reduce the cross linkage between silicon and oxygen. If the modifiers are added in too great a number, however, or if the porcelain is fired too many times, the glass devitrifies or crystallizes. The result is a milky, hard to glaze porcelain.

Porcelain can be classified according to firing temperature. Porcelain which fuses at high temperatures, 2350°F–2500°F (1290°C–1370°C), is used primarily for denture teeth. It is composed of feldspar (70%–90%), quartz (11%–18%), and kaolin (1%–10%). When the feldspar undergoes fusion, it becomes glassy, which gives the porcelain its translucent quality. It serves as a matrix for the high fusing quartz ($SiO_2$), which in turn acts as a matrix for the other materials to fuse around. Kaolin is a clay which holds the particles together before the porcelain is fired.

Low and medium fusing porcelain are similar. They both are made by a process referred to as fritting. In this process, the ingredients of porcelain are fused, quenched, and then ground into a fine powder. When this powder is refined, it fuses at a lower temperature. Some of the constitutents of low and medium fusing porcelain are

|  | Low | Medium |
|---|---|---|
| Silicon dioxide | 69.4% | 64.2% |
| Boric acid | 7.5% | 2.8% |
| Potassium oxide | 8.3% | 8.2% |
| Calcium oxide | 1.9% | |
| Sodium oxide | 4.8% | 1.9% |
| Alumina oxide | 8.7% | 19.0% |

Metallic substances can be added to alter the color or to render the porcelain more opaque. Zirconium oxide, titanium oxide, and tin oxide are used to make the porcelain opaque so that it will mask the metal coping under the porcelain. The metallic substances used to alter the color are indium, which produces yellow; chromium tin, which produces pink; iron oxide, which produces black; and cobalt salts, which produce blue. By varying the combination and percentage of each, shading can be affected.

## Porcelain Jacket Crown

The porcelain jacket crown offers the best aesthetic results of any crown. It achieves that distinction over the ceramic–metal crown because it does not have a metal coping which must be camouflaged. It does not possess the strength of porcelain–metal crowns, how-ever, so anterior teeth with little or no occlusal contact are the best locations for a jacket crown.

The porcelain jacket crown is usually made with an inner core of aluminous porcelain containing 40%–50% alumina. This provides greater strength than high fusing porcelain used alone (28) because the alumina crystals block the propagation of cracks.

The porcelain is made over a matrix of platinum foil. The 0.001 in. thick foil matrix is adapted to the die without wrinkles, then removed and degassed in an oven at 2100°F for 6 min under vacuum. This action removes gaseous impurities and anneals the matrix.

Aluminous porcelain is mixed with distilled water and placed on the matrix in a layer 0.5 mm thick on the labial and incisal surface. It should be thicker on the lingual and proximal surfaces. The porcelain can be condensed by vibrating gently and then blotting to remove excessive moisture. This core is fired at 1500°F–1900°F under vacuum for 6 min. The vacuum is then released and the temperature is raised to 2000°F for 15 min.

The matrix is removed after cooling and translucent porcelain is added. There should be at least 1 mm space for the translucent porcelain on the facial and incisal areas without overcontouring. The jacket crown is dried, set in the oven, and fired at 1500°F–1950°F under total vacuum for 1 min. At this point the jacket crown can be tried in the mouth and the contours adjusted to the final form desired. Special or modifying stains can be added.

The restoration is returned for glazing at a temperature of 1950°F. The temperature is held for 2–4 min without vacuum. Glazing gives the porcelain restoration its smoothness and its lifelike quality.

The matrix is removed from the inside of the crown by grasping a corner of the platinum foil with pliers and twisting it out.

## Porcelain-Fused-to-Metal Restorations

The porcelain-fused-to-metal restoration combines the strength of metal with the cosmetic benefits of porcelain. It consists of a metal coping with porcelain fused over the metal surface. The amount of porcelain depends upon the aesthetic and the functional demands.

DESIGN OF THE METAL FRAMEWORK. The coping should be designed and fabricated so it provides 1) good fit with good marginal integrity; 2) good retention, since the coping is the only part of the restoration in contact with the tooth; 3) proximal contact, unless the contacts are to be restored with porcelain; and 4) support for the porcelain. The metal must be thick enough to resist deformation and have contours which do not cause stress concentration.

The accuracy of the fit of the coping pattern to the die is no different from that sought with any other wax pattern. The outer contours are quite different, however. If the coping is to be covered with porcelain, it should have very little bulk, although it must be at least 0.3–0.5 mm thick to resist deformation. To prevent stress concentration areas to be covered with porcelain must be convex in shape with no sharp corners. No undercuts should be present. The junction of the porcelain to the area not covered by porcelain should be at right angles; this avoids burnishing of the metal and fracture of the porcelain.

The porcelain veneer consists of three layers: 1) the opaque layer which serves to obscure the metal coping; 2) the body porcelain, which constitutes most of the restoration and provides the basic shading to the porcelain (Fig. 5–19); and 3) the incisal porcelain, which is quite translucent and is blended to gradually fade out gingivally.

The occlusal contacts should be in metal because they are more precisely controlled and because metal lends itself better to adjustments if necessary. If porcelain is to be carried onto the occlusal surface, the junction between the porcelain and the metal must not be placed in an area of occlusal contact. If the contact cannot be placed on metal, it should be placed well onto the porcelain. Contact at the junction may produce flow of the metal leading to fracture of the porcelain.

The proximal contact on anterior teeth is made in porcelain because the proximal surface should be translucent. The best stress distribution occurs if the porcelain–metal junction is located lingual to the contact areas.

**PORCELAIN-FUSED-TO-METAL FIXED PARTIAL DENTURES.** Porcelain-fused-to-metal restorations serve well as units in a fixed partial denture because the metal is strong enough to withstand the increased stresses placed upon them. The porcelain must be an even thickness to avoid weakening of the porcelain through uneven stress concentrations.

The pontics are designed in the normal manner (see Pontics). The junction between the porcelain and the metal should not be in an area next to the soft tissues. Preferably the tissue contacts should be in porcelain only to avoid a potentially rough surface.

QUESTIONS

50. Low and medium fusing porcelain are made by a special process called
  1. bisque baking
  2. devitrification
  3. crystallization
  4. fritting
  5. fusion

51. Metallic substances such as indium and cobalt are added to porcelain to
  1. add strength to the porcelain
  2. increase the translucency of the porcelain
  3. provide a matrix around which the other materials fuse
  4. lower the fusion temperature
  5. alter the color or shade

52. What is the chief advantage of the porcelain jacket crown over the porcelain–metal crown?
  1. It is generally more aesthetic.
  2. It is less expensive.

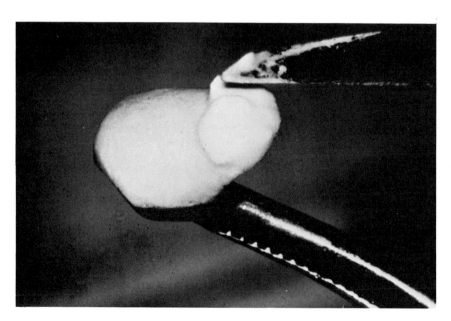

**FIG. 5-19.** Additional layers of the body or gingival porcelain are placed to provide the subtle shadings needed in the veneer.

3. It is easier to adjust and repolish.
4. It usually achieves better marginal fit.

53. What are the layers of porcelain that are fused over the metal coping of a porcelain–metal crown?
    1. Coping, incisal, and body layers
    2. Opaque, body, and incisal layers
    3. Devitrified layer and opaque layer
    4. Body layer and incisal layer
    5. Body layer and devitrified layer

54. How thick must the metal coping be to resist deformation under occlusal pressures?
    1. 0.1–0.3 mm
    2. 0.3–0.5 mm
    3. 0.5–0.75 mm
    4. 0.75–1.1 mm

55. For greatest retention of the porcelain veneer, the coping design should be
    1. convex with undercuts to retain porcelain
    2. convex with no undercuts
    3. convex with sharp angles to distribute stresses
    4. concave on facial surface to provide room for porcelain

56. Occlusal contact should never occur at the junction of the porcelain and the metal of the unveneered area because
    1. prematurities are hard to detect in this area so adjustments are difficult
    2. contact produces flow or burnishing of the metal leading to fracture of the porcelain
    3. bonding in this area is usually weaker
    4. the metal layer is considerably stronger than the porcelain so stress distribution is uneven

## CEMENTATION

### Types of Cement

There are several types of "permanent" cement available. They differ in chemical make-up and in physical characteristics (Table 5–1).

Zinc phosphate cement, first introduced in 1878, has a good compressive strength and film thickness but is not high in tensile strength. Another undesirable trait is that it has a very low pH (3.5) initially and is potentially quite injurious to the pulp. Two layers of cavity varnish applied to the preparation prior to seating the casting minimizes the penetration of the acid into the tubules, however.

Polycarboxylate cement has adequate compressive strength and excellent tensile strength, and it is not too soluble in oral fluids. While its pH is low (4.8), the large size of the polyacrylic acid molecule seems to prevent its penetration into the dentinal tubules. It seems therefore to cause very little, if any, irritation to the pulp, in contrast to zinc phosphate cement (41).

The orthoethoxybenzoic acid (EBA) cement has good compressive strength and adequate tensile strength, and it is not too soluble. However, its film thickness may be great enough to prevent adequate seating of the casting (17).

Zinc oxide–eugenol with polymer reinforcement is not a good permanent cement because of its limited strength.

It appears that the zinc phosphate cement and the polycarboxylate cement represent the two best choices. Zinc phosphate cement is the stronger and also has a long history of reasonable success. In situations where pulpal health is of no concern (endodontically treated teeth or teeth with amalgam or composite build-ups), it is the cement of choice. Polycarboxylate cement is the cement of choice for teeth with large pulps. It is strong enough for fixed partial dentures as well as single crowns.

Neither cement is truly adhesive and both are soluble in oral fluids. Therefore the restoration must supply its own retention via frictional resistance to removal. The marginal fit must be tight to minimize the loss of the soluble cement.

### Cementation of the Restoration

ZINC PHOSPHATE CEMENT. The area must be kept dry during cementation. Cavity varnish can be placed over the dentinal surfaces to prevent penetration of the acid with resultant postoperative sensitivity. A lubricant can be added to the outside of the crown to aid in removal of the cement after the cement has set.

The cement is mixed on a glass slab with a metal spatula. Cooling the glass slab delays the setting reaction so that a maximum amount of powder can be incorporated. No moisture should be present as it produces premature setting of the cement. The powder is set at one end of the slab and divided into several small increments. Several drops of liquid are placed near the other end. A *very* small increment of powder is brought into the liquid and mixed slowly over a wide area for a few seconds. The cement is allowed to sit for several seconds. This incorporation of a small amount of power followed by a delay decreases the speed of the setting reaction.

The mixing process is then continued by adding small increments one at a time. Each increment is mixed for approximately 10–15 sec. The cement is mixed slowly in a circular motion over a wide area of the glass slab. This delays the setting reaction and helps to dissipate some of the heat generated by the exothermic reaction occurring. It also makes it possible to add more power, which decreases the acidity of the cement (23).

Powder is added to the liquid until the desired con-

**Table 5-1.  Commonly Used Cements**

| TYPE | COMPOSITION | COMPRESSIVE STRENGTH (PSI) | FILM THICKNESS (μm) | SOLUBILITY IN DISTILLED WATER (%) | TENSILE STRENGTH (PSI) |
|---|---|---|---|---|---|
| Zinc phosphate | Calcined zinc oxide, magnesium oxide, orthophosphoric acid, water, aluminum phosphate, zinc phosphate | 14,000–16,000 | 25 | 0.20 | 640 |
| Polycarboxylate | Zinc oxide, magnesium oxide, polycarboxylate acid, water | 9900 | 25–48 | 0.05 | 980 |
| EBA zinc oxide and eugenol | Zinc oxide, alumina, eugenol, orthoethoxy benzoic acid | 10,000–15,000 | 50 | 0.02–0.04 | 660 |
| Zinc oxide–eugenol with polymer | Uncalcined zinc oxide, white rosin, zinc acetate, polymethylmethacrylate, eugenol, mineral or vegetable oil | 5600 | 36 | 0.08 | 620 |

sistency is obtained. This is determined by touching the cement with the spatula blade and then raising it. Correctly mixed cement is thick enough to follow the spatula up approximately ¾–1 in. above the slab before falling away.

The cement is applied in a thin layer over all the internal walls of the restoration, and the walls must be dry and clean for best results. Excessive amounts of cement may prevent complete seating of the restoration. Some authorities suggest placing a small amount of cement into the retentive grooves, etc. on the preparation prior to seating the casting to assure cement gets into all the areas.

The restoration should be seated slowly on the tooth. Pressure is applied until the restoration is almost seated. The pressure is eased momentarily to decrease hydraulic pressure and then reapplied to seat the restoration completely. The margins should be checked to assure the restoration is properly placed. If not, it must be immediately removed, cleaned, and then recemented. Failure to remove the restoration quickly may make it very difficult to remove it without damaging it or the preparation.

If the casting is seated completely, the patient can close on an orangewood stick, cotton roll, or inlay seater until the cement has set (10). The cement should be set enough in 5 min to remove excess cement. The explorer tine can be used to see if the cement has hardened. The cement loses its luster when it has set.

Any cement beyond the margins of the restoration must be removed with the explorer tine or some other suitable instrument, because any particle of cement left may serve as a nidus for plaque accumulation. Care must be taken to avoid damaging a margin.

**POLYCARBOXYLATE CEMENT.**  The area must be dry for the cementation process. No debris should be pres-

ent in the casting. The outside of the restoration can be coated with a lubricant to prevent adherence of cement.

The power:liquid ratio for polycarboxylate cement is 1.5:1. The power is measured by a scoop provided. Three drops of liquid are used for each level scoopful of powder. The spatulation time is approximately 30 sec. (9). The consistency of correctly mixed polycarboxylate cement appears rather viscous, especially when compared with zinc phosphate cement. It flows readily enough, however.

The procedures for coating the internal surfaces of the casting and seating the casting are identical with those used with zinc phosphate cement. The tests of whether it has set are its hardness and the loss of surface luster.

**EBA ZINC OXIDE–EUGENOL CEMENT.**  The area to be cemented with EBA zinc oxide–eugenol cement is prepared in the same way as areas to cemented with zinc phosphate and polycarboxylate cements.

The liquid:powder ratio for EBA cement is 4 drops of liquid to 1 level scoop of powder. The powder is quickly incorporated into the liquid and mixed for 60 sec. The inside of the restoration is coated and then seated with pressure. Excess cement is wiped off with a cotton roll or gauze 2 × 2 and allowed to set.

### QUESTIONS

57. The chief advantage of zinc phosphate cement is its
    1. good compressive strength
    2. lack of irritation to the pulp
    3. film thickness
    4. low solubility

58. The biggest advantage of polycarboxylate cement is its
    1. good compressive strength
    2. lack of irritation to the pulp

3. low film thickness
4. low solubility
5. ease of mixing and using

59. The setting reaction of zinc phosphate cement can be delayed by
    1. adding less powder to the liquid
    2. mixing slowly
    3. adding 2–3 drops of water
    4. cooling the mixing slab
    5. 2 and 4 above

60. Even correctly mixed zinc phosphate cement is irritating to the pulp. How can this irritation be minimized?
    1. Place 2 coats of cavity varnish over the preparations.
    2. Add 1 drop of eugenol to the cement after mixing.
    3. Apply eugenol with a cotton pellet to the preparation.
    4. Decrease the liquid:powder ratio of the cement.

## POSTCEMENTATION CARE AND INSTRUCTIONS

No matter what the cement used, all excess must be removed. Dental floss must be pulled through the contact areas. It may be helpful to tie a knot in the floss and pull it through the embrasure area to help remove the cement.

The occlusion is checked to assure that cementation has not left the restoration in premature occlusion (Fig. 5–20). The patient should be asked to report any discomfort, sensation of pressure, or perceived alteration of the bite, because the occlusion may require further adjustment. Premature occlusion may result in

1. premature wear of the restoration and/or its antagonist
2. alteration of the occlusal relationships resulting in premature wear of other teeth or restorations
3. excessive stresses on the periodontal tissues resulting in changes in the periodontal membrane and loss of bony support
4. stress upon the temporomandibular joint and the muscles of mastication leading to pain in the joint and muscles, popping, and/or trismus
5. hypersensitivity of the tooth itself

The patient should be instructed that postoperative sensitivity is possible. Sensitivity is more likely to occur with zinc phosphate cement than with polycarboxylate or EBA cements.

QUESTION

61. The patient complains of sensitivity a few days after cementation of a fixed partial denture with polycarboxylate cement. What is the most likely cause?
    1. Irritation from the cement
    2. A loose retainer
    3. Premature occlusion
    4. An open margin
    5. None of the above

## REFERENCES

1. ASGAR K: Elastic impression materials. Dent Clin North Am 15 (1):93, 1971
2. BAUM L: Advanced Restorative Dentistry Modern Materials and Techniques. Philadelphia, WB Saunders, 1973, p 199
3. BEHREND DA: The mandibular posterior fixed partial denture. Prosthet Dent 37 (6):622–638, 1977

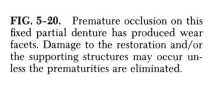

FIG. 5-20. Premature occlusion on this fixed partial denture has produced wear facets. Damage to the restoration and/or the supporting structures may occur unless the prematurities are eliminated.

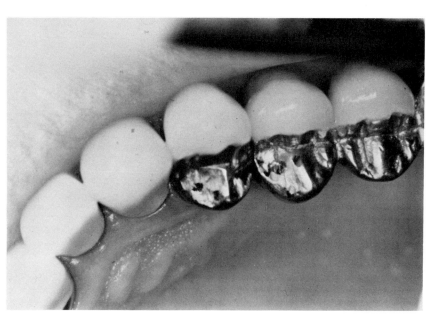

4. BELL BH, GRAINGER DA: Basic Operative Dentistry Procedures. Philadelphia, Lea & Febiger, 1971, p 319

5. BERRY TG: Tissue response to pontic materials and design. Tenn Den Assoc 51 (4) p 283–288, 1971

6. BINON P: Restorative impression techniques. In Clinical Dentistry, Vol 4. New York, Harper & Row, 1976, p 1–16

7. CHARBENEAU GT et al: Principles and Practice of Operative Dentistry. Philadelphia, Lea & Febiger, 1975, p 390

8. COLMAN H: Selection of retainer designs. In Clinical Dentistry, Vol. 4. New York, Harper & Row, 1976

9. EAMES WB et al: Proportioning and mixing cements: a comparison of working times. Operative Dent 2 (3):97–104, 1977

10. EAMES WB et al: Technique to improve the seating of castings. Am Dent Assoc 96 (3):432–437, 1978

11. FISHER DW: Conservative management of gingival tissues for crowns. Dent Clin North Am 20 (2):273–284, 1976

12. GEIGER A, HIRSCHFELD L: Minor Tooth Movement in General Practice. St Louis, CV Mosby, 1974, p 9

13a,b GILMORE HW et al: Operative Dentistry. St. Louis, CV Mosby, 1977; a, p 263; b, 278

14. GLICKMAN I: Clinical Periodontology, Philadelphia, WB Saunders, 1964, p 75

15. GREENER EH et al: Materials Science in Dentistry. Baltimore, Williams & Wilkins, 1972, p 204

16. GUYER SE: Multiple preparations for fixed prosthodontics. Prosthe Dent 23:529–546, 1970

17. HEMBREE JH et al: Film thickness of cements beneath complete crowns. J Prosthet Dent 39 5:533–538, 1978

18. HENRY PJ et al: Tissue changes beneath fixed partial dentures. J Prosthet Dent 16:937–947, 1966

19. HOOD JAA et al: Stress and deflection of three different pontic designs. J Prosthet Dent 33 (1):54–59, 1975

20. JOHNSTON JF et al: Modern Practice in Crown and Bridge Prosthodontics. Philadelphia, WB Saunders, 1971, p 11

21. KANTOR ME, PINES MS: A comparative study of restorative techniques for pulpless teeth. J Prosthet Dent 38 (4):405–412, 1977

22. KAUFMAN EG et al: Factors influencing the retention of cemented gold castings. J Prosthet Dent 11:487–502, 1961

23. KAUFMAN EG et al: Factors influencing the retention of cemented gold castings: the cementing medium. J Prosthet Dent 16:731–739, 1966

24. KORNFELD M: Mouth Rehabilitation, Vol 1. St. Louis, CV Mosby, 1974, p 48

25. LAU VMS: The reinforcement of endodontically treated teeth. Dent Clin North Am 20 (2):313–328, 1976

26. LUND MR: Current findings for spruing the cast gold restoration. Curr Ther Dent 6:263–266, 1977

27. MALONE W, MANNING J: Electrosurgery in restorative dentistry. J Prosthet Dent 20:417–425, 1968

28. MCLEAN J: The alumina reinforced porcelain jacket crown. J Am Dent Assoc 75 (3):621–628, 1967

29. MITCHELL P: Selection of abutment teeth. In Clinical Dentistry, Vol 4. New York, Harper & Row, 1976, pp 1–11

30. PARKINSON EF: Excessive crown contours facilitate endemic plaque niches. J Prosthet Dent 35:424–429, 1976

31a,b PHILLIPS RW: Science of Dental Materials. Philadelphia, WB Saunders, 1973; a, p 110; b, 393

32. RAMFJORD SP, ASH MM: Occlusion. Philadelphia, WB Saunders, 1966, p 67

33. REISBICK MH, SHILLINGBURG HT: Effect of preparation geometry on retention and resistance of cast gold restorations. J Calif Dent Assoc 3(4): 51–59, 1975

34. ROSS IF: Problems connected with combined periodontal therapy and fixed restorative care. Dent Clin North Am 16:47–57, 1972

35. SCHLUGER S et al: Periodontal Disease. Philadelphia, Lea & Febiger, 1977, p 590

36. SELLERS WR: Selection and accuracy of impression materials for the indirect procedure. Curr Ther Dent 6:263–266, 1977

37. SHILLINGBURG HT: Fundamentals of Fixed Prosthodontics. Chicago, Bach-Und Zeitschriften-Verlag "Die Quintessenz," 1976, p 304

38. SHILLINGBURG HT: Conservative preparations for cast restorations. Dent Clin North Am 20 (2):259–271, 1976

39. SHILLINGBURG HT et al: Preparations for Cast Gold Restorations. Chicago, Bach-Und Zeitschriften-Verlag "Die Quintessenz," 1974, p 43

40. SHILLINGBURG HR et al: Fundamentals of Fixed Prosthodontics. Chicago, Bach-Und Zeitschriften-Verlag "Die Quintessenz," 1976, p 9

41. SMITH DC: Dental cements. Dent Clin North Am 15 (1):28, 1971

42. STEIN RS: Pontic-residual ridge relationship: a research report. J Prosthet Dent 16:251–285, 1966

43. STEIN RS, GLICKMAN I: Prosthodontic considerations essential for gingival health. Dent Clin North Am:177–188, 1960

44. STURDEVANT CM et al: The Art and Science of Operative Dentistry. New York, McGraw-Hill, 1968, p 314

45. WAGMAN SS: The role of coronal contours in gingival health. J Prosthet Dent 37 (3):280–287, 1977

46. WILLEY RL: Retention in the preparation of teeth for cast restorations. J Prosthet Dent 35 (5):526–531, 1976

## ANSWER KEY

| | | | |
|---|---|---|---|
| 1. 1 | 17. 5 | 32. 3 | 47. 4 |
| 2. 5 | 18. 4 | 33. 4 | 48. 2 |
| 3. 4 | 19. 4 | 34. 1 | 49. 1 |
| 4. 4 | 20. 3 | 35. 5 | 50. 4 |
| 5. 1 | 21. 4 | 36. 1 | 51. 5 |
| 6. 1 | 22. 3 | 37. 2 | 52. 1 |
| 7. 5 | 23. 1 | 38. 1 | 53. 2 |
| 8. 1 | 24. 1 | 39. 4 | 54. 2 |
| 9. 2 | 25. 2 | 40. 5 | 55. 2 |
| 10. 1 | 26. 3 | 41. 1 | 56. 2 |
| 11. 3 | 27. 2 | 42. 4 | 57. 1 |
| 12. 5 | 28. 1 | 43. 5 | 58. 2 |
| 13. 3 | 29. 2 | 44. 4 | 59. 5 |
| 14. 1 | 30. 1 | 45. 3 | 60. 1 |
| 15. 2 | 31. 5 | 46. 3 | 61. 3 |
| 16. 3 | | | |

# 6
# REMOVABLE PROSTHODONTICS

## PART I
## PARTIAL REMOVABLE
## PROSTHODONTICS

### Gerald S. Weintraub

Proper design of the removable partial denture in concert with a well thought out and properly executed treatment plan to prepare the oral cavity for receiving the prosthesis contributes to the preservation of remaining natural teeth, osseous structure, and gingival tissues. The partial denture also aids in the maintenance of tooth position and occlusion; at the same time it restores the patient's ability to masticate, improves phonation, and enhances appearance. The preservation of oral tissues, in conjunction with the improvement and/or restoration of function, points out the legitimacy of the concept of the removable partial denture as a prevention oriented treatment modality. The partial denture included in a well-planned oral health care program is not simply a device with which missing teeth are replaced.

Mandel (33) stated that "all dental procedures must be considered not only in terms of dealing with past or present disease but in terms of preventing future disease as well." Included in these dental procedures are those involving removable prosthodontics. Prosthetic dentistry may prevent loss of function and therefore should be considered tertiary prevention. Specific objectives of prevention can be related to removable partial dentures, factors of the prosthesis design, and treatment involving it (Table 6–1). All phases of removable prosthodontic therapy (Table 6–2), from examination and diagnosis through postinsertion adjustments and recall appointments, have preventive implications. Some are obvious, some subtle, but all are important in the overall maintenance of remaining oral

tissues in a state of health. For the purpose of this discussion, the assumption is made that primary preventive therapy (prevention of initiation of disease) and secondary preventive therapy (prevention of recurrence and progression of disease) have been performed and are being maintained by the dentist and the patient. Obviously tertiary preventive therapy such as prosthetic dentistry is dependent upon successful primary and secondary controls.

It is important to note that many factors of removable partial denture design are dictated by the nature of the support offered to the prosthesis, that is, by the position and number of remaining natural teeth and edentulous areas in the involved arch. Two distinct types of removable partial dentures reflect the support systems. The first is the all-tooth-supported denture, used when natural teeth border the edentulous area or areas. The second is the distal extension denture, used when natural teeth are present only at the anterior border of the edentulous area or areas.

The removable partial denture has no routinely available alternatives in a situation such as a partially edentulous arch with only six or eight anterior natural teeth remaining, which is commonly seen. The restoration of this situation with a bilateral distal extension removable partial denture using extracoronal direct retainers (clasps) offers a formidable challenge to the prothodontist. The challenge lies in the dentist's ability to create a restoration that satisfies the criterion paramount in any phase of removable prosthodontics: to preserve the remaining tissues in a state of health.

**Table 6-1.** Design Factors of Removable Partial Dentures Related to Disease Prevention

A. Prevention of the lesion of occlusal traumatism
   1. Clasp assembly design
   2. Proximal guiding planes
   3. Rest seat preparation and location
   4. Occlusal scheme
   5. Anatomic vs. functional form of residual ridge
   6. Resistance of the prosthesis to rotation-producing forces
B. Controlling resorption of residual ridges
   1. Denture base extension and adaptation
   2. Anatomic vs. functional form of residual ridge
   3. Rest seat location
   4. Occlusal scheme
   5. Major connector design
   6. Recall and maintenance regimen
C. Prevention of tissue injury
   1. Proximal guiding planes
   2. Indirect retainers
   3. Major connector design
   4. Minor connector design
   5. Laboratory technique
   6. Resistance of prosthesis to rotation-producing forces
D. Prevention of carious lesions
   1. Clasp assembly design (minimal tooth contact)
   2. Reinforcement of primary and secondary prevention
   3. Care of the prosthesis
   4. Framework design (minimal tooth contact)
   5. Recall and maintenance regimen

The tissues involved include the abutment teeth, periodontium, mucoperiosteum, and osseous structure of the residual ridge.

Mechanically the problem is one of equitable stress distribution to the abutment teeth and supporting residual ridge. Lack of proper stress distribution is manifested as abutment tooth mobility and/or increase of the resorptive process of the residual ridge. This is indicative of failure of partial denture therapy.

## DIAGNOSIS AND TREATMENT PLANNING

Diagnosis is the systematic investigation of an unnatural condition, the identification of this condition, and the determination of its cause. Data are obtained from dental and medical histories, extraoral and intraoral examination, roentgenographic survey, and analysis of articulated diagnostic casts.

### Visual Examination

The number of restored teeth, signs of recurrent decay, and evidence of decalcification should be noted before a decision is made on the use of unrestored teeth as potential abutment selections. Evidence of periodontal disease and mobility of teeth should also be noted and further investigated by roentgenographic examination, because they affect the selection of suitable abutments.

Visual and digital examinations of the edentulous areas reveal the quality of the residual ridge, which influences to a great extent the treatment planning and design phase of therapy with a removable partial denture. Examination also reveals palatal and mandibular tori and other conditions which may require surgical intervention to prepare the mouth for the prosthesis.

### Oral Examination

A complete oral examination should be preceded by a thorough oral prophylaxis, excavation of carious lesions, and placement of treatment restorations. A complete series of diagnostic roentgenograms, periodontal charting including pocket depth and mobility, and impressions to obtain accurate diagnostic casts are also necessary. The data derived from these procedures enable the operator to formulate a total treatment plan which will provide the appropriate foundation for the replacement of missing teeth with a removable partial denture.

### Roentgenographic Analysis

In addition to examining the teeth for pathology, it is important to measure roentgenographically the quality of the alveolar support of potential abutment teeth, because these teeth will be called upon to withstand increased forces in their role as abutments for the removable prosthesis. A more critical evaluation must be made regarding the support offered to abutment teeth adjacent to distal extension edentulous areas. Need for splinting to an adjacent tooth, selection of clasp assembly design, and selection of impression materials and technique are among the many considerations of therapy directly related to the amount of alveolar support present.

### Medical and Dental Histories

A procedure that has gained attention and importance over the past few years is the recording of a thorough medical history. Serious illness, past and present, should be noted since such an illness might necessitate prophylactic or remedial medications before and after dental treatment. Allergies, current medication, family history, tobacco and alcohol habits all play a role in constructing a treatment plan that is correct for the individual.

Past dental history, particularly past experiences with removable prostheses, contributes valuable data which, if overlooked, can result in treatment failure. The patient should be encouraged to describe what is right and what is wrong with any existing dentures. Refinement of these dentures into "treatment prostheses" based upon the patient's complaints and the operator's

**Table 6-2.** Flow Chart of Removable Partial Denture Clinic and Laboratory Procedures

I. Examination and diagnosis

Oral surgery   Endodontics   Periodontics   Survey and design   Diagnostic casts

II. Restorative therapy

Single tooth restorations   Fixed prosthodontics   Abutment tooth restorations

III. Removable partial prosthodontic therapy

A. Preliminary impression
   1. Survey cast to determine need for tooth modification
   2. Construct final impression tray
B. Final impression
   1. Modify tooth contours as indicated
   2. Prepare rest seats in natural tooth structure
   3. Make impression
   4. Pour cast
C. Preparation of final cast for duplication
   1. Survey and design on final cast
   2. Place ledges, parallel block out, relief wax
   3. Duplicate, wax, invest, cast, finish and fit framework
D. Initial seating of framework, intermaxillary records, tooth selection
   1. Adjust framework
   2. Evaluate occlusion
   3. Alter cast impression (if indicated)
   4. Make face-bow transfer
   5. Take centric occlusion/relation record
   6. Transfer cast to articulator
   7. Select artificial teeth
   8. Arrange artificial teeth and wax denture bases

E. Trial denture appointment
   1. Evaluate vertical dimension of occlusion and vertical dimension of rest
   2. Evaluate centric relation/occlusion
   3. Evaluate aesthetics and phonetics
   4. Take eccentric records as indicated and set articulator
   5. Refine set up in centric occlusion
   6. Refine set up to desired eccentric occlusal scheme
   7. Refine waxing of denture bases
   8. Invest denture and process bases
   9. Remount and equilibrate after processing
   10. Preserve face-bow record if indicated
   11. Finish and polish prosthesis
F. Insertion of prosthesis
   1. Evaluate seating of framework
   2. Evaluate and refine base extensions
   3. Evaluate occlusion, remount on articulator, and equilibrate if indicated
   4. Reinforce home care instructions of restoration
   5. Reinforce oral hygiene procedures
   6. Reappoint for postinsertion evaluation
G. Postinsertion adjustments
H. Recall appointments

clinical interpretation of these complaints is a valuable diagnostic and therapeutic tool in the determination of the final treatment plan.

## Diagnostic Casts

Impressions for diagnostic casts may be taken with irreversible hydrocolloid. They should accurately reproduce the remaining teeth, residual ridge, and adjoining structures. All tissues to be contacted by the finished prosthesis (framework and bases) must be captured in the impression. Maxillary landmarks include the hard palate, buccal and labial vestibules, muscle attachments, hamular notches, and tuberosities. Mandibular landmarks include the buccal, labial and lingual vestibules, retromolar pads, buccal shelf areas, and muscle attachments.

Articulated diagnostic casts serve a number of purposes. Since they disclose conditions as they existed at the start of the rehabilitative procedure, it is prudent to maintain an unaltered set of diagnostic casts to serve as a future reference. The casts also make it possible to evaluate the occlusal scheme of the natural teeth so that the need for any restorations or any occlusal correction in preparation of the mouth for the removable partial denture can be determined. In a preliminary survey analysis diagnostic casts provide information regarding the need for abutment tooth recontouring by either the placement of a restoration or intraoral adjustments. Diagnostic casts can also be used in the

construction of individualized impression trays and as visual aids in patient education.

It is impossible to design a prosthesis for a dental arch without a determination of how that arch relates to the opposing arch. Therefore opposing casts should be articulated with the use of a face-bow, a centric relation and/or a centric occlusion record, and eccentric records that allow a close approximation of the dynamics of the patient's occlusion to be simulated on the articulator. Stable and retentive record bases and occlusion rims are frequently required for this procedure.

## Indications for a Removable Partial Denture

The method of preference for replacing missing teeth is by means of a fixed partial denture. When the criteria for a fixed restoration are not met or when other reasons contraindicate a fixed partial denture, the removable partial denture becomes the restoration of necessity.

DISTAL EXTENSIONS. Removable partial dentures are indicated to restore edentulous areas posterior to the natural teeth (distal extension). Careful analysis is necessary to determine if edentulous areas distal to first molars need to be restored. Replacement of first molars with a cantilevered fixed prosthesis (generally involving the canine and two premolars as abutments) rather than a removable denture may at times satisfy the restorative requirements of selected patients.

**LENGTH OF EDENTULOUS SPAN.** Ante (1) stated that "in fixed bridges the combined pericemental area of the abutment teeth should be equal to or greater than the tooth or teeth to be replaced." Long unilateral fixed bridges do not meet this criterion and subject the abutment teeth to excessive forces. A removable partial denture in this same situation derives support from abutment teeth on the opposite side of the arch and provides cross arch stabilization, thus making the removable prosthesis the restoration of choice.

**NEED FOR BILATERAL BRACING AND SUPPORT.** Unilateral or bilateral posterior tooth-bordered edentulous spaces may be more effectively restored with a removable partial denture than with unilateral fixed restorations in the presence of abutment teeth that have lost significant support as a result of periodontal disease. A properly designed removable partial denture provides a splinting effect by cross arch stabilization, thus supporting the weakened abutment teeth. Combinations of fixed and removable components are frequently employed to treat these difficult situations.

**RESTORATION OF FACIAL CONTOURS.** It is often necessary to restore facial contours when there is a large anterior edentulous space. Residual ridge morphology following resorption seldom allows for a fixed restoration to replace the anterior teeth in a labiolingual position which will provide adequate lip support for a good aesthetic and functional result. The denture base of a removable prosthesis with a fully extended flange allows the placement of the artificial teeth in a natural position.

Restoration of facial contours is less frequently an indication for a removable prosthesis to replace posterior missing teeth, except where defects have been caused by trauma or surgery.

**TEMPORARY RESTORATIONS.** Interim, transitional, and treatment partial dentures can play an important role in the treatment plan leading either to a fixed prosthesis or a "definitive" removable partial denture.

### Surveying and the Initial Survey Analysis

No treatment plan for the partially edentulous patient is complete without an initial survey analysis of diagnostic casts. A surveyor determines the relative parallelism of two or more surfaces of the teeth or other parts of the diagnostic cast. Surveying the diagnostic cast identifies the most favorable path of prosthesis placement by locating tooth surfaces that are or can be altered to be parallel. These parallel tooth surfaces can then function as guiding planes during the placement and removal of the prosthesis. Also during the initial survey analysis potential retentive areas on abutment

teeth are located and measured so that these teeth can be restored in a way that will allow as ideal a crown morphology as possible for the selected clasp assembly design. Exostoses, lingual tori, severely lingually inclined mandibular posterior teeth, and questionable osseous or soft tissue contours of edentulous areas are also analyzed at this time to determine if tooth recontouring, extraction, preprosthetic oral surgery, or selection of a different path of insertion is required as part of the overall rehabilitative procedure.

## REMOVABLE PARTIAL DENTURE DESIGN

### Classification of Partially Edentulous Arches

A widely accepted classification system of partially edentulous arches was proposed by Kennedy (28a). Kennedy's system (Fig. 6–1) places any partially edentulous arch into one of four groups. Each class, except

**FIG. 6–1.** Classification of partially edentulous arches, according to Kennedy. A. Class I. B. Class II. C. Class III. D. Class IV. E. Class III, modification 1. F. Class I, modification 1. (Weintraub G S, Goyal B K: J Prev Dent 3:30–42, 1976)

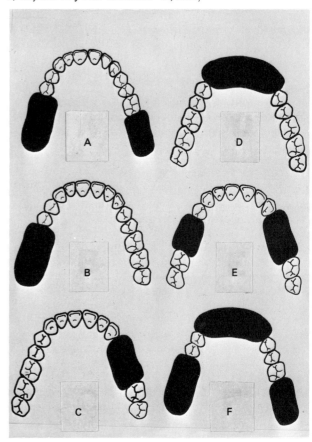

Class IV, contains subdivisions based on additional edentulous areas (Figs. 6–1E and 6–1F). This classification system does not and should not dictate design of the prosthesis, but it does facilitate communication. Anyone who is familiar with the classification is instantly aware of factors that should be considered in the design of a prosthesis for a particular class. For example, the presence of one (Class II) or two (Class I) edentulous areas that have no posterior teeth to lend support to the planned prosthesis is a feature common to Classes I and II (Figs. 6–1A, 6–1B, and 6–1F). Contrast this with the common feature of Classes III and IV (Figs. 6–1C, 6–1D, and 6–1E) in which all edentulous areas are bordered anteriorly and posteriorly by remaining teeth. This classification identifies the system of support offered by the arch to the prosthesis.

A major problem in removable partial denture design is that of the distal extension removable partial denture (Classes I and II). The support for this type of prosthesis is based upon two functionally different systems (1) the remaining teeth and associated periodontal structures and (2) the residual ridge and mucoperiosteum. The finished prosthesis should use both systems of support without placing one or the other under excessive stress. If this is accomplished, the residual hard and soft tissues are more likely to remain healthy.

### Components of the Typical Removable Partial Denture

Several components are generally included in the typical removable partial denture (Fig. 6–2). The base supports the artificial teeth and effects the transfer of occlusal forces to the supporting structures. The major connector unites the parts of the prosthesis located on one side of the arch with those located on the opposite side. The minor connectors join the major connector with all other components of the removable partial denture. Direct retainers (clasps) limit the displacement of the removable partial denture in an occlusal direction. Indirect retainers limit the movement of a denture base away from the tissues. Indirect retention is a feature of design in an all-tooth-supported prosthesis if one abutment bordering an edentulous span is not clasped. Artificial teeth prevent further disorganization of the dental arch, restore function, and improve appearance and phonation. Occlusal and/or cingulum rests support the prosthesis upon the abutment teeth and transfer occlusal forces to the abutment teeth.

CLASP ASSEMBLY DESIGN.    A clasp assembly consists of an occlusal or cingulum rest, a retentive clasp arm, and a reciprocal component (Fig. 6–3). The rest, which maintains the prosthesis in its planned location in relation to teeth and soft tissues, should be designed to transmit forces along the long axis of the abutment tooth. This is best accomplished by carefully planning the size (39) and the slope (34) of the floor of rest seat preparations (Fig. 6–4). The objectives of rest seat preparations can best be met when the rest seats are placed in a cast restoration.

The contribution of the retentive clasp arm design to the overall retention of the prosthesis must be placed in its proper perspective. Retention for the removable partial denture is achieved by 1) placing retentive elements (clasps) on the abutment teeth and 2) by the accurate adaptation of denture bases and, at times, major connectors to the underlying tissues. A good rule of thumb to follow is that, as the partially edentulous state of any given patient approaches the completely edentulous state, primary retention of the prosthesis should

FIG. 6-2.   Components of the typical removable partial denture. **a.** Denture bases. **b.** Major connector. **c.** Minor connector. **d.** Direct retainer. **e.** Indirect retainer. **f.** Artifical teeth. **g.** Occlusal rest. (Weintraub G S, Goyal B K: J Prev Dent 3:30–42, 1976)

FIG. 6-3.   Typical clasp assembly consisting of **(a)** an occlusal rest, **(b)** a retentive clasp arm, and **(a)** a reciprocal clasp arm. (Weintraub G S, Goyal B K: J Prev Dent 3:30–42, 1976)

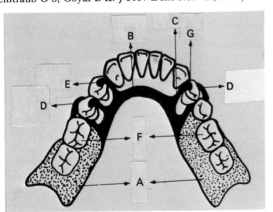

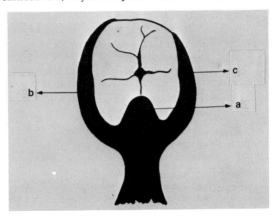

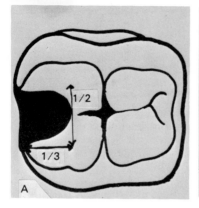
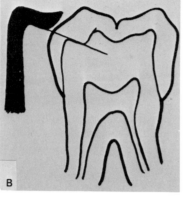

**FIG. 6-4.** Rest seat preparation. A. The rest seat prepared on posterior teeth should extend one-third of the mesiodistal dimension of the tooth and one-half of the buccolingual dimension of the tooth measured between cusp tips. B. The angle formed by the floor of the rest seat preparation and the proximal tooth surface should be 90° or less. (Weintraub G S, Goyal B K: J Prev Den 3:30–42, 1976)

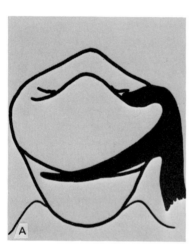
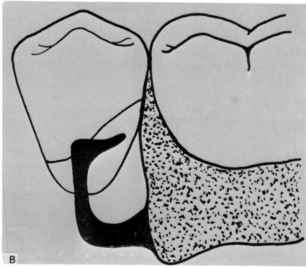

**FIG. 6-5.** A. Retentive terminus of the circumferential clasp arm positioned on gingival one-third of the abutment tooth. B. Retentive terminus of the bar clasp arm positioned on the gingival one-third of the abutment Tooth. (Weintraub G S, Goyal K B: J Prev Dent 3:30–42, 1976)

be achieved through the relationship between denture base–major connector components and the supporting tissues. This can be accomplished by using direct retainers such as clasps to support and stabilize the abutment teeth and to augment retention of the prosthesis rather than to serve as the sole retaining mechanism. Translation of this concept into clinical practice helps to prevent loss of remaining natural dentition. To consider clasp retention as the only mechanism of removable partial denture retention can lead to a potentially destructive situation.

Two commonly selected retentive designs used on abutments bordering all-tooth-supported edentulous spans are the circumferential (Akers) and bar (Roach) clasp arms. Their selection for use on abutment teeth on all-tooth-supported removable partial dentures depends primarily on the survey analysis, the need for abutment tooth restorations, and aesthetic considerations. More critical factors come into play when a clasp assembly is designed for abutment teeth adjacent to distal extension edentulous spans.

An important factor in clasp design and selection that has preventive implications is clasp location on the abutment tooth. The circumferential arm requires a survey line that allows placement of the retentive terminus on the gingival one-third of the crown and placement of the rigid portion of the arm no further occlusally than the junction of the gingival and middle thirds (36) (Fig. 6–5A). The bar clasp arm, regardless of its design modification, also requires a survey line that allows placement of the retentive terminus on the gingival one-third of the crown (Fig. 6–5B).

The planned low positioning of clasp arms permits

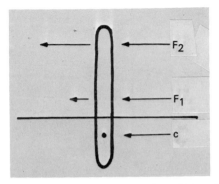

**FIG. 6-6.** The pole can better resist the force ($F_1$) applied closer to its rotation (c) than the same magnitude of force ($F_2$) applied further away. (Weintraub G S, Goyal B K: J Prev Dent 3:30–42, 1976)

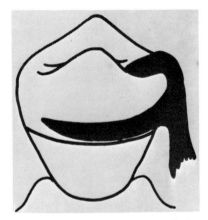

**FIG. 6-7.** Planned positioning of a reciprocal clasp arm at the junction of the gingival and middle thirds of the abutment tooth. (Weintraub G S, Goyal B K: J Prev Dent 3:30–42, 1976)

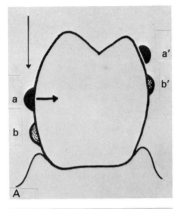

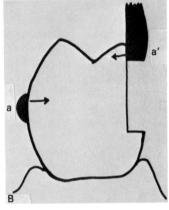

**FIG. 6-8.** A. Generally natural tooth contours permit the retentive clasp arm (a) to contact the tooth well before contact is made by the reciprocal arm (a'). Not until the retentive arm is fully seated (b) does the reciprocal arm (b') contact the tooth. B. A cast restoration with a lingual wall prepared parallel to the path of insertion allows simultaneous contact of the reciprocal component (a') and the retentive clasp arm (a) with the abutment tooth. (Weintraub G S, Goyal B K: J Prev Dent 3:30–42, 1976)

the abutment teeth to resist horizontal and torquing forces better than if the retentive components were located further occlusally. The physical principle involved can be illustrated by applying the same magnitude of force on different locations to a pole driven into the ground (Fig. 6–6). Properly planned positioning of retentive clasp arms can be achieved by a thorough understanding of survey analysis in conjunction with selective recontouring of the abutment teeth or by placement of cast restorations.

There are two factors important in the design of the reciprocal component of the clasp assembly. First, when fully seated on the abutment tooth, the reciprocal clasp arm should be located no further occlusally than the junction of the gingival and middle thirds of the crown (Fig. 6–7). The same rationale applies to the location of the reciprocal arms as was described for the retentive arms. Second, the reciprocal arm must be

placed on a tooth surface prepared parallel to the path of insertion of the prosthesis in order to fulfill its function, which is to resist the force exerted on the abutment tooth as the retentive clasp arm flexes over the height of contour during placement and removal of the prosthesis. Generally the reciprocal arm does not resist the force created by the flexing retentive arm when the clasp assembly is placed on natural unrestored tooth contours (Fig. 6–8A). Reciprocation can be more effectively created by the use of cast abutment restorations (Fig. 6–8B).

**PROXIMAL GUIDING PLANES.** The term, guiding planes, is defined as two or more parallel vertical surfaces of abutment teeth so shaped as to direct a prosthesis during placement and removal (19) (Fig. 6–9). Guide planes decrease the transmission of destructive forces

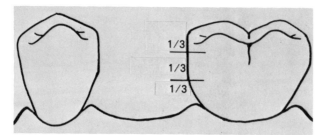

**FIG. 6–9.** Guiding plane surfaces prepared on teeth bordering an all-tooth-supported span can extend to the junction of the gingival and middle thirds of the teeth. (Weintraub G S, Goyal B K: J Prev Dent 3:30–42, 1976)

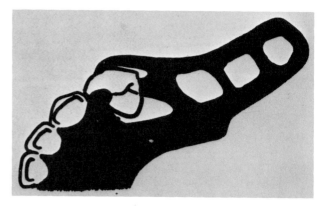

**FIG. 6–10.** Linguoplate, a commonly used mandibular major connector. (Weintraub G S, Goyal B K: J Prev Dent 3:30–42, 1976)

on abutment teeth during the placement and the removal of the prosthesis. They allow the patient to use tactile ability to insert the removable partial denture along the correct and repeatable path. Because using this path ensures that the reciprocal and retentive components function as planned, the chances of soft tissue injury during placement and removal are minimized.

Guiding plane surfaces should extend no further gingivally than the junction of the gingival and middle thirds of the crown for all-tooth-supported removable partial dentures (Fig. 6–9). To extend them the entire length of the proximal tooth surface would cause the minor connectors of the framework to impinge on the gingival tissues.

A key factor in using preventive concepts in clasp assembly design is tooth contour. Therefore, if during the treatment–planning phase it is found that the abutment tooth contours do not permit the application of these concepts, proper restorative procedures should be prescribed to alter unfavorable contours by selective grinding or by cast restorations. This approach toward removable partial denture therapy is consistent with the role of the removable partial denture in comprehensive dental care.

MAJOR CONNECTORS.     Proper stress distribution is important for the preservation of remaining teeth and residual ridges. Therefore major connectors must be rigid so that stresses applied to any one portion of the denture may be distributed effectively over the entire supporting area, including abutment teeth and mucoperiosteum. Soft tissue injury can be prevented by locating the major connectors in a favorable relation to moving tissues and, at the same time, avoiding impingement of gingival tissues. Areas of nonsupporting tissue underlying major connectors must be relieved from the connector to prevent settling and subsequent tissue injury.

*Mandibular Major Connectors.* The most frequently used mandibular major connector is the lingual bar. Features of design that contribute to tissue health include adequate relief from underlying nonsupporting tissues, proper cross-sectional form, and proper location in relation to gingival tissues and tissues on the floor of the mouth. The superior border of the lingual bar should be positioned at least 4 mm below the lingual gingival margins, while the inferior border must not interfere with the functional activity of the tissues on the floor of the mouth.

The second most frequently used mandibular major connector is the linguoplate, also referred to as a Kennedy Blanket (Fig. 6–10). In removable partial denture design no component should be included unless it has a specific function and rationale; the linguoplate should not be used routinely or indiscriminately, but only when indicated. There are several indications for the linguoplate, however (18):

1. Insufficient room for the placement of a conventional lingual bar.
2. Class I partially edentulous arches in which the residual ridges have undergone excessive vertical resorption. Little resistance to horizontal displacement is offered by flat residual ridges, and coverage of the lingual vertical tooth surfaces with a linguoplate provides this resistance. (Fig. 6–11).
3. Questionable prognosis of one or more of the remaining mandibular anterior teeth. If a linguoplate is used as major connector, an extracted tooth can be easily replaced without remaking the prosthesis.
4. Need for indirect retention in Kennedy Class I and II arches. An indirect retainer is mechanically most effective when placed as far anteriorly as possible and at right angles to the fulcrum line drawn between the two primary abutment teeth. Therefore, a linguoplate is effective as an indirect retainer only when there is a distinct arc of the anterior teeth (Fig. 6–12). To direct forces transmitted by the linguoplate along the long axis of the teeth contacted rest

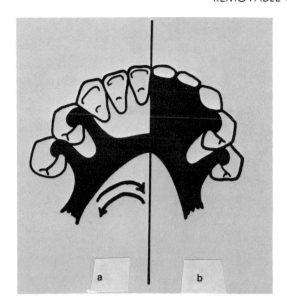

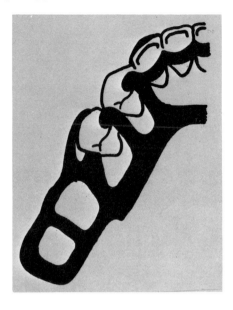

**FIG. 6-11.** The lingual bar (**a**) offers no resistance to horizontal rotational forces as does the linguoplate (**b**) by virtue of its contact with vertical tooth surfaces. (Weintraub G S, Goyal B K: J Prev Dent 3:30–42, 1976)

**FIG. 6-13.** The continuous bar retainer incorporates design features of the lingual bar and the linguoplate. (Weintraub G S, Goyal B K: J Prev Dent 3:30–42, 1976)

**FIG. 6-12.** A. A linguoplate placed on teeth that present little or no curve does not serve as an effective indirect retainer. B. A linguoplate placed on teeth with a marked curve is effective. (Weintraub G S, Goyal B K: J Prev Dent 3:30–42, 1976)

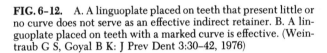

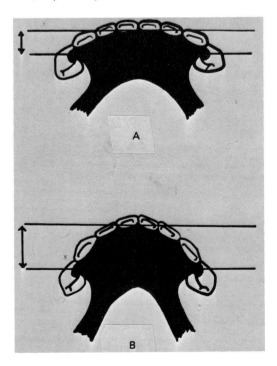

seats must be prepared on all teeth or at least on the terminal teeth supporting the plate.

5. Need to stabilize periodontally weakened mandibular anterior teeth. If the linguoplate is used for stabilization, each tooth involved must have a properly prepared rest seat. Otherwise it is conceivable that the forces exerted by the linguoplate will further aggravate the condition that it is intended to alleviate.

A relatively infrequently used mandibular major connector is the continuous bar retainer (Fig. 6–13). The inferior portion of this connector is a lingual bar, and it should meet the criteria of design and location of any lingual bar. The superior portion is included to provide indirect retention or tooth stabilization. If its function is indirect retention, minimally the terminal supporting teeth should receive rest seats. If its function is stabilization, each tooth contacted should receive a rest seat.

Two circumstances indicate the choice of a continuous bar rather than a linguoplate. Where the axial inclinations of the anterior teeth are such that excessive block-out of the interproximal undercuts would be required for the placement of a linguoplate, a continuous bar would be more acceptable since its placement and design is not interfered with by these undercuts. Where wide embrasures exist beneath contact areas, the continuous bar would be more acceptable aesthetically than the linguoplate, which would allow visibility of the metal from a labial view (Fig. 6–14).

The continuous bar minimizes tooth coverage and

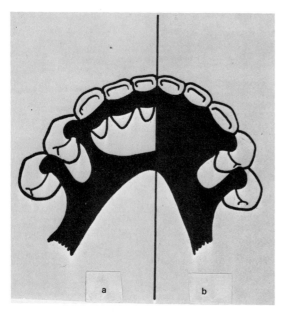

**FIG. 6-14.** The continuous bar retainer (**a**) allows no visibility of metal from a labial view in the presence of wide embrasure spaces, but the linguoplate does. (Weintraub G S, Goyal B K: J Prev Dent 3:30–42, 1976)

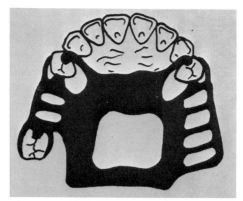

**FIG. 6-15.** Anterior and posterior palatal bar connector illustrated on a Kennedy Class II, modification 1 arch. It is also commonly used in Class IV situations. (Weintraub G S, Goyal B K: J Prev Dent 3:30–42, 1976)

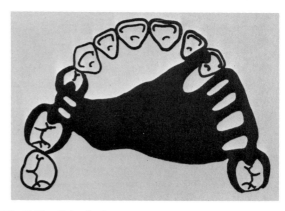

**FIG. 6-16.** Palatal plate connector illustrated on a Kennedy Class III, modification 1 arch. It is also favored for Class I arches to provide support and retention to the prosthesis. (Weintraub G S, Goyal B K: J Prev Dent 3:30–42, 1976)

gingival coverage, in contrast to the linguoplate. This is a distinct advantage and should be considered in the selection of the mandibular major connector when indirect retention and/or tooth stabilization are to be provided by the major connector.

*Maxillary Major Connectors.* There are basically three designs of maxillary major connectors widely in use. They are the U-shaped connector, the combination anterior and posterior palatal bar connector (Fig. 6–15), and the palatal plate connector (Fig. 6–16). In general the borders of all maxillary major connectors should be placed 4–6 mm from gingival tissues. Relief should be provided between the tissue surface of the major connector and a prominent median palatine raphe to prevent tissue injury. The posterior extension of maxillary major connectors must terminate anterior to the soft palate. To minimize interference with the tongue they should have only enough bulk to provide sufficient rigidity. Maxillary major connectors that have anterior components should follow the contour of the rugae, and their borders should be placed in the depression between rugae to minimize entrapment of food and debris between the connector and tissue in this area.

The U-shaped connector is generally unacceptable for Kennedy Class I and II situations. Its flexibility contributes to the potential for increased ridge resorption. It may be the connector of choice, however, in the presence of an inoperable palatal torus that extends pos-

teriorly to the junction of the hard and soft palates, because such a torus precludes the use of the combination anterior and posterior palatal bar connector. If used, the U-shaped connector should be cast with a cobalt chromium alloy rather than a gold alloy to obtain the necessary rigidity. The U-shaped connector is acceptable for use in the Kennedy Class IV situation, which entails an all-tooth-supported prosthesis.

The combination anterior and posterior palatal bar major connector meets the criterion of rigidity and can be used in all four Kennedy classes. Specifics of design include location of the posterior bar on the hard palate just anterior to the junction of hard and soft palates, and a broad and thin anterior bar that does not impinge upon the incisive papilla (Fig. 6–15). To minimize the bulk of the anterior component an "anatomic replica" pattern is used. This provides a corrugated effect which permits adequate rigidity and minimal bulk. The combination anterior and posterior bar design is most commonly used in Kennedy Class II and IV situations where maximum support gained from more extensive palatal coverage is not needed.

Another maxillary major connector that can be used in all four Kennedy classes is the palatal plate (Fig. 6–16). The palatal plate varies in width from the relatively narrow plate used in Kennedy Class III, modification I arches to the full palatal coverage used in Kennedy Class I situations. The palatal plate contributes to the support and retention of the prosthesis directly proportional to its area and intimacy of contact with underlying tissues. Achieving a more equitable stress distribution between abutment teeth and other supporting tissues is an important function of the palatal plate in Kennedy Class I maxillary arches.

The palatal plate can also contribute to indirect retention (as can the combination anterior and posterior bar connector) when placed on two planes (Fig. 6–17). This design is commonly used in Kennedy Class III arches and Kennedy Class I arches. Its use in the Class III situation reflects its simplicity of design and comfort. In the Class I situation the factors of support, stress distribution, and augmentation of retention are important considerations in selection of the maxillary major connector design.

MINOR CONNECTORS. Minor connectors unite direct retainers, indirect retainers, occlusal and cingulum rests, denture bases, and artificial teeth to the major connector. To promote tissue health there should be a slight amount of relief where the minor connector crosses gingival tissue to a vertical tooth surface, and the connector should cross gingival tissues at right angles to minimize gingival coverage. Rigidity is required to provide stress distribution and to stabilize the prosthesis against horizontal rotational forces. For comfort the bulk of the minor connector should be kept to the minimum consistent with the need for rigidity.

A minor connector which is difficult to design and difficult for the patient to contend with is the connector placed along a lingual embrasure to unite an occlusal rest or a direct retainer to the major connector. It should be triangular in shape from both the lingual and occlusal views with the apices of the triangles toward the tooth surface and toward the occlusal surface (Fig. 6–18). Contact should be made between the minor connector and the distolingual line angle of the mesial tooth involved and the mesiolingual line angle of the distal tooth involved. This contact minimizes food impaction in the embrasure area. However, the cervical third of the minor connector stands away from the tooth, making it mandatory to clean the teeth and prosthesis after each meal.

DENTURE BASES. Denture bases in removable partial dentures support the artificial teeth, transfer occlusal forces to abutment teeth, and enhance aesthetics. In contrast to the importance of the denture bases for the tooth-and-tissue-supported edentulous span, the denture base for the all-tooth-supported edentulous span need only extend buccally, labially, or lingually to provide a seal between it and the tissues to prevent impaction of food (Fig. 6–19). Where maximum exten-

**FIG. 6–18.** The minor connector located interproximally is triangular in shape. A. Occlusal view. B. Lingual view. (Weintraub G S, Goyal B K: J Prev Dent 3:30–42, 1976)

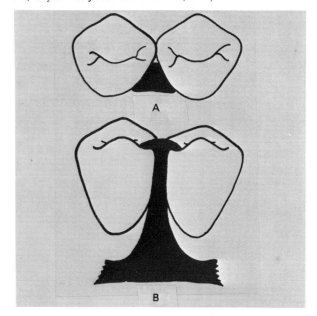

**FIG. 6–17.** Indirect retention is provided by contact of the major connector with the maxilla in two planes (**a–a, b–b**). Little or no indirect retention is provided by a flat palate (**c–c**). (Weintraub G S, Goyal B K: J Prev Dent 3:30–42, 1976)

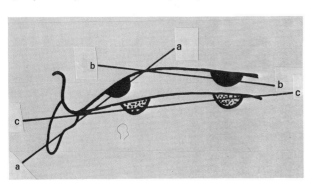

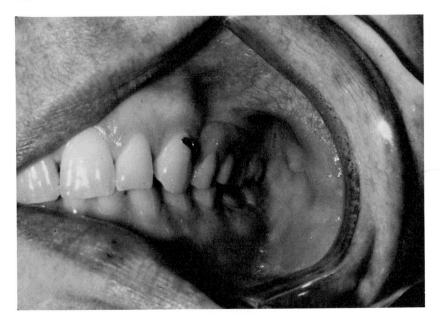

**FIG. 6-19.** The borders of an all-tooth-supported posterior denture base need not be extended maximally. (Weintraub G S, Goyal B K: J Prev Dent 3:30–42, 1976)

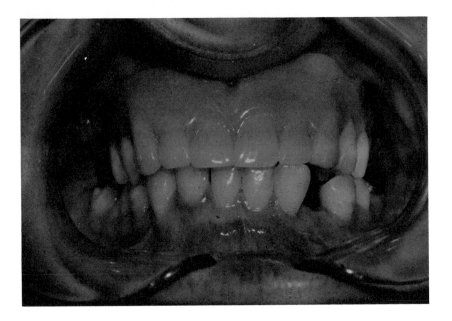

**FIG. 6-20.** In a Kennedy Class IV situation maximum extension is generally required for aesthetics and support. (Weintraub G S, Goyal B K: J Prev Dent 3:30–42, 1976)

sion into the vestibular fornix is needed to provide adequate lip and cheek support and enhance aesthetics, however, this extension must be compatible with the functional muscular activity of the bordering tissues (Fig. 6–20). Adequate relief should be provided for frenal attachments. The selection of the base material (acrylic resin versus cast metal) depends upon the length of the span and aesthetic considerations.

**ARTIFICIAL TEETH.** Artificial teeth prevent further disorganization of the dental arch, restore and maintain

the vertical dimension of occlusion, restore masticatory efficiency, improve phonation, and enhance aesthetics. Artificial teeth alone must not be used to increase or restore the vertical dimension of occlusion in the presence of natural tooth contacts maintaining the vertical dimension of occlusion. The result of this rather arbitrary increase is a loss of support of abutment teeth, and/or destruction of residual ridge, and/or destruction of the prosthesis in the patient's attempt to reestablish natural tooth contacts (Fig. 6–21).

To minimize the work load upon the abutment teeth

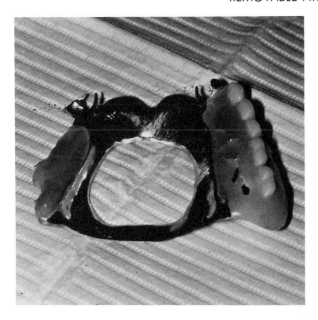

**FIG. 6-21.** Often the result of an arbitrary increase in the vertical dimension of occlusion supported by artificial teeth is destruction of the prosthesis or the residual ridge. (Weintraub G S, Goyal B K: J Prev Dent 3:30–42, 1976)

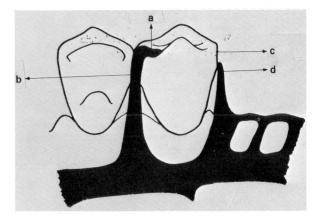

**FIG. 6-22.** Lingual view of the RPI clasp illustrating the mesial rest (**a**), the interproximal minor connector (**b**), the prepared guide plane (**c**), and the proximal plate (**d**). (Weintraub G S, Goyal B K: J Prev Dent 3:35–50, 1976)

induced by the presence of the artificial teeth, the buccolingual width of the occlusal surfaces should be narrowed. For this same reason clasp arms must be placed away from the occlusal one-third of the abutment tooth. Clasp arms located on the occlusal one-third create a wider occlusal table, thus increasing the work load placed upon that tooth.

## Distal Extension Removable Partial Denture Design

Those features of design that are influenced by the dual nature of support required by a distal extension prosthesis are 1) clasp assembly design, 2) rest seat preparation and location, 3) guiding plane preparation and extension, 4) indirect retention, 5) resistance to rotational forces, 6) denture base extension and contour, 7) impression technique and materials, 8) denture base material, and 9) occlusion.

CLASP ASSEMBLY DESIGN. The importance of the clasp assembly design for a Class I or II removable partial denture increases in situations where the soft tissues overlying the distal extension ridge exhibit a high degree of displaceability. Since movement of the denture base as it functions is transmitted as stress to the abutment tooth via the clasp assembly, the clasp assembly must be designed in such a fashion that the amount of stress transmitted is minimized. The objective of clasp design for the distal extension abutment

tooth is twofold (29). First, the clasp assembly at rest must have a passive relationship to the abutment tooth. Second, when occlusal forces are directed to the denture base, the clasp assembly should allow the supporting mucoperiosteum to assume its functional form without transmitting potentially destructive forces to the abutment tooth. During functional movement of the prosthesis it is desirable for the clasp assembly to have a small amount of movement independent of the abutment tooth.

Many concepts of clasp design have been proposed to meet the unique problem offered by these objectives. One recent approach involves the rest-proximal plate-I bar (RPI) clasp retainer and its modifications. The RPI clasp described by Krol (31) approaches the problem of clasp design for the distal extension abutment tooth from three aspects. This design 1) minimizes tooth coverage by the clasp assembly, 2) minimizes gingival coverage by the clasp assembly, and 3) theoretically minimizes stress transmitted to the abutment tooth by the clasp assembly when the denture moves in function. The concept of minimal tooth and gingival coverage is intended to minimize plaque accumulation under clasps and minor connectors in order to maintain the health of the periodontium.

The RPI clasp includes a mesially located rest placed in a well-rounded rest seat that allows rotation when the distal extension base is displaced by occlusal forces. The minor connector that carries the rest to its position is located interproximally. Care must be taken during the preparation of the final cast and subsequent waxing of the framework to design a minor connector that allows this slight rotation. The minor connector should not be in contact with the distolingual line angle of the tooth located just mesially to the connector (Fig. 6-22).

The proximal plate is designed to disengage the

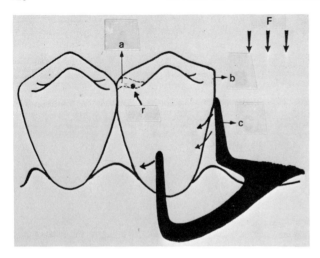

**FIG. 6–23.** As an occlusal force (**F**) is applied to the distal extension base, the mesially placed rest (**a**) serves as the point of rotation (**r**). The proximal plate (**c**) disengages the proximal guiding plane (**b**). The plate and the retentive I-bar clasp arm move downward and forward. (Weintraub G S, Goyal B K: J Prev Dent 3:35–50, 1976)

prepared proximal guiding plane as the base moves tissueward. This is accomplished by having the superior border of the proximal plate contact the inferior border of the short guiding plane. This contact is broken as the base is displaced. The rest serves as the point of rotation, allowing downward and forward movement of the proximal plate (Fig. 6–23).

The retentive arm is of the I-bar design. Its retentive terminus should be located at or mesial to the greatest mesiodistal prominence on the buccal surface (Fig. 6–23). This position is a critical consideration since placement of the retentive area distal to the prominence will not allow the intended action of the clasp design, that is, disengagement between the retentive clasp arm and the tooth when the base is displaced toward the tissue.

It is apparent that in many instances a cast abutment restoration will be required if this clasp assembly is to be used. This is not a contraindication for consideration of the design, however. On the contrary, it emphasizes the responsibility of the dentist to determine the best possible design of a prosthesis and then to make that design feasible by creating abutment contours that satisfy its demands.

Other designs are also suitable for clasping a distal extension removable partial denture, for example, cast circumferential clasps, combination clasps, bar clasps and their variations, and others can be and are used successfully in various situations. In light of the fact that no long-term in vivo study has definitely identified a clasp design or designs of choice for the distal exten-

sion restoration, the dentist cannot simply rely on clasp design as a solution to the problems inherent in the treatment with this restoration. Many other design features of the distal extension removable partial denture must be considered in the attempt to achieve the desired equalization between the two supporting systems.

**REST SEAT PREPARATION AND LOCATION.** Rest seats can be prepared in cast restorations, amalgam restorations, or natural tooth structure. A rest seat which supports the clasp assembly of a distal extension prosthesis must meet the same criteria of design in regard to size and form described previously in Clasp Assembly Design section. The rest seat must be well rounded and polished to permit some rotation to occur between the rest and its seat when depression of the distal extension base takes place. In contrast, an all-tooth-supported prosthesis can use internal rest seats (boxlike preparations) in abutment restorations for support and stabilization against horizontal movement; at times such rest seats eliminate the need for facial clasp arms, which gives them an aesthetic advantage in the all-tooth-supported restoration. To prevent a possible transfer of horizontal stress to the abutment tooth, the occlusal rest and prepared rest seat for the distal extension prosthesis should exhibit a relationship similar to that of a shallow ball and socket joint. Its main function is to provide occlusal support.

It may be difficult to adhere to the principle of mesial rest seat location when the abutment tooth is a canine. Describing a mesiolingual rest seat preparation for a canine tooth, Krol (31) points out that it must be deep enough to prevent the rest from slipping gingivally. He indicates that generally the preparation involves penetration into the dentin and advocates further deepening of the preparation and placement of a direct filling gold or amalgam restoration.

Location of the rest seat on the abutment tooth is definitely influenced by the support system offered to the prosthesis. Using the mesial rotation point for the distal extension prosthesis, as described by Kratochvil (30), affects the arc of movement of the denture base. The direction of movement and force application is more nearly perpendicular to the residual ridge underlying the base, allowing the tissues to offer positive support to the prosthesis. Distal placement of the rest leads to a more oblique movement of the base in reference to the residual ridge, and this movement does not take advantage of the supporting qualities of the ridge. Another advantage of the mesial rest is that the more vertical movement of the denture base results in a decreased potential for impingement on gingival tissues adjacent to the edentulous area. In addition a mesial rest tends to tip the abutment tooth anteriorly, a di-

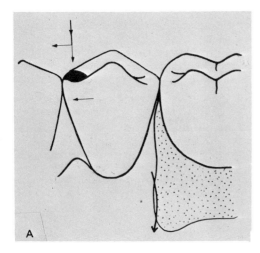

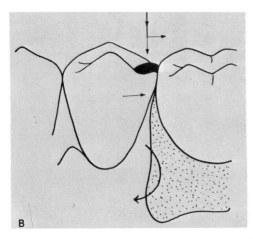

**FIG. 6-24.** Placement of rests. A. A mesial rest allows the extension base to move more perpendicularly to the ridge and transmits a mesial tipping force to the abutment tooth. B. A distal rest allows the extension base to move more obliquely to the ridge and transmits a distal tipping force to the abutment tooth. (Weintraub G S, Goyal B K: J Prev Dent 3:35–50, 1976)

rection which is resisted by adjacent teeth. A prosthesis designed with a distal rest, however, tends to exert a distal pull on the abutment tooth when the base moves toward the tissue, and the minor connector engages the proximal tooth surface. When this force is applied to the tooth, it is not resisted and can lead to mobility and bone loss (Fig. 6–24).

**GUIDE PLANE PREPARATION AND EXTENSION.** Miller (36) emphasized that it is important to distinguish between guiding planes on abutment teeth that bound an edentulous space anteriorly and posteriorly and guiding planes on abutment teeth that support a distal extension base. A pronounced guiding plane on the distal

surface of the abutment tooth next to an edentulous space magnifies the stress which the denture base transmits to the abutment as the base moves during function. The relation between the prepared guiding plane and the minor connector should be such that a slight degree of movement of the base and the clasp assembly is permitted without transmitting stresses to the abutment tooth.

Robinson (40) describes a short guiding plane, involving approximately the occlusal one-third of the tooth surface, in conjunction with a mesial rest. This design shifts the fulcrum from the contact area between the guiding plane and minor connector to the rest, allowing the minor connector to disengage from tooth contact when the denture base moves toward the tissue. This concept is incorporated in the RPI clasp assembly design in which the prepared guiding plane surface is contacted only at its inferior border by the proximal plate of the framework when the clasp assembly is in a passive relation to the abutment tooth (Fig. 6–23).

**INDIRECT RETENTION.** Indirect retention is needed on Class I and II removable partial dentures and should be considered for all-tooth-supported dentures when a distal abutment tooth with a guarded prognosis stands alone, because the loss of this tooth would create a distal extension edentulous area. Indirect retainers minimize the rotational movement of extension bases away from the tissue, thus preventing tissue injury that could occur if the major connector impinged upon underlying tissues during this rotation. Generally, strategically located rests in prepared rest seats serve as indirect retainers, although indirect retention can be provided by other features of partial denture design. For example, complete palatal coverage in a maxillary Class I situation provides both direct and indirect retention. Placing the retentive terminus of a clasp assembly adjacent to an extension base in a distobuccal location also provides direct and indirect retention.

Steffel (45) describes the axes of rotation that pass through abutment teeth in various partially edentulous situations. In the Kennedy Class I arch the axis of rotation that aids in the determination of indirect retainer position passes through the rests on the abutment teeth. In the Kennedy Class II arch the axis of rotation is diagonal, passing through the occlusal rest on the abutment on the distal extension side and the occlusal rest on the most posterior abutment on the other side. For maximum effectiveness the indirect retainer should be placed at right angles to, and as far anterior to, the axis of rotation as possible, depending on the ability of the tooth upon which the indirect retainer will lie to accept the additional stress (Fig. 6–25). Occlusal or cingulum rest seats must be placed in prepara-

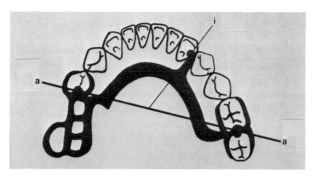

**FIG. 6–25.** A prosthesis placed on a Kennedy Class II arch is able to rotate around a diagonal axis (**a–a**) that passes through the abutment teeth. Rotation of the base away from the ridge is reduced by the indirect retainer (**i**). (Weintraub G S, Goyal B K: J Prev Dent 3:35–50, 1976)

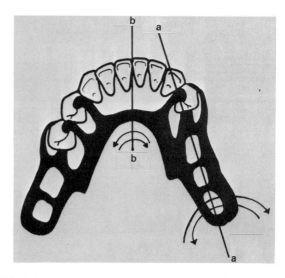

**FIG. 6–26.** Rotation about the longitudinal axis (**a–a**) is controlled primarily by the rigidity of the major connector. Rotation about an imaginary axis (**b–b**) perpendicular to the center of the dental arch is resisted by components of the prosthesis that contact vertical tooth and ridge surfaces. (Weintraub G S, Goyal B K: J Prev Dent 3:35–50, 1976)

tion for an indirect retainer to help the teeth contacted to withstand the forces directed to them.

**RESISTANCE TO ROTATIONAL FORCES.** The application of the triangular or quadrangular concept of clasping for the all-tooth-supported prosthesis provides the resistance of the prosthesis to rotational forces. This is not the case, however, when unilateral or bilateral distal extension dentures are involved. Such dentures are subjected to rotational forces that allow three possible movements, all of which must be considered in the design of the restoration to minimize them and their destructive effect upon the residual soft and hard tissues.

The first of these movements is the rotation about an axis formed by the two principal occlusal rests. Although movement of the base away from the supporting ridge can be controlled with the placement of indirect retainers, the denture base can also rotate towards the ridge. This degree of rotation is controlled by maximum extension, accuracy of adaptation to the tissue, and the nature of the impression of the supporting ridge (anatomic form or functional form). In the maxillary arch the design of the major connector is an important factor in resisting the tissueward movement of a distal extension prosthesis. A properly designed maxillary major connector contributes to the support, stability, and retention of the prosthesis, thereby relieving the abutment teeth of much stress.

The second movement is described as rotation about a longitudinal axis as the extension base moves about the residual ridge (Fig. 6–26). This is controlled primarily by the rigidity of the major connector.

The third movement is rotation about an imaginary perpendicular axis located near the center of the dental arch (Fig. 6–26). This is resisted by components of the framework that contact vertical tooth surfaces, i.e., re-

ciprocal clasp arms, minor connectors, guiding plates, and major connectors such as the continuous bar and the linguoplate. Maximum extension and adaptation to the vertical walls of the residual ridge also contribute to the ability of the denture base to resist forces causing this rotational movement.

Of utmost importance in the control of these rotational movements is the implementation of an occlusal scheme that is in harmony with the opposing dentition and free of lateral interferences during eccentric jaw movements.

**DENTURE BASE EXTENSION AND CONTOUR.** Maximum adaptation and extension of distal extension bases is of primary importance in the effort to distribute stresses among the support systems and the residual ridge. The greater the area covered by the denture base, the less the force per unit of area. The extension must not be arbitrary, but planned to be in harmony with the functional activity of the surrounding tissues. One of the most glaring discrepancies observed in both removable partial and complete dentures is the failure to use all the areas available for support and stress distribution, and failure to take advantage of the activity of the surrounding tissues to aid in the retention and stability of the removable prosthesis.

There are three distinct areas of importance in the denture base extension and contour for the distal extension removable partial denture: 1) the tissue surface of the base, 2) the borders of the base, and 3) the pol-

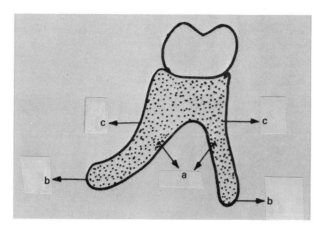

**FIG. 6-27.** Cross section of a mandibular distal extension base illustrating the tissue surface (**a**) the borders (**b**) and the polished surface (**c**). (Weintraub G S, Goyal B K: J Prev Dent 3:35–50, 1976)

ished or "muscular" surface of the base (Fig. 6–27). All three should be determined in a planned fashion. There is no question that a single impression procedure with irreversible hydrocolloid in a stock tray or even an individualized tray is insufficient. A double impression allows the operator to consider each phase of the extension–base impression independently in a step-by-step procedure. The advantage of using materials such as modeling plastic and impression wax is stated quite simply as "correctability." With these materials the operator can manipulate the tissues to the advantage of the prosthesis.

To describe proper border extensions for the mandibular distal extension prosthesis, an arch with only the six anterior teeth remaining will be considered (Fig. 6–28). The posterior border of the base must cover the retromolar pad area to support the prosthesis and to prevent rapid resorption of the residual ridge. The distobuccal border should reflect the activity of the mas-

seter muscle upon the buccinator muscle. This is generally seen as a notching effect; if not incorporated in the impression and subsequent base, it can lead to discomfort for the patient and displacement of the base.

Located between the masseter area posteriorly and the buccal frenum area anteriorly is the extremely important buccinator area. This is also referred to as the buccal shelf because of its broad surface which extends laterally to the external oblique ridge of the mandible. The buccal shelf is the primary supporting area of the mandibular distal extension base and should be fully covered. Some impingement can occur between the base and the attachment of the buccinator muscle since the action of this muscle is in an oblique direction in relation to the base and therefore has little displacing action on the denture.

The distolingual border of the base is involved with the retromylohyoid area. Maximum vertical and posterior extension is desirable here to aid in retention of the prosthesis. This extension must be in harmony with the function activity of the tongue, and tongue exercises are indicated when this border is formed during the impression-taking procedure. Anterior to the retromylohyoid area is the mylohyoid area. The extension of the base can be inferior to the mylohyoid ridge since the greatest activity of the mylohyoid muscle is not at its attachment but medially. Again, tongue exercises during the impression procedure identify the maximum extension.

The contour of the polished surface should improve the retention of the prosthesis. A horizontal concavity located bucally and lingually on the mandibular distal extension base takes advantage of the tissues in seating the denture. Lingually this concavity must not extend further laterally than the lingual wall of the artificial teeth to prevent the creation of an undercut (Fig. 6–27).

The maxillary arch distal extension base will also be

**FIG. 6-28.** Anatomic landmarks that influence the extension of the mandibular base include the mylohyoid ridge (**a**), the buccal shelf (**b**), the masseter muscle (**c**), the retromolar pad (**d**), and the retromylohyoid space (**e**). (Weintraub G S, Goyal B K: J Prev Dent 3:35–50, 1976)

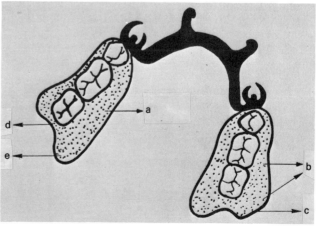

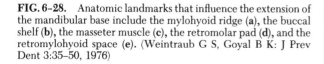

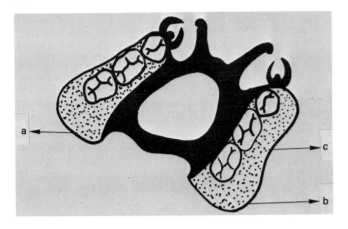

**FIG. 6–29.** Anatomic landmarks that influence the extension of the maxillary base include the hamular notch (**a**), the coronoid process and buccal pouch (**b**), and the zygomatic process (**c**). (Weintraub G S, Goyal B K: J Prev Dent 3:35–50, 1976)

described by using the example of an arch with only six remaining natural teeth (Fig. 6–29). If there is a maxillary major connector of full palatal coverage in cast metal, it is not necessary to create a posterior palatal seal on the soft palate as indicated for a complete maxillary denture. The posterior border should be located slightly anterior to the junction of the hard and soft palates. Slight scoring of the final cast prior to its duplication provides an intimate seal between the major connector and the underlying tissue. The lateral posterior border should be placed in the hamular notch between the maxillary tuberosity and the hamulus of the medial pterygoid plate. The distobuccal border is considered to include that area located between the hamular notch posteriorly and the zygomatic process anteriorly. It should be filled in both height and width by the denture base. However, allowance must be made in the base contours for the downward, forward, and medial movements of the coronoid process into the vestibule during eccentric movements of the mandible. The zygomatic process must not be impinged upon by the denture base. Generally the border of the denture base should exhibit a concavity corresponding to the contours of the process.

On the buccal side the polished surface should exhibit a horizontal concavity located between the periphery of the base and the simulated zone of attached gingiva. Palatally no undercuts should be presented to the tongue. Fish (14) writes in great detail concerning the most advantageous form of the polished surface of a denture base, equating its importance with that of the impression and occlusal surfaces. Indeed, Beresin's (3) neutral zone complete denture technique, in which the polished surface contours are determined by the patient's muscular activity rather than by arbitrary carving, might be effectively applied to the polished surface contours of the distal extension base, especially in situations that present advanced ridge atrophy.

QUESTIONS

1. A high survey line that allows placement of the retentive terminus of a clasp arm on the gingival one-third of the abutment tooth indicates that
   1. the angle of cervical convergence is small
   2. the angle of cervical convergence is large
   3. the abutment tooth must be recontoured
   4. a bar clasp is the clasp design of choice

2. True reciprocation infers that the reciprocal component of a clasp assembly
   1. lies on the middle one-third of the clinical crown
   2. is a lingual blanket rather than a lingual arm
   3. contacts the abutment tooth simultaneously with the retentive arm
   4. contacts the tooth immediately after the retentive arm assumes its passive position on the retentive area

3. Which of the following is not a function of occlusal rests?
   1. Maintenance of the correct occlusal relation of the artificial teeth
   2. Guiding of prosthesis along planned path of insertion
   3. Stabilization of clasp arms in their planned position
   4. Resistance to cervical movement of prosthesis

14. Aesthetics is an important consideration when deciding between a fixed or a removable partial denture for which of the following Kennedy classifications?
   1. Kennedy Class I
   2. Kennedy Class II
   3. Kennedy Class III
   4. Kennedy Class IV

5. All of the following statements related to the RPI clasp assembly are false except one. Which one?
   1. The rest may be placed on the distal aspect of the occlusal surface.
   2. A boxlike rest seat is desirable to promote stability of the prosthesis.
   3. Proper depth of the rest seat may require an amalgam or a direct filling gold restoration.
   4. Contact between the mesial minor connector and the adjacent tooth is desirable.

6. Which of the following is (are) not a valid criterion(a) of incisal rest seat design?
   1. The deepest portion (mesiodistally) is toward the center of the tooth.
   2. Sharp line angles are desirable.
   3. Contact area is involved in the preparation.
   4. Small bevels are placed labially and lingually.
   5. 1 and 4
   6. 2 and 3

7. When surveying a diagnostic cast, the selection of a suitable anteroposterior tilt is to
   1. indicate the greatest available support for the removable partial denture
   2. provide relative parallelism among proximal tooth surfaces
   3. provide suitable reciprocation for retentive clasp arms
   4. eliminate soft tissue undercuts in the retromylohyoid areas

8. Which of the following statements regarding the design of minor connectors is (are) true?
   1. The minor connector must be rigid.
   2. The minor connector must engage an undercut low on the tooth.
   3. The minor connector should present minimal interference to the tongue.
   4. The minor connector should cover the minimum of gingival tissue possible.
   5. 1, 3, and 4
   6. All of the above

## MOUTH PREPARATION

In reference to treatment with removable partial dentures the term "mouth preparation" has evolved to take on a limited meaning. Mistakenly mouth preparation is thought to include only those procedures carried out to modify abutment tooth contours by intraoral recontouring or the placement of restorations. In fact these procedures represent only one phase of mouth preparation for a removable prosthesis. A better phrase that describes procedures to prepare the mouth for a removable partial denture is preliminary oral rehabilitation. This term signifies that removable partial denture therapy begins at the diagnosis and treatment planning stage and that all dental treatment required by a patient influences or is influenced by the need for a removable partial denture. Periodontal preparation and surgical preparation for the partially edentulous mouth are among the most important phases of preliminary oral rehabilitation.

### Preparation of Abutment Teeth

Three classifications of abutment teeth can be identified: those that are to be used as they exist (recon-

touring if needed of natural tooth structure or existing restorations), those that are to receive partial coverage restorations, and those that are to receive full crowns.

One objective of recontouring tooth structure or existing restorations is the modification of the height of contour (survey line) to allow more ideal placement of a properly designed clasp assembly. An acceptable height of contour places the rigid portion of the retentive clasp arm at the junction of the gingival and middle thirds of the clinical crown and the retentive clasp terminus on the gingival third of the clinical crown. The reciprocal clasp arm should be positioned no higher than the middle one-third of the clinical crown. Other objectives of recontouring natural tooth structure or existing restorations include the preparation of guiding planes and the creation of occlusal, cingulum, or incisal rest seats. The nature of the support offered to the prosthesis influences the extent (occlusogingivally) of the guiding planes prepared on proximal tooth surfaces adjacent to edentulous areas. The form of the rest seat and its position (mesial or distal) on the tooth also are influenced by the type of prosthesis being constructed (all-tooth-supported or tooth-and-tissue-supported).

All intraoral recontouring procedures must be accomplished in a conservative fashion with the diagnostic cast as a guide. Additional diagnostic casts should be made for survey analysis to determine if additional modification of tooth contour is necessary. In most cases the ideal tooth contour for a well-designed clasp assembly can best be achieved by means of cast restorations prepared on a full arch cast on a dental surveyor.

### Indications for Restoring Abutment Teeth

An obvious indication for restoring abutment teeth as a prophylactic measure is the presence of caries or a high caries index. In addition, when the survey analysis reveals that the anatomic crown forms do not harmonize with an appropriate clasp assembly design, prescribing restorations to achieve optimal contours is considered better treatment than providing an unacceptable clasp design to fit the existing contours of the abutment tooth.

Tipped or tilted abutment teeth, which are frequently encountered adjacent to the posterior border of an edentulous span, should be provided with suitable guiding planes to minimize potential food trap areas. Extruded abutments require correction to provide a proper plane of occlusion. The treatment depends upon the degree of extrusion. A mildly extruded tooth may require occlusal recontouring only, while a more severely extruded tooth may require a cast restoration (inlay–onlay, three-quarter crown, or full crown) to correct the discrepancy (Fig. 6–30). Prior to the making

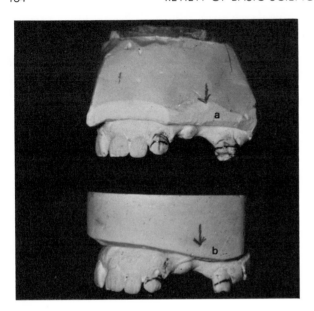

**FIG. 6-30.** Extruded molar (**a**) corrected with a full gold crown (**b**) allowing ideal survey line for circumferential clasp with mesiobuccal retention.

of a cast restoration for a severely extruded tooth it may be necessary to perform intentional endodontics and place a coping if there is insufficient interarch space for a cast anatomic crown. This is preferable to extracting a tooth that would convert the prosthesis from a tooth-supported to a tooth-and-tissue-supported partial denture. This coping will provide support and stability for the prosthesis, as well as contribute to the preservation of the residual ridge.

Additional indications for restorations include the necessity of using a nonvital tooth as an abutment, compromised alveolar support which may require splinting of an abutment tooth to an adjacent tooth, and anterior modification spaces which should be eliminated whenever possible by restoration with a fixed prosthesis.

There are general considerations that apply to both intraoral recontouring of abutment teeth and carving wax patterns for abutment restorations. A definite regimen should be followed related to the tooth surfaces involved. Guiding planes should be established first, followed by preparation of the buccal and lingual contours. After these are correct, rest seats are prepared. When waxing an abutment tooth restoration, normal crown contours should be established first and then modified so that they can accept a well-designed clasp assembly. Waxing normal anatomic contours first eliminates the possibility of exaggerated tooth contours that are not biologically compatible with the supporting tissues. All cast restorations must be waxed on a full

arch cast on the surveyor to allow continued reference to the contours of the teeth being restored in their association with the selected path of insertion and degree of undercut required.

QUESTIONS

9. Which of the following is an (are) indication(s) for recontouring natural tooth structure in preparation for a removable partial denture?
   a. Need to create rest seats
   b. Need to prepare guiding planes
   c. Need to lower a survey line
   d. Need to raise a survey line

   1. a and b
   2. a, b, and d
   3. a, b, and c
   4. c
   5. All of the above

10. As part of the preliminary oral rehabilitative phase of removable partial denture therapy, an isolated mandibular second premolar should ideally be
    1. extracted
    2. used for support only
    3. used as a primary abutment
    4. splinted to a canine with a fixed prosthesis

11. All of the following are indications for restoring abutment teeth with the exception of
    1. as a prophylactic measure where a low caries index is present
    2. when the abutment tooth is nonvital
    3. when the abutment tooth has undergone significant extrusion
    4. when survey analysis reveals that crown form must be significantly altered to allow proper clasp assembly design
    5. 1 and 4

12. Which of the following treatment approaches should be considered for a severely extruded abutment tooth, the loss of which would create a distal extension area?
    1. Extraction
    2. Occlusal recontouring
    3. Endodontic therapy and coping placement
    4. Cast restoration

## IMPRESSIONS AND FINAL CASTS

Elastic materials are used for the final impressions from which the final casts are made. The final cast, after being prepared for duplication, is copied in a hydrocolloid mold to create the refractory cast on which the framework is waxed and then invested for casting (Fig. 6–31). The final cast must be an accurate reproduction of the partially edentulous arch.

Experience has shown that hydrocolloids (reversible and irreversible), mercaptan rubber base impression materials, and silicone impression materials are suffi-

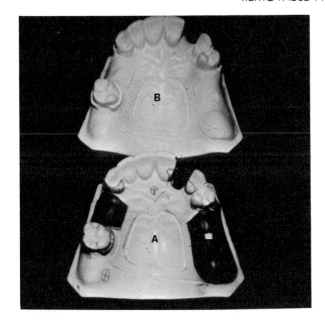

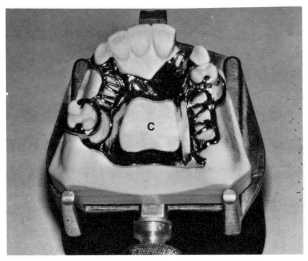

**FIG. 6-31.** A. Final cast prepared for duplication. B. Duplicate refractory cast. C. Finished framework on final cast.

tion of an all-tooth-supported prosthesis, as long as handling characteristics of the selected material are understood and respected.

## INFLUENCE OF THE SUPPORT SYSTEM

A clear distinction has been made between the philosophy of design of the all-tooth-supported prosthesis and the tooth-and-tissue-supported prosthesis. This divergence of philosophy is related to the impression procedures as well.

### Literature Review

In 1899 Bonwill (5) described his method of partial denture construction formulated to prevent injury to the remaining natural teeth. Many authors, including Blatterfein (4), DeVan (12), Kabcenell (24), McCracken (35), Robinson (40), Steffel (46), and Weinberg (48), have since proposed clasp assembly designs for the bilateral distal extension removable partial denture, each claiming a design which causes less tipping, tilting, torquing, and stressing of the abutment teeth. There is, however, a lack of long-term experimental data to either substantiate or negate these claims. The problem of abutment teeth and residual ridge preservation was approached differently by Holmes (22), who advocated reduction of denture base movement by recording the functional form of the mucoperiosteum, and by Yalisove (49), who described a technique involving construction of tapered copings on the abutment teeth and secondary crowns that are incorporated into the partial denture to fit over the copings, thus avoiding the use of clasps. Kratochvil (30) and Krol (31) have designed a clasp assembly for the distal extension abutment tooth that has received wide acceptance.

Laboratory investigations by Frechette (15), Cecconi (8), Clayton (9), Kaires (25, 26), Weinberg (48), and Shohet (43) have contributed greatly to an understanding of the forces and their effects on removable partial denture abutment teeth, but the results have not been validated in vivo. Kaires (27, 28), in two studies with patients, compared stress distribution when the framework was altered, but he maintained a constant clasp assembly design. No in vivo study was found in which a comparison was made of the effect of various clasp assembly designs upon abutment tooth mobility.

Carlsson (6) and associates in a 4-year investigation reported destructive effects of the distal extension denture on the periodontium. Fenner et al. (13) demonstrated that a significant increase in abutment tooth mobility was produced by treatment with removable partial dentures, but they did not describe the design of the clasp assembly. Seeman (42) demonstrated a correlation between periodontal disease and the wearing of

ciently accurate to produce a final cast on which a prosthesis that fits accurately in the mouth can be fabricated. In most instances an acrylic resin individualized final impression tray is constructed on a diagnostic cast, with an appropriate amount of relief incorporated to accommodate the impression material. At times carefully modified stock trays can be used successfully to take a final impression of a partially edentulous arch that is to be restored with an all-tooth-supported prosthesis. In fact, a single final impression with an individualized tray using one of these materials (Biomaterials chapter) produces an accurate final cast for the fabrica-

removable partial dentures. Muhlemann (37, 38) measured tooth mobility produced through artificial trauma and concluded that changing the magnitude and direction of functional forces produced definite modifications of mobility patterns. Such clinical studies and observations led Waerhung to warn against the use of removable partial dentures in periodontal therapy and to question "whether partial dentures in many cases cause more harm than good."

## Methods of Treatment

Most treatment approaches currently used to provide optimal stress distribution for the distal extension removable partial denture generally fall into three categories. First, stress-breaking devices may be incorporated to allow denture base movement under occlusal forces independent of movement by the direct retainers. Various types of nonprecision and precision stress breakers are available, and they are an effective means to gain support from the edentulous ridges. Whether or not increased resorption of the ridge is caused by this treatment technique is widely debated. Second, a multiple clasping and multiple rest design may be used with fully extended denture bases. This method is intended to minimize the amount of stress applied to any one point in the partially endentulous arch. Third, the functional rather than the anatomic form of the mucoperiosteum of the residual ridge in relation to the abutment teeth may be recorded. Applegate (2) accomplished this by using an impression wax which flows at mouth temperature. Hindels (20) describes a double impression procedure to relate the anatomic form of the residual ridge to the remaining teeth. Another approach was that of Steffel (44), who used a functional reline impression procedure. The goal of all three approaches is to insure that neither the support offered by the teeth nor that offered by the residual ridge is overstressed when the prosthesis is fully seated under occlusal loading forces.

## Obtaining the Functional Ridge Form

It is conceivable that a prosthesis constructed on a cast reflecting the anatomic ridge form will not be supported by the residual ridge when the denture is subjected to occlusal loading forces, and if there is no residual ridge support, all the stresses are taken up by the abutment tooth as if the distal extension base were simply cantilevered from that tooth. The objective of using the functional ridge form is to ensure that the prosthesis, in function, is supported by both systems in an equitable fashion. Generally this cannot be achieved by a single impression procedure with irreversible hydrocolloid in a stock rim lock tray or an individualized resin tray.

Hindels (20) describes a double impression technique in which an acrylic resin custom tray involving only the edentulous ridges and peripheral tissues is fabricated from a diagnostic cast. The tray which does not include the teeth is then used to take an accurate impression of the extension base tissues in a passive (anatomic form) state. The impression is evaluated for accuracy and lack of pressure areas and, if considered satisfactory, is reinserted in the mouth. The second impression is made with irreversible hydrocolloid in a stock perforated tray in which two circular openings (each approximately ¾ in. in diameter) in the first molar region have been prepared. The loaded perforated tray is then inserted over both the teeth and the acrylic resin tray. The operator passes the index fingers through the prepared openings in the perforated tray and places positive pressure on the acrylic resin tray. Pressure is maintained until the irreversible hydrocolloid is set, then the impression is removed as one unit. This technique does not record the functional form of the residual ridge, but it reveals the relationship of the passive or anatomic form of the ridge to the teeth as it exists when the denture base is displaced during mastication. Questions that arise concerning this technique involve the arbitrary degree of pressure exerted by the operator and the fact that the position of the initial tray cannot be seen during the secondary impression.

The second method, described by Steffel (44), involves a functional relining procedure in which modeling plastic is initially used to establish the impression of the ridge and identify border extensions. This is further refined by relieving the modeling plastic along the ridge crest and the mylohyoid ridge, placing vents through the base, and painting an impression wax over the entire impression surface. The denture is inserted and the patient is instructed to simulate mastication and perform facial exercises. This allows the functional form of the tissues covering the ridge to be recorded while molding the periphery of the impression in harmony with functional muscular activity. The prosthesis is then invested to convert the impression material to acrylic resin.

The third method also uses a secondary impression made after seating and refinement of the framework. This technique, described by Holmes (22), is referred to as the altered cast impression procedure. In an earlier publication Holmes (21) described the influence of impression procedures on occlusal loading and partial denture movement. Three identically designed removable partial dentures were constructed for each of three subjects who were missing mandibular molars. The variable in treatment involved the nature of the tray and the impression technique. A stock rim lock tray with irreversible hydrocolloid was used for the first denture, an individualized acrylic resin tray with irreversible hydrocolloid for the second denture, and the altered cast technique with irreversible hydrocolloid for the third denture. Movement of the denture bases under simulate occlusal forces was measured and found to decrease as the accuracy of the impression technique involved increased; the altered cast technique produced the least movement.

Four dentures identical in design were then constructed for each of the three subjects using the altered cast technique but varying the impression materials. The following materials, listed in order of decreasing magnitude of movement observed in the distal extension base of the finished prostheses, were used: 1) irreversible hydrocolloid, 2) rubber base, 3) metallic paste, 4) impression wax. It was clearly demonstrated that the magnitude of movement of extension denture bases under occlusal forces is related to the impression technique and impression material selected.

The altered cast impression procedure involves the following steps:

1. Routine construction and intraoral refinement of framework
2. Preparation of acrylic resin tray attached to framework and relieved from tissue
3. Recording the functional form of the residual ridge, border molding with modeling plastic to perfect border extensions and refinement of impression with fluid wax (Fig. 6–32A)
4. Laboratory procedures; alteration of master casts by removing edentulous ridge areas, securing framework and ridge impression to altered cast, boxing and pouring of ridge areas to complete new final cast (Fig. 6–32B)

All the techniques described have merit in that they take into consideration the two systems of support offered to the distal extension removable partial denture. The need to relate the extension base functionally to the supporting teeth increases when examination reveals weak abutment teeth and/or badly resorbed residual ridges covered by soft movable tissues. Other factors include the strength of the patients musculature, the length of the edentulous span, and the nature of the opposing dentition (natural teeth or removable restoration).

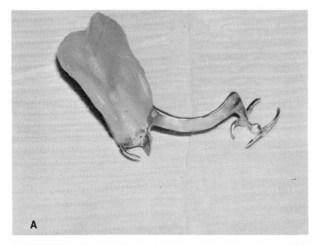

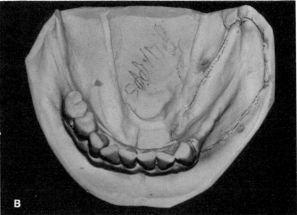

FIG. 6–32. A. Altered cast impression maintaining existing framework. B. Completed altered cast. Left edentulous area reflects functional ridge form.

### QUESTIONS

13. The altered cast technique can be used to obtain
    1. a functional impression of the edentulous ridge area
    2. an anatomic impression of the edentulous ridge area
    3. a functional impression of selected supporting areas and an anatomic impression of nonsupporting areas
    4. 1 and 2
    5. All of the above

14. Identify the proper sequence of procedures to arrive at an altered cast for a distal extension removable partial denture.

    a. Fitting of framework (intraoral)
    b. Removal of distal extension portion of final casts
    c. Making altered cast impression
    d. Final impression for framework construction
    e. Construction of impression trays on framework

    1. a, b, c, d, e
    2. b, d, c, a, e
    3. d, a, e, b, c
    4. d, b, c, a, e

## JAW RELATIONS

All removable partial dentures require the following intermaxillary records to allow the mounting of the casts on a suitable articulator: 1) face-bow transfer to mount the maxillary cast, 2) a determination of the vertical dimension of occlusion if not supported by natural tooth contacts, and 3) a centric occlusion or centric relation record taken at the vertical dimension of occlusion to transfer the mandibular cast to the articulator.

### The Face-Bow Record

Semiadjustable articulators allow a face-bow mounting that is at a reasonably accurate distance from the true axis of condylar rotation. If the radius from the axis of condylar rotation of the articulator to any point on the mounted cast compared to the patient's radius from the center of rotation to the corresponding point in the partially edentulous arch is not within a reasonable deviation, errors of occlusion develop; the degree of the error depends upon the magnitude of the mounting error. The face-bow orients the maxillary cast to the opening and closing axis of the temporomandibular joint, and it orients the elevation of the maxillary cast in relation to the Frankfort horizontal plane. This permits the maxillary cast to be oriented in the articulator space comparable to the relationship of the maxilla to the Frankfort horizontal plane identified on the patient. In order to transfer the angle of elevation of the maxillary cast, three reference points are needed. The two posterior reference points are close to the center of rotation of the condyles. The anterior reference point is quite frequently either the nasion or the inferior border of the orbit (Articulator also discussed in chapter on Fixed Prosthodontics).

When mounting a partially edentulous maxillary final or diagnostic cast with a face-bow record, it is important to determine whether a record base and an occlusion rim are needed. Quite frequently the framework may be used rather than a record base to support the occlusion rim. In general, Kennedy Class I or II partially edentulous arches require both a record base (framework) and an occlusion rim. Kennedy Class III and IV partially edentulous arches generally contain sufficient well-positioned natural teeth to allow stability of the maxillary cast in the wax index, eliminating the need for a record base (framework) and occlusion rim. A split cast mounting technique is required to allow subsequent remount of the prosthesis for occlusal equilibration.

### Horizontal Position of the Mandible

A decision must be made early in the treatment planning stages regarding the horizontal position of the mandible, centric relation or centric occlusion. The centric relation position is required when a mandibular removable partial denture opposes a maxillary complete denture. To record this relationship accurately the maxillary arch requires a record base and occlusion rim, and the mandible requires either a record base or framework with an occlusion rim if the partially eden-

tulous arch is a Kennedy Class I or II. Like the maxillary cast, the mandibular cast may be used alone if the partially edentulous arch is a Kennedy Class III or IV where sufficient posterior teeth are present to provide an accurate and stable record of the centric relation position. The centric relation position is also required in the restoration of a fully edentulous mandible opposed by a partially edentulous maxilla. The mandibular arch requires a record base and occlusion rim, and the maxillary arch requires either a framework or record base supporting an occlusion rim if the arch is a Kennedy Class I or II or the maxillary cast alone if it is a Kennedy Class III or IV.

When opposing removable partial dentures are to be constructed or when a partial denture is to oppose natural dentition, centric relation is used in the following situations:

1. Where there are no natural opposing tooth stops or insufficient ones, to provide centric occlusion or to support the vertical dimension of occlusion (Fig. 6–33)
2. Where posterior teeth are to be restored (crowns, inlays, onlays, etc.)
3. Where the existing occlusal scheme is evaluated as pathologic

Centric occlusion may be used when there is sufficient natural tooth contacts to maintain centric occlusion and vertical dimension of occlusion. In addition the occlusion must be evaluated as "physiologic" for the individual patient (Fig. 6–34). This may occur in situations which require opposing removable partial dentures or where a single removable partial denture opposes an intact arch.

### Vertical Dimension of Occlusion

When natural tooth contacts support the vertical dimension of occlusion, the opposing contacts with and without the prosthesis in place must be identical. In situations where insufficient or poorly positioned teeth do not support the vertical dimension of occlusion, the vertical dimension of occlusion must be established and evaluated. Engaging the patient in casual conversation is a valuable aid in the determination of vertical dimension of occlusion, particularly if the patient has previously worn a removable prosthesis. The patient's neuromuscular perception, the appearance of the extraoral facial landmarks, and a comparison with the existing denture are all guides that should be used in the evaluation of the vertical dimension of occlusion presented by the new prosthesis.

### QUESTIONS

15. Which of the following maxillary partially edentulous arches does not generally require record bases and oc-

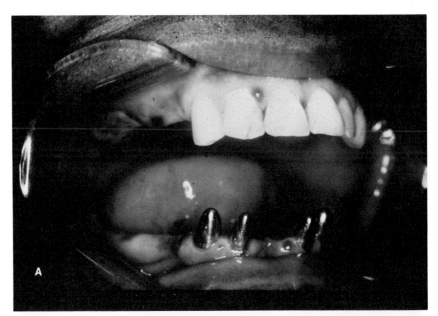

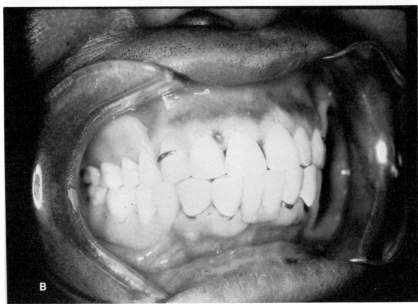

**FIG. 6-33.** Centric relation may be the only repeatable reference position. A. Mouth restored with a conventional maxillary removable partial denture. B. Mandibular removable partial denture of the crown and sleeve coping design.

clusion rims (or framework) for an accurate face-bow record?

1. Kennedy Class I, modification 1
2. Kennedy Class III, modification 1
3. Kennedy Class II
4. Kennedy Class II, modification 2

16. The horizontal mandibular position recorded for a maxillary complete denture opposing a Kennedy Class III, modification 1 removable partial denture should provide
    1. centric occlusion coincident with centric relation
    2. maximum intercuspation anterior to centric relation

3. 1 and 2
4. 1 or 2

## OCCLUSAL FACTORS

A review of removable partial dentures cannot be complete without mention of occlusal factors and their relationship to health in the restored partially edentulous mouth. Coleman (10) writes that "the two main functions of a removable partial denture are to restore lost functional parts and to preserve the remaining oral

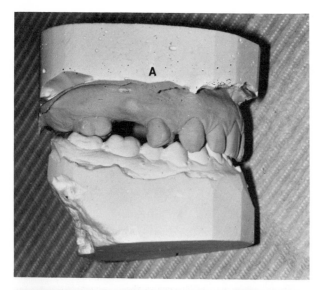

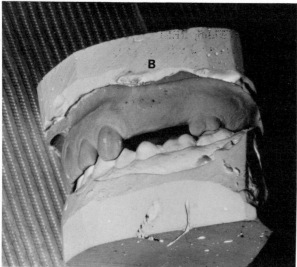

**FIG. 6–34.** Diagnostic cast for which a maxillary Kennedy Class III, modification 1 removable partial denture will be constructed in harmony with existing centric occlusion A. Right side. B. Left side.

remaining natural teeth must be analyzed and imbalances corrected by occlusal adjustment or restorative procedures to place the remaining natural teeth in harmony with the occlusal scheme that is determined to be physiologic for the patient. The removable partial denture is then constructed in harmony with this planned occlusal scheme. If occlusal imbalances are not corrected prior to the placement of the removable partial denture, it is conceivable that the additional loading of the abutment teeth by the denture would render these teeth incapable of supporting and retaining the prosthesis.

Many all-tooth-supported removable partial dentures (Kennedy Class III and IV) are constructed in centric occlusion or maximum intercuspation anterior to the centric relation position. For such restorations it is essential that the patient's jaw be guided into the more retruded position to detect any imbalances created by the removable partial denture; this imbalance must be corrected.

## Guidelines for Occlusal Schemes

Coleman (10) summarized the occlusal requirements of the all-tooth-supported removable partial denture:

When natural teeth provide and are suitable for anterior guidance, the artificial teeth of the removable partial denture should provide centric occlusion contacts in harmony with those of the natural teeth with disocclusion of the posterior segments during eccentric movements.

When natural teeth provide working side contacts without anterior guidance and in the presence of strong abutment teeth, the artificial teeth of the removable partial denture should provide centric occlusion contacts and working side contacts in harmony with those of the natural teeth.

When natural teeth provide working side contacts without anterior guidance and in the presence of weak abutment teeth, the artificial teeth of the removable partial denture should provide centric occlusion contacts in harmony with those of the natural teeth and disocclusion of the artificial teeth during eccentric movements.

When a complete denture opposes an all-tooth-supported removable partial denture, the artificial teeth of the removable partial denture should provide centric occlusion contacts in harmony with those of the natural teeth and be coincident with centric relation. Bilateral balance is desirable in eccentric positions to maintain the stability of the complete denture.

The importance of occlusal factors for the all-tooth-supported prosthesis to the maintenance of tissue

structures. Unless scrupulous attention is paid to the details of restoring function, the very function that is restored may destroy that which remains." Thorough analysis and planning of a desired occlusal scheme and/or proper rehabilitative restorative procedures preliminary and prerequisite to removable partial denture therapy are essential.

Accurately mounted diagnostic casts are essential for occlusal analysis, which is part of the treatment planning phase. Factors such as extrusion, intermaxillary space, plane of occlusion, etc. can be evaluated best by means of mounted casts. The occlusal relationship of health applies no less to the tooth-and-tissue-supported denture. The positive effect of proper design of this most difficult restoration upon the equitable distribution of stress can be totally negated by an improper occlusal scheme in the finished restoration.

Coleman (10) also summarized the occlusal requirements of distal extension prostheses:

When natural teeth provide and are suitable for anterior guidance, the artificial teeth of the removable partial denture should provide centric occlusion contacts in harmony with those of the natural teeth with disocclusion of the posterior segments during eccentric movements.

When no anterior tooth guidance is provided by the natural teeth, or if the anterior teeth are not suitable to provide anterior guidance, the artificial teeth of the removable partial denture should provide centric occlusion contacts and working side contacts.

When a complete denture opposes a distal extension base removable partial denture, the artifical teeth of the removable partial denture should provide centric occlusion contacts in harmony with those of the natural teeth and be coincident with centric relation. Bilateral balance is desirable in eccentric positions to maintain the stability of the complete denture.

## Occlusal Equilibration of Completed Removable Partial Dentures

All-tooth-supported removable partial dentures are equilibrated preferably on the articulator following processing. Equilibration is intended to reestablish the vertical dimension of occlusion to maintain natural tooth contacts, to achieve a tight centric occlusion, and to refine the eccentric occlusal scheme. Although equilibration of the all-tooth-supported prosthesis can be accomplished intraorally, intraoral equilibration is more difficult and less accurate.

Frequently final casts are destroyed when they are removed from investments after processing. If this occurs, the removable partial denture can be remounted on the articulator by using a mounting model. Such a model is constructed by seating the prosthesis intraorally, "pulling" the prosthesis in an overall impression, and then blocking out the prosthesis where indicated prior to pouring the casts. The next step is to make the appropriate intermaxillary records and mount the prosthesis with the mounting cast. After the records have been verified, the occlusion is refined by equilibration.

Like the all-tooth-supported prosthesis, the finished distal extension partial denture must be equilibrated after processing to reestablish the vertical dimension of occlusion, obtain a tight centric occlusion, and refine the eccentric occlusal scheme. The occlusal equilibra-

tion of tooth-and-tissue-supported removable partial dentures (Kennedy Class I and II) requires an equilibration on the articulator. If the final cast has been destroyed or injured, it is imperative that a mounting cast be constructed so that the prosthesis can be mounted on the articulator via new intraoral records, because a tooth-and-tissue-supported removable partial denture cannot be accurately equilibrated intraorally. Displaceability of the mucoperiosteum can hide occlusal discrepancies of significant magnitude that will be translated clinically as irritation of the underlying ridge, destruction of the artificial teeth and/or denture base, and subsequent potential rapid resorption of osseous support (Fig. 6–21).

## QUESTIONS

17. Maxillary and mandibular removable partial denture frameworks have been independently adjusted for occlusion to allow natural tooth contacts. With both frameworks seated it is noted that the natural teeth are in slight hyperocclusion. The premature contact exists between
    1. the mandibular framework and the natural maxillary teeth
    2. the maxillary framework and the natural mandibular teeth
    3. opposing frameworks
    4. Any of the above; all are possible

18. In order to achieve maximum intercuspation in centric occlusion when setting posterior artificial teeth for a removable partial denture, the artificial teeth are first set in hyperocclusion and then equilibrated back to the original vertical dimension of occlusion. This procedure must be accomplished for all of the following situations with the exception of setting
    1. maxillary artificial posteriors against mandibular natural posteriors
    2. maxillary artificial posteriors and mandibular artificial posteriors
    3. mandibular artificial posteriors against a maxillary posterior fixed prosthesis

19. A distal extension removable partial denture with natural anterior teeth that are capable of anterior guidance requires the posterior artificial teeth to provide
    1. centric occlusion and working contacts
    2. centric occlusion contacts only
    3. balancing and working contacts

20. The occlusal requirements of a mandibular bilateral distal extension removable partial denture against a maxillary complete denture are
    1. centric occlusion
    2. centric occlusion and working contacts
    3. centric occlusion and balancing contacts
    4. centric occlusion, working contacts, and balancing contacts
    5. balancing and working contacts

## AESTHETIC CONSIDERATIONS

### Anterior Tooth Selection

The selection of artificial anterior teeth is facilitated by the presence of remaining natural anterior teeth which serve as an accurate guide in the determination of size, shape, shade, labiolingual placement, and arrangement of the artificial anterior teeth. It is important to maintain the gingivoincisal length of the artificial teeth in harmony with the anterior natural teeth during the setting of the teeth in the laboratory. Spacing, incisal wear, and individualization of both position and rotation should be accomplished as a chairside procedure during the trial denture appointment to allow the patient to evaluate the anterior appearance. After the patient has given approval, no change should be made in this arrangement other than refinement of

the waxing of the denture base in preparation for completion and insertion of the prosthesis.

If all the natural anterior teeth are to be restored with the prosthesis, the selection process for the anterior teeth parallels that for complete dentures (Fig. 6–35). Midline, high lip line, and distal surface of the canine lines should be scribed on the occlusion rim, supported either by a record base or the framework. The occlusion rim should be adjusted initially to establish the anterior plane of occlusion parallel to the interpupillary line. In order to be sure there will be adequate lip support labial positioning of the occlusion rim is accomplished; extraoral landmarks such as the philtrum, the vermilion border of lip, the nasolabial sulcus, and the mentolabial sulcus as well as intraoral landmarks such as the incisive papilla, are used as guides. The initial height of the occlusion rim is determined by phonetic evaluation, harmony with the pos-

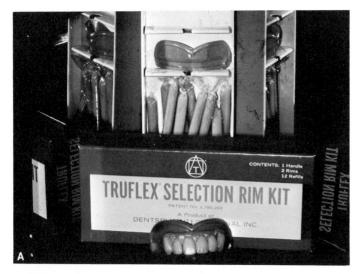

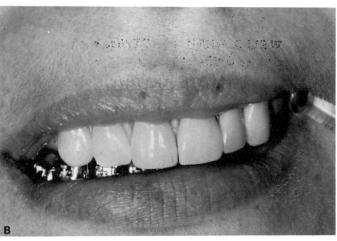

**FIG. 6–35.** A. The Truflex Selection Rim Kit serves as an excellent aid in the selection of artificial anterior teeth. B. A full complement of artificial anterior teeth.

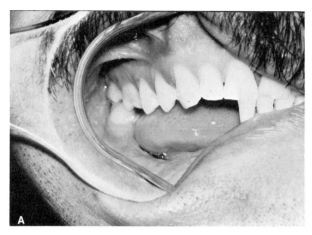
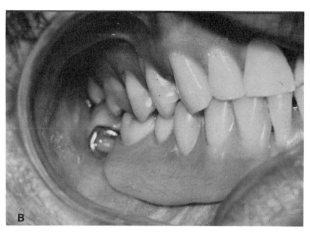

**FIG. 6-36.** A. Mandibular defect following surgical removal of ameloblastoma restored with an interim removable partial denture B. Note harmony in appearance aspects between artificial and natural teeth.

terior plane of occlusion, and consultation with the patient to find out how much tooth structure the patient wants visible when the lips are separated in a relaxed position.

The selection of the shade, which must harmonize with the remaining natural teeth, generally poses no great difficulty. The patient's face form, in conjunction with photographs, may provide a guide in the selection of the size and shape of the anterior teeth. Obviously available space is a limiting factor in the selection of artificial tooth size. Individualization and characterization of tooth arrangement must be accomplished as a chairside procedure and evaluated by the patient prior to completion of the prosthesis. An excellent review of the common problems associated with artificial tooth arrangement is presented by Lombardi (32). Although the paper addresses complete dentures, it is no less relevant to removable partial dentures.

### Posterior Tooth Selection

Posterior tooth selection is also facilitated by the presence of natural teeth. Shade, size, buccolingual position, and degree of cuspation should be in harmony with the remaining natural teeth (Fig. 6-36). A common unsightly error is failure to maintain sufficient gingivoocclusal height of artificial teeth adjacent to natural teeth. This is seen when posterior teeth must be ground to fit a limited interocclusal space and also to adapt to the imposition of framework components in this space. Careful ridge lap grinding of the artificial teeth can generally allow for adequate gingivoocclusal height to be maintained.

### Denture Bases

Acrylic resin for denture bases is available in a variety of shades. Shade selection is particularly important when the prosthesis includes an anterior denture base flange, and the distal termination of an anterior base must not contrast in shade with the adjacent mucosa. Individual characterization of denture bases can be accomplished as a laboratory procedure or as a chairside procedure by adding pigmentation with self-polymerizing acrylic resins to the denture base.

Proper extension of denture bases contributes to the overall aesthetic result of the restoration. One must keep in mind that the denture base, in addition to supporting the artificial teeth, also replaces lost osseous structure which supported the cheeks and lips. Indeed, the fact that it may be necessary for the base and artificial anterior tooth position to provide lip support is sometimes an indication for a removable partial denture rather than a fixed partial denture to restore a Kennedy Class IV partially endentulous arch (Fig. 6–37). Visible denture base borders should be thinned, beveled, and contoured in such a fashion that they blend with the adjacent mucosa and thereby do not attract attention. See also Restoration of Facial Contour.

### Path of Insertion

When anterior teeth are to be included in a removable partial denture, the path of insertion determined during the initial survey analysis may influence the aesthetic aspects of the restoration. A mediolateral tilt should be identified that does not cause severe undercuts to be presented by proximal tooth surfaces adjacent to the anterior edentulous space. Such undercuts would not allow the creation of normal-appearing interproximal embrasures between the natural tooth and the adjacent artificial tooth.

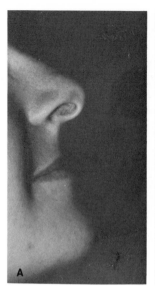
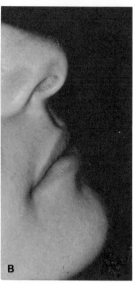

**FIG. 6-37.** Profile of patient for whom a Kennedy Class IV removable partial denture was indicated. A. Without the prosthesis in place. B. With the prosthesis in place.

QUESTIONS

21. The final path of insertion may affect aesthetics by permitting
    1. the most suitable size and shape of anterior tooth replacements
    2. less clasp metal to be displayed
    3. Both of the above
    4. Neither of the above

22. Aesthetic considerations related to the selection of posterior artificial teeth and waxing of the denture base include
    1. maintenance of artificial tooth height (gingivoocclusal)
    2. placement of gingival papillae above contact areas
    3. harmony of artificial tooth size with adjacent natural teeth size
    4. 1 and 3
    5. All of the above

## INSERTION AND POSTINSERTION ADJUSTMENTS

### Preparation of Prosthesis for Insertion

If time and effort are devoted to anticipating the causes of patient discomfort at the time the removable partial denture is inserted, many of the problems associated with the adjustment phase can be minimized or prevented. A definite regimen should be followed in the evaluation of a finished prosthesis prior to an insertion appointment. The tissue surface of the denture base should be examined for imperfections and minute projections. These should be removed conservatively, and sharp or angular borders of the denture base should be well rounded, smoothed, finished, and polished. An examination should be made of the polished surface of the denture base for proper contour and finish. Border extensions can be verified and corrected, if necessary, following intraoral evaluation. If a distal extension base is involved and its borders have been created with an altered cast technique, generally few border alterations are required.

A common problem that can prevent seating of the finished denture is a flash of acrylic resin lying between a proximal minor connector and the adjacent natural tooth surface. The proximal guiding planes of the framework should be examined and freed of any acrylic resin that has encroached between the plane and the adjacent tooth. Also, to promote gingival health, the acrylic resin lying cervical to the guiding planes should be slightly relieved so that the gingival papilla can assume a resting position with no resulting impingement by the removable partial denture. These procedures should be done routinely prior to the patient's appointment. Besides preventing subsequent patient discomfort, they can save valuable chairside time.

### Insertion of Prosthesis

Interferences by the removable partial denture framework should not be a factor at the time of insertion of the prosthesis, if interferences were corrected during the trial insertion of the framework. One of the objectives at the trial insertion of the framework was to maintain identical occlusion with and without the framework placed intraorally. Frequently bilateral soft tissue undercuts prevent seating of the finished denture, but the operator must be conservative when relieving these areas on the denture bases. Once seated, the denture bases should be evaluated for proper border extension buccally, labially, and lingually, as well as for proper relief of muscle attachments. Obvious overextensions must be shortened, refined, and repolished. Indicating pastes or indicating waxes are useful for this purpose. Overextensions of a mandibular denture base posterior to the retromolar pads should be identified and corrected, as well as overextensions beyond the hamular notches of a maxillary posterior distal extension prosthesis.

Although the fit of the framework was evaluated and refined at its initial seating, at the insertion visit it is prudent to verify again the fit of the direct retainers, indirect retainers, rests, and the relationship of blanket areas of the framework to the underlying teeth. Excessive force should not be required to either seat or remove the finished prosthesis. Clasps must be treated with extreme care, because distortion of clasps may necessitate remaking of the entire prosthesis. Cast clasps, due to their one-half round cross sectional form are extremely difficult to return to their original position in relation to the tooth if they are distorted. Frequently the presence of saliva on rests and rest seats may mask an inaccuracy in the fit of the rest. Therefore an air spray should be directed to the occlusal rests so that any discrepancy in their relation to the rest seats can be clearly identified.

## Evaluation of Framework Finish

The completed framework should be evaluated for correct finishing and polishing. Both surfaces of the mandibular lingual bar, the nontissue surface of maxillary major connectors, the nontissue surface of all clasp arms and blanket areas, both surfaces of vertical connecting arms of No. 2 clasp designs, and the nontooth surface of minor connectors not to be imbedded in denture base material are to receive a high finish and polish.

## Occlusal Analysis

After the removable partial denture has been fully seated and necessary refinements made, the occlusion must be evaluated. When natural tooth contacts dictate centric occlusion and vertical dimension of occlusion, the occlusion with and without the partial denture in place must be identical. No matter what eccentric occlusal scheme has been planned for the restoration, all restorations must allow simultaneous bilateral posterior contact in centric occlusion at times coincident with centric relation. The "final equilibration" may have been accomplished after processing via a laboratory remount procedure. Quite frequently additional intraoral records are required during the insertion visit, the construction of mounting casts accomplished, and the prosthesis placed back on the articulator for additional refinement of the occlusion.

## Patient Education

Although patient education is at times a neglected phase of treatment in removable prosthodontics, patient understanding of the role of oral hygiene and care of the restoration has been shown to be an important factor in the success of treatment with a removable partial denture. At the insertion appointment the patient must be instructed in the proper procedure for insertion and removal of the prosthesis and must demonstrate the ability to place and remove the prosthesis with no difficulty before being dismissed. To seat the prosthesis the patient should align the clasps with the appropriate abutment teeth and engage the guiding plates on the guiding planes. Firm bilateral pressure is then applied through the path of insertion until the prosthesis is completely seated. It should be emphasized that the partial denture must not be seated by biting forces from the opposing teeth, because this could cause clasp distortion, as well as tissue injury. The patient should learn to remove the partial denture by grasping the clasps as close as possible to the minor connector where the clasps are more rigid and less likely to distort.

Home care is critical for proper maintenance of a dental arch restored with a removable partial denture and should be emphasized at the insertion visit. Clinical studies have indicated that satisfactory home care can maintain healthy supporting tissues while lack of home care can lead to gingival inflammation and progressive periodontal breakdown of the abutment teeth. Instructions should be provided for the patient regarding cleansing of the prosthesis. Generally it is preferable that the dentures not be worn continuously; the supporting tissues need an opportunity to rest. The patient should select a convenient time during which the prosthesis may be removed from the mouth for 4–6 hours without any embarrassment. While the prosthesis is out of the mouth, it should be immersed in a commercially available cleansing solution such as an oxygenating cleanser which effectively cleans areas not readily reached by a denture brush. The patient should maintain a soft diet for the first 1 or 2 days following insertion. Most patients, depending on previous experience with a removable partial denture, are able to return to a normal diet within a short period of time.

The patient should be given sufficient time to digest all this material and to ask any questions regarding the maintenance of the prosthesis and care of the supporting tissues. A definite postinsertion regimen should then be established and the patient appointed to return within 24–48 hours for the first postinsertion visit.

## Postinsertion Phase

During the first postinsertion visit the dentures are removed and the supporting tissues examined. Soreness of the denture-bearing area generally falls into one of four categories. First, a localized, well-circumscribed area of irritation is generally caused by an irregularity on the tissue surface of the acrylic resin. To correct this, mark the irritation with a gentian violet marking stick and seat the denture accurately. The violet mark is transferred to the internal surface of the base, indicating the area of irritation, which is then conservatively relieved. Second, generalized redness of the mucosa is usually due to an occlusal error, quite frequently hyperocclusion. If this is determined to be the cause, an equilibration must be accomplished, preferably by a remount procedure on the articulator. Third, irritation on the lingual or buccal aspects of an edentulous ridge of a distal extension prosthesis is generally caused by occlusal interferences in lateral excursions which allow some rotational movement of the distal extension base; this is also corrected by a remount and equilibration of the prosthesis on the articulator. Fourth, redness or ulceration of the mucosa at the periphery of the denture base is generally the result of an overextended base or a rough angular periphery of a denture border. Disclosing or indicating pastes are used to pinpoint the overextension, which is then relieved, finished, and polished.

If during subsequent recall visits abutment tooth mobility is present, its cause can be attributed to 1) insufficient clasp flexibility, 2) occlusal disharmony, 3) movement of the distal extension base, or 4) a distorted framework. Clasp flexibility can be increased by reestablishing the taper of the clasp arm or reducing the inferior border of the clasp arm, thus decreasing the amount of horizontal undercut engaged by the retentive terminus. Occlusal disharmony, frequently seen with a distal extension base, may lead to abutment tooth mobility. To correct this, new intraoral records should be made, the denture mounted on an articulator with the aid of mounting casts, and refinement of the occlusal scheme in centric occlusion and excursive movements accomplished. Excessive movement of a distal extension base, which increases the destructive force transmitted by the lever arm to an abutment tooth adjacent to an edentulous area, can be caused by resorption of the underlying osseous support or initial failure to ensure accurate adaptation of the denture base to the underlying tissues via a functional impression technique. To correct this and to gain support from the residual ridge, a functional reline or rebase is indicated. Mobility of an abutment tooth can develop due to a flexing of a major connector or a distorted framework. Such flexibility can generally be traced to inaccuracies in fabrication of the prosthesis or careless handling by the patient. The results of these errors can be quite destructive and necessitate remaking of the partial denture framework.

### Removable Partial Denture Failures

Failure of removable partial denture therapy can be traced to several sources. Unfortunately, one of the most common sources of partial denture failure is improper diagnostic and treatment planning procedures. All too often a partial denture is placed in the mouth simply to fill a space created by the loss of several natural teeth, or the proper preliminary rehabilitative restorative procedures are not planned and accomplished. Hasty and laboratory oriented planning or lack of good laboratory technique supervision can lead to failure of the prosthesis. Close control and supervision

can and should be maintained over laboratory procedures. If the dentist employs a laboratory technician or uses a commercial laboratory, specifically worded work authorizations and good communication with the technician are necessary. When establishing a relationship with a commercial laboratory, it is advantageous initially to request that certain phases of laboratory procedures be returned to the dentist for evaluation until confidence is gained in the laboratory. For example, the return of the final cast prepared for duplication along with the refractory cast with the wax framework in place prior to the casting, finishing, and polishing of the framework allows the dentist to point out any inconsistencies between the design and the laboratory technician's execution of the design.

Partial denture therapy may fail in spite of proper diagnostic and planning procedures, good laboratory supervision, well-executed mouth preparations, excellent framework design, and excellent technical results if the patient does not understand his or her role in the postinsertion and maintenance phase of the use of the prosthesis. Indifferent patient education on the part of the dentist or disinterest on the part of the patient, in conjunction with insufficient insistence on periodic maintenance of the prosthesis by the dentist or lack of response on the part of the patient, may mean the difference between success and failure of therapy with a removable partial denture.

QUESTION

23. If careless handling of the prosthesis has distorted the major connector, the steps taken in the corrective procedure are to
   1. reestablish the taper of the clasp arm
   2. accomplish a functional reline
   3. remake the prosthesis
   4. remount and equilibrate the prosthesis
   5. adjust the major connector

## DENTAL MATERIALS

### Denture Bases

Bases for removable partial dentures may be constructed of cast metal, acrylic resin, or a combination of the two (Fig. 6–38). As a denture base material, metal has properties which are superior to those of acrylic resin. Metal is a thermal conductor, while resin is a thermal insulator. In addition, metal exhibits considerably greater accuracy and permanence of form, is more easily cleaned than acrylic resins, and is light in weight while possessing strength and rigidity. Metal is comparatively unaesthetic and not easily correctable when a reline or rebase is needed, however. The main advantages of acrylic resin as a denture base material are

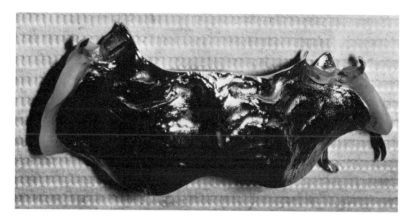

**FIG. 6–38.** Cast metal base with buccal veneer and periphery of acrylic resin.

correctability (readily relined or rebased) and aesthetics.

Because the all-tooth-supported prosthesis directs all forces to abutment teeth and not to ridge, selection of the base material is not as critical as that for the tooth-and-tissue-supported restoration. The base for the all-tooth-supported restoration for anterior replacement is generally metal for small edentulous spans (in conjunction with an artificial tooth form such as the Steel's facing) and acrylic resin for large anterior edentulous spaces where restoration of atrophied ridge areas is a consideration. The same considerations apply to the selection of base material for the all-tooth-supported posterior edentulous span: metal for small spans with little ridge atrophy, acrylic resin or a combination of resin and metal for large spans with significant ridge atrophy.

An important factor to be considered in the selection of material for a distal extension base is the potential for change in the form of the edentulous ridge. Because of the observed need for subsequent rebasing or relining, the material of choice in these situations is one that is easily correctable, generally acrylic resin. From a preventive point of view, however, cast metal bases might be more beneficial because they help to preserve the residual ridge. The advantages of metal bases may outweigh in selected cases the only obvious advantage of acrylic resin—better correctability. The use of cast metal distal extension bases (generally in combination with acrylic resin) may be considered in the following circumstances (19): 1) favorable age and general health of the patient and 2) remaking of a distal extension prosthesis when the edentulous ridge has changed little in form over a significant period of time.

### Artificial Teeth

Materials available for the artificial teeth of a removable partial denture include gold, porcelain, and acrylic resin. Gold is the material of choice to occlude against natural teeth or teeth restored with gold (Fig. 6–39). Porcelain teeth are generally not compatible with opposing surfaces of gold or natural tooth structure. Also, technical problems may be encountered in the arrangement of porcelain posterior teeth while recontouring these teeth to conform to various components of the framework. Acrylic resin teeth offer the technical advantages of ease of recontouring and finishing and they also can be used to create custom occlusal surfaces when opposed by natural teeth or existing restorations. Indeed acrylic resin teeth in such situations should be thought of as nothing more than a block material out of which an appropriate occlusal form can be created. In addition, acrylic resin teeth do not wear away opposing gold or natural tooth surfaces.

### Metal Alloys for Removable Partial Denture Frameworks

Base metal alloys have largely replaced gold alloys for the fabrication of removable partial denture frameworks, despite the fact that Type IV gold alloys possess advantages in terms of physical and mechanical properties. When the physical properties of gold are compared to those of the base metal alloys, a significant difference can be noted in modulus of elasticity; base metal alloys possess values approximately twice those of the gold alloys. This means that the base metal alloys are twice as stiff as gold alloys. Therefore, when space is limited, the base metal alloys have a distinct advantage for the major connectors and other components of the partial framework that require rigidity. When flexibility is desired, as for a retentive terminus of a clasp, gold alloys offer the advantage. If a base metal alloy is used, generally the undercut on the abutment tooth must be correspondingly reduced or the retentive portion of the clasp assembly must be constructed of gold alloy wrought wire.

An important comparison between the two metals for selection of frameworks concerns hardness. Base

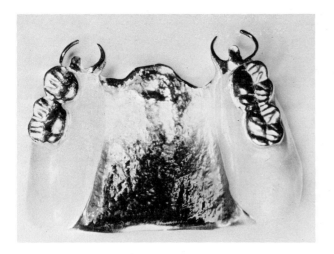

**FIG. 6–39.** Cast gold occlusal surfaces on a maxillary Kennedy Class I removable partial denture which opposes fixed partial prostheses. (Courtesy of Dr. Daniel Isaacson).

metal alloys are about 30% harder than the gold alloys, making finishing and polishing procedures more difficult. In fact, special laboratory instruments and equipment are required to accomplish the procedures.

The most significant comparison of mechanical properties of the two alloys is that of casting shrinkage. The base metal alloys shrink more than the gold alloys when solidification occurs. Clinically this means that the fit of gold alloy removable partial denture frameworks is more accurate. The poorer fit of base metal alloys is most apparent on the more complex designs generally seen in maxillary castings. For this reason, whenever multiple clasp assemblies and multiple contacts on vertical tooth surfaces by the framework are required, the more accurate material (Type IV gold) better meets the objectives of a partial denture framework.

Cunningham (11) identified factors that may influence the decision in the choice of alloys as 1) the availability of space for the major connectors, 2) the amount and location of undercut on the proposed abutments for retention, 3) the complexity of the framework design, 4) the question of whether intracoronal attachments are to be used, 5) the availability of competent technical assistance, and 6) costs. When space for the major connectors and other rigid units of the framework is limited, the base metal alloys offer an advantage in that rigidity can be maintained with less bulk. These alloys can also be successfully employed when abutment contours can be controlled either by restoring or recontouring. However, because of their physical properties, base metal alloys offer less latitude in the amount of undercut employed. It has already been stated that gold alloys are indicated for the more com-

plex designs which demand greater accuracy. When intracoronal attachments are to be used, gold alloys are also indicated due to the ease of soldering. Some technicians are quite skillful in fitting the base metal alloy framework casting to the master cast during the finishing and polishing procedures. Their availability is a consideration in selecting a base metal for a framework. Although cost of the metal must be a consideration in some cases, this is a relatively small differential as compared to the cost of the total service and therefore should be a secondary consideration.

QUESTIONS

24. Theoretically the best combination for a partial denture framework is
    1. chromium alloy for the clasps, gold alloy for framework and connectors
    2. gold alloy for the clasps and connectors, chromium alloy for the framework
    3. chromium alloy for the clasps and connectors, gold alloy for the framework
    4. gold alloy for the clasps, chromium alloy for the framework and connectors
    5. None of the above

25. Which of the following is (are) considered to be (an) advantage(s) of metal denture bases compared to acrylic resin denture bases?
    1. Metal acts as a thermal insulator.
    2. Metal is easily relined or rebased.
    3. Metal exhibits greater accuracy.
    4. Metal is more aesthetic.
    5. 1 and 3

26. Acrylic resin artificial teeth rather than porcelain artificial teeth are generally used as posterior tooth replacements in a removable partial denture because
    a. acrylic resin teeth are easily adjusted to accommodate the retentive meshwork and the minor connectors
    b. acrylic resin teeth maintain the vertical dimension of occlusion over a longer period of time
    c. the occlusal surfaces of acrylic resin teeth need no modification to occlude against natural teeth
    d. acrylic resin teeth are potentially less destructive when opposed by natural teeth or gold restorations
    1. a, c, and d
    2. a and d
    3. b and c
    4. All of the above

## INTERIM, TRANSITIONAL, AND TREATMENT REMOVABLE PARTIAL DENTURES

### Interim Prosthesis

An interim prosthesis is one used prior to the construction of a fixed prosthesis or a definitive removable partial denture. It may be an immediate replacement

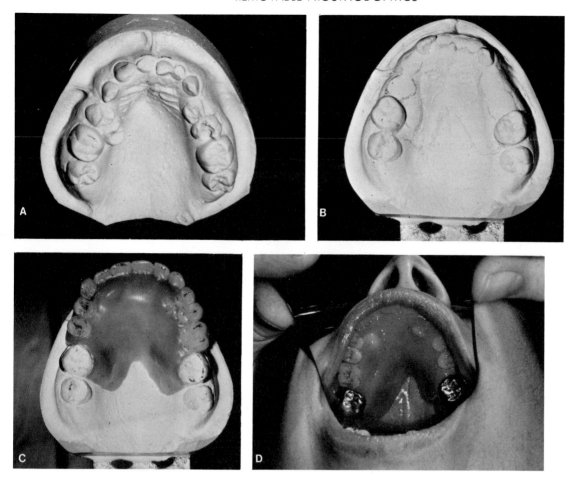

**FIG. 6-40.** A. Cast for interim immediate removable partial denture. B. Cast after teeth to be extracted have been removed. C. Prosthesis waxed on final cast. D. Insertion of immediate interim removable partial denture.

or one that is replacing already missing teeth (Figs. 6-40 and 6-41). Indications for its use include insufficient time for complete rehabilitative procedures, poor health of the patient, prematurely lost teeth in a young patient where the maintenance of space and aesthetics are considerations, and recent extractions when time is required for complete healing of the tissues but occlusion and appearance must be maintained. The interim removable partial denture can also be used as a "training" prosthesis. This is particularly important for patients who feel that they will be unable to adapt to a removable partial denture.

### Transitional Prosthesis

A transitional removable partial denture is a prosthesis to which teeth are added as natural teeth are lost.

The prosthesis then becomes either an interim removable partial denture or an interim complete denture, depending upon the number of teeth to be extracted during its use as a transitional prosthesis (Fig. 6-42).

A transitional removable partial denture is indicated for a patient who is to receive a complete denture and who has had no previous removable prosthodontic experience. For this patient it is wise to construct a transitional removable partial denture replacing the posterior teeth first. In this way the vertical dimension of occlusion can be established and verified, and the patient can be given an adjustment period before wearing the full prosthesis. This procedure also allows the occlusal scheme to be refined, thus eliminating some of the inaccuracies that may develop with a complete immediate prosthesis. The use of the transitional partial denture in these circumstances improves the prognosis of the eventual immediate complete denture since only the anterior teeth are involved in the immediate pros-

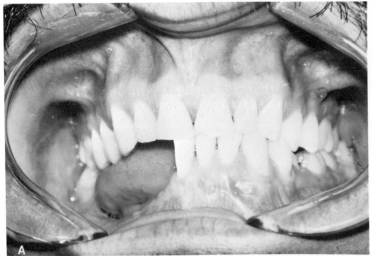

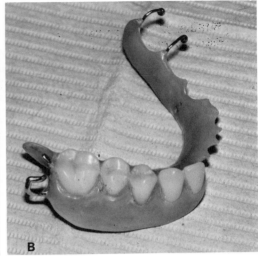

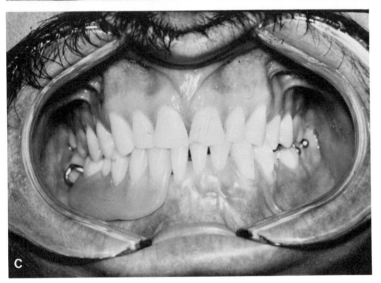

FIG. 6-41. A. Mandibular interim removable partial denture required. B. View of prosthesis. C. This interim prosthesis serves multiple functions such as vertical dimension of occlusions and prevention of extrusions.

thesis and the patient has already adapted to the transitional removable partial denture for posterior teeth.

### Treatment Prosthesis

A treatment prosthesis is one used to establish a new occlusal relationship or to restore vertical dimension (Fig. 6–43). A treatment prosthesis is also indicated to condition abused tissues prior to the construction of the definitive prosthesis.

It is imperative that the patient understand the distinction between the interim, transitional, or treatment partial denture and the definitive prosthesis for which the oral cavity has been prepared. If these temporary prostheses are worn beyond the time of their intended purpose, they may be destructive to the supporting tissues.

### Construction

The use of an all acrylic resin denture with wrought wire clasps is not always synonymous with the construction of interim, transitional, or treatment removable partial dentures. The materials of construction are not inferred in the definition of the restoration; the definition of these restorations identifies simply their function and indications for their use. Therefore, if it is anticipated that an interim, transitional, or treatment removable partial denture will be worn for an extended

*(Continued)*

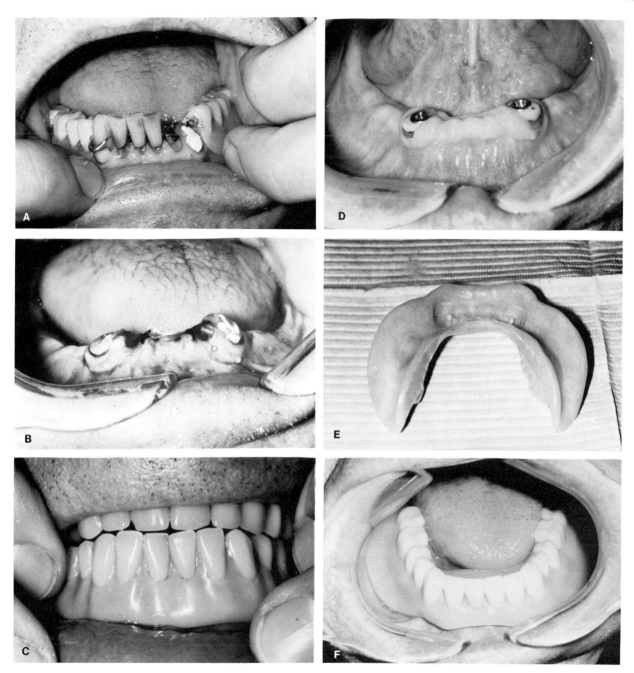

**FIG. 6–42.** A. Existing mandibular removable partial denture to be used as a transitional prosthesis. B. Conversion to an interim immediate tooth-supported complete denture. C. Converted denture. D. Placement of intraradicular attachments. E. New tooth-supported complete denture. F. Inserted denture.

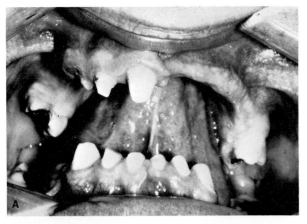

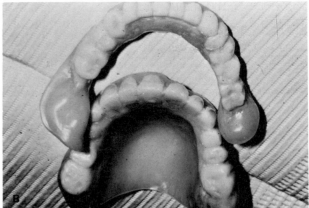

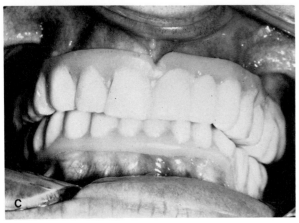

**FIG. 6-43.** A. Remaining teeth do not provide a vertical dimension of occlusion. B. Treatment dentures were constructed to determine the vertical dimension of occlusion and the mandibular horizontal position. C. Inserted dentures. (Courtesy of Dr. I. Yalisove)

period of time, it is suggested that a cast framework be used in the temporary prosthesis to provide rigidity, cross-arch stabilization, and stress distribution.

## DISCUSSION

The conventionally clasped removable partial denture is a much maligned restoration. Heintz (17) points out that failure of treatment with a removable partial denture is the result of inadequate diagnosis and poor planning; he summarizes the unfavorable results as follows: 1) unnecessary trauma contributing to a loss of natural teeth, 2) trauma to soft tissue, 3) unjustified extractions of third molars and moderately malposed teeth, 4) cantilever and torquing forces imparted by poor design, 5) poor aesthetics, and 6) premature edentulousness.

Despite the prevailing gloom contributed to by the current state of abuse of the removable partial denture, many experts in this matter are in agreement that the removable partial denture can and should make a major contribution to the preventive aspects of den-

tistry. In fact, it is becoming more widely used because of improved preventive and restorative techniques which ensure the retention of teeth previously condemned to extraction.

Carlsson (7) concludes that ". . . under favorable conditions partial dentures can be used for good oral rehabilitation for relatively long periods of time without incurring a major risk or damage to the remaining teeth." Favorable conditions include a high standard of home care and interest on the part of both patient and dentist. Basic principles of denture construction should be observed in addition to a well-planned maintenance and recall regimen. Rudd (41) and Krajicek (28b) also emphasized the need for adhering to basic principles of design. They indict the dentist rather than the restoration for the currently poor reputation of the removable partial denture.

Most experts are in agreement that the profession is delinquent in meeting its responsibility in this important phase of restorative dentistry. Most also agree that the basic principles of design that have evolved over the years are sound and should be followed in the treatment of the partially edentulous patient. The knowledge, experience, and techniques to construct a removable partial denture that contributes to the over-all health of the oral cavity are available to the profession. All that remains is that they be incorporated into daily clinical practice.

# PART II
# COMPLETE DENTURES

## Bal K. Goyal

## DIAGNOSIS AND TREATMENT PLANNING

Diagnosis is the act or process of deciding the nature of a diseased condition by examination. In complete denture therapy, however, it is not always possible to stay within the confines of this definition. The diagnostic procedure becomes a continuing endeavour which runs concomitantly with therapeutic procedures. Each therapy session reveals more information about the patient and frequently makes it necessary to modify the deductions arrived at during the original diagnostic phase. Although the diagnostic procedure continues throughout the treatment phase, it is well to organize and collect the relevant information in order to present a comprehensive treatment plan and well-founded prognosis to the patient.

### General Information

AGE. The age of the patient plays an important part in determining the prognosis of the treatment. A younger patient is generally more adaptable to the drastic change from the dentulous to the edentulous state and finally to artificial dentures. Younger patients also show more rapid tissue healing and good body resistance. At an advanced age patients exhibit poorer adaptation to dentures, which can generally be attributed to lack of coordination, excessive bone resorption, high tissue sensitivity, and poor healing.

SEX. Many women are more exacting in their demands concerning aesthetics than men. They are more aware of their face and lips. During menopause, psychologic problems, dry mouth, burning sensation in the mouth, and general vague pain contribute to the difficulty of treatment.

GENERAL HEALTH. Patients in good general health usually adapt to dentures better and faster than those in poor health. It is a good practice to observe the patients as they walk to the operatory and sit in the chair. Questions regarding health and medications should be carefully worded so that they do not cause embarrassment or loss of confidence. If necessary, the dentist should not hesitate to contact the patient's physician for further information.

OCCUPATION AND SOCIAL STATUS. Knowing the patient's occupation may at times assist the dentist in evaluating the patient's expectations of treatment results. Placement of anterior teeth will certainly be critical for a patient who plays a wind instrument. Similarly the social status of the patient provides important information to the dentist. Patients enjoying higher social positions are usually more demanding regarding aesthetics and comfort, and they are frequently less amenable to accepting the limitations of dentures.

### Mental Attitude and Expectations of Patients

One of the most important factors influencing the outcome of complete denture therapy is the mental attitude of the patient towards treatment. According to House (23), the patient's mental attitude can be classified into four main groups: 1) philosophic, 2) indifferent, 3) critical, and 4) skeptical.

Philosophic patients understand their oral situation and are willing to accept the judgment of their dentists. They take the advice of the dentist and follow it meticulously, making an effort to contribute towards the success of treatment. In contrast, indifferent patients are not motivated enough to seek treatment on their own. Usually they seek dental care due to the insistence of family and friends. Such patients are liable to terminate treatment if problems arise during the course of treatment. Indifferent patients need much specific instruction on the value, use, and care of dentures, and the dentist must be prepared to spend more time with them.

Typically a critical patient is one who possesses a number of sets of dentures, none of which provides satisfaction. Such patients are very unhappy with previous dentists because they did not follow instructions. They insist that they know exactly what they want, and they try to direct the course of treatment. These patients are difficult to manage unless the dentist takes firm control of the treatment phase. It must be made clear from the start that, although their complaints will be carefully evaluated, it is the dentist who will make the decisions and direct the treatment. Sometimes it is possible to revise these patients' attitude by taking time to explain the limitations of dentures. The most important factor in managing critical patients is identifying them early in treatment and then modifying treatment accordingly.

Skeptical patients have lost hope that anything can be done to help them, usually as a result of bad experiences with previous denture treatment and/or unrelated setbacks in life. Typically these patients are hysterical and in poor general health coupled with excessively resorbed ridges and other unfavorable oral conditions. Management of these patients requires a sympathetic approach and an effort to win their confidence. Extra time and patience may be needed at each step to build up their trust so that they can recognize that the dentist is taking care of their dental problems. These patients also must be recognized early and treatment modified accordingly.

It is evident that in complete denture therapy modifying the approach according to the patient's personality is a very important aspect of successful treatment. This is so because the overall success of complete denture treatment depends to a large extent upon the mental acceptance of the dentures by the patient.

## Medical and Dental Histories

The medical history of the patient is an essential adjunct to the diagnostic procedure. A patient who is both physically and emotionally healthy is generally predisposed to successful denture treatment. On the other hand, if the patient has an involved history of chronic illness associated with lowered body resistance, the introduction of a prosthetic appliance is frequently associated with a continuous pathologic process. Therefore, to determine an informed prognosis, it is essential for the dentist to know if the patient is suffering from any systemic illness.

Diabetes, blood dyscrasias, or hypovitaminoses are examples of disorders that affect the mucosal response to denture pressures. It may be possible to delay the prosthetic treatment until the acute phases of these diseases are under control. Similarly hormonal disturbances such as hyperthyroidism, hyperparathyroidism and climacteric changes, if left unattended, may cause problems in the course of treatment. Arthritis may affect the joints and pose problems in obtaining accurate and repeatable jaw relations. Neurologic disorders such as Bell's palsy and Parkinson's disease also complicate the procedure of taking maxillomandibular relations and may cause problems in denture retention. Cardiovascular diseases at times contraindicate denture treatment. In such cases the patient's cardiologist must be consulted to determine when therapy can be initiated.

Oral malignancies must be carefully studied and handled in consultation with the surgeon. If radiation therapy has been instituted, sufficient time must be allowed for the oral mucosa to return to as near normal as possible before subjecting it to the stresses of a denture. Such patients require more frequent postinsertion examinations. In order to evaluate fully the medical status of a patient it is advisable to have the patient complete a medical questionnaire. In doubtful areas the patient's physician should be consulted before starting treatment.

The dental history, including an evaluation of the patient's denture experience, is also necessary to arrive at a comprehensive treatment plan. If the patient has dentures they must be appraised at this stage inside as well as outside the mouth and the findings correlated with the patient's complaints. The main causes of dissatisfaction must be identified so that they can be corrected, if possible, in the new dentures. In addition, if the dentist thinks some alterations of the existing dentures are necessary, they should be noted and presented to the patient in the treatment plan. A note should also be made of the materials and the type of teeth used in the old dentures.

In certain cases the old dentures can be successfully utilized as treatment dentures. They can be altered in many ways, and the response to the alterations appraised. Modification of the basal seat, occlusion, flange extension, or occluding vertical dimension can be effected to provide valuable information prior to the construction of new prostheses.

## Examination

EXTRAORAL EXAMINATION.   A general examination of the patient's face provides a considerable amount of useful information. It is well to pay attention to the features of the face both in their relaxed and functional state. Patients frequently request that facial wrinkles be either elevated or eliminated to make them appear more youthful. The dentist should be careful to point out that, although much can be accomplished to improve appearance, dentures are not a panacea for the natural aging process. However, wrinkles caused by a decreased vertical dimension of occlusion or poor lip support can be improved with a well-made denture.

The form and length of patients' lips vary considerably. Thick lips give the impression of adequate support even when the teeth are not present. Long lips make it difficult for sufficient tooth structure to show, while short lips give the appearance that there is too much tooth structure.

A profile view of the face provides some indication of a prognathous or retrognathic mandible which might pose some future problems in selection and arrangement of teeth.

**INTRAORAL EXAMINATION.** A systematic intraoral examination is necessary to evaluate the oral environment and the health of the hard and soft tissues which are to support the dentures. As the examination progresses, each condition should be carefully noted in the patient's record to keep the information readily available for planning clinical procedures and for discussion with the patient.

The method of examination should be both visual and digital. Digital examination using gentle but firm pressure with the ball of the index finger reveals much about the character of the underlying bone, mucosa, submucosa, glandular tissue, and fat tissue. Visual examination determines the topography, color, and the general contour of the tissues, while digital examination reveals whether the tissues are resistant to displacement, as well as any tenderness and pain. Digital examination also gives the dentist an opportunity to observe the reaction of the patient to a foreign substance introduced into his or her mouth for the first time.

The examination should include a careful survey of all the mucous membranes of the oral cavity, that is, the superior and inferior borders of the tongue, the lining mucosa of lips and cheeks, the lingual and facial surfaces of the ridges, the hard and soft palate, the anterior pillar of fauces, and the posterior wall of the pharynx. Abnormalities of color, texture, contour, or continuity that may be manifestations of disease are noted. Special emphasis should be placed on the examination of the floor of the mouth and base of the tongue because of the higher incidence of cancer of these areas.

The next step in examination, and a most significant one, is the examination and evaluation of the maxillary and mandibular basal seats. The appraisal of these seats is important since they serve as the foundations for the dentures.

**MAXILLARY BASAL SEAT.** The residual alveolar ridge offers the primary support to the maxillary denture (Fig. 6–44). The most favorable maxillary basal seat is one with an alveolar ridge with enough height to give the denture support and resistance to lateral movement. A broad flat ridge crest offers excellent vertical support. The hard palate also should have a broad and flat surface to offer optimal vertical support and retention.

Frequently a bony enlargement referred to as a torus palatinus is found in the midline of the hard palate (Fig. 6–45). Its size may vary from that of a small pea to a huge enlargement filling the entire palate. The mucosal covering of this bony protuberance is usually thin and less resilient, which leads to problems in denture tolerance. Moreover, it also acts as a fulcrum, leading to instability of the denture. Fortunately, small tori can be managed by providing relief in the denture, but larger tori generally require surgical reduction.

In the midline and slightly to the lingual of the anterior

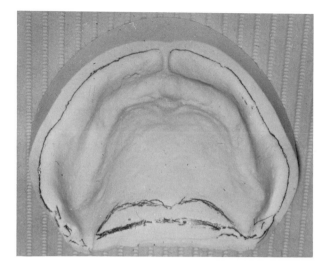

**FIG. 6-44.** Cast of a well-formed maxillary edentulous arch.

ridge crest is the incisive papilla. Since this pad covers a foramen through which blood vessels and nerves emerge, it requires some relief in the denture. The incisive papilla also serves as a landmark in the arrangement of anterior teeth.

Immediately palatal to the upper anterior ridge is the rugae zone, which is tough and hard in the normal state. Although this area does not usually require any relief, the denture must be relieved if the folds are too prominent and exhibit soft tissue undercuts.

In the midline, near the junction of the hard and soft palate, are the fovea palatine, two small depressions representing orifices of minor salivary glands. They often mark the posterior limit of the hard palate but should not be used as landmarks for the posterior limit of the denture, since the posterior border of the maxillary denture can be extended further posteriorly depending upon the type of soft palate.

Usually there are three frenal attachments bordering the maxillary denture bearing area, the superior labial attachment and the two buccal attachments. Adequate relief should be provided to allow them to function without interference by the denture.

The area between the labial frenum and the buccal frenum, the labial vestibule, is nonresistant tissue and provides retention to the denture. Similarly the area between the buccal frenum and the distal aspect of the tuberosity, the buccal vestibule, contributes considerably to retention. The thickness of the denture border in this area is influenced by the coronoid process of the mandible which should be recorded during border molding and impression making. Between the tuberosity and the pterygoid bone is the hamular notch, which determines the lateral posterior border of the denture.

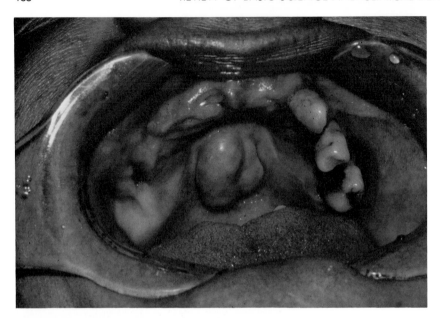

**FIG. 6-45.** Palatal torus scheduled for removal at the time a maxillary immediate complete denture is inserted.

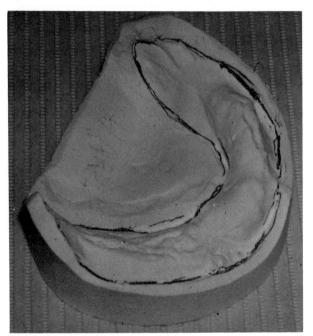

**FIG. 6-46.** Cast of a mandibular edentulous arch exhibiting advanced ridge atrophy of posterior segments.

**MANDIBULAR BASAL SEAT.** The mandibular alveolar ridge is similar to the maxillary ridge except that there is no supporting bone within its arch (due to its horseshoe shape), which makes it less supportive than the maxillary denture foundation (Fig. 6–46). The ridge on its lingual surface frequently presents tori in the region of premolar teeth. The management of mandibular tori involves surgical removal, because it is not possible to relieve them in the denture without jeopardizing the border seal in that area.

The mandibular arch usually has four frenal attachments which are active and need adequate relief to allow functional stability of the denture. These are the labial frenum, the two buccal frena, and the lingual frenum.

The retromolar pad is an easily displaceable soft tissue pad at the posterior extent of the mandibular ridge. This landmark, which should be covered to maintain the integrity of the supporting tissues, serves as a guide in establishing the mandibular plane of occlusion.

The area between the labial frenum and the buccal frenum is the labial vestibule and it must be recorded carefully since a very active lower lip can cause denture instability. The area between the buccal frenum and the retromolar pad, the buccal vestibule, includes the buccal shelf region which is between the ridge and the external oblique line. The buccal shelf is of particular importance since it provides considerable area coverage, thus contributing to the retention of the mandibular denture and distribution of occlusal forces. In addition, the buccal shelf is generally at right angles to the occlusal forces, making it a primary stress bearing area.

The anatomy and function of the floor of the mouth influence the lingual border of the mandibular denture. If the superior spine of the genial tubercle is prominent, for example, it limits the anterior lingual extension of the prosthesis. Similarly the sublingual glands influence the lingual borders in the canine–premolar area. In the mylohyoid area the floor of the mouth may protrude superiorly and eliminate the lingual vestibule entirely. However, the tissues in this area can be manipulated to permit the proper

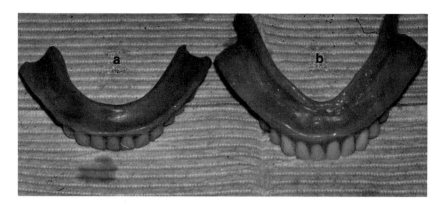

**FIG. 6-47.** Comparison of border extensions of patient's existing denture (**a**) and a new mandibular complete denture (**b**). Surgical preparation of the ridge allowed maximum extension in the retromylohyoid and anterior lingual areas.

extension of the denture. The retromylohyoid area is influenced by the activity of the tongue. Maximum extension is important here for denture retention and stability (Fig. 6–47).

LOCAL FACTORS.    Other factors which must be recognized during the clinical examination of the oral cavity are the local anatomic features which directly or indirectly influence treatment procedures and/or the choice of materials.

*Arch Size.*    The size of the maxillary and mandibular denture bearing areas ultimately determines the total support available for complete dentures. The smaller the size of the jaws, the more problems encountered in obtaining retention, stability, and overall masticatory efficiency.

*Ridge Form.*    Ideal ridges are U shaped in cross section with a flat ridge crest. Ridges which are V shaped, knife edged, or flat offer poor resistance to vertical and horizontal forces, thus reducing the support considerably.

*Ridge Relation.*    An orthognathous ridge relation is best for developing an effective occlusal scheme. The arrangement of teeth in retrognathic and prognathic ridge relations makes it difficult to obtain adequate occlusal contact during eccentric movements, which adversely affects the stability of the dentures.

*Ridge Parallelism.*    Maxillary and mandibular ridges which are parallel to each other offer the best resistance to occlusal forces on the dentures, because they minimize anteroposterior and mediolateral shifting of the bases.

*Interridge Distance.*    The available vertical distance between the two ridges at the rest position is important from many aspects. An excessive distance causes problems in stability because the distance between the teeth and the supporting bone is great. In addition, an excessive distance is usually associated with advanced ridge atrophy. On the other hand, a limited interarch distance, though providing mechanical advantage, may interfere with the proper arrangement of teeth. In extreme situations a small inter-

ridge distance may lead to contact of the maxillary and mandibular denture bases in the posterior region. These cases should be recognized during the diagnosis phase and referred for surgical correction.

*Shape of the Hard Palate.*    The most favorable shape of the palatal vault is one that is medium in depth with a well-defined incline of the rugae area. A flat palate offers good resistance to a vertical force, but it does not resist the dislodgement of the denture by a lateral or anterior force. On the other hand, a V-shaped palate does not offer satisfactory resistance to a vertical force. Management of a palate which is unfavorably shaped for a complete denture requires extra effort in developing the border seal and a balanced occlusion.

*Form of the Soft Palate.*    A gradually sloping soft palate with minimal movement is best suited for developing a wide and effective posterior palatal seal. A soft palate that slopes abruptly and exhibits hypermobility does not allow much extension of the seal area.

*Frenal Attachments.*    Low frenal attachments (closer to the vestibule) indicate a favorable prognosis, while high attachments (closer to the crest of the ridge) reduce the amount of retention. If the frenal attachments are at the crest of the ridge, it is necessary to correct them surgically.

*Osseous Undercuts.*    Osseous undercuts, if present, must be evaluated as to whether they can be useful or whether they should be surgically eliminated. It is a good practice to survey the diagnostic cast prior to reaching a decision. Many times a mild unilateral undercut may be preserved to improve retention.

*Tongue.*    The tongue should be examined for size and position. An excessively large tongue poses problems in impression making and impairs denture stability. A small and narrow tongue, although not interfering with clinical procedures, may jeopardize the lingual seal.

*Pendulous or Flabby Tissues.*    Soft flabby tissue on the ridge is undesirable because it contributes to denture instability. If not excessive, it can be managed with appropriate impression procedures. In extreme cases such tissue should be removed surgically to render the area more suitable for dentures.

*Muscle Tone.*   Normal muscle tone of the facial and masticatory muscles is necessary for several steps in denture contruction and enhancement of denture function.

*Neuromuscular Coordination.*   Successful wearing of dentures is to a large extent dependent upon good neuromuscular coordination of the patient. An effort must be made to determine the patient's ability or inability to execute muscular movements on demand.

*Saliva.*   The success of complete dentures is largely dependent upon a normal amount and normal consistency of saliva. Thick, ropy saliva is likely to interfere with the accuracy of impression procedures, thin ropy saliva can interfere with retention of the prosthesis.

*Temporomandibular Joint.*   The temporomandibular joint should be examined carefully. If there is limitation of movement, it may affect the registration of intermaxillary records. During its acute stage, arthritis of the temporomandibular joint may seriously hinder impression procedures.

### Diagnostic Aids

Diagnostic aids provide considerable assistance in treatment planning. Radiographs are of value in examining the quality of the osseous supporting structures. Dense bone with few medullary spaces and overall opacity provides a very favorable foundation for the dentures. Cancellous bone provides adequate support if occlusal loading forces are well controlled. In addition to the quality of bone, radiographs also provide information concerning retained roots, impacted teeth, bony spicules, cysts, tumors, and various bone diseases.

Study casts provide further information regarding tissue contours, degree of undercuts, etc., and also are used for fabricating custom final impression trays.

Many preoperative (preextraction) records can serve as guides in the construction of dentures, because they contain useful information about the size, shape, color and position of the natural teeth, the vertical dimension of occlusion, the support of the lips, and the relationship of the teeth to the lips.

### Preprosthetic Surgery

Many times unfavorable conditions of the denture bearing areas require surgical correction before dentures can be constructed. Although every effort should be made to avoid unnecessary surgery, it is unwise to neglect it if surgery is definitely indicated.

Alveoloplasty is advocated when the maxillary and/or mandibular ridges cannot be managed by conservative means. Unfavorable features include opposing undercuts, extreme irregularities of the ridge crest, exostoses, sharp spinous ridges, and lack of intermaxillary space.

Certain features should be removed surgically to provide comfort for the patient wearing complete dentures and/or to ensure adequate support for the dentures. For example, palatal and mandibular tori are benign bony outgrowths which should be removed. When a ridge or part of a ridge shows unstable, flabby tissue which is not well-supported by bone, it is advisable to remove such tissue surgically to gain firm support for the denture. Frenectomy is carried out in cases where the frena of maxillary and/or mandibular denture bearing areas are unusually high on the ridge and prevent utilization of adequate area for denture support.

Vestibular extension is indicated if the clinical ridge height is inadequate. By extending the vestibule, the total denture bearing area of the ridge is increased, which improves the retention of the denture and the peripheral seal. However, the success of this procedure is at times limited

**FIG. 6–48.**   Inflammatory palatal papillary hyperplasia commonly seen on the tissue corresponding to a "relief chamber" prepared in the maxillary denture. B. Maxillary denture with such a relief chamber.

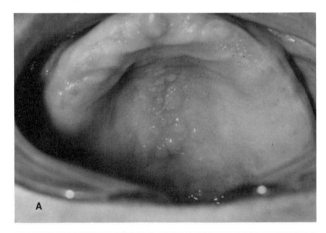

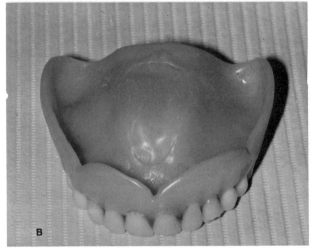

owing to difficulty in maintaining the surgically established depth.

Inflammatory palatal papillary hyperplasia and epulis fissurata (Figs. 6–48 and 6–49) are conditions commonly seen in patients who have worn ill-fitting dentures over a period of time. These soft tissue abnormalities can be treated by discontinuing the use of dentures, applying tissue conditioners or by surgical intervention.

### Presentation of the Treatment Plan and Prognosis

After all the relevant information has been gathered, the dentist arrives at a prognosis and formulates a treatment plan including procedures to be followed, materials to be utilized, and the time schedule required for treatment. The dentist should then present the treatment plan, prognosis, and the fee to the patient for approval. Upon the patient's consent, treatment is initiated.

#### QUESTIONS

27. When a patient needs a complete denture, preprosthetic surgery is generally not indicated when which of the following conditions exist?
    1. Pedunculated torus palatinus
    2. Papillary hyperplasia
    3. Epulis fissurata
    4. Root tips embedded in mandibular bone
    5. Torus mandibularis

28. Which of the following may compromise complete denture retention and stability?
    1. A wide buccal shelf in the mandibular arch
    2. A long gentle slope (drape) of the soft palate
    3. A high, V-shaped palatal vault
    4. Absence of a well-defined mylohyoid ridge
    5. All of the above

29. According to the House classification of mental attitudes of complete denture patients, the least favorable prognosis is offered by the

    1. philosophical patient
    2. exacting patient
    3. indifferent patient
    4. hysterical patient

30. Inflammatory fibrous hyperplasia of the alveolar mucosa (epulis fissurata) is usually a result of denture irritation seen about the anterior vestibule. The treatment consists of
    a. occlusal equilibration
    b. removal of irritant
    c. reduction of the vertical dimension of occlusion
    d. surgical removal of epulis fissurata
    e. only the construction of a new denture
    1. a and b
    2. b and c
    3. b and d
    4. e

31. Mandibular tori
    1. may be compensated for in the final denture base by relieving the base over the tori after spotting the area with a pressure indicating medium
    2. are unilateral in nature, thereby providing the patient with a path of insertion for the denture which involves seating the denture over the torus first then easing the opposite side to place
    3. should be considered for removal prior to denture construction
    4. if surgically removed, require a healing period of 10–12 weeks prior to beginning the preliminary impression

## IMPRESSIONS AND CASTS

An impression is a negative form of the tissues of the denture bearing area in a given static position. It can be safely stated that the success of a complete denture to a large extent depends upon the accuracy of the impression.

### Objectives of a Complete Denture Impression

The main objectives of a complete denture impression include retention, stability, support for the denture, support for the lips and cheeks, and maintenance of the health of oral tissues.

RETENTION. Retention in complete dentures is defined as the ability of a denture to resist the vertical unseating forces which are produced by gravity, the adhesiveness of foods, and the forces associated with opening of the jaws. Denture retention is directly related to the relationship of the denture base to the underlying soft tissues.

It is generally recognized that the physical factors of adhesion, cohesion, and to a certain extent atmospheric pressure play an important part in denture retention. Adhesion is the physical force of attraction between dissimilar molecules, such as between saliva and mucosa, and between saliva and denture base. The closer the adaptation of the denture base to the mucosa, the greater is the force

**FIG. 6–49.** Epulis fissurata caused by an ill-fitting denture flange.

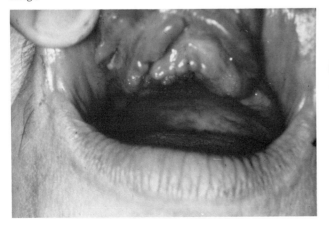

of adhesion, thus providing better retention. The quality of saliva also influences the net retention obtained, a moderate amount of saliva of normal consistency provides effective retention. In cases of xerostomia, when salivary flow is diminished, retention is a problem.

Extension of the denture base is also an important factor in taking advantage of the force of adhesion. The greater the area covered, the greater is the adhesive force developed between the mucosa and the denture base. Hence, to take full advantage of adhesion as a positive force of retention, the impression must be in intimate contact with the tissues and extend fully to the physiologic limit of the tissues.

Cohesion is the physical force of attraction between similar molecules. This occurs in the layer of saliva between the mucosa and the denture base. For the cohesive factor to be effective in denture retention, the layer of saliva must be thin, which implies that the denture base (preceded by the impression) should be in intimate contact with the mucosa.

The retentive force exerted on a denture by atmospheric pressure is directly proportional to the area coverage. For this force to be effective, the denture must have an adequate seal around its entire border, and this border is developed at the time the impression is made.

The oral and facial muscles also contribute to the retention of complete dentures. The external surfaces of the dentures should be contoured in such a way that muscles in contact with these surfaces enhance the stability and retention of the prostheses.

**STABILITY.** Stability is the attribute of a denture which enables it to resist horizontal forces. Stability is enhanced by a favorable residual ridge morphology exhibiting adequate vertical height.

**SUPPORT.** Support is the resistance offered to the vertical forces of mastication applied to the denture. The amount of support available for a denture is related to the area available, the quality of supporting bone, and the ridge morphology. Therefore, the impression should record the maximum area coverage of the basal seat within physiologic limits.

**AESTHETICS.** A well-developed border of an impression restores lip and cheek contours when the denture is in place and provides the required support to the muscles involved. In addition, the peripheral seal of a properly developed border contributes to retention.

**MAINTENANCE OF TISSUE HEALTH.** Maximum area coverage and close adaptation to the tissues are perhaps the two most important factors of impression making related to the preservation of the supporting tissues. Broad coverage reduces the force per unit area delivered to the supporting structures, and close adaptation minimizes the movement of the denture over the basal seat.

## Anatomic Landmarks

In a dentulous mouth the oral cavity is divided into a vestibular area and an oral cavity proper by the presence of the dental arches. However, when teeth are lost, these two subcavities of the mouth communicate freely with each other. Their shape and form influence the extension and thickness of denture borders, and the position of the denture teeth. Therefore it is essential for the dentist to understand the pertinent anatomy of the edentulous jaws and their limiting peripheral structures before making impressions.

The following landmarks should be incorporated in the extension of a maxillary complete denture (Fig. 6–50):

1. Superior labial frenum attachment. Relief must be sufficient, but not excessive, to allow normal functional activity of this muscle attachment.
2. Labial vestibule. The height and thickness of this border area must reflect the activity of the orbicularis oris muscle.
3. Buccinator attachment. Adequate anteroposterior relief must be provided to eliminate interference between the buccinator attachment and the prosthesis.
4. Zygomatic process. The denture border reflects, as a concavity, the presence of the zygoma. Overextension in this region causes discomfort to the patient because the denture then impinges upon the thin mucosal covering over the zygomatic process.
5. Buccal vestibule. Proper extension in height and thickness of the denture border in this region contributes greatly to retention and stability of the prosthesis. Allowance must be made in the thickness of this border for the downward, forward, and medial movement of the coronoid process of the mandible.

**FIG. 6–50.** Maxillary complete denture shows border extensions influenced by labial frenum attachment (**a**), labial vestibule (**b**), buccal frenum attachment (**c**), zygomatic process (**d**), buccal vestibule (**e**), hamular notch (**f**), and posterior palatal seal region (**g**).

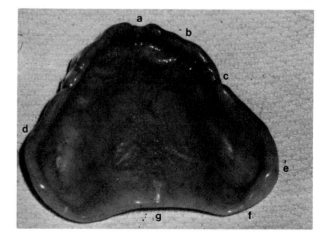

6. Hamular notch (pterygomaxillary raphe). The depression between the tuberosity of the maxillary bone and the pterygoid bone delineates the lateral posterior border of the maxillary denture.

7. Posterior palatal seal area. This region is located between the anterior vibrating line (approximately the junction of the hard and soft palates) and the posterior vibrating line (junction of the aponeurotic and muscular regions of the soft palate).

8. Fovea palatina. The openings of these minor salivary glands are generally located anterior to the posterior palatal seal region. They do not delineate the posterior border of the prosthesis.

9. The incisive papilla, the median palatine raphe, and the rugae, although not landmarks concerned with border extension, also must be recorded accurately in the impression.

The following landmarks should be incorporated in the extension of a mandibular complete denture (Fig. 6–51):

1. Retromylohyoid space. The distolingual flange of a mandibular denture is critical to retention and stability. Tongue movement is required of the patient when the impression is taken to determine the functional depth of this denture border. The functional movement of the glossopalatine arch, which is formed by the glossopalatine muscle and the lingual extension of the superior constrictor muscle, influences the distolingual extension of the lower denture.

2. Genioglossus–geniohyoid muscle attachment. The depth of the anterior lingual border is influenced to a great extent by the muscles attached to the genial tubercle. Tongue movements simulating functional activity serve to identify how deep the anterior lingual denture border should be in order to avoid impinging on the bordering tissues.

3. Mylohyoid ridge. The posterior lingual flange of the denture should extend to, or be slightly inferior to, the mylohyoid ridge. The greatest activity of the mylohyoid muscle, which raises and lowers the floor of the mouth, is medial to its attachment to the mylohyoid ridge. Therefore, the denture is generally not displaced by the normal functional activity of this muscle.

4. Lingual, labial, and buccal frena attachments. Each attachment should be visually and digitally examined to determine its morphology and activity. The denture borders should reflect the attachments' activity without excessive relief.

5. External oblique ridge. The buccal flange located between the buccinator attachment anteriorly and the retromolar pad posteriorly is of critical concern in the mandibular complete denture. The flange should extend laterally to the external oblique ridge, thus allowing the dense cortical bone found between the external oblique ridge and the buccal wall of the residual ridge to assume its role as the primary support of the prosthesis.

6. Masseter muscle. The distobuccal border of the mandibular denture is influenced by the activity of the masseter muscle upon the buccinator muscle. This activity is reflected as a notching effect ("masseter notch") in the distobuccal border and should be incorporated to ensure patient comfort and denture stability.

7. Retromolar pad. The posterior border of the denture should cover the retromolar pad. Failure to achieve adequate posterior extension may increase the rate of ridge resorption. Stability of the prosthesis is enhanced by coverage of the retromolar pad because the pad presents a different plane from that of the remainder of the ridge, thus reducing potential anteroposterior movement of the prosthesis.

## Theories of Impressions

The various techniques of making an impression are related to tissue function and the nature of the materials available. When prosthodontics was in its infancy, denture impressions were made without regard to muscle function. Impression materials such as plaster, gutta-percha, and wax were used without muscle trimming in order to obtain an impression of the basal seat only. As the understanding of tissue function advanced and its effect on the success of treatment became evident, impression procedures were modified to take full advantage of the surrounding anatomic structures. The three main techniques of making complete denture impressions can be identified as the definite pressure, minimal pressure, and selective pressure techniques.

**FIG. 6–51.** Mandibular complete denture shows border extensions influenced by retromylohyoid space (**a**), genioglossus–geniohyoid muscle attachment (**b**), mylohyoid ridge (**c**), frenum attachments (**d**), external oblique ridge (**e**), masseter muscle (**f**), and retromolar pad (**g**).

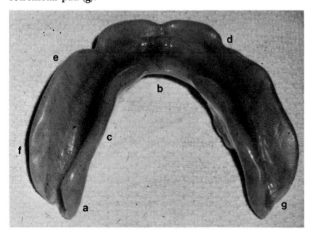

**DEFINITE PRESSURE TECHNIQUE.** Proponents of the definite pressure technique advocate recording the denture bearing areas under occlusal pressure. The rationale is that, since dentures are subjected to occlusal loading forces during function, they will be most easily retained if the tissues supporting them were also recorded in function. The procedure of making such impressions utilizes well-fitting bases with occlusion rims attached. The tissue surface of the bases is filled with the impression material and seated intraorally. The patient then closes the mouth and performs functional movements to mold the impression.

Critics of this concept argue that dentures so made might fit well during function, but when not in function, the dentures will not be as closely adapted to the tissues because of tissue rebound. Furthermore dentures made from closed mouth impressions generally are overextended and must be arbitrarily trimmed.

**MINIMAL PRESSURE TECHNIQUE.** The minimal pressure technique is based on the assumption that a denture should be constructed from a passive impression of the nonmovable soft tissue region of the denture bearing area. Subscribers to this concept base their theory on Pascal's law which states that pressure in a confined liquid will be transmitted throughout the liquid in all directions. Their interpretation is that mucosa, being more than 80% water, will react like a liquid in a closed vessel and thus cannot be compressed. This analogy is thought by some to be untrue since mucosa is not in a closed vessel and the tissue fluids can easily escape under the borders. Since it is supposed to record the static state of mucosa without distortion, this technique is also referred to as "mucostatics" or a non-pressure technique. The technique requires that every minute detail of the mucosa be copied in the impression so that the completed denture will fit all the elevations and depressions of the tissues. Furthermore metal bases are indicated to obtain maximum retention because their dimensional stability is greater than that of acrylic resin.

Adherents of the mucostatic concept consider interfacial tension the primary retentive mechanism for complete dentures. In view of this, they do not use conventional labial, buccal, and lingual flange extensions in the dentures since these do not contribute to the resistance of the dentures to vertical displacement.

Critics suggest several disadvantages to this technique. Most importantly, it deemphasizes the principle of dissipating occlusal forces over a larger area to maintain the health of the basal seat. Moreover, since the dentures do not extend into the labial and buccal vestibules, the necessary lip and cheek support is missing. Also the musculature is not being utilized fully for retention of the dentures.

**SELECTIVE PRESSURE TECHNIQUE.** The selective pressure technique combines the principles of the other two techniques. It is recognized that certain regions of the denture bearing area can tolerate pressure without unto-

ward reaction, while others cannot accept any pressure. The selective pressure technique takes advantage of the relative tolerance of the basal seat to pressure and allows the impression to cover as broad an area as possible, thus obtaining maximum support for the denture within the limits of functional adaptation.

### Impression Procedures

Impressions for complete dentures can be made in a variety of ways using different techniques and materials. A generally accepted technique will be described.

**"MAKING" VS. "TAKING" IMPRESSIONS.** The phrase "taking an impression" suggests that the procedure involves recording an exact negative imprint of the denture bearing area. This phrase would be appropriate if the tissues were static and nondisplaceable, but the tissues of and around the denture bearing areas are resilient and dynamic in nature. Therefore, dentures will not be successful unless these tissues are recorded in a functional position. Tissues are manipulated in various positions to obtain the best support for the dentures during function and the most effective retention possible.

**PRELIMINARY IMPRESSIONS.** Preliminary impressions are usually made with modeling plastic in stock metal trays and are generally slightly overextended due to low flow of the material. These impressions are used for making preliminary casts on which custom impression trays are fabricated for final impressions, or after modifications the preliminary impressions themselves can be used as custom trays for final impressions.

The tissues and denture base can be divided into three distinct zones (Fig. 6–52). Zone 1, the region of firmly attached mucosa, is a relatively static region and presents minimal problems in obtaining an accurate impression. Zone 2 is the region of loosely attached mucosa and may be identified as the mucobuccal, mucolingual, and mucolabial folds. The zone 2 region is a potential space that decreases as the degree of mouth opening increases. In the mandibular arch tongue position influences the lingual zone 2 region. Zone 3 is that portion of the edentulous mouth represented by the mucosa of the lips, cheeks, and tongue that contacts the outer or polished surfaces of the dentures. The morphology of the denture that contacts the zone 3 tissues generally is created somewhat arbitrarily by carving. Techniques which allow the zone 3 tissues to determine the shape of the polished surfaces of the dentures are particularly indicated in the presence of severely atrophied ridges. Zone 3 exhibits extreme changes in shape and dimension according to mouth position (open or closed) and muscle activity.

Considering the potential for change in zones 2 and 3, an impression material must be selected that is correctable, because correctability allows the operator to record

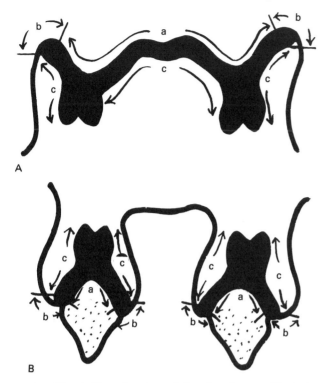

**FIG. 6–52.** A. Frontal section of the edentulous maxilla in the first molar region showing Zone 1 (**a**), Zone 2 (**b**), and Zone 3 (**c**) tissues corresponding to denture base regions. B. Zone 1 (**a**), Zone 2 (**b**), and Zone 3 (**c**) in the frontal section of mandible.

the dynamics of the zone 2 and 3 tissues in a static impression. Use of a correctable material makes it possible to record functional movements in the impression so that the denture will have border extensions in harmony with function, maximum retention and stability, the potential for reducing bone loss.

Although many materials are available for this purpose, modeling plastic is particularly well suited for making preliminary impressions and refining the borders of final impression trays (Figs. 6–53A & B). After obtaining an accurate preliminary impression of the Zone 1 region, the peripheral aspects of the impression are softened. The patient is instructed to simulate functional muscle movements by the following exercises:

1. Alternately and forcibly mouthing the "ooo" and "eee" sounds determines the width of the labial borders, provides relief for the buccal frenum attachments, and influences the buccal extensions in height and width.
2. Sucking action further refines the labial border in width and height, provides sufficient vertical relief for the labial frenum attachments, and influences the buccal border extensions.
3. Moving the mandible to the protrusive and lateral protrusive positions allows the coronoid process of the

mandible to influence the height and thickness of the maxillary buccal border.
4. Biting on the operator's fingers placed over the posterior aspect of the tray causes the masseter muscle to contract. This forces the buccinator muscle to push the softened modeling plastic medially, creating the notch effect on the distobuccal border of the mandibular impression.
5. Moving the tongue from one corner of the mouth to the opposite corner of the mouth activates the palatoglossus muscle, influencing the morphology of the distolingual denture border. This exercise also uses the mylohyoid muscle and the genioglossus muscle to identify the lingual border extension and anterior lingual border extension, respectively.

When the impressions are satisfactory, they are beaded, boxed, and poured with stone to prepare the preliminary casts. The beading wax is placed 2–3 mm inferior and parallel to the height of the borders of the impression so that the height and thickness of the borders are preserved. The impressions should be poured within an hour of the impression making, since modeling plastic flows at room temperature.

Preliminary impressions can also be made with an irreversible hydrocolloid impression material, but such impressions are usually grossly overextended and are not correctable.

**FINAL IMPRESSIONS.** Custom impression trays are used for making the final impressions. Usually they are constructed of autopolymerizing acrylic resin, which provides a rigid and dimensionally stable tray. The casts obtained from preliminary impressions are utilized for making the trays. If large undercuts are present on the cast, they are blocked out with wax. An outline of the tray is drawn on the casts 2–3 mm short of the fold areas all around the denture bearing area to provide adequate relief for the labial, lingual, and buccal frena. A uniform mix of autopolymerizing acrylic resin is then adapted on the cast and trimmed to the outline. A handle which makes approximately a right angle to the ridge crest is provided for the ease of manipulation.

Final impressions for complete dentures are made in two steps. The first step is to establish the accurate height and width of the borders, and the second step is to record tissue detail with a suitable impression material.

The final impression trays are examined in the mouth for retention and also to verify that the tray borders are 2–3 mm short of the folds and muscle attachments. Once the trays are found to be satisfactory, border molding is accomplished with low fusing modeling plastic which possesses the property of staying plastic at lower temperature, by asking the patient to perform the border molding exercises used for the preliminary impression (Fig. 6–54).

The completed border molding of the maxillary and

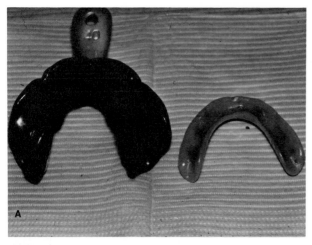

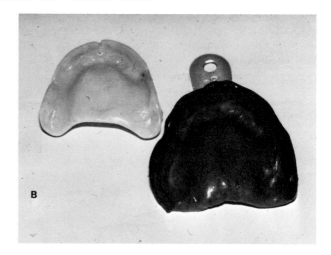

**FIG. 6–53.** A. Comparison of border extensions of previous mandibular denture and mandibular preliminary impression. B. Comparison of border extensions of previous maxillary denture and maxillary preliminary impression.

mandibular trays must be checked carefully. If, in any region, the plastic has flowed onto the zone 1 areas, it must be removed to prevent a pressure area from developing. The borders themselves must show a smooth rolled surface with adequate relief for the frena. The custom trays, after the completion of the border molding, must exhibit satisfactory retention and stability.

The final impression is usually made with one of the following materials: plaster of paris, zinc oxide–eugenol paste, irreversible hydrocolloid, rubber base impression material, or silicon impression material. Plaster and zinc oxide–eugenol paste are excellent materials for complete denture impressions, since they duplicate the tissue details faithfully and are dimensionally stable. In addition, their flow is excellent and they record the tissue surface with minimal displacement (Fig. 6–55). However, since they become rigid after setting, they are not suitable in cases of marked bony undercuts.

The other materials listed are elastic in nature and can be used for recording undercuts in the denture bearing areas. Their ability to duplicate tissue details is excellent, and they exhibit dimensional stability if poured within a reasonable period of time. Hydrocolloids, however, must be poured immediately.

### Final Casts

If the final impressions are acceptable, they are beaded, boxed, and poured with stone. The beading wax is attached about 2–3 mm below and parallel to the borders of the impression to preserve the zone 2 and 3 areas. In the mandibular impression a sheet of wax is attached in the tongue area to obtain a flat surface in that part of the cast. The retromolar pad area also requires special attention. In

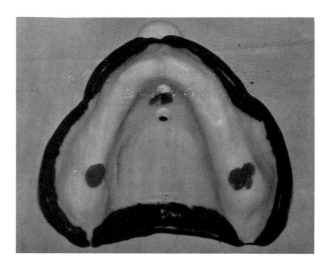

**FIG. 6–54.** Border-molded final impression tray prior to making final impression.

this region the beading wax should follow the slope of the borders and extend well beyond, otherwise the retromolar pad areas of the cast will not have any land and may tend to fracture due to lack of bulk of stone in this area.

Since zinc oxide–eugenol impression pastes do not require a separating medium, the boxed impression can be poured immediately. The material of choice for making the final cast is stone, because the cast will be subjected to considerable pressure during the packing and processing of the denture base material.

Once the stone is set, the final casts are recovered from the impressions and checked. They should reproduce all tissue details without any artifacts. The land areas of the casts, if too high, should be trimmed to within 1 mm of the depth of the sulci. Since these casts will be used for fabricating the dentures, they must be handled carefully.

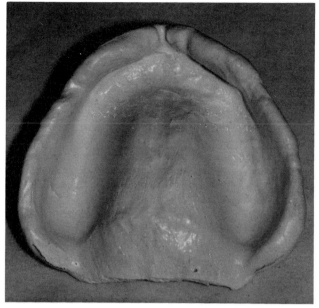

**FIG. 6-55.** Maxillary final impression made with a zinc oxide–eugenol paste.

32. All of the following are landmarks concerned with location of the posterior palatal seal except the

    1. fovea palatina
    2. hamular notch
    3. anterior nasal spine
    4. posterior vibrating line
    5. aponeurotic palate

33. The principal advantage of using modeling plastic rather than irreversible hydrocolloid for endentulous preliminary impressions involves

    1. accuracy of the zone 1 area
    2. accuracy of the zone 2 and 3 areas
    3. ease of manipulation
    4. dimensional stability of material
    5. correctability of impression
    6. 2 and 5
    7. 2, 4, and 5

34. Salivary control is not a significant factor for final impression procedures using rubber base or zinc oxide–eugenol because saliva will be absorbed by these impression materials.

    1. The statement is true and the reason is true.
    2. The statement is true but the reason is false.
    3. The statement is false but the reason is true.
    4. The statement is false and the reason is false.

35. The muscle responsible for elevating the floor of the mouth during swallowing and whose action may impart a characteristic S appearance to the lingual flange of a mandibular complete denture is the

    1. mylohyoid muscle
    2. genioglossus muscle
    3. superior constrictor muscle
    4. digastric muscle

## JAW RELATIONS

Relating the mandible to the maxilla in reproducible relationships is a prerequisite for developing an occlusal scheme which will allow the dentures to function in harmony with the masticatory complex. It is impossible to capture such relationships during function (except with pantographic recording devices) due to the ability of the mandible to execute an infinite number of relationships with the maxilla. However, definite, static relationships, which are repeatable, can be recorded and transferred to an articulator to develop an effective occlusion. In prosthodontic procedures these relationships of the mandible to the maxilla are classified under the broad heading of jaw relations.

All jaw relations are essentially bone-to-bone relations. For the sake of convenience in describing clinical procedures they can be divided into three categories: 1) the spatial relationship of the maxilla to the condylar axis, 2) the vertical relationships of the mandible to the maxilla, and 3) the horizontal relationships of the mandible to the maxilla. These three relationships are recorded to transfer the orientation of the mandible to maxilla in three dimensions onto the articulator. The spatial relationship of the maxilla to the condylar axis (face-bow record) provides the orientation of mandible to the cranium, the vertical relation (vertical dimension of occlusion) locates the mandible in the inferior-superior relation to the maxilla, and the horizontal relation (centric relation record) locates the mandible in the anteroposterior, mediolateral relation to the maxilla.

## Record Bases and Occlusion Rims

Since the accuracy of recording jaw relations is critical for success of complete dentures, it is essential that records are taken with record bases which do not allow movement when the records are being made. Record bases are constructed on casts obtained from final impressions. If a functional posterior palatal seal was accomplished at the time the impression was made (Fig. 6–56), it is on the cast and is automatically incorporated in the record base. However, if a posterior palatal seal is to be cut into the final cast, this should be accomplished before the record base is fabricated. The main difference between the "functional" and "arbitrary" methods of developing the posterior palatal seal is that the depth of the area in the latter method is established according to the estimated displaceability of the tissues, while in the former the depth is established by the interaction between a physiologic type wax and the viscoelastic properties of the tissues.

Usually record bases are fabricated from autopolymerizing acrylic resin, because it is easy to manipulate, adapts well to the final cast, maintains its form, and exhibits adequate dimensional stability. Certain criteria must be met in making record bases. The borders should be extended up to the depth of the labial, lingual, and buccal vestibules of the final casts to obtain maximum retention. Secondly, the labial, lingual, and buccal frena must be relieved in order to provide stability during the movements of the surrounding musculature. Thirdly, the thickness of the bases should not be excessive, lest it interfere with the placement of teeth. In addition, the border width should conform to the width of the vestibule on the casts. If the borders of the bases are too thin, the peripheral seal will be lost. If the borders are too thick, the bases will be displaced by the activity of the peripheral tissues. An ideal record base is one which is processed and stabilized (Fig. 6–57) so that it provides the dentist and the patient with an accurate preview of comfort, stability, and retention of the finished prosthesis.

Once the record bases are formed, their borders are lightly polished for smooth tissue contact and wax occlusion rims are attached on their external surfaces. Since the wax rims represent the future position of the artificial teeth and are necessary in recording jaw relations, they should be carefully constructed. Posteriorly they should terminate anterior to the tuberosity region in the maxillary arch and to the ascending slope of the retromolar area in the mandibular arch. Their width should be narrowed in the anterior incisal region (3–4 mm), gradually increasing (6–8 mm) in the posterior occlusal region to simulate the width of the artificial teeth. The plane of occlusion of the wax rims is kept flat, with a slight tilt towards the ridge in the posterior region of the maxillary arch and at the level of one-half to three-quarters the height of the retromolar pad area of the mandibular arch. The shape, size, form, and position of the occlusal rims, are tentatively determined in the laboratory and are to be recontoured according to individual clinical requirements at the time the jaw relations are recorded (Fig. 6–58).

## Clinical Procedures

For the sake of convenience the procedure of recording jaw relations is carried out in three separate clinical steps: 1) the face-bow record, 2) the vertical dimension of occlusion, and 3) the centric relation record. Although it is possible to record all three relations in one step, making separate recordings maintains the accuracy of each record. Before making any of these records, however, it is necessary to refine the record bases and occlusion rims intraorally.

**MAXILLARY OCCLUSION RIM.** The refinement of the maxillary occlusion rim is carried out in three stages.

**FIG. 6–56.** A. After excess wax is trimmed, the impression is reseated for 5–8 min. This last seating allows tissues in the area of the posterior palatal seal to exert their displacing effect on wax, thereby achieving functional depth of seal. B. Posterior palatal seal (**outlined**) is incorporated in final cast.

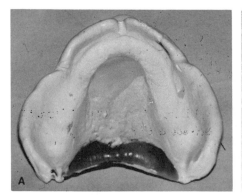
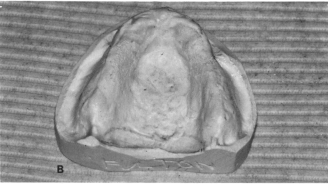

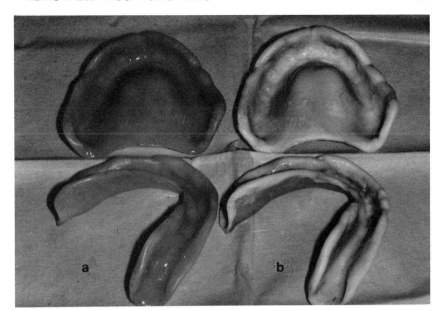

**FIG. 6-57.** Processed record bases (**a**) and stabilized record bases (**b**).

First, the labial fullness is adjusted according to the needs of the profile of the patient, and the wax is contoured in the anterior region to provide adequate support for the upper lip. Second, the vertical length of the anterior part of the occlusion rim is adjusted to allow 1–2 mm of it to be visible below the relaxed upper lip. Finally, the plane of occlusion is adjusted to make the anterior occlusal plane parallel to an imaginary interpupillary line and the posterior occlusal plane parallel to the ala–tragus or Camper's line. The midline of the face is also marked on the occlusion rim at this stage.

**FACE-BOW RECORD.** The face-bow record orients the maxilla to the transverse axis of the mandible in three dimensions and allows the transfer of this orientation to the articulator. The face-bow recording can be made using selected anatomic references or by locating the true hinge axis. The main difference between the two is accuracy of locating the rotational axes of the condyles, the latter being more accurate. The selected anatomic reference type of face-bow record is generally considered to be satisfactory for complete denture therapy, however.

**VERTICAL DIMENSION.** Vertical dimension of the jaws refers to the superoinferior relation of the mandible to the maxilla. The importance of this relationship lies in the fact that it provides a vertical reference for developing the occlusal scheme. The vertical dimension is subdivided into the vertical dimension of occlusion and the vertical dimension of rest. When natural teeth are present, the vertical dimension of occlusion is established by the occlusal contact of the maxillary and the mandibular teeth, and the vertical dimension of rest

is established by muscles and gravity. However, when teeth are lost, the reference position of the vertical dimension of occlusion is also lost; it becomes the responsibility of the dentist to reestablish this position so that the artificial occlusion will be in conformity with the lost natural occlusal pattern. Fortunately the vertical dimension of rest is not affected by the loss of natural teeth and can be effectively utilized for reestablishing the occlusal scheme in edentulous mouths.

The vertical dimension of rest depends upon the physiologic rest position of the mandible, which is a postural position controlled by the muscles which open, close, and protrude the mandible. The physiologic rest position remains relatively constant throughout life and is a repeatable reference, within an acceptable range, which makes it useful for establishing the vertical dimension of occlusion. Physiologic rest position can be measured by the following methods:

1. Facial measurements. Placing two reference points, one at the base of the nose and the other on the chin, then measuring the distance between them when the patient is relaxed, provides an approximate measurement of vertical dimension of rest. The procedure is repeated until a consistent (within a small range) measurement is obtained. This measurement is then used to establish the vertical dimension of occlusion.
2. Phonetics. Speech can also be used for establishing the vertical jaw relations. Under normal conditions there is a clear space of about 1 mm between the incisal edges of the maxillary and mandibular anterior teeth or occlusion rims when words with S sounds are pronounced.

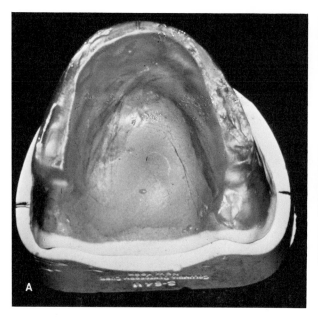
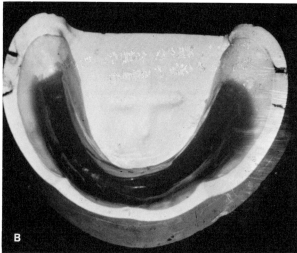

**FIG. 6–58.** Occlusion rims are constructed in the laboratory following general guidelines and then individualized as a chairside procedure.

3. Electromyography. Based on the theory that muscles display the least amount of electrical activity at a rest position, this procedure involves use of an apparatus called the electromyograph which is not routinely available in the dental office.

4. Swallowing. The act of swallowing can be utilized as an aid in determining the vertical dimension of rest. The maxillary and mandibular teeth make contact during swallowing, and after the completion of the act of swallowing, the mandible assumes its rest position.

Although these methods yield satisfactory results individually, it is wise to combine two or more methods to establish the vertical dimension of rest.

The registration of vertical dimension remains a matter of clinical judgment, however, and the accuracy of the record varies within a range rather than a definite measurement. In edentulous mouths the physiologic rest position may be determined first; then the occlusal position is established 2–4 mm less than the rest position. The amount of space between these two relations is referred to as the interocclusal distance. This distance between the two vertical positions is important for denture efficiency, speech, comfort, and aesthetics. Excessive reduction of this space results in an increased vertical dimension of occlusion, and the patient will not only experience soreness and discom-

fort under the dentures due to constant trauma but also may exhibit increased ridge resorption. The appearance of the patient will also be affected since the muscles of facial expression will exhibit a tense, strained appearance. There may also be clicking of the teeth and difficulty in phonation. If, however, the interocclusal space is increased markedly so that the vertical dimension of occlusion is insufficient, there will be an obvious collapse of the lower third of the face, resulting in a typical edentulous appearance. These patients also may develop discomfort in the ears and temporomandibular joints.

The clinical procedure involved in the determination of the vertical dimensions is accomplished with record bases and occlusion rims. After the face-bow record is taken and the maxillary cast mounted, the maxillary occlusion rim is removed from the articulator and refined to its original contour. Next, with both occlusion rims in place, the physiologic rest position is established by one of the methods described. When adequate interocclusal space between the maxillary and the mandibular occlusion rims is allowed, a tentative vertical dimension of occlusion is obtained.

A typical process to establish a tentative vertical dimension of occlusion begins with two marks placed on relatively less mobile tissues of the lower third of the face, usually one at the base of the nose and the other on the chin. The maxillary occlusion rim is inserted in the mouth, and the patient is asked to swallow and relax;

then a measurement is made between the two marks. The procedure is repeated until a fairly consistent measurement is obtained which represents the vertical dimension of rest. The mandibular occlusion rim is inserted, the height of which is then adjusted to allow an interocclusal space of 2–4 mm between the two occlusion rims when the mandible is in its physiologic rest position. This is further confirmed by one or more of the various methods described.

**CENTRIC RELATION.** Centric relation refers to the horizontal relationship of the mandible to maxilla in two dimensions, that is, anteroposterior and mediolateral. Fortunately this relationship can be accurately recorded in edentulous patients and used as a reference point in developing the desired occlusal scheme in the artificial dentures. When an accurately recorded centric relation at the proper vertical dimension of occlusion and a face-bow record are transferred to an articulator, the three dimensional spatial relationship between the mandibular and maxillary casts is the same as that between the two jaws.

In dentulous persons contraction of the muscles moves the lower jaw into centric occlusion which, in the majority of cases, does not coincide with centric relation. Neuromuscular reflexes set up by the proprioceptive elements in the periodontium respond to tooth contacts by deflecting the lower jaw away from centric relation to the centric occlusion position. These two relations can exist in the natural dentition in the form of a minor malocclusion which may or may not contribute to damage of the supporting structures. However, when natural teeth are lost, the proprioceptive element is also lost, rendering the lower jaw incapable of avoiding any deflective occlusal contacts. If deflective occlusal contacts are present in the centric relation of complete dentures, they will cause movement of the denture bases, resulting in damage to the supporting tissues or directing the mandible away from centric relation. Therefore it becomes absolutely essential to record centric relation accurately so that the centric occlusion can be made to coincide with it.

Since centric relation is defined as the most posterior relation of the mandible to the maxilla at the established vertical relation, a definite correlation exists between centric relation and the vertical dimension of occlusion. Therefore, it is well to establish the most desirable vertical relation before taking the centric relation record. Once the records are mounted on the articulator, no changes should be made in the vertical relation. If the vertical relation must be changed, it should be followed by a new centric relation record and a remount of the mandibular final cast. However, if the true hinge axis is used for mounting the maxillary cast on the articulator, minor changes in vertical dimension do not affect the centric relation record.

The various methods used for recording centric relation are classified into three main groups: graphic recordings, functional recordings, and interocclusal recordings.

*Graphic Recordings.* Graphic recordings utilize tracings in the horizontal plane to record the centric relation. In addition, the protrusive and lateral movements of the mandible, which can be used to set the horizontal and lateral condylar indications of the articular, are recorded. The tracing obtained by this method is in the form of an arrow point, referred to as a gothic arch tracing. The apex of the tracing represents centric relation; the two sides of the tracings, originating from the apex, denote the lateral movements; and the straight line in the middle is scribed by the protrusive movement of the lower jaw (Fig. 6–59.) The tracing can be made with intraoral or extraoral instrumentation. An advantage of the extraoral method is that the tracing is enlarged and is visible while being made, thus making it much easier to instruct the patient and evaluate the record.

*Functional Recordings.* Functional methods of recording centric relation utilize functional activity or movement of the mandible at the time the record is being made. Two important methods in this group are those suggested by Needles and Paterson. The Needles method uses four metal styluses placed in a maxillary occlusion rim made of impression compound. The mandibular occlusion rim is also made of compound. During movement, the styluses of the upper occlusion rim cut diamond-shaped tracings in the lower occlusal rim which can then be used for transferring the records to a suitable articulator.

The Paterson method uses wax occlusion rims in which an undercut prepared on the occlusal surface is filled with a mixture which is half plaster and half carborundum paste. The occlusion rims are prepared at a

**FIG. 6–59.** A typical gothic arch tracing made with an intraoral tracing device. The apex represents centric relation.

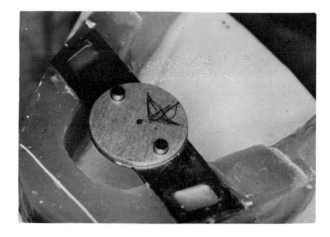

slightly raised vertical dimension and inserted in the mouth; then the patient is instructed to perform various mandibular movements which generate compensating curves on the plane of occlusion of the plaster–wax rims. When the rims are reduced to the predetermined vertical dimension, the patient is instructed to close in centric relation and the occlusion rims are joined in this position. The record is then transferred to a suitable articulator.

*Interocclusal Recordings.* Perhaps the most common method of recording centric relation is with interocclusal records. The main advantages of this method are that it is simple, does not require special devices, and can be accomplished and verified in a short period of time. The procedure involves placing a suitable recording medium between the wax occlusion rims when the jaws are positioned in centric relation. The recording medium can be plaster, wax, zinc oxide–eugenol paste, or autopolymerizing acrylic resin. Each material exhibits its own merits and demerits, but wax is the most commonly used material.

*Clinical Procedure.* The centric relation record is made only after the acceptable vertical dimension of occlusion is established with the wax occlusion rims.

The maxillary and mandibular occlusion rims are inserted in the mouth, and the patient is guided to close in the centric relation position. This procedure is repeated until a consistent centric relation closure is obtained. With the occlusion rims in contact, three reference lines are cut into the upper and lower wax rims. First, the midline on the upper wax rim, which was scored during the face-bow recording, is extended onto the lower rim. Two other lines, usually at the canine positions, are scored on either side of the upper wax rim and extended onto the lower rim. These three lines serve as reference lines for checking the accuracy of the centric relation record to be taken.

The occlusal rims are removed from the mouth. Two v–shaped notches are cut in the maxillary wax rim, one on either side in the first molar region. A 1-mm thickness of wax is removed from the premolar and molar regions on either side of the mandibular occlusion rim and is replaced by a 2-mm thickness of a suitable recording wax. The anterior parts of the opposing rims are left intact to serve as vertical stops (Fig. 6–60).

The maxillary base and occlusion rim is inserted in the mouth. The lower occlusion rim is inserted after softening the recording wax. The patient is then guided into a gentle closure in the centric relation position. With the occlusion rims in contact, the three sets of reference lines are checked. If they do not coincide, a new record is made.

The wax record is chilled, the occlusion rims removed, and the record evaluated. The excess recording wax is removed with a sharp knife, and the occlusion rims are reinserted in the mouth for verification of the record (Fig. 6–61). This tentative record is considered verified if the patient closes smoothly into the index in centric relation without any perceptible movement of either record base. To mount the lower final cast in the correct centric relation on the articulator, first the maxillary base is luted to the maxillary mounted cast. Then the mandibular occlusion rim is luted to the maxillary occlusion rim in its correct position, after which the mandibular cast is luted to the mandibular record base. The lower cast is then mounted to the lower member of the articulator, completing the transfer of jaw relations to the articulator in preparation for the selection and arrangement of the artificial teeth.

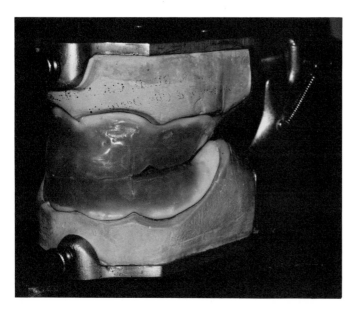

**FIG. 6-60.** Maxillary and mandibular occlusion rims prepared for taking a centric relation record with a wax recording medium.

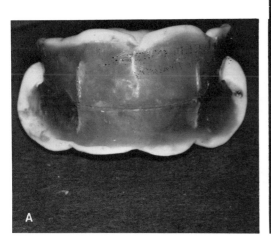
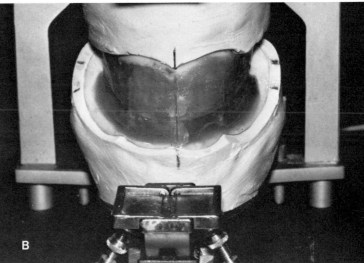

**FIG. 6-61.** A. The wax index (centric relation record) allows the occlusion rims and record bases to be accurately reoriented. B. The reorientation is in preparation for mounting of the mandibular final cast on the articulator.

## QUESTIONS

36. Insufficient interocclusal space for a patient with complete dentures may result in
    1. an annoying "clicking" sound during normal conversation
    2. excessive forces on the denture supporting tissues
    3. potential for increased resorption of the alveolar bone
    4. facial distortion and difficulty in swallowing
    5. 2 and 3
    6. All of the above

37. A face-bow record in complete denture construction is used to
    1. orient the maxillary cast to the centric relation record
    2. facilitate the mounting of the mandibular cast
    3. record the relation of the mandible to the opening and closing axis of the temporomandibular joint
    4. allow for exact determination of the vertical dimension of occlusion
    5. 1 and 3
    6. None of the above

38. Centric relation must be accurately recorded so that the
    1. face-bow record can be accurately taken as the next step in denture construction
    2. centric occlusion can be developed in harmony with centric relation
    3. vertical dimension of rest can be determined
    4. degree of Bennet angle can be measured.

39. When the vertical dimension of occlusion is evaluated for the edentulous patient at the occlusion rim stage of denture construction, the vertical dimension of rest
    1. should be equal to the vertical dimension of occlusion
    2. may exceed the vertical dimension of occlusion if aesthetics are enhanced
    3. is of little significance in the evaluation of the vertical dimension of occlusion because it is subject to variation
    4. must always be greater than the vertical dimension of occlusion

40. Which of the following are criteria pertinent to the fabrication of an acceptable temporary record base?
    1. It must be constructed on the final cast.
    2. It must be constructed on the preliminary cast to preserve the accuracy of the final cast.
    3. Its construction must include the entire vestibular fold portion of the cast.
    4. All surfaces that contact lips, cheeks, and tongue should be finished.
    5. 1, 3, and 4
    6. 2, 3, and 4

## OCCLUSION AND ARTICULATION

After the jaw relations are recorded and transferred onto the articulator, the artificial teeth are arranged in a definite scheme of occlusion planned to be aesthetically pleasing and functionally in harmony with the other components of the masticatory complex.

### Posterior Occlusion and Articulation

The term occlude literally means to close. In dentistry the word occlusion is used in reference to the contact position of the maxillary and mandibular teeth. This is a static position which signifies the specific relationship of opposing teeth when the mandible is not moving, even though contact between the opposing teeth can occur during a variety of positional relationships of the mandible to the maxilla. In complete denture occlusion the occlusal contact between the teeth when the mandible is in centric relation is initially arranged to coincide with centric occlusion. All the other contact relationships between the maxillary and the mandibular teeth, i.e., left lateral, right lateral, and protrusive, are designated as eccentric occlusion.

Articulation is a dynamic contact relationship of the occlusal surfaces of the maxillary and mandibular teeth. It signifies the contact relations of the opposing teeth when the mandible is executing various eccentric movements. Both occlusion and articulation are factors of an artificial occlusal scheme and must be given due importance during the arrangement of posterior teeth. Although the distinction between occlusion and articulation is clear, the two terms are often used interchangeably.

## Posterior Tooth Form

There are various types of posterior tooth forms available, varying from 33° cusps to flat or monoplane artificial teeth. The use of any one of these occlusal forms in a particular situation can be justified as long as it fulfills the objectives of 1) functional harmony, 2) maintenance of the health of soft and hard tissues of the denture bearing areas, and 3) aesthetics. Posterior artificial tooth forms are divided into three groups: anatomic, monoplane, and nonanatomic teeth.

ANATOMIC POSTERIOR TEETH.    Anatomic posterior tooth forms are those that duplicate the anatomy of the natural teeth. The teeth show definite cuspation and well-formed fossae and grooves. The advantages of anatomic posterior teeth, as claimed by their proponents, are that they provide a more natural look to the dentures and are more efficient in mastication, their definite cusp-to-fossa relation provides a well-organized occlusal scheme and resists denture rotation, and their cuspal inclination facilitates the development of bilateral balance in eccentric occlusal positions. Critics of the anatomic posterior tooth forms suggest that serious damage to the supporting tissues of the denture may be caused by inaccuracies in intercuspation that develop as the vertical dimension of occlusion is lost through progressive resorption of the ridges. Another claimed disadvantage of anatomic teeth is that it is difficult to develop an effective occlusal contact when the jaws are in abnormal horizontal relations. The usefulness of anatomic teeth is further restricted in patients whose lack

of neuromuscular coordination makes it difficult to obtain a repeatable centric relation record.

MONOPLANE POSTERIOR TEETH.    Monoplane posterior artificial teeth do not resemble the occlusal surfaces of natural teeth. Instead these teeth have a flat surface with no cuspal angle in relation to a horizontal plane. The advantages claimed for monoplane posterior teeth include reduced horizontal forces delivered to the residual ridges, increased flexibility in buccolingual placement, particularly for abnormal jaw relations, and suitability for patients with compromised muscular coordination. However, they also suffer from certain disadvantages: their aesthetic qualities are inferior to those of the anatomic teeth, they decrease masticatory efficiency, and they make it difficult to obtain eccentric balance.

NONANATOMIC POSTERIOR TEETH.    Artificial posterior teeth which do not copy the natural anatomic form of teeth but still present some cuspal inclinations on their occlusal surfaces are called nonanatomic teeth. A number of nonanatomic occlusal forms of posterior teeth which can be used effectively in a variety of situations are available.

SELECTION.    Although the selection of one posterior occlusal form or another is a matter of personal preference and judgment, certain broad outlines can be defined for tooth selection in a particular situation. Anatomic teeth can be effectively used in the presence of well-formed alveolar ridges, fairly normal horizontal ridge relations, definite and repeatable centric relation records, and good muscle coordination. They are also appropriate for relatively younger patients.

Monoplane posterior teeth are more suitable for patients exhibiting: excessive alveolar resorption resulting in flat or knife edge ridges, extreme retrognathic or prognathous ridge relations, a nonrepeatable centric relation due to temporomandibular joint dysfunction or poor muscle coordination, habitual bruxism, and systemic diseases which may cause an accelerated rate of ridge resorption.

## Concepts of Complete Denture Occlusion

Artificial posterior teeth are arranged in accordance with one of the three basic concepts of occlusion: organic occlusion, spherical occlusion, and neutrocentric occlusion.

ORGANIC OCCLUSION.    The concept of organic occlusion involves posterior teeth with cusps modified to meet the requirements of individual patients. The cusp-to-fossa relationship of upper and lower posterior teeth is developed in centric relation, while the height of the cusps and depths of the fossae are carved in accordance with the mandibular movements. Organic occlusion is developed with the help of three plane pantogram recordings and a fully adjustable articulator or with suitable eccentric records and a semiadjustable articulator.

SPHERICAL OCCLUSION. Spherical occlusion is an arrangement of artificial teeth in which their occlusal surfaces are placed on an imaginary sphere (usually 8 in. in diameter) with its center above the level of the teeth. This concept requires that both the mediolateral and anteroposterior inclines of the posterior teeth be in harmony with a spherical surface.

NEUTROCENTRIC OCCLUSION. In the neutrocentric concept of posterior occlusion the plane of occlusion is identified as a flat plane parallel to the plane of the denture foundation; it is not dictated by the horizontal condylar guidance. The posterior teeth are arranged on this plane without any anteroposterior or mediolateral inclination. The posterior tooth forms are without cusps, and the patient is instructed to avoid incising, which eliminates the need for any horizontal condylar inclination. Since the teeth are not arranged for eccentric balance, the lateral condylar inclination is also kept at zero. The buccolingual width of the teeth is reduced to minimize the occlusal forces, and the working occlusal surfaces are centralized in the area of premolars and first molars. The second molars are either omitted from the arch or kept out of occlusion. The principle behind neutrocentric occlusion is that favorable leverage can be obtained by bringing the occlusal surfaces of the posterior teeth toward the center of the denture foundation, buccolingually and anteroposteriorly.

## Eccentric Balance in Posterior Occlusion

One of the most controversial aspects of posterior complete denture occlusion is eccentric balance. Although prosthodontists unanimously agree that equal contact or balance in centric occlusion is essential, the opinion is not so uniform regarding the desirability of eccentric balance. It is generally considered important, however, to have a balanced occlusion in complete dentures for the retention and stability of the dentures. This is achieved by incorporating anteroposterior and mediolateral compensating curves. Even though it is apparent that a small bolus of food on the working side can eliminate the balance on the nonworking side, balanced occlusion is considered important during eccentric contacts that occur during the various parafunctional excursive movements of the mandible.

BALANCE WITH MONOPLANE TEETH. Monoplane teeth are usually arranged with a flat occlusal plane which does not provide eccentric balance, but balance can be achieved by placing a ramp distal to the mandibular second molar. This ramp is adjusted so that it makes contact with the maxillary second molar during the eccentric movements and thus achieves a three-point contact (third point anteriorly). Another method of obtaining balance with flat plane posterior teeth is to incorporate compensating curves which enable the teeth to maintain contact during the excursions of the mandible.

BALANCE WITH ANATOMIC TEETH. Achieving eccentric balance with anatomic posterior teeth is an elaborate procedure which for convenience of discussion may be divided into the topics of protrusive and lateral balance. To obtain occlusal balance during the protrusive movement of the mandible, the influence of the inclination of the condylar guidance, the inclination of the incisal guidance, the orientation of the occlusal plane, the inclination of the cusps, and the prominence of the compensating curve must be recognized. The first two factors, condylar and incisal guidance, control the movements of the articulator, while the other three are modified to obtain harmony among the five factors. The condylar guidance is obtained from the patient by means of a protrusive or lateral protrusive registration and is not under the control of the dentist. The incisal guidance is determined by the dentist by considering the amount of horizontal and vertical overlap of anterior teeth needed for a favorable aesthetic and functional result. The other three factors are controlled and modified by the dentist to function in harmony with the two end factors, thereby providing balance during the protrusive movement.

Lateral occlusal balance is also governed by five factors. The two controlling end factors for obtaining lateral balance are the inclination of the balancing side condyle and the slope of the working side cuspal inclines. The other three intermediate factors, which can be modified to obtain harmony, are the inclination of the balancing side cuspal inclines, the inclination of the balancing side teeth, and the inclination of the occlusal plane on the balancing side.

## Conclusion

No longitudinal clinical study as yet provides dentistry with a simple solution to the problem offered by complete denture occlusion. Prosthodontists do agree that complete denture occlusion is a significant factor in the long-term success of the prosthesis, and therefore the occlusion should be continually monitored during the postinsertion phases to maintain the objectives of whatever occlusal form and scheme were selected for the patient.

41. The neutrocentric concept of occlusion maintains that
    1. four mandibular molars must be used in every complete set up
    2. the anteroposterior plane of occlusion should be parallel to the plane of the denture foundation
    3. opposing anterior teeth must contact in centric occlusion
    4. the occlusal plane of the mandibular posterior teeth must be aligned to one-quarter the height of the retromolar pads
    5. All of the above
    6. None of the above

42. The dentist controls the following factors of complete denture occlusion with the exception of
    a. occlusal plane
    b. incisal guidance
    c. Bennett movement
    d. compensating curves
    e. condylar path
    1. a and b
    2. c and e
    3. a and d
    4. b and c
    5. None of the above

43. In a completed monoplane denture arrangement
    1. maxillary anterior teeth may exhibit a small degree of vertical overlap in relation to the mandibular anterior teeth when an orthognathic ridge relationship exists
    2. the degree of horizontal overlap of maxillary posterior teeth to mandibular teeth must be small regardless of ridge relationship
    3. central fossae areas of maxillary molars are always aligned over the mandibular crest of ridge line
    4. inadequate buccal overlap of maxillary posterior teeth in relation to mandibular posterior teeth may result in cheek biting

44. Occlusal equilibration for complete dentures should be accomplished by a
    1. laboratory remount after processing
    2. patient remount with new intermaxillary records
    3. Both a and b
    4. Either a or b

## AESTHETICS AND PHONETICS

In addition to fulfilling the needs of masticatory function, complete dentures must fulfill the needs of aesthetics and phonetics. While posterior teeth assume the main responsibility for function, the requirements of aesthetics and phonetics are mainly met by the anterior teeth. The distinction between the function of the anterior and posterior segments is not always clear-cut, however, and frequently a compromise has to be made to achieve the desired balance between functional and aesthetic requirements.

Although definite rules and procedures can be followed to insure that a denture will meet functional and biomechanical needs, there are no strict rules for obtaining an aesthetic result. A different set of factors must be taken into consideration for each patient in order to achieve an acceptable aesthetic result. The dentist has to depend upon artistic sense to select and arrange the teeth in such a manner that they blend with the patient's face and produce a pleasing overall effect. However, even in a subjective area such as aesthetics, certain recognized principles can be used as guidelines for the selection and arrangement of anterior artificial teeth to obtain the desired results.

### Selection of Artificial Anterior Teeth

In the absence of preextraction records selecting anterior teeth for a complete denture is very much dependent upon the aesthetic sense of the operator and to a certain extent upon the preference of the patient, but there are certain principles which can be effectively used as aids to determine which shade, form, and size is best suited in the individual case.

Generally the shade of the artificial teeth is correlated with the color of the skin, hair, and eyes of the patient. The shade should not contrast with the surrounding structures and thus interfere with the harmony of color. At times it is possible to make a minor variation to create a more natural appearance or to satisfy the preference of the patient. Shades should be examined under both artificial and natural light, against the skin of the face, and within the oral cavity.

The form of the artificial anterior teeth selected usually conforms to the general outline of the face, that is, square, tapering, ovoid, or any combination thereof. The form of the teeth may also be influenced by the sex of the patient. Teeth selected for a female patient usually have more pronounced curvatures, rounded point angles, and a more delicate appearance. The curvature of the labial surface of the teeth depends upon the profile of the patient. For example, if the profile is convex, the teeth selected should exhibit more prominent curvature incisogingivally to maintain harmony between the teeth and the facial contours.

A relationship has been demonstrated between the size of the maxillary central incisors and the anthropometric measurements of the face. The mesiodistal width of the central incisor is usually 1/16 of the total bizygomatic measurement, and the gingivoincisal length is 1/16 of the length of the face, measured from patient's hairline to the chin. It is obvious that these measurements cannot be used strictly to select the artificial teeth, but they do provide a general idea of the size of the teeth which will harmonize with the face of the patient. Another aid in selecting the tooth size is marking a high lip line and two canine lines on the occlusion rim at the time the jaw relations are recorded. These guide lines provide information about the gingivoincisal length and total mesiodistal width of the maxillary six anterior teeth. Another widely known concept regarding the selection of anterior teeth is the dentogenic concept of Frush and Fisher, (16) who have integrated the selection of teeth into an aesthetic system governed by the age, sex, and personality of the patient.

### Arrangement of Anterior Teeth

The arrangement of anterior teeth has to fulfill certain biomechanical needs as well as aesthetic ones. Therefore, the placement of the teeth in the anterior segment is generally governed by certain rules to achieve the best mechanical advantage during function.

**HORIZONTAL PLACEMENT.**  The labiolingual or horizontal position of the maxillary six anterior teeth is influenced by the amount of ridge resorption which has occurred since the loss of the natural teeth. The artificial teeth should be positioned in the same general area where the natural teeth were. This position was tentatively established during the clinical refinement of the labial contour of the maxillary occlusion rim to provide adequate lip support and phonetics. Initially this same position is maintained by setting the teeth so that their labial surfaces conform to the labial contour of the wax rim. Another useful guide is the incisive papilla, which is a constant anatomic landmark. The position of the labial surfaces of the natural maxillary central incisors is in the range of 6–8 mm anterior to the incisive papilla. No attempt should be made to standardize normal horizontal overlap between the upper and lower anterior teeth if the ridges are in Class II (retrognathic) or Class III (prognathic) relations. Special care must be exercised to keep the lower anterior teeth close to the ridge in order to obtain best mechanical advantage for the mandibular denture.

**VERTICAL PLACEMENT.**  The vertical position of the maxillary anterior teeth is governed by the low lip line and the smile line of the upper lip. Generally about 1–2 mm of the incisal portion of the maxillary central incisors is visible below the relaxed lip. The vertical position of the anterior plane is also influenced by the available vertical space between the upper and lower ridges. At times a compromise must be made to gain mechanical advantage for one or the other ridge at the expense of aesthetics.

**ARCH FORM.**  The mesiodistal placement of the maxillary anterior teeth follows the general form of the anterior residual ridge to maintain harmony between the artificial teeth and facial contours. If the anterior ridge form is square, the anterior teeth will also be arranged in a square form.

**INDIVIDUAL TOOTH INCLINATIONS.**  **In order to obtain the best individualized aesthetic results, due consideration should be given to the inclina**tion of each tooth in the anterior segment. Within limits a tooth can be inclined or rotated to fulfill certain aesthetic needs. This procedure is used to its maximum potential when accomplished at chairside during the trial denture appointment so that the dentist and the patient can exchange ideas and evaluations. Active patient participation has been shown to enhance the overall prognosis of complete denture therapy.

### Phonetic Considerations

An important function of complete dentures is a phonetic one. In a dentulous person the anterior teeth, as well as the tongue, act as a part of the valving mechanisms which modify the flow of air to produce speech sounds. When the natural teeth are lost, the modifying effect of the anterior teeth on speech is also lost and the patient is rendered incapable of articulation and enunciation of a normal speech pattern. The position of the artificial teeth is critical in the production of some speech sounds, and the ability of the dentures to function phonetically should be evaluated at the trial denture visit.

**LABIAL SOUNDS.**  The sounds "p" and "b" are referred to as labial sounds. If the lips are not supported properly by the artificial teeth, these sounds may be defective. Therefore, the horizontal position of the teeth must be evaluated from the point of view of phonetics as well as aesthetics.

**LABIODENTAL SOUNDS.**  The labiodental sounds "f" and "v" are produced by contact between maxillary incisors and the posterior one-third of the lower lip. If the teeth are set too far labially or lingually, the production of these sounds will be abnormal.

**LINGUODENTAL SOUNDS.**  Linguodental sounds such as "th" are produced by extending the tip of the tongue between the upper and lower anterior teeth. The normal extension of the tongue beyond the incisal edges during this sound is 3–6 mm. If the patient demonstrates excessive variation from this range at the trial denture visit, the labiolingual position of the anterior teeth should be reevaluated.

**LINGUOPALATAL SOUNDS.**  When pronouncing linguopalatal sounds such as "t" and "d" the tip of the tongue contacts the anterior part of the palate or the palatal surfaces of the anterior teeth. If the teeth are placed too far palatally, the "t" sound will resemble "d"; if they are set too far labially, the "d" sound will resemble "t." The necessary correction must be made at the trial stage by moving the anterior teeth. At times excessive thickness of the denture base in the rugae area may affect these sounds in the same manner. Therefore, the base of the trial denture should also be evaluated.

Other linguopalatal sounds, such as "ch," "j," and "s," are influenced by the relationship between the upper and lower anterior teeth. During pronunciation of these sounds the maxillary and mandibular anterior teeth approach each other in an end-to-end relation just short of making contact. The "s" sound is also made by contact between the tip of the tongue and the palate in the rugae area with a small space for the escape of air between the tongue and the palate. If this space is too small, a whistle usually results, and if the space is too broad and thin, the "s" sound is replaced by the "sh" sound somewhat like a lisp. These discrepancies, if found during evaluation, must be corrected at the trial stage by refining the denture base wax-up.

## QUESTIONS

45. When the vertical dimension of occlusion is evaluated by means of phonetics, the occlusion rims should not make contact when the patient pronounces the "s" sound because this demonstrates inadequate free-way space.
    1. The statement is true and the reason is true.
    2. The statement is false and the reason is false.
    3. The statement is true but the reason is false.
    4. The statement is false but the reason is true.

46. The tentative midline on the maxillary occlusion rim can be determined by
    1. referring to the midline of the nose
    2. extending a vertical line from the lingual frenum to the occlusion rim
    3. projecting a line from the middle of the uvula through the middle of the anterior nasal spine on to the maxillary occlusion rim
    4. bisecting the face with an imaginary line and projecting it on to the maxillary occlusion rim

47. The average ratio of maxillary central incisors to the bizygomatic width is
    1. 1:12
    2. 1:14
    3. 1:16
    4. 1:18
    5. 1:20

## INSERTION AND POSTINSERTION

The insertion of complete maxillary and mandibular dentures represents the climax of a carefully planned and executed sequence of clinical and laboratory procedures. Although insertion does not complete treatment, it is a very important and exciting time for most patients. Preparation of the prosthesis for insertion, the insertion visit, and postinsertion adjustments require the same high degree of skill and care that has been devoted to all previous phases of complete denture therapy.

### Preparation for Insertion

After the processed dentures are recovered from the flasks, they are *not* separated from their casts immediately but are first remounted on the articulator using the indices that have been preserved for this purpose (Fig. 6–62).

1 **RESTORING THE VERTICAL DIMENSION.** In most cases the processed dentures exhibit an increase in the vertical dimension which may vary from slight to moderate. The main reason for this change is the introduction of occlusal discrepancies during the processing of the acrylic resin denture base material. These occlusal discrepancies are eliminated when the dentures are prepared for insertion by a remount and equilibration to restore the original vertical dimension of occlusion.

**PRESERVING THE FACE-BOW RECORD.** The positional relationship of the maxillary cast and the denture may be preserved, thereby eliminating the need for taking a new face-bow record at the time of insertion. To accomplish this a remounting jig is attached to the lower member of the articulator. A quick-setting plaster is placed on the jig and a mounting index of the occlusal surfaces of the maxillary teeth constructed (Fig. 6–63). After the plaster has set, the jig is removed from the articulator and maintained for future use. The dentures may then be removed from the final casts for finishing and polishing.

**CONSTRUCTING THE MOUNTING CASTS.** After the dentures are finished and polished, mounting casts are prepared to facilitate the mounting of the dentures for further occlusal equilibration. Undercuts in the dentures are blocked out; then casts are poured using quick-setting plaster. The maxillary denture (on the mounting cast) is seated in the remounting index and attached to the upper member of the articulator (Fig. 6–64). The dentures are then removed from the mounting casts and kept moist until the denture insertion appointment.

### Insertion Procedure

The denture insertion appointment is the most important appointment from the patient's point of view because this is the patient's first opportunity to evalu-

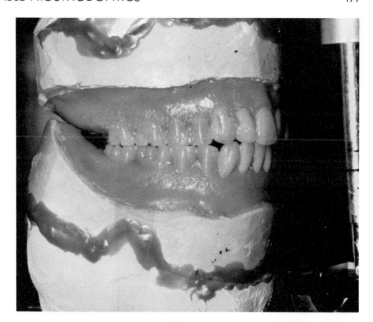

**FIG. 6-62.** Processed dentures are remounted on the articulator to restore the vertical dimension of occlusion before the final casts are destroyed.

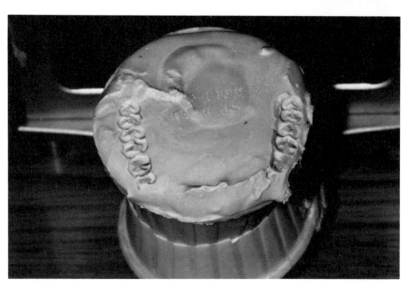

**FIG. 6-63.** Mounting index of the polished maxillary denture on the articulator which eliminates the need for new face-bow record.

ate the finished dentures. Patients who have no previous denture experience may be apprehensive and doubtful regarding what to expect. On the other hand, experienced denture wearers know what they want and are ready to criticize. It is good practice for the dentist to spend time with the patient to allay any anxiety, build confidence, and correct any misinformation before inserting the dentures. A specific regimen should be followed for insertion.

**RETENTION AND STABILITY.** The first step in denture insertion is to evaluate the adaptation, retention, stability, border extensions, and relief areas of each denture

individually. Adaptation may be evaluated with use of pressure disclosing paste. Evaluation of the extension of borders and adequacy of relief is accomplished with a disclosing wax. After the dentures are adjusted individually in the mouth, both dentures may be inserted for evaluation of jaw relations.

**VERTICAL DIMENSION AND CENTRIC RELATION.** An evaluation of the vertical dimension is made first. A variety of modalities should be used because of the subjectivity of the evaluation. Observing the interocclusal space and the facial contours, as well as asking the patient to pronounce "s" sounds in words like sixty-six to

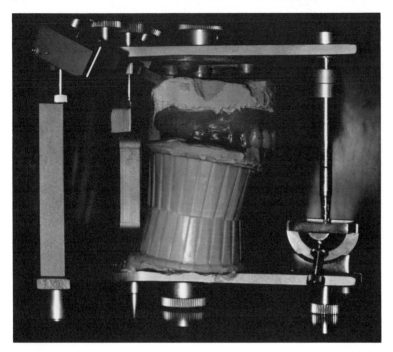

**FIG. 6-64.** Maxillary denture on mounting cast ready to be positioned on the articulator.

evaluate the closest speaking space, are among the techniques employed for this difficult evaluation.

After a clinical evaluation of centric relation, the mandibular denture is mounted on an articulator with a centric relation record to verify that record prior to any equilibration. An evaluation of the occlusion of dentures mounted on an articulator is more accurate than an intraoral evaluation because significant discrepancies may be masked in the mouth. If any interferences or deflective contacts are revealed between the upper and lower occlusal surfaces in centric relation, they are eliminated by selective grinding to obtain a uniform contact. An equilibration to refine the bilateral balance is then accomplished. The equilibrated dentures are then seated in the mouth and evaluated for comfort, aesthetics and phonics.

**INSTRUCTIONS TO THE PATIENT.** It is important that instruction regarding the limitations, the effective use, and the home care of dentures be reviewed. It must be emphasized that dentures do not perform with the same efficiency as do natural teeth but that with experience and intelligent manipulation most patients achieve a satisfactory level of masticatory function. Patients should be discouraged from comparing dentures with those of relatives or friends because dentures are highly individualized and reflect the patients own local and systemic factors.

Initially speech with the dentures may not be absolutely normal. After a relatively short period of time, however, speech becomes clearer due to the adaptability of the tongue. It helps the patient a great deal to practice speech by reading aloud for the first few days following insertion.

Instructions for oral hygiene must be given in writing so that the patient can refer to them when in doubt. It must be emphasized that the dentures are to be cleaned at least twice daily. The dentures should be cleaned over a basin partially filled with water to avoid breakage should they be dropped accidentally.

To maintain the health of the residual ridges, patients should be instructed to remove the dentures daily for an extended period of time. The patients should be strongly advised not to resort to over-the-counter adhesives and home reliner materials to "refit" dentures, these materials can do much harm to the soft tissues of the denture bearing areas. Routine recall of the patient every 6 months will go a long way toward the elimination of this problem if a strong commitment to the recall procedure is made by both the dentist and the patient. Once all the instructions are made clear to the patient and any questions answered, arrangements are made for the first postinsertion visit, in 24 hours.

### Postinsertion Visits

During the first postinsertion visit any complaints regarding the patient's first experience with the dentures are evaluated. Generally at this visit tissue irritations are examined, and appropriate corrective procedures such as simple relief of an irregularity on the denture base, reduction of a slight overextension, or further occlusal refinement by equilibration are initiated.

After the occlusion and the denture bases are adjusted, the patient is instructed to subject the dentures to normal mastication during the subsequent days and arranged for a second postinsertion visit within 3–5 days. This provides time for the patient to become more adept in manipulating the prostheses and allows the dentist to evaluate the functional and aesthetic results of treatment. During the second visit the same procedure is followed in adjusting the occlusion and the denture bases as for the first postinsertion visit. It is advisable to examine the patient again after 3 weeks for further evaluation. Following this appointment, the patient should be instructed to call for an appointment if any problem develops. At the same time a recall appointment should be scheduled within 3 months, although it can be extended to 6 months if the evaluation of treatment is satisfactory.

QUESTIONS

48. Before relieving an area on the denture base which appears to be related to an area of mucosal irritation, the dentist should first
   1. be certain that the patient has worn the denture because the irritation could be due to trauma from hard sharp food
   2. determine the precise area of the base to be relieved by using one of the disclosing materials available
   3. examine the occlusion since occlusal discrepancies may cause tissue irritation
   4. remove the dentures and apply a topical anesthetic ointment
   5. All of the above

49. All of the following procedures are carried out in preparation for the delivery appointment with the exception of
   1. preservation of face-bow record
   2. construction of mounting casts
   3. mounting of the mandibular denture
   4. finishing and polishing of the restorations
   5. mounting of the maxillary denture

50. It is generally accepted that a more accurate method of finally equilibrating complete dentures is on the articulator rather than intraorally because the denture supporting tissues allow a degree of movement of the denture bases that can mask inconsistencies in the occlusion.
   1. The statement is false but the reason is true.
   2. The statement is true and the reason is true.
   3. The statement is true but the reason is false.
   4. The statement is false and the reason is false.

51. Rebasing and relining complete dentures include
   1. restoring the accuracy of denture base fit to supporting tissues
   2. maintaining occlusal relations of teeth
   3. maintaining the vertical dimension of occlusion

4. recording supporting tissues in a resting position
5. 1 and 2
6. All of the above

## DENTAL MATERIALS

A variety of materials are used during the clinical and laboratory phases of construction of complete dentures. If these are not properly manipulated, they can compromise the accuracy of the completed prosthesis. Therefore, it is important to have a thorough understanding of the physical properties, manipulation, and clinical influence of materials in order to achieve accurate results. The different types of materials used in complete denture construction are: impression materials, modeling and investing materials, denture base materials, and artificial tooth materials.

### Impression Materials

Impression materials used for complete dentures are divided into three main groups: rigid, plastic, and elastic.

RIGID MATERIALS. Rigid impression materials include impression plaster and the metallic oxide pastes. Both of them are widely used for making final impressions.

Impression plaster consists of plaster of paris combined with modifiers such as accelerators, binders, and plasticizers to make it more suitable for impression procedures. It is an excellent impression material because its considerable flow enables it to duplicate minute tissue details with minimal pressure. Impression plaster is very stable dimensionally and can be stored for a reasonable time before pouring, but it requires a separating medium before the stone cast can be poured. Another drawback of impression plaster is that it is difficult to use in the presence of undercuts and patients have expressed considerable discomfort, particularly upon removal of a plaster impression from the mouth.

Metallic oxide pastes are also rigid impression materials which have good handling characteristics and reproduce tissue details excellently. It is dimensionally stable and does not require any separating medium. However, being rigid, it is difficult to withdraw from the mouth if undercuts are present.

PLASTIC MATERIALS. The plastic group of impression materials includes modeling plastic and impression waxes. Modeling plastic is commonly used for making preliminary impressions and for establishing the borders of final impression trays. The main advantage of modeling plastic is that it is easy to manipulate and can be corrected repeatedly until a saatisfactory result is obtained. Modeling plastic has a poor flow, however, so impressions made with it are usually overextended and exhibit poor tissue detail. It is therefore unsatisfactory as a final impression material.

The dental waxes which are used for making final impressions are also called mouth temperature waxes or physiologic waxes. The most familiar of these are Korecta wax and Iowa wax. Because the physiologic waxes soften at mouth temperature, they record tissue details without displacing the soft tissues. Although the impression waxes were designed for extension base partial denture impressions, they can also be used successfully in complete denture procedures. In addition, these waxes are effectively used for correcting minor discrepancies of impressions taken with rigid materials, for obtaining functional posterior palatal seal, and for performing various impression procedures in maxillofacial prosthodontics.

ELASTIC MATERIALS. The elastic group of impression materials consists of the hydrocolloids (reversible and irreversible), rubber base impression material, and silicon impression material. These materials exhibit elasticity after setting and thus can be effectively used in the presence of undercuts.

There are two types of hydrocolloids used as impression materials, reversible and irreversible. Both are excellent materials and capture the minute details of the tissues. Reversible hydrocolloid is fluid at high temperature and sets to a gel form upon reduction of temperature. It requires special water-cooled trays for gelatin. Irreversible hydrocolloid impression material is supplied in the form of powder and forms a gel when mixed with water. It is much easier to manipulate than the reversible hydrocolloid.

The hydrocolloid impression materials are mainly used in fixed partial and removable partial prosthodontic procedures. However, in certain cases, such as when undercuts are present in the mouth or when immediate complete dentures are needed, hydrocolloid can be used effectively for complete denture impressions. The main drawbacks of these impression materials are that they show considerable dimensional changes if proper precautions are not observed in storing and pouring the impression and that they are not correctable.

The mercaptan rubber base (Thiokol) impression material is generally used for fixed prosthodontics. However, it can be used in making complete denture impressions, specifically in cases where the bony undercuts on the ridges are severe or when the patient needs immediate dentures. The tissue details obtained with rubber base material are excellent, but since the flow of the material is poor, some displacement of the tissue is unavoidable while making the impression. This disadvantage is reduced by the use of the light body rubber base impression material which exhibits an adequate flow. The dimensional stability is reasonably good if a uniform thickness of the material, not exceeding 1/8 in., is used in the custom tray. The rubber base impression does not need a separating medium, and the stone cast poured against it shows a hard and smooth tissue surface.

The silicon impression materials are similar to rubber base materials in their advantages and disadvantages, but they are more expensive and must be handled more delicately than rubber base material.

## Modeling Materials

The materials commonly used for constructing casts from complete denture impressions are plaster of Paris and dental stone. Plaster of Paris casts are quickly made but are weaker than stone casts. The setting time of stone is much longer than that of plaster, and to obtain the optimum amount of hardness it must be allowed to set for a minimum of 45 min.

Plaster is generally used for making diagnostic and preliminary casts. The final casts are invariably made from dental stone, which is essentially plaster of Paris modified to produce a much harder and denser cast. Plaster and dental stone are also used for investing the trial dentures in the flask in preparation for processing. Other uses of plaster include mounting of casts to the articulator and taking centric and eccentric records (quick-setting plaster).

## Denture Base Materials

Denture bases support the artificial teeth, enhance aesthetics, support the lips and cheeks, and provide support for the denture by maintaining an intimate contact with the mucosa of the denture bearing areas. In order to carry out these functions the denture base material must fulfill certain physical requirements which directly or indirectly influence the performance of artificial dentures in the mouth. The main requisites of an acceptable denture base material include dimensional stability, inertness in the oral environment, natural appearance, low specific gravity, adequate strength, ease of fabrication and repair, and ability to be used with a variety of artificial tooth materials. Unfortunately, none of the materials available is an ideal denture base material. The acrylic resins, which were introduced to dentistry in 1937, come closest to fulfilling all the requirements and are therefore the most commonly used denture base materials. The other materials sometimes used in combination with acrylic resin are gold alloys and chromium–cobalt alloys.

The most common acrylic resin used as denture base material is poly (methyl methacrylate). Although it is not ideal, it exhibits many of the properties required of a denture base material. It is supplied in the form of powder (polymer) and liquid (monomer) which, when mixed together and polymerized, results in a homogenous solid mass. The polymerized resin has adequate dimensional stability and strength and is capable of receiving a high polish. With reasonable care, a denture base made with acrylic resin can provide good service without deterioration for a substantial period of time.

The most commonly used acrylic resin is the heat-curing type. It is a powder–liquid system that uses external heat as the activator. The initiator is benzoyl peroxide which is included in the polymer (powder). The monomer (liquid) is generally pure methacrylate with a slight amount of hydroquinone added to inhibit polymerization during storage. The chemical reaction begins when heat activates benzoyl peroxide, which in turn initiates the reaction (polymerization) which continues until all the monomer molecules are converted into polymer.

Another type of acrylic resin, the chemically activated resin, is generally used for procedures such as repairs and relines. Its composition is similar to that of the heat-curing type except that it utilizes a chemical, usually dimethyl-p-toluidine, as the activator. Although it is more convenient to use the chemically activated and autopolymerizing resin, the physical properties of their end product are inferior to those of the end product of a heat-curing resin.

## Artificial Tooth Materials

The materials most commonly utilized in the manufacture of artificial teeth are porcelain and acrylic resin. At times, metals such as gold alloys and chromium–cobalt alloys are also used in various combinations.

PORCELAIN TEETH. Porcelain material is a mixture of fine particles of feldspar and quartz fused with various pigments. Artificial teeth made from porcelain show excellent qualities of resistance to wear, dimensional stability, masticatory efficiency, and aesthetics. However, they suffer from certain inherent drawbacks such as brittleness and friability, possible clicking sound in use, poor bonding with acrylic denture base material, and difficulty in grinding, which also removes the surface glaze and makes them more abrasive.

ACRYLIC RESIN TEETH. The resin material used for making artificial teeth is an acrylic material modified with pigments and a crosslinking agent which makes it resistant to crazing and wear. The resin teeth are resilient, tough, and natural looking; they bond chemically with the acrylic denture base material. They do not produce clicking sounds in use and can be ground and repolished without affecting the efficiency. However, due to their low resistance to abrasion they show significant wear in the mouth after a period of time, which may lead to an altered occlusion and decreased vertical dimension. In order to minimize the occlusal wear of resin teeth it has been suggested that porcelain teeth be used on the maxillary denture and acrylic resin teeth on the mandibular denture. This combination produces a lower coefficient of wear than that of acrylic resin against acrylic resin. In cases where natural teeth occlude against the artificial teeth, it is a good practice to provide gold alloy or amalgam occlusal restorations in the acrylic resin artificial teeth to maintain the vertical dimension of occlusion.

### QUESTIONS

52. Which of the following combinations of artificial teeth should not be used in complete maxillary and mandibular dentures?
    1. Anterior, plastic; posterior, porcelain
    2. Anterior, porcelain; posterior, plastic
    3. Anterior, plastic; posterior, plastic
    4. Anterior, porcelain; posterior, porcelain

53. Porosity in denture bases is due to all of the following except
    1. placing the packed flask immediately in boiling water
    2. improper finishing and polishing of the base
    3. insufficient resin used during packing
    4. lack of adequate pressure during processing
    5. poor mixing technique of monomer and polymer

54. The final impression materials combination of choice for immediate complete dentures is
    1. heavy body rubber base and irreversible hydrocolloid
    2. irreversible hydrocolloid and stone
    3. plaster of paris and heavy body rubber base
    4. zinc oxide–eugenol and irreversible hydrocolloid

55. Match the tooth material (Column 2) with the appropriate property it exhibits (Column 1).

| Column 1 | Column 2 |
| --- | --- |
| Resistant to wear | 1. porcelain artificial teeth |
| Mechanically retained in the denture base | 2. acrylic resin artificial teeth |
| Relatively easy to restore, finish, and polish after occlusal adjustment | |

## REFERENCES

1. ANTE IH: The fundamental principles of design and construction of crown and bridge prosthesis. D Items Interest 50:215–232, 1928
2. APPLEGATE OC: Essentials of Removable Partial Dentures Prosthesis, 2nd ed. Philadelphia, WB Saunders, 1959

3. BERESIN VE: The Neutral Zone in Complete Dentures. St. Louis, CV Mosby, 1973

4. BLATTERFEIN S: Study of partial denture clasping. J Am Dent Assoc 43:169–185, 1951

5. BONWILL WGA: New methods of clasping artificial dentures to human teeth without injury versus immovable bridges. D Items Interest 21:656–670, 1899

6. CARLSSON GE, HEDEGARD B, KOIVUMAA KK: Studies in partial denture prosthesis. IV. Final result of a four year longitudinal investigation of dentogingivally supported partial dentures. Acta Ondontol Scand 23:443–472, 1965

7. CARLSSON GE, HEDEGARD B, KOIVUMAA KK: Current place of removable partial dentures. Dent Clin North Am 14:533–567, 1970

8. CECCONI BT, ASGAR K, DOOTY E: The effect of partial denture clasp design on abutment tooth movement. J Prosthet Dent 25:44–56, 1971

9. CLAYTON JA, JASLOW C: A measurement of clasp forces on teeth. J Prosthet Dent 25:21–43, 1971

10. COLEMAN AJ: Occlusal requirements for removable partial dentures. J Prosthet Dent 17:155–162, 1967

11. CUNNINGHAM DM: Base metal and type IV gold alloys. Dent Clin North Am 17:719–722, 1973

12. DEVAN M: Preserving natural teeth through the use of clasps. J Prosthet Dent 5:208–214, 1955

13. FENNER W, GERBER A, MUHLEMANN HR: Tooth mobility changes during treatment with partial denture prosthesis. J Prosthet Dent 6:520–525, 1956

14. FISH W: Principles of Full Denture Prosthesis, 6th ed. London, Staples Press, 1964

15. FRECHETTE AB: The influence of partial denture design on distribution of forces to abutment teeth. J Prosthet Dent 6:195–212, 1956

16. FRUSH JP, FISHER RD: Dentogenetics: Its practical application. J Prosthet Dent 9:914–921, 1959

17. HEINTZ WD: Symposium on removable partial dentures. Dent Clin North Am 17:569, 1973

18. HENDERSON D: Major connectors. Dent Clin North Am 17:661–678, 1973

19. HENDERSON D, STEFFEL VL: McCracken's Removable Partial Prosthodontics, 4th ed. St. Louis, CV Mosby, 1973

20. HINDELS GW: Load distribution in extension saddle partial dentures. J Prosthet Dent 2:92–100, 1952

21. HOLMES JB: Influence of impression procedures and occlusal loading on partial denture movement. J Prosthet Dent 15:474–481, 1965

22. HOLMES JB: The altered cast impression procedure for the distal extension removable partial denture. Dent Clin North Am 14:569–582, 1970

23. HOUSE MM: Studies in prosthesis. J Am Dent Assoc 18:827–852, 1931

24. KABCENELL JL: Effective clasping of removable partial dentures. J Prosthet Dent 12:104–110, 1962

25. KAIRES A: Effect of partial denture design on bilateral force distribution. J Prosthet Dent 6:373–385, 1956

26. KAIRES A: Effect of partial denture design on unilateral force distribution. J Prosthet Dent 6:526–533, 1956

27. KAIRES A: Partial denture design and its relation to force distribution and masticatory performance. J Prosthet Dent 6:672–683, 1956

28. KAIRES A: A study of partial dentures design and masticatory pressures in a mandibular bilateral distal extension case. J Prosthet Dent 8:340–350, 1958

28a. KENNEDY E: Partial Denture Construction, 2nd ed. Brooklyn, Dental Items of Interest, 1951

28b. KRAJICEK DD: Why partial dentures fail. Dent Clin North Am 16:145–160, 1972

29. KOTOWICZ WE, FISHER RL, REED RA, JASLOW C: The combination clasp and the distal extension removable partial denture. Dent Clin North Am 17:651–660, 1973

30. KRATOCHVIL F: Influences of occlusal rest position and clasp designs on movement of abutment teeth. J Prosthet Dent 13:114–124, 1963

31. KROL AJ: R.P.I. Clasp retainer and its modifications. Dent Clin North Am 17:631–649, 1973

32. LOMBARDI RE: A method for the classification of errors in dental esthetics. J Prosthet Dent 32:501–513, 1974

33. MANDEL ID: What is preventive dentistry. J Prev Dent 1:25–29, 1974

34. MCCRACKEN WL: Mouth preparations for partial denture. J Prosthet Dent 6:39–52, 1956

35. MCCRACKEN WL: Survey of partial denture designs by commercial dental laboratories. J Prosthet Dent 12:1089–1110, 1962

36. MILLER EL: Removable Partial Prosthodontics. Baltimore, Williams & Wilkins, 1972

37. MUHLEMANN HR: Tooth mobility. V. Tooth mobility changes through artificial trauma. J Periodontol 25:202–208, 1954

38. MUHLEMANN HR: Ten years of tooth mobility measurements. J Periodontol 31:110–122, 1960

38a. NICHOLS IG: Prosthetic Dentistry. St. Louis, CV Mosby, 1932

39. PERRY C: Philosophy of partial denture design. J Prosthet Dent 6:744–784, 1956

40. ROBINSON C: Clasp design and rest placement for the distal extension removable partial denture. Dent Clin North Am 14:583–594, 1970

41. RUDD KD: Tissue injury from removable partial dentures. Dent Clin North Am 16:805–813, 1972

42. SEEMAN S: A study of the relationship between periodontal disease and the wearing of partial dentures. Aust Dent J 8:206–208, 1963

43. SHOHET H: Relative magnitude of stress of abutment teeth with different retainers. J Prosthet Dent 21:267–282, 1969

44. STEFFEL VL: Relining removable partial dentures for fit and function. J Prosthet Dent 4:496–509, 1954

45. STEFFEL VL: Planning removable partial dentures. J Prosthet Dent 12:524–535, 1962

46. STEFFEL VL: Clasp partial dentures. J Am Dent Assoc 66:803–811, 1963

47. WAERHUNG J: Epidemiology of periodontal disease. Ann Arbor, World Workshop in Periodontics, 1966

48. WEINBERG LA: Lateral force in relation to the denture base and clasp design. J Prosthet Dent 6:785–800, 1956

49. YALISOVE IL: Crown and sleeve coping retainers for removable partial prosthesis. J Prosthet Dent 16:1069–1085, 1966

## SUGGESTED READING

### Diagnosis and Treatment Planning

BARONE JV: Diagnosis and prognosis in complete denture prosthesis. J Prosthet Dent 14:207–213, 1964

BOUCHER CO (ed): Swenson's Complete Dentures. St. Louis, CV Mosby, 1962

BOUCHER CO, HICKEY JC, ZARB GA Prosthodontic Treatment for Edentulous Patients, St. Louis, CV Mosby, 1975

ELLINGER CW, RAYSON JH, TERRY JM, RAHN AD: Synopsis of Complete Dentures. Philadelphia, Lea & Febiger, 1975

NAGLE RJ, SEARS VH: Denture Prosthetics, 2nd ed. St. Louis, CV Mosby, 1970

PERRY C: Examination diagnosis and treatment planning. J Prosthet Dent 10:1004–1014, 1960

SHARRY JJ: Complete Denture Prosthodontics, 3rd ed. St. Louis, McGraw-Hill, 1974

YOUNG HA: Diagnosis of problems in complete denture prosthesis. J Am Dent Assoc 39:185–200, 1949

## Impressions and Casts

BOUCHER CO, HICKEY JC, ZARB GA: Prosthetic Treatment for Edentulous Patients. St. Louis, CV Mosby, 1975

COLLET HA: Complete denture impressions. J Prosthet Dent 15:603–614, 1965

DEVAN MM: Basic principles of impression making. J Prosthet Dent 2:26–35, 1952

ELLINGER CW, RAYSON JH, TERRY JM, RAHN AO: Synopsis of Complete Dentures. Philadelphia, Lea & Febiger, 1975

FISH WW: Principles of Full Denture Prosthesis, 4th ed. London, Staples Press Ltd, 1948

FRIEDMAN S: Edentulous impression procedures for maximum retention and stability. J Prosthet Dent 7:14–26, 1957

HEARTWELL CM: Syllabus of Complete Dentures. Philadelphia, Lea & Febiger, 1968

NAGLE RJ, SEARS VH: Denture Prosthetics, 2nd ed. St. Louis, CV Mosby, 1962

SHARRY JJ: Complete Denture Prosthodontics, 3rd ed. St. Louis, McGraw-Hill, 1974

## Jaw Relations

BOUCHER CO, HICKEY JC, ZARB GA: Prosthodontic Treatment for Edentulous Patients. St. Louis, CV Mosby, 1975

ELLINGER CW, RAYSON JH, TERRY JM, RAHN AO: Synopsis of Complete Dentures. Philadelphia, Lea & Febiger, 1975

HEARTWELL CM: Syllabus of Complete Dentures. Philadelphia, Lea & Febiger, 1968

MOYERS RE: Some physiologic considerations of centric and other jaw relations. J Prosthet Dent 6:183–194, 1956

NICHOLS IG: Prosthetic Dentistry. St. Louis, CV Mosby, 1932

SAIZAR P: Centric occlusion and centric relations. J Am Dent Assoc 67:505–512, 1963

SHARRY JJ: Complete Denture Prosthodontics, 3rd ed. St. Louis, McGraw-Hill, 1974

TRAPAZANO VR: Occlusal records. J Prosthet Dent 5:325–332, 1955

TURRELL AJW: Clinical assessment of vertical dimension. J Prosthet Dent 28:238–246, 1972

## Occlusion and Articulation

BOUCHER CO, HICKEY JC, ZARB GA: Prosthodontic Treatment for Edentulous Patients. St. Louis, CV Mosby, 1975

ELLINGER CW, RAYSON JH, TERRY JM, RAHN AO: Synopsis of Complete Dentures. Philadelphia, Lea & Febiger, 1975

FELDEMANN EE: Tooth contacts in denture occlusion—centric occlusion only. Dent Clin North Am 15:875–887, 1971

HEARTWELL CM: Syllabus of Complete Dentures. Philadelphia, Lea & Febiger, 1968

SEARS VH: Thirty years of nonanatomic teeth. J Prosthet Dent 3:596–617, 1953

SEARS VH: Selection and management of posterior teeth. J Prosthet Dent 7:723–737, 1957

SHARRY JJ: Complete Denture Prosthodontics, 3rd ed. St. Louis, McGraw-Hill, 1974

## Esthetics and Phonetics

BOUCHER CO, HICKEY JC, ZARB GA: Prosthodontic Treatment for Edentulous Patients. St. Louis, CV Mosby, 1975

ELLINGER CW, RAYSON JH, TERRY JM, RAHN AO: Synopsis of Complete Dentures. Philadelphia, Lea & Febiger, 1975

FRUSH JP, FISHER RD: The dynesthetic interpretation of the dentogenic concept. J Prosthet Dent 8:558–581, 1958

GOYAL BK, BHARGAVA K: Arrangement of artificial teeth in abnormal jaw relations, maxillary protrusion and wider upper arch. J Prosthet Dent 32:458–461, 1974

LOMBARDI RE: A method for the classification of errors in dental esthetics. J Prosthet Dent 32:501–513, 1974

SHARRY JJ: Complete Denture Prosthodontics, 3rd ed. St. Louis, McGraw-Hill, 1974

## Insertion and Post Insertion

LUTES MR, HENDERSON D, ELLINGER CW et al: Denture modification during adjustment phase of complete prosthesis. J Prosthet Dent 28:572–579, 1972

NAGLE RJ: Post insertion problems in complete denture prosthesis. J Am Dent Assoc 57:183–187, 1958

SHARRY JJ: Complete Denture Prosthodontics, 3rd ed. St. Louis, McGraw-Hill, 1974

WOODS V: Management of postinsertion problems. Dent Clin North Am 8:735–748, 1964

## Dental Materials

ASGARZADEH K, PEYTON FA: Physical properties of corrective impression materials. J Prosthet Dent 4:555–567, 1954

Council on Dental Materials: Guide to Dental Materials, 5th ed. Chicago, American Dental Association, 1970

MAHLER DB: Plaster of paris and stone materials. Int Dent J 5:241–254, 1945

PEYTON FA, CRAIG RG: Restorative Dental Materials, 4th ed. St. Louis, CV Mosby, 1971

PHILLIPS RW: Skinner's Science of Dental Materials, 7th ed. Philadelphia, WB Saunders, 1973

# ANSWER KEY

| | | | |
|---|---|---|---|
| 1. 1 | 15. 2 | 29. 4 | 43. 4 |
| 2. 3 | 16. 1 | 30. 3 | 44. 3 |
| 3. 2 | 17. 3 | 31. 3 | 45. 3 |
| 4. 4 | 18. 2 | 32. 3 | 46. 4 |
| 5. 3 | 19. 2 | 33. 6 | 47. 3 |
| 6. 6 | 20. 4 | 34. 4 | 48. 3 |
| 7. 2 | 21. 3 | 35. 1 | 49. 3 |
| 8. 5 | 22. 4 | 36. 6 | 50. 2 |
| 9. 3 | 23. 3, 4, 2, 1 | 37. 6 | 51. 6 |
| 10. 4 | 24. 4 | 38. 2 | 52. 2 |
| 11. 1 | 25. 3 | 39. 4 | 53. 2 |
| 12. 3 | 26. 2 | 40. 6 | 54. 4 |
| 13. 5 | 27. 4 | 41. 2 | 55. 1, 1, 2 |
| 14. 3 | 28. 3 | 42. 2 | |

# 7

# PEDODONTICS

**J. Bernard Machen   /   Henry W. Fields, Jr.   /   F. Thomas McIver**

This chapter is an overview of pedodontics that focuses upon eight aspects of dentistry for children: 1) child behavior guidance, 2) preventive dentistry, 3) developmental disturbances in dentition, 4) diagnosis and correction of minor irregularities of the dentition, 5) pulp therapy, 6) traumatic injuries, 7) restorative dentistry, and 8) oral tissues of children with disease.

## CHILD BEHAVIOR GUIDANCE

Possibly the most useful service a dentist performs is preparing a child for a lifetime of continuing dental care. The anxiety often associated with visiting the dentist can be seen in the numerous stories and jokes told about a visit to the dentist. Many words have been written and spoken on the stress accompanying dental care and how the dentist can better manage the behavior of patients undergoing this stress. A review of the literature reveals a number of individual approaches to the problem of child behavior guidance. At times these various approaches appear to conflict with each other; there is some degree of argument as to the preferable manner of child behavior guidance.

Many professionals working in the field of child behavior management seem to be directing their efforts toward reducing or eliminating fear. Others concede that going to the dentist is an anxiety-producing event and will probably remain so for most people. Rather than seeking to eliminate fear, they seek to help patients learn ways of coping with their anxiety in a way that allows the dentist to perform quality dental services. Anxiety in the proper amount is viewed as a positive and necessary emotion which serves to alert the individual to danger. Certainly most children associate going to the dentist with some danger and therefore display variable degrees of anxiety.

The child behavior guidance techniques that appear most useful focus on the dentist and the dentist's staff as teachers who help the child learn to cooperate during dental treatment even though he or she is experiencing a significant amount of anxiety. In addition, and of equal importance, the child should be willing to return for further treatment as a result of learning experiences at the dentist's office.

### Learning in Relation to Dental Care

Learning can be defined as a relatively permanent change in behavior resulting from experience. Some amount of learning probably accrues as a result of every experience. Much of the behavior a child exhibits in the dental office is the result of learning experiences in the past. For example, the 4-year-old child who willingly leaves his mother in the waiting room and engages in conversation with the dentist has probably had many pleasant experiences with other people and is therefore willing to enter into new relationships.

There are four general means of controlling learning for dental care: 1) expectation, 2) modeling, 3) association, and 4) reinforcement, both positive and negative. Each of these means is very powerful and is interwoven in the entire experience of a child. Often several means of learning are at work during a single experience.

**EXPECTATION.** It is evident that an individual tends to perform in a way that is expected. This concept leads a football coach to spend a great deal of effort to make the players understand that certain qualities are expected of them, and the players tend to acquire these qualities through learning of the expectations of their coach. Similarly, children tend to learn helpful behavior in the dental office if they understand what is expected of them. It is the function of the dentist and the dental auxiliaries to define precisely the helpful behavior that is expected of the child.

**MODELING.** Children learn a great deal by imitating the behaviors of a model. It is important to remember that a child will model an emotion, i.e., anxiety, as well as a clearly observable behavior.

The child is very sensitive to any anxiety which can be observed through the nonverbal communication of others. It is especially true that there is a strong relationship between any anxiety that a mother exhibits regarding a dental appointment for her child and the anxiety a child feels toward the appointment. In the same way, a child tends to model any anxiety in the dentist and auxiliaries. Therefore, it is imperative that the treatment be carried out in the presence of helpful models. This is a primary reason for treating the child in the absence of the parent. Since children with a great deal of anxiety frequently have mothers with similar feelings, these mothers are not useful as models in the dental operatory.

A child may model the other children in the dental office. It is sometimes useful to allow a new child patient, especially a young child, to sit quietly and watch a sibling or another child being treated. This is assuming, of course, that the model child is cooperating with the treatment since the new patient may model uncooperative behavior as well as desirable behavior.

ASSOCIATIONS. It is merely common sense to predict that a person who experiences pain at a dental office will associate going to the dentist with unpleasantness and will feel increased anxiety at subsequent dental appointments. However, association can be used to guide behavior by replacing unpleasant associations with more positive and useful associations. This use of association is one reason for arranging the treatment sequence for a child in a way that places the least stressful treatments first (examination, prophylaxis, etc.) and delays the more unpleasant treatments (extractions and restorations) until after the child has been able to make some pleasant associations with visits to the dentist.

REINFORCEMENT. Learning through reinforcement has the advantage that the dentist is in relatively direct control of the reinforcements (rewards) that are provided in the office to increase the frequency of desirable behavior. There are two types of reinforcement that play a part in behavior guidance—positive and negative. Positive reinforcement is the process of providing a reward immediately after a particular behavior. The rewards most often used in the dental office are words of praise, hugs, and other direct demonstrations that the child has done something admirable. A long list of common, useful statements could be made, but each dentist must use the rewards that suit his or her personality and the specific situation. A few statements that are usually rewarding to children are

"You are a good helper."
"I'm proud of the way you help."

"Mom and Dad will be proud of the way you helped."
"Good."
"You are my best patient today."
"We like for you to come to see us."

Children, as well as most adults, thrive on the knowledge that they are doing a good job and that others appreciate it. A dentist is not likely to make rewarding statements too often. It is more common for the dentist to become so engrossed in the technical aspects of the treatment that he or she fails to reinforce the child's desirable behaviors.

Since reinforcement is such a powerful means of learning, it is essential to good behavior guidance that only desirable behavior be reinforced. Through the use of negative reinforcement, a dentist may unwittingly reinforce undesirable behaviors. Consider, for example, the excessively anxious child who chooses to avoid dental care by not cooperating with the dentist. Because of this behavior, the decision is made to delay treatment until the child feels more willing to accept it. Since the child's behavior has led to an escape from an unpleasant and anxiety-producing situation, the child will probably employ similar tactics on future visits to the dentist. This is a clear example of negative reinforcement in the dental office; the child has learned undesirable behavior.

The child's departure from the dental office is an extremely important event; it may be the most rewarding aspect of going to the dentist. The child should believe that something beneficial has happened during the appointment and that some dental care (even though the amount may be small) has been accomplished. Leaving is then a reward for helping with the accomplishments.

Gifts may be provided for children as they leave. It is necessary, however, to point out the reason for the gift. It may be that the child has been "a good helper." Even if the child has not been a very good helper, a gift may be given. To keep the child from thinking of the gift as a reward for uncooperative behavior, it is essential for the dentist to point out to the uncooperative child some behaviors that were helpful. There is seldom a child who does absolutely nothing that could be rewarded. The child who has been less than cooperative can be told that the dentist enjoyed the child's visit and believes that the child will be able to help much more at the next visit. This child receives a gift because the dentist wants to give a token of friendship, and the gift is given in this instance primarily to promote positive associations with visits to the dentist.

## Emotional Status of Children

The dentist must always consider the pattern of behavior and the degree of development that can be expected at a given age and must try to determine whether the child is developing according to the so-called norm.

**PRESCHOOL CHILDREN.** At 2 years of age, children differ greatly in their ability to communicate, primarily because of considerable variations in vocabulary development at that age. According to Gessell (3), the vocabulary of 2-year-olds ranges from 12–1000 words. If communication is limited, cooperation is likely to be limited. For this reason work can be successfully completed for some 2-year-old children, but not for others.

The 2-year-old child is often referred to as being in the "precooperative stage." The child is too young to be reached by words alone and must handle and touch objects in order to grasp their meaning fully. The dentist must allow the child at this age to handle the mirror, to smell the toothpaste, or to feel the rubber cup. Doing these things gives the child a better idea of what the dentist is attempting to do. Since a child this young is shy around new people and places and finds it difficult to be separated from his or her parents, almost without exception a parent should accompany the 2-year-old to the treatment room.

The dentist can usually communicate and reason with the 3-year-old child more easily during the dental experience. The 3-year-old has a great desire to talk and will often enjoy telling stories to the dentist. At this stage dental personnel can begin to use the positive approach with the child. It is well, however, to point out the positive rather than the negative factors of behavior because a child at this age is likely to do the things that have been forbidden.

It has been reported by Hymes (4) that when they are hurt, fatigued or frightened children 3 years of age and under automatically turn to their mothers for comfort, support, and assurance. They therefore feel more secure if a parent is allowed to remain with them until they become fully acquainted with the personnel and the procedures in the dental office.

The 4-year-old child usually listens with interest to explanations and is normally quite responsive to verbal directions. A child at this age usually has a lively mind and may be a great talker. In some situations the 4-year-old may become quite defiant and may resort to name-calling. In general, however, the 4-year-old child who has had a happy home life with a normal amount of training and discipline is a very cooperative patient.

The 5-year-old is ready to accept group activities and community experience. Personal and social relationships are better defined, and the child usually has no fear of leaving one of the parents for the dental appointment. The 5-year-old child who has been properly prepared has no fear of new experiences such as a visit to the dentist's office. A child in this age group is usually very proud of possessions and clothes, and comments about the child's personal appearance can often be effectively used to establish communication with a new patient.

**THE CHILD DURING THE EARLY SCHOOL YEARS.** In the period 6–11 years of age the child learns about the outside world and becomes increasingly independent. He develops a conscience or a sense of responsibility about matters that to him seem important. These are the years when closely knit groups are formed such a clubs and gangs. During this period the child is introduced to the culture of his society through the public or private school. They are important years for learning how to get along with other people and to abide by the rules of society.

The child's independence of his parents is manifested by his gaining a feeling of individuality and by his desire to be treated as a person rather than as a possession. He is apt to show some impatience toward his parents who keep telling him the right things to do. Although he loves them as much as ever, he dislikes emotional display about himself. Joining a club is simply another means of showing his ability to accomplish things independently of adults.

His sense of responsibility is manifested in competitive types of games or ones that require some skill. He becomes a small businessman by setting up a lemonade stand or by starting a garden. He may not carry many of these enterprises through to completion, but the urge to do them is present.

Toward the end of this period he thinks in terms of cause and effect and acquires an insight into the actions of machines and some of the fundamental human relationships. The desire to accomplish great things occupies his mind when he is not doing school- or homework. He dreams of bold adventures, and one of his favorite heroes may well be a character in a comic strip or story where right always wins. Besides the comics, books, radio, television, and motion pictures furnish him with his ideals.

Because of his desire for independence he may be irritating to his parents and present a problem in discipline. The adult must try to overlook some of his less serious bad habits, and when giving orders, try to be matter of fact and friendly. Most obnoxious to the child is the "bossiness" or the nagging voice, which one should strive to avoid. School problems are best taken up with the teacher or school authorities. Poor work in school may be due to many causes—for example, physical defects, such as poor eyesight or hearing and extreme nervousness. The highly intelligent child may be bored with his schoolwork, while the child with a low intelligence cannot comprehend his studies. Finally the school system may be at fault. One should carefully examine and eliminate any or all possible causes instead of punishing the child.

## Child Behavior Guidance in the Dental Office

PRIMARY PROCEDURES IN BEHAVIOR GUIDANCE

*Development of Trust.* Parents who have a high regard for the professional competence of their dentist and believe he or she is sincerely interested in the welfare of their child are supportive in the dentist's treatment of the child. If the parents do not trust the dentist, they may undermine the treatment of the child. Parents tend to trust the dentist who

1. Listens to their concerns
2. Gives information about what is going to be done for their child
3. Explains why certain treatments are necessary
4. Praises the parents and the child
5. Is friendly
6. Appears confident of his or her ability to provide dental care for children

Developing the child's trust depends on the credibility of the dentist. The dentist must never make statements which are later found to be untrue. The child should not be told that a certain procedure does not hurt when it may turn out to be uncomfortable in the child's opinion. The child should be told that the procedure may be uncomfortable ("feel bad," "pinch," etc.) but that it will not last long. Words that unnecessarily evoke fear in the child, such as "pain," "shot," "needle," etc., should be avoided. The words used, however, must be understood by the child. For example, it is better to use a term such as "hurt a bit" rather than "mosquito bite" if the child does not clearly understand that a mosquito bite hurts. Remember also that the best management efforts can be undermined by inadequate anesthesia.

*Helping the Child Learn about Dental Treatment*

*Types of Communication.* Verbal communication between any adult and child is more effective if the adult physically gets down to the child's eye level. It must be remembered that communcation is continual and occurs in many ways, regardless of intention.

Explicit communication is information that is intentionally transferred verbally. Positive statements describing what a child is to do are preferable. The dentist should avoid asking questions such as "Will you open your mouth, please?" Questions like that offer the child the option of a yes or no answer. Since "no" is really an unacceptable answer in the dental situation, it is preferable to make a statement such as "Open your mouth, please," rather than to pose a question.

Implicit communication is information that is transferred nonverbally, e.g., facial expression, office decor, tone of voice, etc. Extremely sensitive to information transferred implicitly, children sense the emotions of the dentist and other dental personnel. Any excessive anxiety in the office is readily communicated to the child through implicit channels.

*Tell–Show–Do.* If carefully and constantly used, the method called tell–show–do is very effective in helping the child learn to be a dental patient. The dentist should tell the child what is to be done, show the child what is to be done, and then proceed to do exactly what the child has been led to expect. The approach used varies according to the developmental level and previous experiences of the child. Children in the 3–5-year-old group often do not understand many of the objects in the dental office and consequently may fear such things as dental instruments, dental chairs, strange rooms, x-ray equipment, and even unknown dental personnel. Unfamiliar odors, sounds, and touch sensations may also be feared and should be included in tell–show–do.

The child should be allowed to sense the object in a variety of ways. If possible the child should see, smell, hear, and touch a new object or material. Often it is desirable to demonstrate an object outside of the child's mouth. For example, when the explorer is introduced, it may be helpful to touch the child on the fingernail with it before using it in the mouth.

In general it is preferable to present the most familiar instruments and procedures to the child (mirror, toothbrushing, etc.) first and proceed to the most novel (drill, forceps, etc.). Since the most unfamiliar procedures are likely to produce the most anxiety, placing them later in the treatment experience allows the dental staff to develop rapport with the child prior to presentation of the unfamiliar instruments.

There is some debate regarding the extent to which tell–show–do should be used in the administration of local anesthetic. Experience at the University of North Carolina indicates that the child who does not actually see the anesthetic syringe accepts the procedure best. All other aspects of tell–show–do should be included in the administration of local anesthetic.

The dentist or the auxiliaries should never assume that certain procedures or instruments are so simple and harmless that they will be of no concern to the child. Any experience may be new to the child and therefore should be included in the tell–show–do process.

*Limiting Unacceptable Behavior.* The child should be immediately informed of behavior that is not helpful in accomplishing the dental treatment. The most convenient and effective means of making a child aware that certain behavior is unacceptable is the dentist's voice. The use of the voice in guiding child behavior is referred to as voice control.

In general a child is quite sensitive to voice intonation, and a statement with the proper inflection can very effectively let the child know the limit of acceptable behavior has been passed. Although a tone of voice which is different from the normal one is employed in setting a limit, voice control does not mean that the dentist shouts or yells at the child. On the contrary, lowering the pitch of the voice, shortening or clipping the words, and raising the voice volume only moderately are usually sufficient. Statements such as "No," "Stop that now," and any other appropriate statement spoken in a very firm manner can turn what begins as an unpleasant experience into a rewarding experience for both the child and the dentist.

*Understanding the Child's Fears.* The dentist can help the child identify fears and show empathy for the child's point of view. A child should not be told that there is nothing to fear, but rather that other children have the same feelings and are often afraid of going to the dentist.

Often the child's primary fear is not the fear of being hurt. It is more likely that the child is afraid of the new environment and the new people involved in this experience. The child can be helped by being assured that others understand these feelings and that the dentist will help him or her learn enough about dental treatment to overcome these fears.

SECONDARY PROCEDURES FOR CHILD BEHAVIOR GUIDANCE. The secondary procedures for child guidance in no way eliminate the need to continue the primary behavior guidance procedures in the dental treatment experience.

*Hand Over Mouth Exercise.* Hand Over Mouth Exercise (HOME) is a very controversial and much debated means of guiding behavior (2, 5). HOME is another means of setting limits to behavior and is also very effective in helping establish communication with a child. The technique is indicated only occasionally and should never be considered a routine measure. It is used when the child has become quite uncooperative and may be crying hysterically, when there is no useful communication occurring between the child and the dentist.

The HOME technique involves placing one hand over the child's mouth, without restricting breathing, while the other hand and arm cradle the child's head and restrain its movements. The noise the child was making is stopped in this way, making it possible for the dentist to talk to the child and establish useful communication. The dentist can stress that it is important that the child begin to help and that the hand will be removed from the child's mouth if he or she will sit quietly and still. At this point it is essential to employ all the primary behavior guidance procedures. In some instances it may be necessary to repeat HOME to help the child understand that the limit of acceptable behavior has been passed and to establish communication.

It is imperative that HOME not be used as a punitive measure and that the dentist be kind in approach and words. Furthermore a dentist who uses HOME needs complete self-control lest anger toward the child interfere with effective behavior guidance. The dentist must remember that a child who is in such an emotional state that HOME is indicated is a frightened, anxious child.

*Drugs.* In some cases it may be helpful to premedicate a child with a variety of sedative, analgesic, or tranquilizing drugs. If the child's mental development is normal, drugs are most valuable when relatively traumatic procedures must be performed early in the treatment experience. For example, a 4-year-old who must have teeth removed at the first dental appointment may be able to make more positive associations with dental treatment if effective drugs are used.

No drugs or combination of drugs have proven to be universally effective in child behavior guidance. Because drug actions vary from child to child, it is important to avoid routine use of drugs and reserve the drugs for very specific indications.

*Nitrous Oxide-Oxygen Psychosedation.* Nitrous oxide–oxygen psychosedation is a drug administered by inhalation. Like drugs administered by other routes, it affects children in a variety of ways. It is helpful for some children, while it seems to make other children uncomfortable.

Nitrous oxide–oxygen psychosedation may provide the extra boost some children need to cope with the dental treatment experience. It has been the author's clinical experience that the drug may be of particular benefit to children who have excessive fear of anesthetic injections or very short attention spans making them restless after only a few minutes of treatment. The gases should be presented with the tell–show–do technique, and all of the other primary behavior guidance measures must be utilized. Nitrous oxide–oxygen psychosedation can be used only for children who cooperate with the procedure. It is not a measure to overcome a child who is uncooperative at the inception of treatment.

The authors' philosophy regarding the use of any drug, including nitrous oxide–oxygen, is that it is preferable for a child to cope with life's experiences, i.e., dental care, without the aid of drugs if possible. For this reason drugs should be withdrawn as soon as the treatment becomes tolerable to the child. Certainly the child should not be expected to endure pain, so it is necessary to use local anesthetics for almost all tooth preparation and surgical procedures. It may be possible, however, to eliminate the use of nitrous oxide–oxygen after the child has made several visits to the dentist. By then the child may have learned enough to endure the minor discomforts of dental treatment without drugs.

## QUESTIONS

1. A child's behavior problem in the dental office can be handled by familiarization if the basis of the problem is
   1. the parents
   2. pain
   3. emotional
   4. fear

2. An understanding of the development of human behavior requires a knowledge of the basic concepts of
   1. generalization and facilitation
   2. dependence and independence
   3. maturation and learning
   4. masculinity and femininity

3. A 3-year-old child is frightened by sudden noises, bright lights, loss of support; this behavior is described as anxiety related to
   1. abstract thinking
   2. slow mental maturation
   3. concrete fears
   4. reflex reaction

4. The dentist can favorably alter or extinguish the child's anticipation of a fearful experience by
   a. telling the child what to expect before the procedure is performed
   b. demonstrating any unfamiliar equipment to the child before using it
   c. allowing the child to feel at home
   d. being permissive and accepting all behaviors

   1. a
   2. a and b
   3. a and c
   4. b and c
   5. b and d

5. A boy and girl of the same age are at the same physical and intellectual level but their behavior is extremely different in the dental office. Which of the following is probably most significantly related to this difference?
   1. Maturation
   2. Learning
   3. Sex
   4. Dental health requirements
   5. Parents

6. A behavior problem in the dental office is traced to the fact that a 3-year-old girl heard about dental difficulties from her mother; the most satisfactory method of handling the situation is to
   1. use firmness
   2. modify the fear by familiarization, using tell–show–do techniques
   3. use nitrous oxide–oxygen analgesia
   4. introduce another child as a good example
   5. administer very small doses of barbiturates

7. During the first appointment the dentist can begin to train a nervous child to be a good dental patient by
   a. maintaining a quiet, controlled office
   b. showing, telling, and doing with each instrument and piece of equipment
   c. making sudden unexplained adjustments in the dental chair
   d. separating the child from the mother without warning
   e. expressing appreciation of good behavior by means of a gift

   1. a and b
   2. a, b, and e
   3. b, d, and e
   4. c and d
   5. d and e

8. In a dental situation the basic fear of most children under 2 years of age is concerned with
   1. separation from the parent
   2. injections of local anesthetics
   3. the reason for dental treatment
   4. the instruments to perform dental treatment

## PREVENTIVE DENTISTRY IN PEDODONTICS

Even though major advances in research have made prevention of dental disease a realistic possibility, studies show that by 3 years of age 50% of children in communities with nonfluoridated water have a carious tooth and by adulthood more than 95% of people have carious teeth and/or periodontal disease. This discrepancy between what is known about prevention and what has been accomplished is a result of many psychosocial factors, but evidence is mounting that comprehensive preventive programs are narrowing the gap (see Ch. 4, Community and Preventive Dentistry).

There are a number of important differences between the adult patient and the child patient in regard to preventive care, and it is important for the dentist to recognize and remember these differences when dealing with children.

### Dental Plaque Removal

The aim of plaque removal procedures is to disrupt the bacterial plaque that accumulates on the teeth and to remove food debris from tooth surfaces. These procedures result in better periodontal health and to some extent a reduction in dental caries. The most effective approach is still frequent mechanical disruption of the plaque material by means of toothbrushing and flossing. In infants plaque can be removed by gently scrubbing the teeth with a clean cloth or gauze.

It is important to begin cleansing procedures as soon as the primary teeth erupt. The parent must assume this responsibility until the child is able to accomplish this task independently. In most children this stage of development is reached between 6 and 8 years of age. Even after that time it is important for the parent to evaluate the quality of cleansing and to assist if necessary.

When a parent or other adult performs the cleansing procedure for a small child, proper positioning of the child is crucial. The position chosen must provide support for the child's head and body, must be comfortable for all involved, must provide adequate visibility, and must be near a good source of light. Cleansing can usually be accomplished in a bathroom, but occasionally a room with a soft chair or couch and plenty of space is better. The dental professional who is teaching the procedure should evaluate the abilities of each person involved and recommend an appropriate position. Frequently it is necessary to experiment with several positions before settling on one.

When the child can stand and is cooperative, the adult may find it convenient to stand behind the child, stabilize the child's head against his or her side, and open the child's lips with one hand while brushing with the other. The head is further stabilized by the hand which keeps the child's lips open to provide visualization of the mouth. Another useful position is to have the child seated on the floor and the person brushing seated behind and straddling the patient. The child should look up in order to increase visibility for the person performing the cleansing.

The techniques for brushing and flossing are the same regardless of whether the child or someone else performs the task. Since there is no evidence that one toothbrushing method is clearly superior to others, it seems that the technique used should be the most simple method that is effective in the hands of the individuals performing the brushing. Several studies involving children indicate a horizontal scrub method is superior to other techniques, and this method appears to be the one that is used naturally by children who have been given no brushing instructions (2, 18, 25). In this method the brush is placed horizontally on the facial, lingual, or occlusal surfaces and is merely moved back and forth in short strokes until all surfaces of the tooth have been scrubbed. There is some evidence that, when properly used, the Bass technique may provide superior plaque control for patients with gingival inflammation. This technique differs from the scrub method in that the brush is held at a 45° angle to the facial and lingual tooth surface and the bristles are pushed gently into the gingival crevice. The brush used in both techniques should be soft, multitufted nylon with rounded tips. The size of the brush should be appropriate for the size of the individual's mouth.

The effectiveness of toothbrushing depends to a great extent on the amount of time each tooth is brushed, and a primary objective of any brushing technique must be systematic coverage of all areas of the dentition. It has been demonstrated that 8-year-old children who brush for 3 min are more likely to remove plaque than children who brush for shorter durations (18). To help the child judge how much time to spend on toothbrushing, it can be useful to time the brushing with a 3-min sandglass timer.

Unwaxed dental floss has a permanent place in effective plaque control programs. It has been demonstrated that normal 8-year-old children can be taught flossing skills if the procedure is broken down into small steps which can be taught independently (32). The most difficult part of flossing for some individuals is holding the dental floss with their fingers, but there are a number of floss holders available which can facilitate this part of the task.

The role of dentifrices in plaque removal is not clear. It is apparent that dentifrices with fluoride significantly reduce dental caries, but it has not been established that any dentifrices improve plaque removal. On the contrary, there is some evidence that dentifrices deter plaque removal because they stimulate salivary production, which greatly increases the volume of fluid in the patient's mouth. This fluid, combined with the foaming action of the dentifrice, interferes with the vision of the person doing the brushing and can cause the patient to gag. In fact, parents often complain that their child gags on the dentifrice and use that as a reason for not brushing the child's teeth. If a choice has to be made between brushing with no dentifrice or not brushing at all, the choice is obvious.

The recommended frequency of oral hygiene procedures is a matter which has received considerable attention in the literature. There is support for the position that thorough cleaning once a day significantly improves oral health. If one brushing per day is considered sufficient, it should occur before the child goes to bed at night.

## Fluorides

BASIC FLUORIDE PROGRAMS.    Fluoride is recognized as the most effective agent for preventing dental caries. Recommendations for the use of fluorides to reduce dental decay are continually changing with new discoveries, but current evidence suggests that children who are exposed to either naturally fluoridated or community water to which fluoride has been added should also include brushing with an effective fluoride-containing dentifrice in their daily oral hygiene procedures. At semiannual recall appointments these children should receive topical fluoride applications following either a professional prophylaxis using a very fine agent or a supervised self-cleaning. Techniques of applying fluoride may have to be altered to fit patient behavior.

According to recent estimates, the water supply for more than half the population in the United States is not fluoridated. When the level of fluoride in a child's drinking water is unknown, the water should be analyzed to determine the amount of fluoride in it. Most state health departments maintain laboratories that perform this service, and such an analysis is a mandatory first step in establishing a fluoride program for the patient who is exposed to an unknown amount of fluoride.

In addition to drinking water, other potential sources of fluoride exposure must be carefully checked. School mouth rinse programs and fluoridation of school drinking water increase the exposure of patients to fluoride, for example. Children may attend school in a fluoridated area and live in a nonfluoridated area. In this situation it can be assumed that one-third of the necessary fluoride is obtained at school, and a supplement should be prescribed to supply the remainder. Also, it must be remembered that these children need a full supplement in the summer months when school is not in session.

Once the level of fluoride exposure has been determined, the amount and type of supplement can be determined (Table 7–1). Supplements are usually administered in drops, tablets, or rinses. Drops are incorporated in the patient's food. Tablets require the most patient cooperation, while rinses can either be applied by the patient or brushed on the teeth by parent or guardian. It is important that the dentist prescribing a fluoride supplement program consider preferences of the adult responsible for implementing it. The best fluoride program does no good unless it is carried out regularly!

In addition to these daily fluoride supplements, a fluoride-containing dentifrice should be used in conjunction with regular home care. Semiannual topical fluoride applications should be administered by the dentist after professional prophylaxis or a supervised self-cleaning.

**MODIFICATIONS OF THE BASIC FLUORIDE PROGRAM.** A careful monitoring of the basic program is essential during the first few months of treatment. Is the child, parent, or responsible adult carrying out the program as prescribed? If it appears that the program is

feasible as prescribed, further evaluation can be delayed until the next regular recall appointment. Frequently, however, the initial program may not be satisfactory. The most common problem involves the dietary supplement. In many instances the child can masticate adequately but refuses to take the daily tablet or is unreliable in taking it. If this is the case, the program must be revised and the fluoride supplied in either drops or a rinse that is brushed onto the teeth. Both of these alternatives require more involvement of the parent or responsible adult, however.

**THERAPEUTIC FLUORIDE SUPPLEMENTS.** The patient with rampant decay or the patient who is not progressing adequately under a basic fluoride program should be given a more intensive, therapeutic fluoride program. Such a program may be needed only until oral hygiene and diet are improved or it may be needed for extended treatment periods. These therapeutic regimens are in addition to the basic systemic supplement. The patient is not to swallow or ingest these doses; they are topical. Accepted therapeutic regimens include

1. Daily rinsing with 0.05% NaF solution
2. Weekly rinsing with 0.1%–0.2% NaF solution
3. Brushing with either 0.5%–1.23% acidulated phosphate gels five times a year

These therapeutic fluoride regimens must be carefully and closely monitored by means of frequent recalls because of the potential risk of fluorosis.

### Sealants

Occlusal sealants are a valuable adjunct to preventive dentistry because they help to prevent pit and fissure caries. Research indicates that caries reduction does occur when properly placed sealants are used to cover the occlusal surfaces of posterior teeth. It is also apparent that a thoroughly dry field is necessary to place sealants properly. This is sometimes difficult to achieve with child patients.

### Diet and Nutrition

There are three ways diet and nutrition influence the rate and extent of dental caries and periodontal disease. First, they affect the resistance of the tooth and supporting structures to disease; second, they can affect the type and virulence of the bacteria in dental plaque; and third, they influence the salivary properties of the oral environment.

Dental caries is fundamentally a dietary and bacterial disease. Epidemiologic study (32) has demonstrated that foods high in sucrose increase the incidence of

**Table 7–1. Fluoride Supplement Schedule**

| PATIENT'S AGE (YEARS) | LEVEL OF WATER FLUORIDE | | |
|---|---|---|---|
| | 0–0.3 PPM | 0.3–0.7 PPM | 0.7+ PPM |
| 0–2 | 0.25 mg | 0 mg | 0 mg |
| 2–3 | 0.50 mg | 0 mg | 0 mg |
| 3–8 | 1.00 mg | 0.50 mg | 0.25 mg |
| over 8 | 1.00 mg | 1.00 mg | 0.50 mg |

(Adapted from *Accepted Dental Therapeutics*, 37th ed. Chicago, American Dental Association, 1977, p. 294)

dental caries and that the more the sucrose adheres to the surface of the tooth, the greater the susceptibility to decay. In other studies diet counseling was used to restrict sucrose intake on subjects with rampant caries, and the results were significant improvements in dental health.

The influence of nutrition on the development of periodontal disease is not as clearly defined as its influence on the development of dental caries. It is thought that nutritional deprivations affect the rate and degree of periodontal disease rather than its initiation (21).

## Motivation

Motivation is a very complex and elusive concept, which differs greatly among individuals. Although a low level of dental disease through prevention is a realistic goal for everyone, the actual application of the preventive measures available depends primarily on the motivation of patients and those who care for them. It has been stated that people are motivated to change health habits when they hold three beliefs: 1) that they are susceptible to a disease, 2) that the disease will have severe consequences for them if it occurs; and 3) that there is an action they can take which will be effective in eliminating the disease or reducing its severity.

For children, however, other factors may play a significant role. Young children may be very much motivated by the suggestions and urging of parents or other authority figures. Their desire for approval of activities such as toothbrushing may be very positive factors in the development of an effective preventive program. Because they are eager to help their children, parents are often highly motivated to help in the home care of their children's teeth.

A major component of motivation is the communication of meaningful information about dental disease to those involved in the care of a child. The information and preventive plan must be tailored to the specific needs of the patient, and these needs can be determined only after careful evaluation of the patient and the people caring for him or her. The rationale for performing preventive measures must be based on factors that are important to those involved. In addition, the demonstration of sincere concern for the well-being of the child patient by dental health professionals will likely stimulate others to improve their efforts toward preventive measures. Furthermore, frequent praise of these efforts will pay dividends in better dental health.

### QUESTIONS

9. The anticariogenic effect of fluoride is related principally to the
   1. bacteriocidal action on oral flora
   2. bacteriostatic action on oral flora
   3. buffering effect on acids produced by cariogenic bacteria
   4. alteration in the composition of the enamel
   5. inhibition of oral bacterial fermentation of carbohydrates

10. Systemic fluoridation may be accomplished by means of
    a. water fluoridation
    b. tablet supplement
    c. drop or liquid supplement
    d. mouth wash
    1. a, b, and c
    2. b and c
    3. b, c, and d
    4. All of the above

11. Which of the following statements are true?
    a. The oral hygiene techniques taught the child are partially determined by age and neuromuscular coordination.
    b. Waxed dental floss is carried through the contact areas of the teeth to remove debris and provide clean, polished proximal surfaces in preparation for topical fluoride application.
    c. Topical fluoride application is not indicated for patients receiving the optimal concentration of systemic fluoride.
    d. Sodium fluoride tablets are recommended as a supplement when the daily water supply has an insufficient concentration of fluoride.
    1. a and b
    2. b and c
    3. a and d
    4. All of the above

12. Which of the following is the most effective way to combat dental disease?
    1. Establishing a community fluoridation program
    2. Careful dietary control emphasizing elimination of sweets
    3. Incremental dental care coupled with community water fluoridation
    4. Use of a program composed of community water fluoridation and additional topical fluoridation
    5. Regular prophylaxis followed by topical applications of fluoride

13. The use of which of the following adjunctive aids is necessary to check on the efficacy of an oral prophylaxis for a young patient?
    1. Disclosing solution
    2. Sandpaper strip
    3. Snyder test
    4. Unwaxed floss

14. The final responsibility for the performance of preventive and control dental treatment techniques rests with
    1. parents
    2. community programs
    3. practicing dentists
    4. school dental clinics
    5. public health departments

# DEVELOPMENTAL DISTURBANCES OF THE DENTITION

Like some of its cellular components, the dentition has a definite life cycle. Initially there is tooth formation, which is followed by eruption and then function. These stages are similar for the primary and permanent dentitions, but the primary dentition life cycle also includes resorption and exfoliation, conditions which are observed only in pathologic states of the permanent dentition. This life cycle is well ordered but easily disturbed by genetic and environmental factors (Table 7–2). Anomalies may occur due to either to much or too little activity at each stage.

## Formation

Disturbances which occur during tooth formation lead to problems with the number of teeth, their structure, form, and amount of calcified tissue and its degree of hardness. The quantity or quality of damage to the dentition is dependent upon the time that the disturbances arise.

NUMBER. Problems involving increased or decreased numbers of teeth usually arise during the initiation or proliferation of tooth development. The successional dental lamina proliferates lingual to the primary tooth bud and initiates all succedaneous teeth. It is reasonable to assume that a missing primary tooth signals the absence of the permanent successor. The permanent molars bud from the dental lamina at a point distal to the primary second molar. This developmental sequence enables the dentist to predict, in some cases, absence of permanent teeth.

A decrease in the number of teeth present most frequently occurs due to the congenital absence of one tooth. Most commonly this is the third molar. Although there is some difference of opinion concerning the incidence of missing teeth, maxillary lateral incisors, mandibular second bicuspids, and maxillary second bicuspids are also frequently absent. It is apparent that the most distal tooth in a class of teeth (e.g., incisors, premolars) is the most frequent congenitally absent tooth of that class of teeth. There appears to be a dominant pattern of inheritance involved with this anomaly. When several teeth are missing, the condition is labeled oligodontia. This is frequently encountered in conjunction with ectodermal dysplasia (Fig. 7–1). Complete absence of teeth, known as anodontia, is a rare occurrence.

It is possible for an increased number of teeth to be present in the dentition. Many times they appear as cysts which originate during the initiation or proliferation stage of tooth development. Although many of these cysts occur as intraosseous lesions, some are found on the epithelium of the alveolar ridges. Odontomas are more highly organized structures than cysts and consist of dentin and enamel components. When the organization and structure of these proliferations are normal or nearly normal they are labeled supernumerary teeth. Most supernumerary teeth occur in the maxillary anterior region (Fig. 7–2).

STRUCTURE. Problems of atypical structure usually arise during the histodifferentiation stage of tooth growth. Dentinogenesis imperfecta is an autosomal dominant trait which results in narrow roots, bulbous crowns, and pulp chambers and canals which are nearly obliterated upon radiographic examination. This condition is sometimes seen in conjunction with osteogenesis imperfecta. The quality of change at the dentinoenamel junction allows the enamel to abrade easily. This may be due to a different configuration of the junction or a defect in the dentin matrix.

Dentin dysplasia is another autosomal dominant

**Table 7–2. Life Cycle of Dentition and Associated Developmental Disturbances**

| STAGES | ASSOCIATED DEVELOPMENTAL DISTURBANCES |
|---|---|
| Formation | Number: congenitally absent teeth, oligodontia, anodontia, cysts, odontomas, supernumerary teeth<br>Structure: dentinogenesis imperfecta, dentinal dysplasia, shell' teeth, odontodysplasia<br>Form: peg lateral, microdontia, dens in dente, macrodontia<br>Amount: Hypoplasia (localized and generalized), amelogenesis imperfecta, intrinsic stains<br>Hardness: hypocalcified (enamel and dentin), interglobular dentin, amelogenesis imperfecta |
| Eruption | Natal tooth; Neonatal tooth; Eruption Hemotoma; Generalized early eruption; Localized early and late eruption, Generalized late eruption, Ankylosis |
| Function | Occlusal attrition; Abrasion from other disease states |
| Exfoliation | Premature exfoliation of primary teeth |

Adapted from Schour I, Massler M: Studies in tooth development: The growth pattern of human teeth, Part I. J Am Dent Assoc 27:1778–1973, Nov 1940.

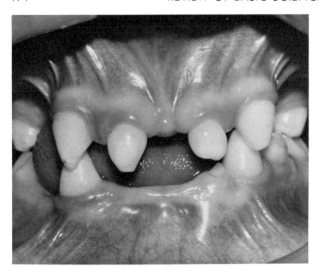

**FIG. 7-1.** Lack of primary teeth and conical shaped crowns of those anterior teeth in a patient with ectodermal dysplasia.

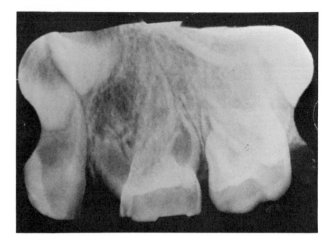

**FIG. 7-3.** Periapical radiograph of a primary posterior segment showing the ghostlike appearance associated with odontodysplasia. The teeth are hypoplastic and hypocalcified. Note also the poorly defined root structure. (Courtesy Dr. T. R. Oldenburg)

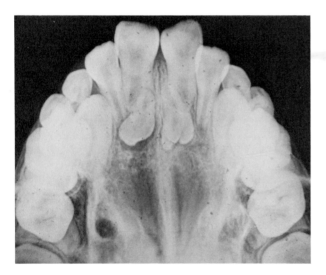

**FIG. 7-2.** Occlusal radiograph demonstrating two supernumerary teeth in the maxillary anterior region. (Courtesy of Dr. T. R. Oldenburg)

anomaly which occurs during histodifferentiation. Again there is obliteration of the pulp chamber and canals with associated short roots and periapical radiolucencies.

Rushton (8) described an entity called "shell teeth." These teeth have normal enamel, but the associated dentin is nearly nonexistent, contributing to large pulp chambers. The roots of these teeth are also very short.

Odontodysplasia (Fig. 7-3) is a bizarre developmental anomaly which shows histologic aberrations in all tissues of the affected teeth. The teeth are small and upon radiographic examination have a ghostlike appearance. The dentin and enamel are thin with associated large pulp chambers. There are short roots and often periapical radiolucencies. The teeth are hypoplastic, hypocalcified, and late erupting. Most likely the entire mineralization mechanism is defective due to the histologic changes.

FORM. Alterations in the form and size of teeth usually occur during morphodifferentiation. The most common example of an isolated decrease in size is the peg shaped lateral incisor. Multiple peg shaped teeth may be associated with ectodermal dysplasia. In microdontia all the teeth are decreased in size.

Increased cellular activity during the morphodifferentiation stage may lead to dens in dente. This entity may range from a small hard tissue invagination to a nearly complete tooth within a tooth. These teeth, which are very susceptible to decay, also exhibit pulpal anomalies. The term macrodontia denotes an entire dentition of large teeth.

AMOUNT OF CALCIFIED TISSUE. During the apposition stage of tooth growth the matrix for the hard tissue is laid down. Enamel hypoplasia may be either localized or generalized. Local enamel hypoplasia (Fig. 7-4A) appears only on isolated teeth and may be due to infection from the primary tooth or supporting structures during the time of permanent tooth formation or traumatic insult to the primary tooth or jaws during the formation period. Enamel hypoplasia of the generalized variety (Fig. 7-4B) may be due to illness, nutritional deficiencies, drug therapy or fluoride in the

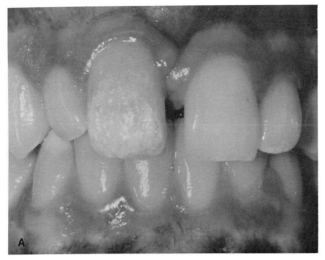
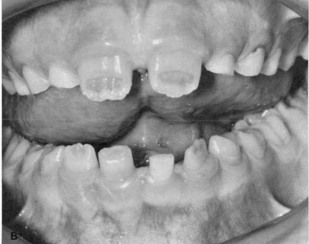

FIG. 7-4   A. Maxillary right central incisor exhibiting local enamel hypoplasia due to local pathology during tooth formation. Generalized enamel hypoplasia present on all teeth which were formed at the time of the systemic disruption. Note the unaffected retained primary incisor which has no permanent successor.

drinking water in excess of 1 PPM. These etiologic factors affect all teeth developing at one time. The length of time the etiologic factor is active determines the extent to which any tooth is affected.

Amelogenesis imperfecta, which may be either a dominant or sex-linked dominant trait, may be manifested as a hypoplastic defect. In this type of amelogenesis imperfecta the quantity of enamel is the variable while the quality of the enamel is within normal limits. The enamel may be pitted, wrinkled, or smooth. Radiographic examination reveals enamel of normal radiopacity but deficient in amount.

The appositional stage of tooth formation is also the point at which intrinsic stains, such as those encountered in porphyria or caused by tetracycline, are incorporated into the tooth matrix. The enamel of the first bicuspid, which is the most posterior tooth that presents an aesthetic problem, normally is completely formed by 6–7 years of age. After this time tetracycline staining should not be a problem. Fluoride concentration in the water in excess of 1 PPM may similarly stain primary and permanent teeth during their formation.

DEGREE OF HARDNESS.   The most common problem of hardness relates to hypocalcification. This may be manifested as hypocalcified enamel and/or dentin. The disturbance of the calcification process leads to soft, caries-susceptible enamel and dentin. Failure of dentin globules to coalesce may also lead to defective interglobular dentin.

Amelogenesis imperfecta has been observed as a hypocalcified autosomal dominant anomaly. This soft,

easily abraded enamel appears more radiolucent than normal on radiographs. It is not uncommon for amelogenesis imperfecta to result in aesthetic problems and loss of vertical dimension, factors which must be remembered when this entity is treated.

## Eruption

Although the evidence is not conclusive at this time, the mobility of the cells of the periodontal ligament appears to be responsible for tooth eruption (20). Normal eruption of teeth usually begins when one-half to two-thirds of the root is formed. The tooth generally erupts to the plane of occlusion when three-quarters of the root is developed, but approximately 3 years is necessary for completion of the apex.

Tooth eruption is often accompanied by a raised, fluctuant, translucent eruption hematoma. This blood filled tissue space, usually observed in the molar area, requires no treatment and resolves with tooth eruption.

EARLY AND DELAYED ERUPTION.   In several instances early eruption has been noted. The natal tooth is sometimes present in the mandibular anterior area of a newborn or appears during the neonatal period. This tooth may be a supernumerary tooth, or more likely, a mandibular primary incisor. It may present one of several problems: looseness with the risk of aspiration, sharpness which may lacerate the tongue, or irritation of the mother's breast during nursing. An occlusal radiograph (Fig. 7–5) will reveal if the tooth is supernumerary. If the tooth causes no problem and is not supernumerary, it should be maintained.

Generalized early eruption of teeth may be due to a familial pattern or an endocrine disturbance, most probably hyperthyroidism or hyperpituitarism. In both

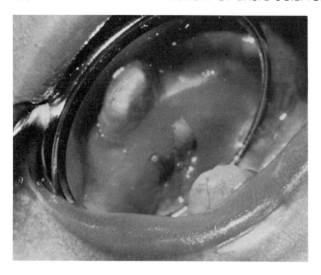

**FIG. 7-5.** Lower primary incisor (natal tooth) erupted at the time of birth. (Courtesy of Dr. F. T. McIver)

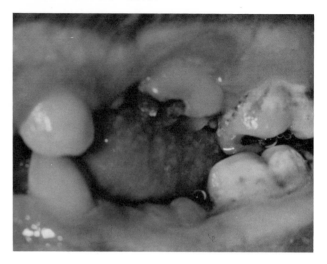

**FIG. 7-6.** Gross vertical occlusal discrepancy due to the ankylosed primary molars. Soft and hard tissue pathology was evident upon radiographic examination.

instances the sequence of eruption would be normal although accelerated. Loss of a primary molar after 7 or 8 years of age may accelerate the eruption of the succeeding premolar. Conversely, primary molar loss prior to 7 or 8 years may delay the eruption of the permanent bicuspid. Aside from premature extraction of primary teeth, several systemic entities may cause delayed eruption of teeth. Most common among these disturbances are hypothyroidism, hypopituitarism, Down's syndrome, and cleidocranial dysostosis. All of these disturbances, except cleidocranial dysostosis, generally result in a delayed pattern of eruption. In cleidocranial dysostosis the permanent teeth may never erupt, even after extraction of primary teeth.

**ANKYLOSIS.** In some instances one or two primary or permanent teeth in a quadrant fail to erupt; this is due to ankylosis (Fig. 7–6). The clinical manifestations of this entity are 1) location of the occlusal portion of the questionable tooth below the occlusal plane, 2) no detectable mobility of the tooth, and 3) a firm sound upon percussion. Occasionally a lack of periodontal ligament space can be discerned on a radiograph. Many times this is impossible, however, since the area in which cementum and alveolar bone are joined is very small. Although ankylosed primary teeth usually exfoliate in a normal fashion, it is possible to have delayed exfoliation and deflection of the erupting permanent tooth. The opposing tooth may supererupt to maintain contact with the ankylosed tooth, which can lead to occlusal irregularities. It is reasonable to maintain an ankylosed tooth unless teeth distal to the ankylosed tooth begin to tip mesially with resultant loss of arch length or unless the ankylosed tooth is submerged to the

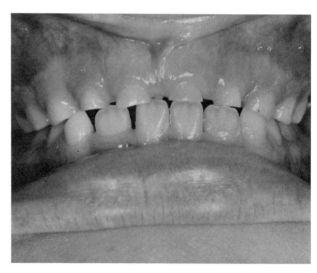

**FIG. 7-7.** Occlusal attrition of primary teeth. Although extensive, it is not remarkably severe. (Courtesy of Dr. F. T. McIver)

point that it causes a periodontal and alveolar bone defect. In some cases an oversized stainless steel crown may maintain occlusal contact and prevent distal teeth from tipping mesially. If it becomes necessary to remove an ankylosed tooth, routine extraction procedures usually prove successful. Rarely is bony dissection necessary. Following the extraction, space maintenance is usually indicated.

### Function

The primary dentition often displays marked occlusal attrition due to bruxism and general wear (Fig. 7–7).

Complete obliteration of primary posterior occlusal anatomy and cuspid form is not uncommon. Patients with dentinogenesis imperfecta and amelogenesis imperfecta exhibit an increase in occlusal abrasion. The hypocalcified form of amelogenesis imperfecta makes the teeth very susceptible to abrasion, and the resultant loss of vertical dimension presents an aesthetic and functional problem. Restoration of the affected teeth with occlusal coverage is desirable.

## Exfoliaton

Resorption and exfoliation of primary teeth are presently attributed to a combination of factors. The presence of an erupting permanent tooth, occlusal forces, and varied amounts of inflammation have all been identified as participants in this intermittent process. The systemic causes of increased and decreased rates of eruption can also affect the rate of exfoliation of primary teeth.

When premature exfoliation of the primary teeth is observed, several other conditions must be considered. Vertical bone loss caused by periodontosis may result in premature loss of primary teeth. Precocious periodontosis (Papillon–LeFèvre syndrome), a periodontal dermatologic entity which also results in severe horizontal bone loss, occurs in conjunction with hyperkeratosis of the palms and soles of the feet. The permanent as well as the primary dentition may be affected in either of these forms of periodontosis.

Other systemic entities such as cyclic neutropenia, fibrous dysplasia, or histiocytosis X diseases may also lead to premature exfoliation of primary teeth. Hypophosphatasia is an autosomal recessive trait associated with early loss of primary teeth. This condition has classically been diagnosed by low levels of serum alkaline phosphatase. Unfortunately this test sometimes leads to false-negative results. A more reliable diagnostic method is to assess the urine for increased levels of phosphoethanolamine.

Loss of alveloar bone and primary teeth sometimes accompanies mercury poisoning (acrodynia). Current measures to reduce mercury in the environment should reduce this problem.

### QUESTIONS

15. Which oral abnormality is commonly found in children with cleidocranial dysostosis?
    1. Alveolar clefts
    2. Premature loss of primary teeth
    3. Micrognathia
    4. High caries incidence
    5. Multiple supernumerary and unerupted teeth

16. A supernumerary tooth results from a deviation during
    1. initiation
    2. differentiation
    3. apposition
    4. calcification

17. Ectodermal dysplasia is characterized by
    1. marked salivary deficiency
    2. missing deciduous teeth but normal number of permanent teeth
    3. missing deciduous and permanent teeth
    4. moist skin

18. Following premature loss of the second primary molar, an unerupted first permanent molar will migrate and cause space loss in
    1. the mandible or the maxilla
    2. the maxilla only
    3. the mandible only
    4. neither the mandible nor the maxilla

19. Clinical features of dentinogenesis imperfecta are
    a. a high susceptibility to caries
    b. translucent or opalescent color
    c. normal development of enamel
    d. abnormal development of dentin
    e. obliterated pulp canals, small chambers
    1. a and d
    2. b, c, and d
    3. a and c
    4. b, c, d, and e
    5. All of the above

20. Amelogenesis imperfecta (hypocalcification type) is an hereditary abnormality. The radiographic appearance of these teeth is characterized by
    1. a sharp contrast in enamel and dentin density
    2. no sharp contrast in enamel and dentin density
    3. Neither of the above
    4. Amelogenesis imperfecta is only apparent as a hypoplastic defect.

21. Hypoplastic defects of the incisal one-third of the incisors and occlusal one-half of the first permanent molars can be traced to
    a. metabolic disturbances
    b. trauma
    c. severe illness
    d. infection of primary teeth
    1. a and b
    2. b and c
    3. a and c
    4. b and d
    5. c and d

22. A primary second molar is in infraocclusion and its occlusal surface is level with the gingival margin of the permanent first molar which is beginning to tip mesially. Radiographs indicate a developing permanent second premolar is present. The dentist should
    1. extract the primary molar and place a space maintainer
    2. extract the primary molar
    3. maintain the primary molar, since it will not drift
    4. maintain the primary molar since they occasionally reerupt

23. Extremely early loss of primary teeth results in
    1. no change in the time of eruption of the permanent teeth
    2. early eruption of the permanent teeth
    3. delayed eruption of the permanent teeth
    4. ankylosis of the permanent tooth

24. Disturbances in the morphodifferentiation stage of the development of the tooth germ results in
    1. an abnormal number of teeth
    2. ameloblastomas
    3. abnormal forms and sizes of teeth
    4. All of the above

25. A 5-year-old child with a massive cellulitis of dental origin did not respond to penicillin therapy, and a broad spectrum tetracycline antibiotic was prescribed. It is possible that side-effects of tetracycline administration will later be seen in which of the following permanent teeth?
    1. Canines and second molars
    2. Premolars
    3. Incisors and first molars
    4. Both 1 and 2
    5. Both 2 and 3

26. In premature exfoliation of primary teeth one should expect
    a. neutropenia
    b. hypophosphatasia
    c. hyperthyroidism
    d. histiocytosis X disease
    e. Papillon–LeFèvre syndrome
    f. leukemia
    1. a, b, c, and f
    2. a, b, d, e, and f
    3. a, c, and f
    4. a, b, c, d, and e
    5. All of the above

## MINOR OCCLUSAL IRREGULARITIES OF THE DENTITION

Many tooth position irregularities occur in the developing dentition. Some irregularities are self-correcting, some require short- or long-term treatment, and others are manifestations of larger problems. Selected problems are discussed in this section according to the Proffit–Ackerman (7) technique of problem recognition. This system organizes problem into profile, perimeter, anteroposterior, tranverse, and vertical categories which facilitates diagnosis.

### Perimeter Problems

**SPACE MAINTENANCE IN PREMATURE LOSS OF PRIMARY TEETH.** When primary teeth are lost due to caries, ectopic eruption, or trauma, the occlusion must be carefully assessed to determine if space maintenance therapy is necessary. Patients who superimpose profile and anteroposterior problems (Class II and III occlusions) on the space maintenance equation demand thorough evaluation of the developing dentofacial complex rather than reflexive space maintenance. It may or may not be advantageous to control space if these problems are present. Reasonable judgments regarding space maintenance, whether or not to use it and which technique (space closure, prosthetic dentistry, or retention of primary teeth) to use if space maintenance is appropriate, must be made on an individual basis. Data collected by investigators from cephalometric radiographs, casts, and intraoral measurements have revealed interesting, although limited, information concerning space management (22).

Generally it can be concluded that space maintenance is appropriate when Class I skeletal and dental relationships are present, when adequate space as determined by a space analysis is available, and when the facial profile is well balanced with appropriate lip posture. Even in the presence of these qualifications, poor patient cooperation and poor oral hygiene may ultimately contraindicate space maintenance.

### Space Closure
*Posterior Space.* The longer a primary tooth has been missing, the greater the incidence and amount of space closure. Closure is more rapid during the first 6 months following tooth loss in either arch, and closure occurs more rapidly in the maxillary arch than in the mandibular arch. Posterior space closure has been noted before and after eruption of first permanent molars. Although space closure is multidirectional, it occurs predominantly from the posterior in the maxillary arch and predominantly from the anterior in the mandibular arch.

*Anterior Space.* The small amount of evidence available indicates little space loss occurs in the anterior region. Commonly there is an adjustment of space in the anterior segment following primary tooth loss, and in the case of mandibular cuspid loss lingual movement of the anterior teeth has been noted. The site in the arch of the missing tooth or teeth is therefore important.

The need for space maintenance in the anterior segment has not been clearly resolved. Space maintenance in the maxillary anterior segment and the mandibular incisor area is not generally necessary. The mandibular canine area usually merits space maintenance.

The time of eruption is another factor to weigh in the space maintenance decision. A primary molar lost prior to 7 or 8 years of age may delay the eruption of the permanent bicuspids. Primary molar loss at a later time may accelerate eruption of the premolar teeth. Only by attention to the individual case can one make reasonable judgments.

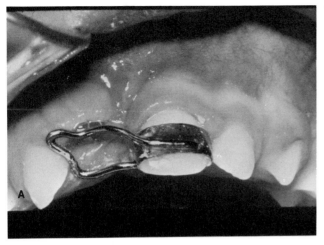

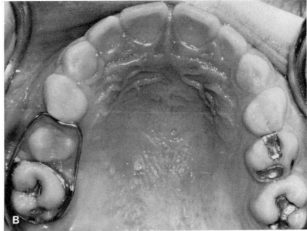

FIG. 7–8.   A. Band and loop space maintainer used in the maxillary anterior segment. (Courtesy of Dr. D. C. Dilley) B. Well-designed band and loop space maintainer used in the maxillary posterior segment. Note that the buccolingual dimension of the loop allowed eruption of the permanent tooth. (Courtesy of Dr. G. J. Dilley)

### Appliances for Space Maintenance

*Band and Loop.*    The band and loop may be used for anterior (Fig. 7–8A) or posterior (Fig. 7–8B) space maintenance. Although the appliance is fixed and therefore requires no patient manipulation, patient cooperation is necessary to maintain oral hygiene. This

FIG. 7–9.   A. Soldered maxillary lingual arch incorporating a palatal acrylic button to maintain molar symmetry and space. The palatal acrylic button may pose hygiene problems. B. Removable mandibular lingual arch. Note that the arch rests on the cingula of the incisors and is designed to allow eruption of the premolars without interference.

appliance should be designed with growth and development of the dental arches and eruption of succedaneous teeth in mind. Careful study of the eruption sequence is necessary, and a replacement or modified appliance may be needed at a later date. This appliance is both nonfunctional and nonaesthetic.

*Lingual Arch Type.*    The lingual arch appliance may be used in either the maxillary (Fig. 7–9A) or mandibular (Fig. 7–9B) arch and offers anterior, posterior, unilateral, or bilateral solutions to space maintenance. Since this is a fixed appliance, little manipulation by the patient is necessary, but again oral hygiene is a necessity. Long-term use of the lingual arch may lead to decalcification of the abutment teeth. Therefore, it may be advisable to consider banding primary molars instead of permanent molars. This appliance is both nonfunctional and nonaesthetic.

*Acrylic Partial Denture.*    Acrylic partial dentures

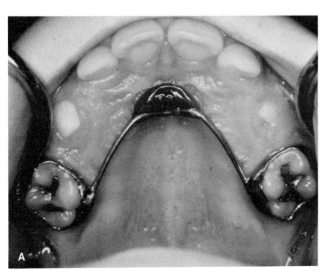

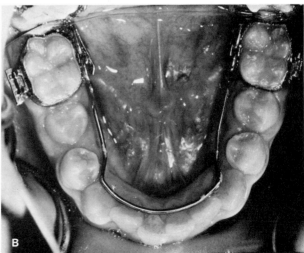

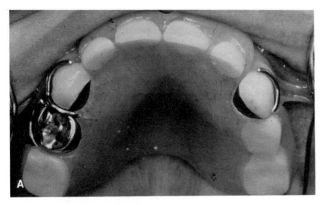
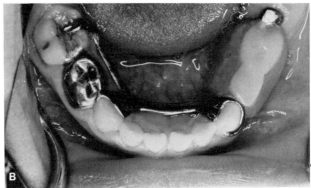

**FIG. 7-10.** A. Acrylic partial denture replacing teeth bilaterally anteriorly and posteriorly. Continued eruption of permanent teeth makes modification of this appliance necessary. (Courtesy of Dr. E. F. Howden) B. Partial denture with a cast framework which provides unilateral posterior space maintenance and incorporates a distal shoe intraalveolar extension to guide the erupting first permanent molar. Alteration of the intercanine width due to permanent incisor eruption demands attention to the clasps on the primary canines. (Courtesy of Dr. E. F. Howden)

are extremely versatile. They may be used for space maintenance in either the maxilla or the mandible, either anteriorly or posteriorly, either unilaterally or bilaterally (Fig. 7-10). These appliances may be constructed so that they are both functional and aesthetic. Since they are removable, they do demand patient cooperation, but their removable nature also facilitates tooth and appliance cleaning.

*Distal Shoe.* The distal shoe is usually the appliance of choice when primary second molars are lost due to caries or ectopic eruption prior the the eruption of the first permanent molar. The orientation of the alveolar portion of the appliance may be used to maintain or regain space. The distal shoe may be constructed as a fixed (Figs. 7-11A and 7-11B) or removable (Figs. 7-11C and 7-11D) appliance; it may be functional or nonfunctional depending upon both the appliance design and material of construction. This appliance is probably contraindicated in cases where a bacteremia could debilitate the patient since complete epithelialigation of the tissue surrounding the intraalveolar portion has not been demonstrated.

**SPACE REGAINING.** Therapy to regain lost space is indicated when the magnitude of space loss is 1–3 mm. It may be a necessary first step toward space maintenance. After space regaining there should be a Class I skeletal dental relationship, adequate space, and a good facial profile. The appliances which are the most reliable and controllable for limited space regaining are maxillary (Fig. 7-12) and mandibular Hawley appliances with helical springs, if adequate retention is incorporated in the design of the appliance.

**ECTOPIC ERUPTION.** Eruption is ectopic when a permanent tooth causes resorption of a primary tooth other than the one it is to replace, or in the case of the erupting permanent molars, resorption of the adjacent primary teeth. Ectopic eruption of the first permanent molars presents a most interesting problem. This painless and often undiagnosed condition occurs more often in the maxilla than in the mandible. The lack of timely intervention may cause space loss and simultaneous tooth loss. Because of the frequent self-correction of this condition, a period of watchful waiting is probably indicated when small amounts of resorption have occurred (Fig. 7-13).

Several methods of intervention are available if they are needed. When a first permanent molar is erupting ectopically, brass ligature (0.025 in.) wire may be looped around the contact between the first permanent molar and the second primary molar. By tightening the ligature, pressure can be transmitted to the ectopically erupting molar, which causes it to move distally and allows it to erupt freely. This technique is also useful when treating impacted second permanent molars (Fig. 7-14). When the occlusal surface of the erupting first permanent molar is accessible, an appliance may be fabricated to apply a distal force to the tooth (Fig. 7-15). In cases exhibiting gross resorption of the primary second molar, removal of the tooth may be the treatment of choice. This procedure should be followed by placement of a distal shoe and guidance of the erupting first permanent molar to a more distal position.

Ectopic eruption also occurs in the anterior segments of the mouth. Most notably, the maxillary or mandibular permanent lateral incisors may cause resorption and loss of the primary cuspids. This may be due to transient anterior crowding caused by the

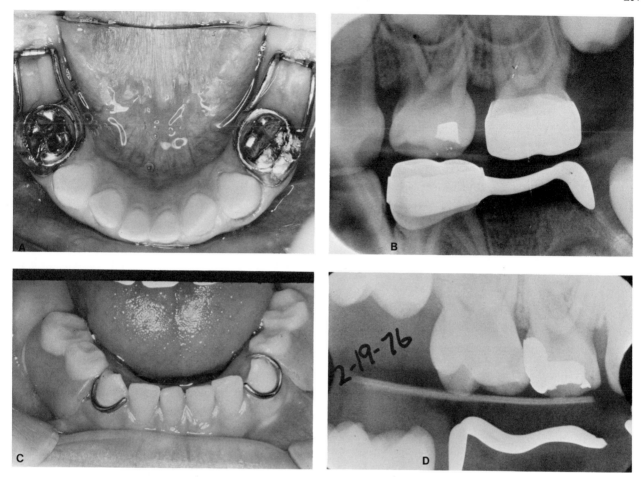

**FIG. 7-11.** A. Bilateral fixed distal shoe space maintainer with the bands cemented to the stainless steel crowns. Removal of the distal shoes is simple and leaves an intact crown. B. Radiograph demonstrating the relationship of the intraalveolar extension of the distal shoe and erupting first permanent molars shown in A. Note the supereruption of the maxillary molar due to the non-functional nature of the appliance. C. Bilateral removable distal shoe space maintainer. The distal shoe stainless steel intraalveolar extensions are incorporated in the acrylic saddle areas. Alternatively, these extensions could be made of acrylic. (Courtesy of Dr. T. R. Oldenburg) D. Radiograph demonstrating the intraalveolar extensions of the bilateral removable distal shoe space maintainer shown in C. (Courtesy of Dr. T. R. Oldenburg)

eruption of the larger permanent incisors, or it may be symptomatic of a significant perimeter problem that will need to be resolved by later permanent tooth extraction.

**ANTERIOR SPACING.**   Spacing is often observed in the maxillary anterior segment during eruption of the permanent incisors and canines. Many times this condition is eliminated when the canines have completely erupted and no longer place a mesial force on the lateral incisor roots. Therefore treatment of this spacing should be delayed until eruption of the canines is completed. If this problem persists, however, and if hard or soft tissue anomalies and the occlusion can be eliminated as the etiologic agent, the spaces may be closed with a removable appliance. Although space closure in these cases may be relatively easy, maintaining the correction is often a problem. Many times a fixed retaining appliance must be used.

### Anteroposterior Problems

The anterior crossbite is probably the most often encountered minor anteroposterior problem in developing dentition. If the etiology of the anterior crossbite is dental and if space is available, this condition should be corrected. Common dental etiology include arch length deficiencies, aberrant eruption direction, unresorbed or traumatized primary teeth or supernumerary teeth. If the anterior crossbite is due to a skeletal

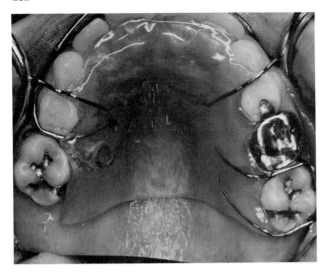

**FIG. 7-12.** Maxillary Hawley appliance with a helical spring to move the permanent first molar distally. Note that good retention is provided by the labial bow and the molar clasp. (Courtesy of Dr. E. F. Howden)

problem, however, its correction may not be advisable due to the amount of dental compensation required. A skeletal problem should be evaluated carefully by someone prepared to deal with continued abnormal skeletal growth. Uncorrected anterior crossbites often lead to continued functional shifts, tooth abrasion or gingival stripping on the opposing incisor.

A pseudo-Class III malocclusion exists when centric

**FIG. 7-13.** (Figs. 7-13, 7-14, and 7-15 are one series and so are labelled in one alphabetical sequence.) A. Radiograph of an ectopically erupting maxillary first permanent molar. Note that the resorption is limited at this time. B. Radiograph of the same ectopically erupting maxillary first permanent molar nearly 17 months later, following self-correction. Note that the resorption is greater than that observed in A. (Courtesy of G. J. Dilley)

relation is not coincident with centric occlusion. Patients with this type of malocclusion occlude with the anterior teeth in an edge-to-edge relationship in centric relation (Fig. 7–16). An anterior slide of several millimeters is necessary for them to reach a comfortable centric occlusion position. Correction of the axial inclination of the anterior teeth often resolves this situation.

The axial inclination of an anterior tooth may be corrected by use of a tongue blade. This is best used when minimal tooth movement is required and when the tooth in crossbite is already mobile. Adequate overbite to retain the correction is necessary. By applying moderate, continuous force with the tongue blade to the offending tooth, the correction should be effected within 30–45 min, preferably in the office, because this allows the dentist to monitor the tooth movement and reinforce the child's behavior. The discomfort can be withstood easily by some children, not by others.

There are numerous appliances which can be designed to effect the desired tooth movement. For example, a Hawley appliance with finger springs may be used to correct anterior axial inclinations. The major considerations are simplicity, adequate retention, and desired force and range of the finger springs. An effective design incorporates a helical spring for tooth movement, combined with Adams clasps for retention (Fig. 7–17). If the overbite exceeds 1.5 mm, a posterior biteplate may be necessary to open the bite and allow the tooth in crossbite to be moved labially without interference from the occlusion.

### Transverse Problems

The transverse problem most commonly encountered in developing dentition is the posterior crossbite.

(*Text continues on p. 205.*)

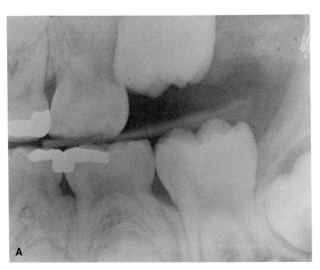

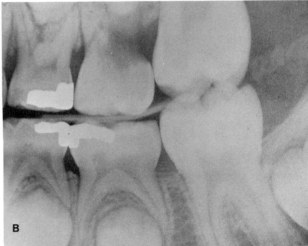

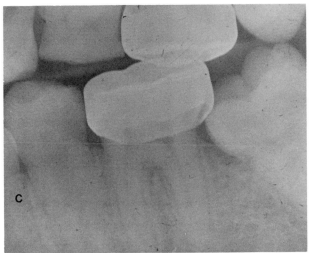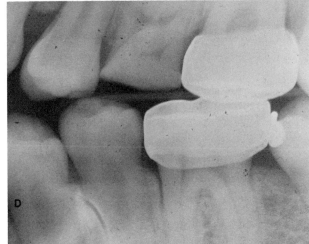

**FIG. 7-14.** (Fig. 7-14 is the continuation of a series begun in Fig. 7-13.) C. Impaction of the erupting second permanent molar which may be due to the eruption pattern or an open stainless steel crown margin. D. Placement of a brass wire ligature has allowed the second permanent molar to continue to erupt.

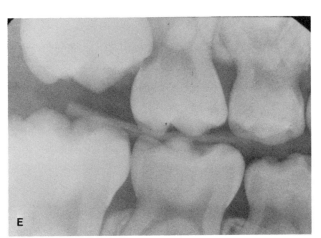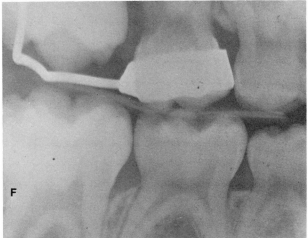

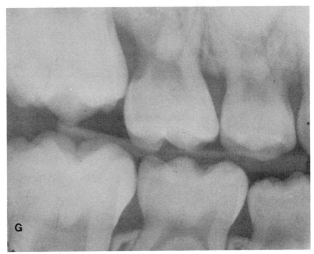

**FIG. 7-15.** (Fig. 7-15 concludes the series of figures begun in Figs. 7-13 and 7-14.) E. Ectopic eruption of a maxillary first permanent molar. F. The ectopically erupting tooth has been moved distally with a spring attached to a band on the second primary molar. G. Continued eruption of the permanent molar.

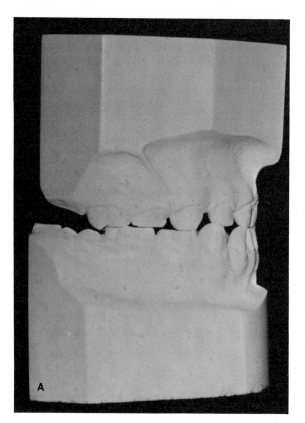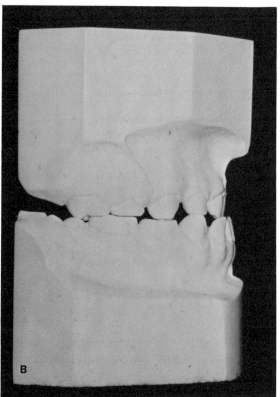

**FIG. 7–16.** A. Pseudo-Class III relationship. In centric relation the anterior teeth are edge to edge. B. Negative overjet in centric occlusion due to the anterior shift of the mandible to a comfortable position.

**FIG. 7–17.** A. Anterior crossbite of the maxillary right central incisor. Note the root prominence of the mandibular right central incisor due to labial movement from the force of occlusion. B. The maxillary right central incisor has been moved labially with a finger spring. The appliance incorporated retention from the multiple Adams clasp on the right and left in lieu of a labial bow.

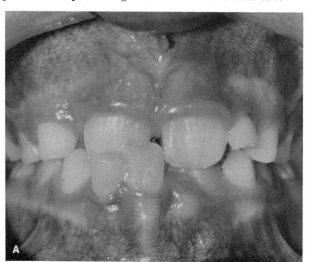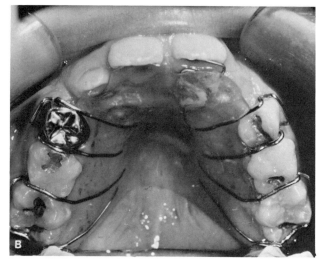

This problem may have a skeletal and/or dental component. When the arches are grossly constricted because of the skeletal structures, rapid palatal expansion with separation of the midpalatal suture is indicated. When the dental structures are at fault, the constriction may be unilateral or bilateral. In a true unilateral crossbite the constriction affects only one side of the occlusion. A bilateral crossbite affects both sides of the occlusion, although the degree of constriction on each side may not be equal.

Due to a shift of the mandible from centric relation to centric occlusion, that which appears to be a unilateral crossbite may in reality be caused by bilateral constriction. To distinguish the difference a careful clinical examination is necessary. By guiding a patient's mandible to the centric relation position and closing the teeth to initial contact, the dentist can observe the buccolingual relationships of the posterior teeth and the canines, as well as the maxillary and mandibular midline relationships. When the patient closes to the centric occlusion position, the relationships of the posterior teeth, the canines, and the midlines are again observed. If there is a bilateral crossbite in centric relation and centric occlusion, the patient has a bilateral constriction (Fig. 7–18). If there is a bilateral crossbite in centric relation accompanied by a lateral shift of the mandible, a change in midline relationships, and a unilateral crossbite in centric occlusion, the patient also has a bilateral constriction (Fig. 7–19). Facial asymmetry and excessive muscle tension on one side of the face may also be clues to a mandibular lateral shift. If the patient has a unilateral crossbite in centric relation and centric occlusion, the patient has a true unilateral constriction (Fig. 7–20).

Correctly trimmed study casts are a necessity for the final diagnosis of a crossbite. Since the transverse problem may be caused by true skeletal asymmetry, occasionally a posteroanterior headplate can also provide useful information in this diagnosis.

Dental crossbites usually involve teeth with axial inclinations that are not consistent with the rest of the dentition. Crossbites in the primary and mixed dentitions are best treated when they are discovered. This will reduce dental alveoli, possibly result in better permanent tooth positions, and eliminate potentially harmful functional patterns. However, when succedaneous teeth or first permanent molars will erupt within 1 year and may also be in crossbite, it is usually best to delay treatment. In a few cases abnormal primary cuspid morphology which causes the patient to occlude in crossbite to eliminate interference may be the etiology of the crossbite. In select cases simple equilibration of the cuspids rectifies this situation.

There are several reliable appliances to correct posterior dental crossbites. The cemented W arch, which is fixed, offers reliable correction of the crossbite with little patient cooperation. When used with lingual arms of equivalent length (Fig. 7–21A), this appliance is very useful in correcting bilateral constrictions. Alternatively the lingual arms may be of unequal length (Fig. 7–21B), thereby making it possible to control the anchorage of the posterior segment and allowing differential or in some cases unilateral movement of the teeth. Three months of retention is usually adequate to maintain the correction.

A split plate acrylic appliance may also be utilized in the correction of posterior crossbites (Fig. 7–22). This removable appliance demands patient cooperation,

**FIG. 7–18.** (Figs. 7–18, 7–19, and 7–20 form a series of illustrations and so are labelled in one alphabetical sequence.) A. Bilateral posterior crossbite in the centric relation posterior with midlines coincident. B. The same relationship occurs that occurred in centric relation. Therefore the crossbite is due to a bilateral maxillary constriction.

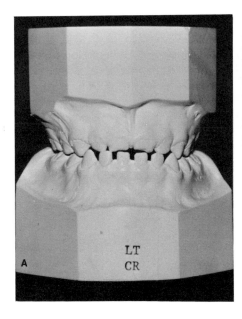
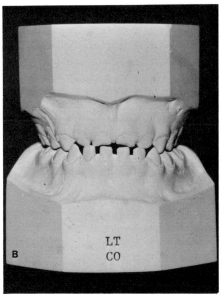

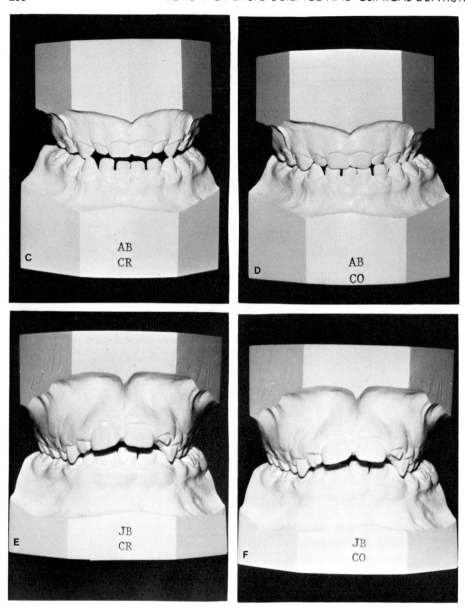

**FIG. 7-19.** (Fig. 7-19 is the continuation of a series of illustrations begun in Fig. 7-18.) C. Bilateral posterior crossbite in the centric relation posterior with the midline coincidents. D. In the centric occlusion position there is a unilateral posterior crossbite, since the mandible has shifted to the left. This is evident from the shift of the mandibular midline to the left. This patient has a bilateral maxillary constriction accompanied by a functional mandibular shift.

**FIG. 7-20.** (Fig. 7-20 concludes the set of illustrations begun in Figs. 7-18 and 7-19.) E. Unilateral posterior crossbite in the centric relation position. F. In the centric occlusion position there is no change in midline relationships and a unilateral posterior crossbite. Therefore this patient has a true unilateral posterior crossbite.

careful adjustment, and excellent retention for continued tooth movement. Dissatisfaction with this appliance most often arises from lack of patient cooperation or overactivation which frequently dislodges the appliance. A 3-month retention period is also recommended with this appliance.

Cross elastics may be used to correct posterior crossbites when alteration of both maxillary and mandibular tooth axial relations is indicated (Fig. 7-23). Since heavy cross elastics must be worn full-time by the patient to effect the necessary change, this method demands patient cooperation. It may cause extrusion of the teeth due to the horizontal and vertical direction of force and should be used for rapid, limited treatment.

Retention provided by the occlusion should be adequate to maintain the correction.

If ectopic eruption of the permanent lateral incisor occurs unilaterally, the mandibular midline may shift to the side where the primary cuspid was prematurely lost. In order to prevent this transverse problem it is advisable to remove the remaining primary cuspid, and it may be necessary to use a lower lingual holding arch. If the mandibular midline has shifted, it may be corrected by the use of a lower lingual holding arch with an auxiliary finger spring or a mandibular Hawley appliance and a finger spring. Overcorrection and retention of the midline provide greater stability. Generally, transverse problems need to be corrected early in the

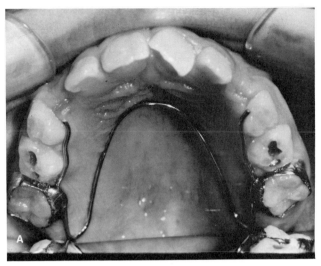

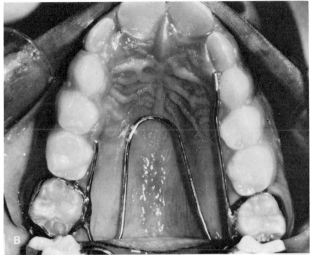

**FIG. 7-21.** (Figs. 7-21, 7-22, and 7-23 are one series and so are labelled consecutively with one alphabetical list.) A. Soldered maxillary W arch with equal length lingual extension arms used to correct a bilateral posterior dental constriction. B. Soldered maxillary W arch with unequal length lingual extension arms used to correct a unilateral posterior constriction affecting only the second primary molar and the first permanent molar.

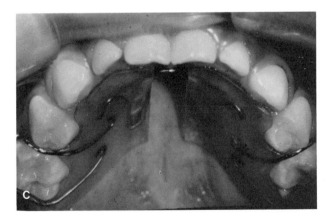

**FIG. 7-22.** (Fig. 7-22 continues the series begun in Fig. 7-21.) C. Removable maxillary split plate appliance used to correct a bilateral posterior constriction.

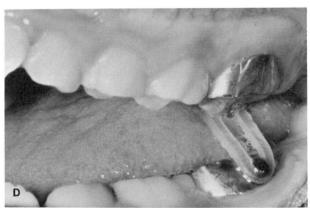

**FIG. 7-23.** (Fig. 7-23 concludes the series begun in Figs. 7-21 and 7-22). D. Cross elastics in place to correct a posterior crossbite of the permanent first molars.

developing dentition since they may cause abnormal growth and development or confuse the diagnosis of other conditions.

QUESTIONS

27. A corrected anterior crossbite is best retained by
   1. the overbite achieved during treatment
   2. overtreatment and anticipated relapse
   3. using a maxillary Hawley retainer for stabilization
   4. using a mandibular acrylic guide plane

28. Crossbite of one maxillary permanent incisor may be the result of
   a. an unerupted labial maxillary supernumerary
   b. a maxillary arch length deficiency
   c. trauma to the primary incisor and surrounding structures
   1. a
   2. a and b
   3. a and c
   4. b
   5. b and c
   6. c
   7. a, b, and c

29. A possible result of not correcting a simple anterior crossbite is
   a. loss of maxillary arch length
   b. gingival stripping of mandibular incisors

*(Continued)*

   c. excessive incisal abrasion of upper and lower incisors

   d. facets on the labial surface of the malposed incisor

1. a and b
2. b and c
3. c and d
4. All of the above

30. The treatment of choice for ectopic eruption of the first permanent molar with minor resorption of the second primary molar is

1. arch expansion
2. extraction of the second primary molar and placement of a distal shoe appliance
3. disking of the distal surface of the second deciduous molar
4. placement of a brass ligature wire to move the first molar distally

31. Posterior crossbites in the primary dentition

   a. should not be corrected unless there is a functional shift associated with the crossbite

   b. may be corrected in some cases by occlusion equilibrium and training in a new mandibular closure path

1. a is true; b is false.
2. a is false; b is true.
3. Both a and b are true.
4. Both a and b are false.

32. A common finding in a child with a unilateral buccal segment posterior crossbite in centric occlusion is

1. a tooth-sized arch discrepancy
2. the mesial migration of the permanent molars
3. a bilateral constriction of the maxillary arch in centric relation
4. a widening of the mandibular arch

33. When a mandibular second primary molar is lost a year or more before its normal exfoliation time, a space maintainer should be constructed to prevent the

   a. mesial drifting of the permanent first molar

   b. distal drifting of the first primary molar

1. a and b
2. None of the above

34. An 8-year-old girl has a diastema between her maxillary central incisors. The maxillary lateral incisors are erupted and in the proper position. The diastema can be caused by

   a. an abnormal frenum attachment

   b. a mesiodens

   c. the normal developmental process

1. a and c
2. a and b
3. All of the above

35. In designing a space maintainer to replace the first primary molar which of the following criteria should be considered?

   a. Facial profile

   b. Available space

   c. Eruption timing

   d. Eruption sequence

   e. Molar and canine relationships

1. b, c, and d
2. b, c, d, and e
3. a, b, c, and d
4. All of the above

36. When deciduous teeth have been lost prematurely, it is most important to hold space for

1. an upper incisor
2. a lower bicuspid
3. a lower incisor
4. All of the above

## PULP THERAPY

The objective of pulp therapy is conservation of the tooth so that it can remain an integral component of the dentition. Preserving the tooth helps to maintain arch integrity, provides for better mastication and speech, and prevents aberrant tongue habits. It also avoids the psychologic effects sometimes associated with tooth loss.

Factors other than the condition of the pulp which must be considered before pulp therapy is performed on a tooth include

1. Length of time the tooth will be in the mouth
2. General health of the patient
3. Extent of coronal breakdown
4. Use intended for the tooth
5. Cooperation of the patient
6. Cost of treatment

The biggest problem for the clinician is predicting the amount or the extent of pulpal damage, but a history, clinical examination, radiographic examination, vitality tests, thermal tests, and percussion tests can all facilitate this determination. The five definitive types of pulp therapy most often used in dentistry for children are 1) indirect pulp cap, 2) direct pulp cap, 3) pulpotomy, 4) partial pulpectomy, and 5) extraction (Fig. 7–24).

### Indirect Pulp Cap

INDICATIONS. This procedure is indicated in either the primary or permanent dentition for deep carious lesions where the pulp has not been seriously or directly involved. Clinical experience has shown that the primary dentition responds less favorably to this procedure, however, because the healing capacity of primary teeth is restricted by the limited vascular supply in the primary dentition. It is also difficult to es-

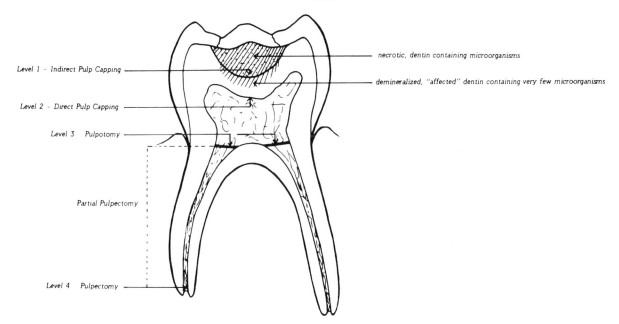

Level 1 – Indirect Pulp Capping

Level 2 – Direct Pulp Capping

Level 3   Pulpotomy

Partial Pulpectomy

Level 4   Pulpectomy

necrotic, dentin containing microorganisms

demineralized, "affected" dentin containing very few microorganisms

**FIG. 7-24.** Levels of pulp therapy in dentistry for children. (University of North Carolina Pedodontic Syllabus. Chapel Hill, University of North Carolina, 1978)

tablish the status of the pulp in primary teeth. Another factor is the fact that the layers of enamel and dentin in primary teeth are thinner so the carious process has less distance to travel before it involves pulpal tissue.

There are several definite contraindications for indirect pulp capping: a history of spontaneous pain (pain occurring without the application of a stimulus), a sharp tenderness to percussion, presence of swelling of the surrounding alveolar gingiva mucosa, presence of a fistula or purulent exudate in the gingival crevice, mobility of the tooth, radiographic evidence of periapical or furcal pathology, radiographic evidence of internal resorption, resorption of more than two-thirds of the root, radiographic evidence of calcified masses in the pulp chamber and/or root canal orifices in either primary or permanent teeth, extensive carious involvement of the root, and any hemorrhaging which indicates exposure of the pulp.

**PROCEDURE.** The procedure for indirect pulp therapy involves removing all soft, necrotic dentin with a large bur in the slow handpiece. A spoon excavator may be used, but there is a tendency with this instrument to gouge out large hunks of leathery dentin and expose the pulp inadvertently. The dentist should remove dentin from the periphery of the lesion first and then gradually move toward the center of the lesion. The peripheral dentin must be sound around the entire circumference of the lesion or an indirect pulp cap is not indicated.

Once a periphery of sound dentin is obtained, the surface layer of necrotic dentin remaining over the pulp chamber is removed, leaving only the soft "affected" dentin over the pulp. This is the dentin that, if removed, would result in an obvious pulp exposure. When the limits of caries removal have been reached, a medicament of calcium hydroxide or zinc oxide–eugenol is placed over the entire exposed dentinal area. It is important to establish an hermetic seal in order to promote a healing response. Over the medication a temporary restoration of zinc oxide–eugenol or amalgam alloy is placed. After a 6–8 week healing period so that sufficient reparative dentin can be formed, the temporary filling and treatment medication can be removed for examination of the remaining dentin. If the treatment was successful, the remaining dentin should be sclerotic in appearance and feel hard to touch. At this time a base can be placed over the sclerotic dentin and the tooth restored with a final restoration.

## Direct Pulp Capping

This procedure is used almost exclusively for permanent teeth with small, vital carious exposures. The procedure is contraindicated in the same situations that contraindicate use of an indirect pulp cap or when the pulp exposure is greater than 1 mm in diameter.

The treatment involves placing calcium hydroxide medicament over the exposure site in order to stimulate secondary dentin and then restoring the tooth with a final restoration. It is not necessary to reopen the tooth at recall visits, but a radiographic examination for vitality is recommended. These teeth can become nonvital and a source of infection.

## Pulpotomy

A pulpotomy is defined as complete removal of the coronal portion of the dental pulp. There are two types of pulpotomy; they are classified according to the medicament used—the formocresol and the calcium hydroxide pulpotomy. Only the formocresol pulpotomy is used on primary teeth since clinical studies consistently show it has a higher success rate in the primary dentition than the calcium hydroxide procedure. Calcium hydroxide pulpotomies are used primarily on young permanent teeth with open apices.

INDICATIONS. This procedure is indicated when there is irreversible inflammation in the coronal portion of the pulp, but not in the pulpal canals usually as a result of carious exposures, large traumatic injuries, or prolonged mechanical exposures. If there are indications of extensive inflammation in the pulp chamber, if there is a history of spontaneous or elicited pain, if the radiograph indicates probable carious involvement beyond that which could be treated by indirect pulp capping, or if there is radiographic evidence of dystrophic calcification in the pulp horn area, then a pulpotomy is indicated. A common indication for a formocresol pulpotomy is a large carious exposure of a primary molar tooth. One common indication for a calcium hydroxide pulpotomy is the management of a fractured young permanent central incisor with a large exposure of the pulp. Another indication is the treatment of a young first permanent molar with a large carious exposure and profuse hemorrhage at the exposure site. This treatment allows for continued apical development so that later endodontic procedures can be performed if necessary.

The pulpotomy procedure is contraindicated when there is evidence that the tooth is nonvital. Swelling of the surrounding alveolar gingiva mucosa, presence of a fistula or purulent exudate in the gingival crevice, lack of hemorrhage from the pulp canals upon opening into the pulp chamber, or radiographic evidence of periapical or furcal pathology are all contraindications.

PROCEDURE. The first step in the pulpotomy procedure is opening the tooth with a fissure bur and establishing outline form. In order to gain access to the pulp, the outline should be wider than that for the Class II cavity preparation so that the roof of the entire pulp chamber can be exposed. All soft necrotic dentin must be removed before the pulp chamber is entered to avoid unnecessary contamination of the pulp. Then the roof of the pulp chamber is opened with a fissure bur and air and water spray, and the preparation is extended to include all pulp horn extensions. A slowly revolving No. 4 or No. 6 round bur in the slow handpiece is used to remove the pulp chamber contents. Frequent flushing of the pulp chamber with water aids visibility and prevents debris from being embedded in the pulp canals. The operator must be careful not to perforate the chamber floor. After pulp chamber contents have been removed, moist sterile cotton pellets are placed over the root canal orifices to control hemorrhage. If there is difficulty controlling bleeding, the operator should check to be sure all pulp remnants have been removed from the pulp areas. If necessary, a #2 round bur can be used to remove more pulp tissue at the root canal orifices. Steps to this point are the same for both the calcium hydroxide and formocresol pulpotomies.

For the calcium hydroxide pulpotomy, once bleeding is controlled a creamy mix of calcium hydroxide is allowed to flow over the floor of the pulp chamber so that it completely covers the root canal orifices. For the formocresol pulpotomy a small pellet of cotton slightly dampened with formocresol is placed over each root canal orifice. (A common mistake is to use cotton pellets saturated with formocresol. This is not only unnecessary but also runs the risk that this very caustic fluid may seep out of the cavity preparation onto the gingival tissues.) A large dry cotton pellet should be lightly pressed over the small pellets to soak up any excess formocresol, and the medicament is allowed to sit for 5 min. After the 5-min treatment, the pulp chamber and root canal orifices should appear dark brown. There should be no bleeding. If bleeding is noted, the areas should be retreated for 3 min with formocresol. After the formocresol treatment, a creamy mixture of zinc oxide mixed with one drop of formocresol and one drop of eugenol is allowed to flow over the floor of the pulp chamber. A thickness of 1 mm is sufficient to seal the orifices.

From this point steps for completing the pulpotomy are the same for calcium hydroxide and formocresol pulpotomies. The pulp chamber is filled with a thick zinc oxide–eugenol mixture and the tooth permanently restored. Restorations for pulpotomized teeth should be either stainless steel crowns for posterior teeth or composite resins for anterior teeth.

Follow-up procedures are essential for pulpotomized teeth. Young permanent teeth treated with calcium hydroxide should be followed periodically by periapical and bite-wing radiographs to check for dentin bridging and to watch for possible calcific metamorphosis. Bridging may become evident after a few months. The prognosis is very good for pulpotomized primary teeth which showed evidence of healthy pulp tissue in the root canals. Experience suggests that 80%–90% of such teeth respond favorably to treatment. Pulpotomized primary teeth should periodically be checked with periapical radiographs, however, because failure of the treatment rarely elicits painful symptoms. Failures are most often detected by radiographs which show periapical or furcal radiolucencies in root resorption.

There are no health hazards for the healthy child who receives formocresol pulpotomy. However, caution should be observed with children who have a chronic illness such as rheumatic fever or nephritis. Some clinicians feel such children should not be subjected to even the remote possibility of a bacteremia from an acute infection resulting from failure of pulp therapy. If this is a concern, the tooth in question should be extracted.

## Partial Pulpectomy

The treatment for a nonvital primary tooth is either partial pulpectomy or extraction. Partial pulpectomy is a very difficult procedure in primary teeth because the canals in primary teeth are thin and tortuous. If the canals cannot be properly cleansed of necrotic material, sterilized, and adequately filled, root canal therapy of this type will not be successful. This procedure is indicated when a primary tooth is essential, for example, when a second primary molar becomes nonvital before eruption of the first permanent molar or when retaining the natural tooth is preferable to placing a space maintainer. This procedure is also indicated when hemorrhage is a problem with a formocresol pulpotomy because of extensive inflammation in the root canal pulp tissue. It is definitely contraindicated when there is advanced periapical bone destruction and pathologic root resorption, when more than two-thirds of the root has been resorbed and the tooth is near exfoliation, when a tooth is unrestorable, when the canals are inaccessible, or when there is a history of chronic illness such as rheumatic fever or nephritis.

Determining the appropriate treatment for primary teeth requires careful consideration of the periapical and bifurcation area of the tooth. If radiolucencies are present which indicate encroachment of the infection onto the developing permanent tooth, extraction is the usual course of treatment. Evidence is accumulating that even after crown development in the succedaneous tooth an infection in the area can cause white spot lesions in the permanent enamel.

The treatment procedure requires a good pretreatment periapical radiograph, and the initial opening into the tooth should be large enough to allow good access to the pulp canals. The periapical radiograph is used to establish a working length, and very fine files are used for gentle débridement of all canals. The files must not be forced because the canals are easily perforated. The operator continues to file until meeting resistance. The canals must be irrigated frequently to flush out necrotic material. Then they are swabbed with a paper point dampened with formocresol. After a small cotton pellet slightly dampened with formocresol or Cresanol is placed over the root canal orifice, a temporary filling is used for 4–7 days.

If the tooth has remained asymptomatic by the second appointment, it is opened and the pulp chamber cleansed. Biomechanical cleansing of the canals is performed by enlarging them with very fine files. Again, the operator must not force the files because of the risk of perforation. In general primary molar canals should be enlarged to at least the size of the No. 30 reamer. The canals are dried with paper points and then filled with a resorbable cement such as zinc oxide–eugenol mixed to a creamy consistency. The pulp chamber is filled with a thickened zinc oxide–eugenol mix, and the tooth is restored with a stainless steel crown in the posterior segment or a composite resin buildup in the anterior segments.

Primary teeth treated with partial pulpectomy should be followed by means of periapical x-rays at periodic recalls. The success rate for this procedure is good if the diagnosis was carefully obtained. Making an accurate diagnosis of the extent of inflammation or determining whether pathologic resorption is present is most difficult, however, and these factors mitigate against success. Nevertheless, in those situations in which maintaining the tooth is essential this procedure is the treatment of choice.

### QUESTIONS

37. While excavating carious dentin in a permanent first molar of a 7-year-old child, a pulp exposure about the size of a No. 6 bur is discovered. There is no periapical involvement of the tooth. The pulp is vital. The treatment of choice is to
    1. cap the exposure
    2. perform a pulpotomy
    3. perform a pulpectomy
    4. extract the tooth and place a space maintainer

38. Following amputation of the coronal portion of the pulp of an immature permanent first molar, the stump should be capped with
    1. formocresol
    2. calcium chloride
    3. thymol zinc oxide
    4. calcium hydroxide

39. Indirect pulp capping procedures on primary molars are indicated when
    1. removal of decay has exposed the pulp
    2. a tooth has a large, long-standing lesion with a history of continuous pain
    3. the carious lesion has just penetrated the dentinoenamel junction
    4. the carious lesion is suspected of producing an exposure of the pulp

40. A 4-year-old child has severe, acute dental pain. So many teeth are carious that the determination of the offending tooth is difficult. The best diagnostic tool to be used is
    1. percussion
    2. radiographs
    3. electric pulp testing
    4. the patient's identification of the offending tooth

41. The cotton pellet applied to the pulpal stumps in the formocresol pulpotomy technique should be
    1. slightly dampened with formocresol
    2. saturated with formocresol
    3. left in place for 15 min
    4. left in place after the second visit

42. The most important criterion of success in a pulpotomy in a young permanent central incisor would be whether
    1. the uncompleted root end would complete its development
    2. the root end remained open if not fully developed when treatment was started
    3. a bridge of secondary dentin became radiographically demonstrable
    4. pulp stones were in evidence several months after treatment

43. A deciduous second molar with a necrotic pulp in a 4-year-old child should be
    1. allowed to remain in the mouth unless it is creating pain for the patient
    2. allowed to remain but treated with an antibiotic to eliminate the infection
    3. extracted to prevent damage to the surrounding bone and the developing permanent tooth
    4. drained through an opening through the crown into the pulp chamber but allowed to remain in the mouth to serve as a space maintainer
    5. treated with a partial pulpectomy

## TRAUMATIC INJURIES

Dental injuries are complex problems which require thorough, rapid handling. The child with a fractured tooth is one of the most challenging cases for the dentist. It is one of the few times in dentistry where time is critical. Even though such traumatic injuries are not regularly scheduled occurrences, it is usually helpful to have a specific office routine for them. Many dentists utilize a specific traumatic injury sheet which outlines the necessary procedures (Fig. 7–25).

### History

Regardless of how soon the patient seeks treatment for an injury, it is important to begin with a history. The dentist should determine when the injury occurred and the amount of time that has elapsed since the injury. This is a critical factor in treatment as the prognosis usually becomes worse as time elapses after an accident. The dentist should also attempt to determine the cause of the injury, as well as to estimate the direction and magnitude of the forces that were involved. This information may suggest injury to the mandible, other facial bones, and/or teeth. It also is important to determine where the injury occurred. The risk of tetanus is higher in the outdoors, where soil is more likely to enter the wound. Any history of previous injuries should be checked to facilitate analysis of the clinical and radiographic picture.

It is always important to obtain a relevant medical history. A standard medical questionnaire should be completed by the parent to identify the patient with bleeding disorders, allergies, or subacute bacterial endocarditis.

An inquiry concerning the status of tetanus immunization is essential. Most children have active immunization with tetanus toxoid as part of the DPT series in the first 2 years of life and a booster at the time they enter school. A further booster of the toxoid is then administered at 14–16 years of age and every 10 years thereafter. Following an injury it is the practice to give the patient a booster dose if more than 10 years have elapsed since the previous booster dose and if there is a clean, minor wound; if it has been more than 5 years since the last booster dose and the wound is contaminated, a booster dose should also be given.

### Radiographic Examination

A periapical film should show the injured tooth, its associated alveolar bone, and the adjacent uninjured contralateral tooth for reference purposes. If this is not possible on one film, an additional film should be exposed. In the young child an anterior occlusal view using standard adult size periapical film is the most practical. When root fracture is suspected, a second film at a different angulation sometimes can display the fracture. The incisors in the opposing arch must be checked for damage also, which may require another film. Where lip lacerations are present, particularly in the full thickness of the lip from the mucosa to the skin has been perforated, there is a possibility that tooth fragments have been retained within soft tissue. By placing a periapical size film in the buccal vestibule and reducing the exposure time, a radiograph of the soft tissue can be obtained. When a fracture of the mandible is suspected, a panoramic radiograph or lateral jaw film should be exposed.

When analyzing the films, the dentist must consider the following points at the initial and follow–up appointments:

1. Pulp size. If the pulp chamber in an injured tooth ceases developing at the same rate as the adjacent

teeth, pathologic changes in the pulp may be inferred. When inflammation of the pulp is chronic, a partial or total obliteration of the chamber may occur. This has also been reported following calcium hydroxide pulpotomy.

2. Root development. The presence of an open apex indicates a greater possibility of continued vitality following injury.
3. Root fracture. It may be difficult to identify root fractures on a wet film. When suspected, perhaps because of mobility of the crown with a fulcrum short of the apex, a second periapical film with different angulation is very valuable. Location of the root fracture has considerable bearing on the prognosis and treatment, and the possibility that the root is involved in a vertical fracture of the crown must be considered.
4. Periapical pathology. It is important to record the extent of radiolucency at the time of injury so that on follow-up examinations the dentist can continue looking for periapical pathology. Pulpal death may occur months after the traumatic injury.
5. Sequelae. When the injury involves total displacement of the tooth from its socket, it is important to have regular radiographic follow-up in order to watch for internal and/or external resorption. Ankylosis is another sequela of such an injury. Absence of a periodontal membrane space is sometimes visible on the radiograph but is usually not detectable until there is infraocclusion of the suspected tooth.

### Clinical Examination

When examining the patient, the dentist must be very gentle and look before touching. First, the tissues are examined by means of light digital palpation. Lacerations to the tongue and lips may cause extensive bleeding and may necessitate urgent first aid measures. Displacement of the tooth may be indicated by changes in the surrounding gingival cuff. Hemorrhage from the gingival crevice indicates severance of major periodontal fibers. Although a full scale analysis of the occlusion is not required, evaluation of the overbite and overjet may reveal intrusion, extrusion, dislocation, and interference with closure.

Limitation of movement of the mandible, anterior openbite, or marked deviation upon opening and closing could point to fracture of the mandible. It is important to determine the cause of any swelling. Usually this is due to the trauma but it may be due to superimposed infection.

On the initial and on each subsequent examination pulpal response should be recorded. The tests currently available for pulp status are not very reliable individually; therefore, several tests are needed. It is preferable to see a pattern of response emerging over a period of time. Pulp testing is usually not indicated on primary teeth or on fractured incisors assessed immediately after injury. The usual pulp response in these situations is negative, but this does not necessarily indicate death of the pulp. If no response is elicited in permanent teeth several months after the injury, however the usual diagnosis is pulpal death. A final determination can sometimes be made by preparing a test cavity into dentin without using an anesthetic agent. The tests most frequently recommended for pulpal response are the electric vitalometer test and the thermal test using a heated stick of gutta percha or a piece of ice. Prolonged response to either stimuli indicates pulp damage.

To assess the degree of mobility, two metal instruments are place facially and lingually and the dentist attempts to move the tooth in a facial-lingual direction. Physiologic mobility is graded at 0, grade 1 is slightly more than that, grade 2 is moderately more than physiologic mobility, and grade 3 is severe facial-lingual or mesiodistal movement with or without a vertical component.

Next, the injured teeth may be percussed. The response to percussion could be characterized as either normal; tender, if the patient responds to the impact of the mirror handle; or very tender. The percussion test can also be assessed on the quality of the sound. If ankylosis has occurred, a more resonant sound may be heard.

Finally, the color of the tooth must be considered. A darker color may indicate extravasation of red cells from the vessels immediately following injury or it may indicate active internal resorption. A lighter color might indicate internal calcification of the pulp chamber. If the tooth is painful during mastication or if the occlusion is disturbed, damage to the tooth supporting structures and/or displacement should be suspected. Spontaneous pain may indicate damage to the supporting tissues such as hyperemia or extravasation of blood in the periodontal ligament.

### Treatment

Determining a course of treatment depends upon careful analysis of the information gained in the history, radiographic examination, and clinical examination. Each case must be assessed individually, and the final disposition of a traumatic injury may not be decided for many months after the initial injury. It is essential to collect accurate data at the first appointment, since these data will serve as a baseline for comparison of subsequent information. Table 7–3 provides a general framework from which to develop a specific treatment for a traumatic injury.

(Text continues on p. 216.)

## CLINICAL EVALUATION SHEET FOR TRAUMA

Patient Name_____Chart #_____Date and time_____

Medical History_____

Allergies_____Date of last tetanus inoculation_____

1. **History of Trauma:**    Date and time of trauma_____

   How & where occurred_____

   Was consciousness lost (time)?_____Headache or vomiting_____

   Bleeding from nose or ears_____

2. Any previous history of trauma?_____Dates_____

   Describe_____

   Previous symptoms_____

3. **Radiographic Examination:**

   Pulp size & variations_____

   Root development & variations_____

   Root fracture_____

   Alveolar fracture_____

   Periapical pathology_____

   Periodontal spacing_____

Number & indicate amount
of root development of
involved teeth.
Draw injury in black,
Draw pulp in red.
Indicate displacement
and amount by arrow.

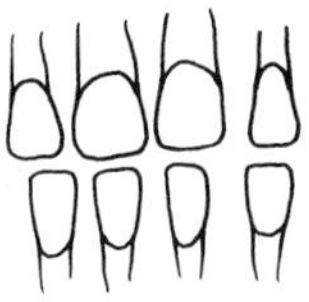

Other_____

Teeth & fragments
accounted for:_____

4. **Clinical Exam:**

   Soft tissues_____

   Teeth & Involvement (including posterior & opposing)_____

   Ant. Occlusion:_____overbite_____overjet_____

                       (tooth # and amount)       (tooth # and amount)

   Displacement_____

   Mandibular movement & symmetry_____

   Other_____

(Please turn to back of page)

**FIG. 7-25.** Clinical evaluation sheet for trauma. (Chapel Hill,
University of North Carolina, 1978)

Indicate tooth # and results

|  | Initial Exam | Sub Exam<br>Date_____ | Sub Exam<br>Date_____ |
|---|---|---|---|
| Sensitive to HOT | _____ | _____ | _____ |
| Sensitive to COLD | _____ | _____ | _____ |
| Sensitive to PERCUSSION | _____ | _____ | _____ |
| Mobility (in mm) | _____ | _____ | _____ |
| Discoloration<br>(indirect lighting) | _____ | _____ | _____ |
| Pain (Masticatory)<br>     (Spontaneous) | _____ | _____ | _____ |
| Electric Pulp Test | _____ | _____ | _____ |
| Evidence of periapical<br>pathology | _____ | _____ | _____ |

SIGNED_____

University of North Carolina
School of Dentistry
Revised 5/78
GJD:rgm

**Table 7-3. Treatment of Traumatic Injuries**

| TYPE OF INJURY | TREATMENT | |
| --- | --- | --- |
| | *Primary* | *Permanent* |
| Enamel crazing | None | None |
| Crown fracture without exposure | Protective dressing and observe | Protective dressing and observe |
| Crown fracture with exposure | If vital, formocresol pulpotomy or pulpectomy; if nonvital, partial pulpectomy or extraction | If vital, calcium hydroxide pulp cap or pulpotomy; if nonvital, apexification or pulpectomy |
| Root fractures | Extraction | Stabilization, pulpectomy, or extraction |
| Intrusion | Allow to reerupt | Reposition, stabilize, and observe |
| Extrusion | Reposition and observe *or* extract | Reposition, stabilize, and observe |
| Avulsion | No treatment | Reimplant and stabilize |

**ENAMEL CRAZING.** Enamel crazing is a very common finding that is often overlooked. When light is deflected through the tooth perpendicular to its long axis, the enamel substance appears to have split lines which do not cross the dentinoenamel junction. When this is the only finding, no treatment is indicated.

**FRACTURES.** Uncomplicated crown fractures involving enamel only or enamel and dentin are initially treated by placing a protective dressing of calcium hydroxide over any exposed dentin and restoring the tooth with a composite resin (Fig. 7-26). If the tooth is badly broken down, it may be necessary to use a stainless steel crown or a welded piece of matrix material to keep the protective dressing in place (Fig. 7-27). Teeth with either enamel crazing or crown fractures should be followed for several months because studies indicate that up to 13% of such cases can develop necrotic pulps.

The treatment of crown fractures when there is exposure of the pulp is either pulp capping, pulpotomy, pulpectomy, or extraction. Pulp capping is primarily indicated in the permanent dentition when the pulp exposure is confined to a small area. At this time, however, the relationship of the size of the pulpal exposure and the probability of pulp survival has not been accurately determined. The pulp should not have been exposed for more than a few hours, but the maximum time limit in this regard is not known. A conservative approach suggests that exposure should have occurred no more than 1 or 2 hours prior to treatment, but successful cases have been recorded with exposures of up to 18 hours. Associated injuries to the supporting tissues should not be present.

In nonvital primary teeth the treatment is either a partial pulpotomy or extraction. Non-vital permanent teeth should be treated with pulpectomy if the root has completely developed or with apexification if the root is not fully developed. See the chapter on Endodontics for further discussion of apexification and pulpectomy.

Root fractures in the primary dentition are treated with extraction, but in the permanent dentition there is frequently the opportunity for stabilization and complete endodontics (see Ch. 9, Endodontics).

**INTRUSION AND EXTRUSION.** The treatment of intruded teeth differs in the primary and permanent dentitions. In the primary dentition, if intrusion does not encroach upon the developing permanent tooth bud, the primary teeth should be allowed to reerupt (Fig. 7-28). They should be carefully monitored by the dentist, however. In the permanent dentition intruded teeth are usually repositioned, stabilized, and then observed for further developments. Current thinking concerning stabilization of any loose teeth suggests that stabilization should be for no longer than 7-10 days, after which splints or other stabilizing mechanisms should be removed. This has been shown to reduce the possibility of ankylosis. A popular stabilization technique involves acid etch resin procedures in conjunction with orthodontic wire.

Extruded primary teeth can be repositioned if there is no danger of damaging the developing permanent successor. If a primary tooth is likely to impinge on the permanent tooth bud, it is usually better to extract the primary tooth. In the permanent dentition, extruded teeth are usually repositioned in the socket, stabilized with some splinting technique, and observed for further developments. Again, stabilization should be for no longer than 7-10 days.

**AVULSION.** When the tooth has been completely displaced from its socket, it is called an avulsed tooth or a completely avulsed tooth. In the primary dentition it is rare that such teeth are reimplanted, but in the permanent dentition definitive action on the part of the dentist is critical. Avulsed permanent teeth are found predominantly in the age group of 7-10 where the permanent incisors are in some stage of eruption; however, this type injury has been known to occur in older individuals (Fig. 7-29).

The most critical factor in the success of reimplantation is the extraoral time period, that is, the period of time the tooth is out of the socket. Whenever possible, an avulsed permanent tooth should be reimplanted within 30 min. of the injury. Reimplantation should be accomplished even if it has to be done by a parent or other available adult without the direct supervision of a

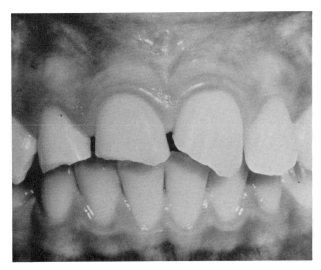

**FIG. 7-26.** Uncomplicated crown fracture of both maxillary central incisors and maxillary right lateral incisor.

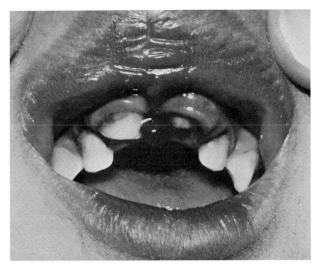

**FIG. 7-28.** Intruded primary maxillary central incisors.

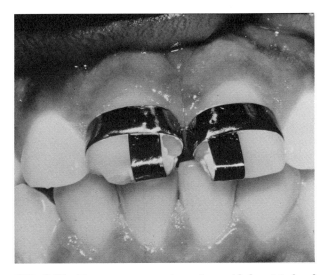

**FIG. 7-27.** Temporary restoration using welded matrix band material.

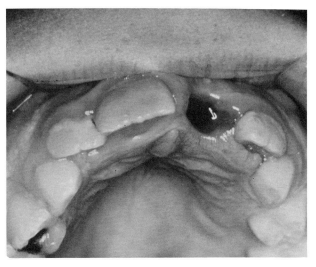

**FIG. 7-29.** Avulsed permanent maxillary central incisor.

dentist. If the tooth cannot be reimplanted at the site of injury, it should be placed in the oral cavity either in the buccal vestibule or underneath the tongue and the patient dispatched to the dentist immediately. No effort should be taken to sterilize the tooth surface because such procedures may damage or destroy vital periodontal tissue and cementum.

Before reimplantation is undertaken, the alveolar socket should be examined for fracture or other damage. A firm blood clot should be removed by irrigation, not by curettage, because curettage may damage the residual periodontal tissue in the socket. The tooth can

be reimplanted with finger pressure and no local anesthesia unless gingival lacerations require suturing. After reimplantation a radiograph is taken to verify that the tooth is in its normal position. The tooth should be stabilized and, if appropriate, tetanus prophylaxis should be given. In most instances root canal treatment should not be performed at the time of the reimplantation procedure. This only increases the extraoral time period for the tooth and involves additional handling of the tooth which may damage or destroy the attached periodontal tissues.

In the case of a closed apical foramen, endodontic

treatment should be carried out within 1–2 weeks after reimplantation because total necrosis of the pulp is anticipated and the endodontic procedure decreases the probability of external resorption. When the apical foramen is wide open and reimplantation is performed within 2 hours after injury, postponing endodontic treatment and awaiting possible revascularization of the pulp can be justified. Radiographic examination should be accomplished 2–3 weeks after reimplantation, because the first evidence of root resorption and periapical infection can usually be seen at this time. Any abnormal radiographic signs dictate immediate endodontic therapy in order to minimize the possibility of external resorption. Repeated successive radiographic examinations should be performed in order to monitor conditions surrounding the reimplanted tooth.

## QUESTIONS

44. A primary central incisor may be allowed to reerupt after it has been traumatically intruded if
   1. splinting is impossible
   2. there is no danger to the permanent successor
   3. it cannot be extracted
   4. None of the above

45. An 8-year-old girl sustains an injury to her maxillary left permanent central incisor. The fracture is well into the dentin. The tooth, however, is not sensitive. A radiograph reveals no root damage. Immediate treatment should involve
   1. disking the roughened enamel margins
   2. treating the exposed dentin with a stannous fluoride
   3. advising the patient to return in 3 months
   4. protecting the tooth with a sedative treatment under a temporary covering

46. The change in color of a traumatized primary incisor usually results from all the following except
   1. laceration of periodontal fibers
   2. diffusion of biliverdin into the dentinal tubules
   3. development of a heavy layer of secondary dentin
   4. internal resorption of dentin within the crown

47. A child 9 years of age received a traumatic fracture without exposure to his central incisor. The pulp test 2 days after the injury was negative. The dentist should consider the condition of the pulp as
   1. nonvital
   2. hypoemic
   3. hyperemic
   4. requiring retesting in 2 weeks

48. A severe blow to a permanent anterior tooth, not causing fracture, frequently leads to
   1. permanent looseness
   2. immediate pulpal death
   3. pulpal death, but only if treatment is delayed too long
   4. pulpal death regardless of treatment
   5. None of the above

49. The radiograph of a traumatized tooth is necessary to
   1. assess the stage of root development
   2. determine the presence or absence of root fractures
   3. have a base from which comparisons can be made with future radiographs
   4. All of the above

50. If a vitality test taken immediately after a traumatic blow to a tooth is negative, this indicates that the tooth should be
   1. immediately considered for a pulpectomy
   2. observed for a period of 10 days to 2 weeks and then another vitality test taken
   3. ignored unless it becomes symptomatic
   4. given a test cavity preparation without anesthesia to determine vitality

51. A 4½-year-old child has fallen within the past 2 hours and traumatized both maxillary central incisors to the point that they are extremely mobile. The treatment of choice would be to
   1. extract them because they would be lost soon anyway
   2. do nothing and observe periodically
   3. immobilize them with a splint and do nothing more
   4. check radiographically for root fractures, and if none, proceed with a splint and periodic examination

## RESTORATIVE DENTISTRY

Maintaining the integrity of the primary dentition is important in order to eliminate disease, pain, and tooth loss with its accompanying space loss. It is obviously preferable to maintain the dentition by instituting preventive measures (oral hygiene, fluoride supplementation, and diet control) rather than by relying on restorative therapy. However, restorative procedures are an important adjunct for the dentist in preserving the dentition.

Epidemiologic data have revealed a pattern of decay in the primary dentition which is partially attributable to occlusal and proximal morphology. The occlusal surface of the second primary molar is more often carious than the first primary molars because of the more defined groove pattern of second primary molar teeth.

The proximal surfaces of the primary dentition display a logical gradient of caries involvement. Adjacent contact areas exhibit similar caries incidences. The incisor–incisor and incisor–cuspid contacts are usually carious only in rampant decay situations, which are generally attributable to poor tooth cleaning and a cariogenic diet (e.g., high sucrose intake) or deleterious diet pattern (e.g., nursing caries). The first primary molar–second primary molar contact is the most susceptible interproximal area due to a large contact area.

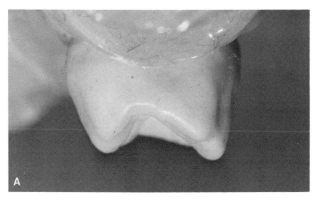

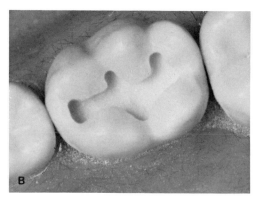

**FIG. 7–30.** (Figs. 7–30 and 7–31 belong to one series of illustrations and so are labelled consecutively with one alphabetical list.) A. Maxillary first primary molar viewed from the mesial. Note the convergence of the labial and lingual surfaces which gives rise to a small occlusal table.

**FIG. 7–31.** (Fig. 7–31 concludes the series begun in Fig. 7–30.) B. Occlusal preparation on a mandibular second primary molar. The necessary grooves provide good extension, while remaining narrow enough to conserve tooth structure.

The distal surface of the second primary molar exhibits few carious lesions until contact is established with the first permanent molar. Therefore, after the primary dentition has erupted and interproximal contacts have been established, adjacent contacts exhibit similar decay with more distal contacts having higher decay rates.

Restorative techniques similar to those employed in the permanent dentition are used in the primary dentition. The significant modifications are based upon morphologic considerations.

### Class I Amalgam Restoration

The occlusal groove pattern of primary molars, especially second primary molars, demands extension of the preparation to remove these potentially carious areas. Isolated shallow enamel grooves may be eliminated by enamelplasty with a bur or stone; followed by a topical fluoride application. This technique eliminates caries-susceptible areas and concerves tooth structure.

While extension is important, the reduced occlusal table of primary molar teeth dictates a limited width for the occlusal portion of any preparation (Fig. 7–30). A narrower preparation also lessens the chances of pulp exposure. The primary pulp is easily exposed mechanically or cariously since it is relatively larger than the permanent pulp. The primary pulp follows the enamel surface, and the thickness of primary enamel is uniformly 1 mm, which is thinner than the enamel layer of the permanent dentition. Rounded line angles within the preparations decrease the likelihood of mechanical exposure (Fig. 7–31).

### Class II Amalgam Restoration

In addition to the considerations required for the Class I preparation, the involvement of one or more proximal surfaces demands attention to other anatomic features of primary teeth. The broad and flat primary tooth proximal contact area requires more proximal (buccolingual) extension in order to place the margins in a cleansible area. The gingival extension of the proximal preparation, on the other hand, must be conservatively placed (Fig. 7–32). Although opening the gingival portion of the contact is essential, the cervical constriction of the primary posterior teeth means that over extension of the gingival portion of the preparation will place the gingival seat dangerously close to the pulp. The enamel of the gingival seat need not be trimmed since the enamel rod configuration is occlusally directed and therefore not likely to be unsupported.

In order to restore the original broad and flat contact, the Class II matrix material may be placed with less contour than in the permanent dentition. Buccal and lingual proximal retentive grooves may be used in the primary dentition, but must be used with care when the preparation extends past the ideal. Again, the relatively large pulp is very susceptible to mechanical exposure. This is especially true of the large mesiobuccal pulp horn encountered in the posterior teeth.

The isthmus of the preparation should remain one-third of the intercusp width (Fig. 7–32A). To increase the bulk of this area and lessen the risk of fracture, the pulpal–axial line angle should be rounded. If all these factors are considered, both Class I and Class II lesions can be prepared and restored in the primary dentition in a biologically sound manner.

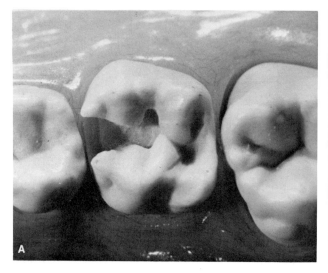

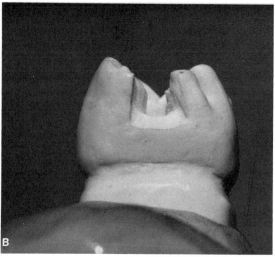

**FIG. 7–32.** Class II preparation extended gingivally, proximally, and occlusally to allow finishing and to eradicate the susceptible grooves. Note the isthmus width is not more than one-third the intercusp dimension. B. Convergence of the labial and lingual walls of the proximal box in Class II preparation viewed from the proximal.

## Class III Restoration

Although the preparation for a Class III restoration in the primary dentition is very similar to that performed in the permanent dentition, the large pulp chamber in a primary tooth makes preparation for bulk and retention of the restoration very difficult. Incisal and gingival retention points help to circumvent the

**FIG. 7–33.** (Figs. 7–33 and 7–34 are one series of illustrations and so are labelled consecutively with one alphabetical list.) A. Class III distal preparation on a mandibular primary canine. Note that the labial dovetail does not cross the center of the labial surface and does not undermine the incisal edge. B. The Class III distal preparation with a labial dovetail viewed from the distal.

retention problem. A labial dovetail may be utilized on anterior teeth in the less visible mandibular arch to augment retention and bulk (Fig. 7–33). A lingual dovetail is recommended in the visible maxillary arch (Fig. 7–34). These methods are both simple and effective modifications which should be included in the restorative regime for primary teeth. The dovetail should be limited to the gingival half of the tooth so the incisal edge is not undermined. If undermined, the incisal edge should be removed and labial *and* lingual dovetails placed simultaneously for increased retention (Fig. 7–35).

## Acid Etch Restoration

When the tooth to be restored has more extensive destruction than can be managed with the conventional or modified Class III preparation, the procedure of

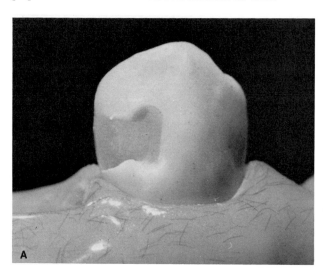

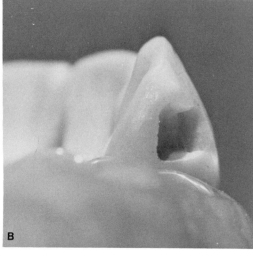

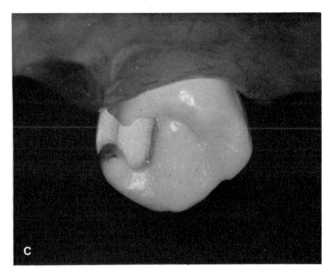

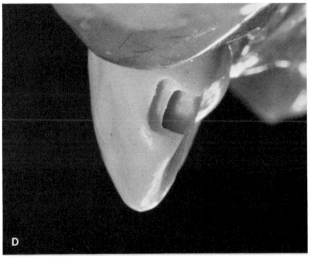

**FIG. 7–34.** (Fig. 7–34 concludes the series begun in Fig. 7–33.) C. Class III distal preparation on a maxillary primary canine. Note that the lingual dovetail is limited to the distal half of the lingual surface and does not undermine the incisal edge. D. The Class III distal preparation with a lingual dovetail viewed from the distal.

choice is to augment the mechanical retention by acid etching the enamel surface. Results are best when the enamel thickness 1 mm lateral to the area to be restored is reduced by one-half with a bur and the enamel margin is scalloped or beveled (Fig. 7–36). This provides a better etch, margins which can be finished while maintaining a bulk of restorative material, and improved aesthetics. Exposed dentin should be protected by a calcium hydroxide material prior to etching. Due to the enamel configuration some clinicians recommend etching primary-enamel with 30% unbuffered phosphoric acid for 2 min, others suggest reducing the enamel thickness by half. Nothing has solved all retention problems. The enamel etch should extend to a depth of approximately 30–50 $\mu$m. The same technique is recommended for restoration of fractured young permanent teeth except that a 1-min etch with 30% unbuffered phosphoric acid is sufficient.

### Resin Crown

The most reasonable restoration for the grossly broken down anterior primary tooth is the resin crown. This technique utilizes mechanical retention augmented by acid etching of the available enamel. Margins should be placed on sound enamel which has been reduced to one-half thickness. All other enamel should be roughened with a stone to enhance the etching (Fig. 7–37A). A plastic crown form similar in size to the unprepared tooth is fitted, trimmed (Fig. 7–37B), and vented (Fig. 7–37C) to allow excess resin to escape. The

exposed dentin is protected by a calcium hydroxide preparation, and the primary enamel is etched for 2 min with 30% unbuffered phosphoric acid. The acrylic crown form is filled with resin and replaced on the tooth during polymerization (Fig. 7–37D). After removal of the acrylic crown form, the resin is shaped and finished (Fig. 7–37E).

### Stainless Steel Crown

A stainless steel crown is indicated when the carious involvement of a tooth is extensive, when an amalgam restoration would have compromised strength, when vertical dimension is being lost due to excessive abrasion of anomalous enamel or dentin, or when pulp therapy has been performed.

Teeth are prepared for a stainless steel crown by first reducing the occlusal surface 1–2 mm (Fig. 7–38A). The proximal surfaces are reduced in order to open the contacts to accept the steel crown and place a feathered margin at the gingival surface. Lingual and buccal surface reduction should be limited to the occlusal portion. This helps to maintain the buccal cervical bulge which is important in crown retention. The line angles and general crown contour should also be maintained during preparation to give the stainless steel crown stability during fitting and cementation. (Fig. 7–38B). A well-contoured stainless steel crown provides better margin adaptation and retention. Occasionally, the crown is extended more than 1 mm below the crest of the gingiva. In this case, crown length should be reduced unless it is necessary to cover deeply prepared tooth structures. The crown is then polished and cemented (Fig. 7–38C).

Difficult situations arise when space has been lost. A crown with appropriate mesiodistal dimension does

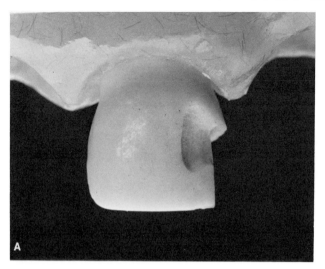

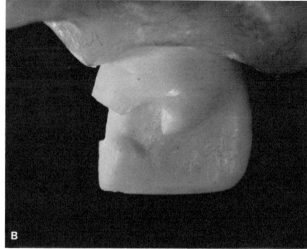

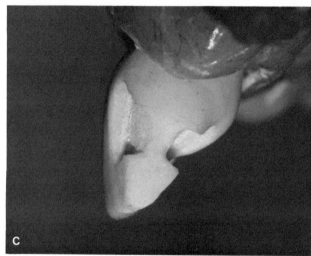

**FIG. 7–35.** A. Doyle preparation utilizing labial and lingual dovetails to improve retention after removal of the mesial portion of the incisal edge. This view demonstrates the labial dovetail. B. The lingual dovetail of the Doyle preparation. C. From the proximal perspective it can be seen how easy it is to undermine the incisal edge by poor placement of the dovetails.

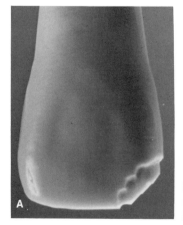

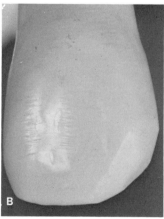

**FIG. 7–36.** A. Mesioincisal fracture of a permanent maxillary central incisor prepared for an acid etch resin restoration. Note that the enamel is prepared to one-half thickness and scalloped. B. The mesioincisal fracture of a permanent maxillary incisor prepared for an acid etch resin restoration. Note that the enamel is beveled to provide a feathered margin.

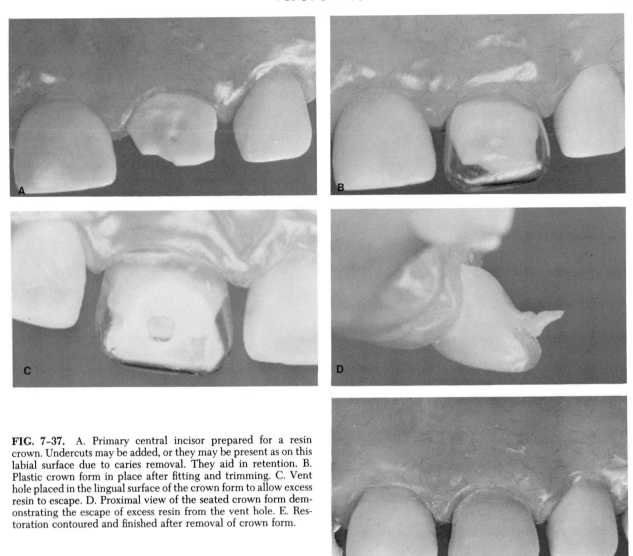

**FIG. 7-37.** A. Primary central incisor prepared for a resin crown. Undercuts may be added, or they may be present as on this labial surface due to caries removal. They aid in retention. B. Plastic crown form in place after fitting and trimming. C. Vent hole placed in the lingual surface of the crown form to allow excess resin to escape. D. Proximal view of the seated crown form demonstrating the escape of excess resin from the vent hole. E. Restoration contoured and finished after removal of crown form.

not accommodate the buccolingual dimension of the tooth. To alleviate this problem, the lingual surface of the tooth must be reduced to fit the crown. When several crowns are to be placed adjacent to one another and slight space loss has occurred, each crown should be prepared individually. The crowns are then cemented simultaneously. This increases the arch length by a small amount.

## Occlusal Sealants

Occlusal sealants are indicated to protect deep, retentive pits and fissures and decalcified or hypoplastic areas. This technique, which is recommended to eliminate these potentially carious areas, is becoming more reliable. The sealants are aesthetic and able to reduce caries incidence. Before sealing, the teeth must be carefully inspected for caries. The etching time and technique used is the same as that for acid etch resin, but attention to moisture control must be increased. Even when the sealants are no longer clinically visible, tags extend into the enamel and continue to protect the teeth.

QUESTIONS

52. In festooning and trimming a stainless steel crown, special attention must be paid to the greater length necessary in the region of the mesiobuccal bulge in the

    1. primary first molar
    2. primary second molar

*(Continued)*

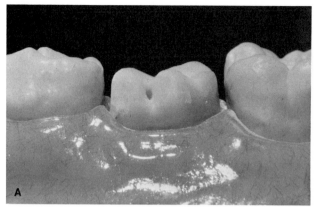

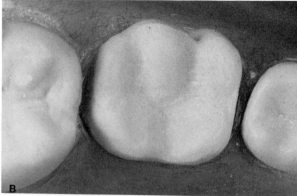

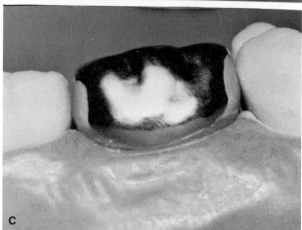

**FIG. 7-38.** A. Primary second molar prepared for a stainless steel crown. Note the amount of occlusal reduction and the minimal convergence of the proximal walls. B. Occlusal view of the primary second molar preparation demonstrating that some occlusal contour is maintained and that the line angles are rounded only to a limited extent. C. Seated stainless steel crown with mesial and distal contact as well as good marginal ridge relationships with the adjacent teeth.

  3. maxillary primary canine
  4. maxillary lateral primary incisor

53. What single morphologic characteristic of the permanent first molar necessitates early restorative procedures in most children?
  1. Mesial proximal contact
  2. Deep grooves and fissures
  3. Large pulp chamber
  4. Early beginning of calcification
  5. Presence of an auxiliary cusp

54. In tooth preparation for a steel crown, the surface requiring the least amount of reduction is the
  1. distal
  2. buccal
  3. mesial
  4. lingual
  5. occlusal

55. In placing an alloy in the Class II preparation on a primary tooth, much consideration is given to the placement of the matrix band and wedging because the contact point is
  1. broad and flat
  2. narrow and close to the marginal ridge

  3. closer to the buccal, and the wedge should be placed from the lingual
  4. closer to the lingual, and the wedge should be placed from the buccal

56. The pulp horn which is most likely to be exposed during cavity preparation on a primary molar is the
  1. mesiobuccal horn of the primary first molar
  2. distobuccal horn of the primary first molar
  3. mesiolingual horn of the primary second molar
  4. distobuccal horn of the primary second molar

57. The outline form for an occlusal Class I cavity preparation should insure that
  a. all unsupported enamel is removed to prevent lateral spread of caries at the dentinoenamel junction
  b. it goes around cusps to conserve tooth structure and avoid exposing pulp horns
  c. margins are not in stress-bearing areas
  d. if a weak enamel wall (2 mm) separates two outlines they are joined together

  1. a, b, and c
  2. b, c, and d
  3. a, b, and d
  4. All of the above

58. The isthmus of a Class II cavity preparation in the primary molar is broad and shallow to
    1. provide for adequate bulk of restorative material
    2. assist in achieving a right angle cavosurface margin at the lateral walls of the proximal box
    3. minimize the possibility of pulp horn exposure
    4. All of the above
    5. 1 and 2

59. When the proximal portion of a Class II cavity preparation in a primary molar extends rather deeply gingivally, a satisfactory gingival seat may not be obtained because the
    1. enamel rods in the gingival third of the primary tooth extend occlusally
    2. buccal and lingual surfaces of primary molars converge occlusally
    3. proximal contact of primary molars is broad and flat
    4. primary teeth have a marked cervical constriction

60. The dovetail on a modified Class III cavity preparation in the primary dentition should be accentual toward the
    1. gingival
    2. incisal
    3. midline
    4. crest of the contour of the tooth

61. In the preparation of a primary molar tooth for a stainless steel crown
    1. the mesial and distal contact areas must be broken
    2. the buccal surface must be reduced
    3. the occlusal surface must be reduced
    4. all angles must be rounded
    5. All of the above

62. The gingival seat cavosurface margin of a Class II preparation in a primary tooth should be
    1. left unbeveled because of the angle of the enamel rods
    2. beveled to reduce occurrence of caries
    3. beveled to remove unsupported enamel rods
    4. beveled about the same as for a permanent tooth

63. Dental restorations involving the proximal surfaces in the primary dentition, particularly molars, should restore the full mesiodistal diameter for
    1. the appearance of the child
    2. maintenance of arch length
    3. proper bulk of restorative material to minimize fracture
    4. aid in the digestion of food

# EFFECT OF DISEASE ON THE ORAL TISSUES OF CHILDREN

## Gingival Manifestations of Disease

### SYSTEMIC DISEASE

*Leukemia and Lymphoma.* The intraoral lesions seen in children with leukemia or lymphoma offer diagnostic supporting evidence as well as a therapeutic problem to be solved. Most commonly, gingival hyperplasia and gingivitis associated with bleeding are encountered. Occasionally a rapidly growing soft tissue mass may be evident. Treatment is most often aimed at symptomatic relief and prevention of subsequent infections. Oral hygiene measures combined with débridement usually provide relief.

*Neutropenias.* Either the cyclic, familial, or drug-induced neutropenia is associated with a clinical picture of hyperplastic bleeding gingiva and possibly early exfolitation of primary teeth. As with the leukemias, symptomatic relief is best provided by means of plaque control, curettage, and scaling.

*Sturge–Weber Syndrome.* Sturge–Weber syndrome is characterized by an intracranial angioma, possible seizures and mental retardation, facial nevus in the area supplied by the trigeminal nerve, and intraoral hemangioma of the tongue, gingiva, or mucosa. The hemangioma may be treated by surgical or electrosurgical excision, but it commonly recurs.

### LOCAL GINGIVAL DISEASE

*Marginal Gingivitis.* The young patient often exhibits inflammation limited to the marginal gingiva. Most often the result of local microorganisms associated with poor oral hygiene, it can be identified by the red, edematous, enlarged gingiva. The resiliency of the young patient makes this type of lesion readily reversible with improved oral hygiene and only slowly progressive without care.

*Eruption Gingivitis.* At times marginal gingivitis may be associated with the exfoliation of primary teeth and/or the eruption of permanent teeth. A mobile, exfoliating primary tooth may cause impaction of food debris or exposure of pulp therapy medicaments, either of which can be irritating to the gingiva. The inflammation generally resolves rapidly upon exfoliation or removal of the offending tooth, although pericoronitis may develop around the most distal erupting tooth. Again this condition is due to the debris and bacterial accumulations. Vigorous cleansing of this area often relieves this condition.

*Acute Herpetic Gingival Stomatitis.* Acute herpetic gingival stomatitis usually appears in the 1–3 year age group and is extremely contagious. It is manifested by tender, inflamed gingiva and mucosa, vesicular lesions, fever, and malaise. Although this condition is self-limiting, for the 7–10 day duration problems can occur due to limited fluid intake. Nonirritating, room temperature liquids usually provide the necessary hydration and nutrition. Analgesics may also be necessary for relief of the intense pain.

*Acute Necrotizing Ulcerative Gingivitis.* Acute necrotizing ulcerative gingivitis (ANUG) is usually manifested by destruction of the interdental papilla and painful bleeding lesions which rarely involve the mucosa. Lymphadenopathy, malaise, fever, and foul breath usually accompany this entity. ANUG is believed to have a bacterial etiology, but it may have psychologic components. Débridement of the lesions, curettage, and scrupulous oral hygiene usually lead to rapid resolution.

**Acute Periodontal Abscess.** Acute periodontal abscesses in the primary and young permanent dentitions are usually associated with debris lodged in the gingival crevice. Swollen red lesions associated with vital teeth commonly exhibit exudate upon probing. Removal of the food debris and general débridement of the area lead to resolution of the abscess, which is generally rapid and uneventful.

**Phenytoin Gingival Hyperplasia.** One possible sequela of the use of phenytoin sodium for seizure control is gingival hyperplasia. The gingival enlargement is fibrotic in nature. Individuals exhibit variable sensitivity to the drug, but careful attention to oral hygiene usually limits the extent of the gingival hyperplasia. Surgical removal of grossly enlarged tissue is indicated.

**Gingival Fibromatosis.** Enlargement of the attached gingiva in gingival fibromatosis, which is an idiopathic disease, may cause deformation of the alveolus or delayed eruption. Excision of tissue may be necessary to allow the eruption of permanent teeth covered by the firm dense tissue. In some cases recontouring of the alveolus may also be necessary.

**Pyogenic Granuloma.** The pyogenic granuloma which is an elevated, smooth, and easily bleeding lesion, is often ulcerated. It is essentially granulation tissue from an overactive response to trauma. Local excision is generally successful but a small percentage do recur.

**Peripheral Giant Cell Reparative Granuloma.** The lesions of peripheral giant cell reparative granuloma resemble the pyogenic granuloma in appearance but often occur in the adolescent age group. These lesions are usually limited to the gingiva and often follow some traumatic injury. In contrast to the pyogenic granuloma, these lesions may exhibit some osseous radiolucency on a radiograph. Multinucleated giant cells and hemosiderin are diagnostic in the histologic sections of this lesion. Surgical excision is the treatment of choice and is not followed by recurrence.

**Peripheral Ossifying Fibroma.** The peripheral ossifying fibroma appears in the gingiva and is clinically similar to the pyogenic granuloma and peripheral giant cell reparative granuloma. Microscopically, however, there are inclusions of osteoid and bone. These lesions often recur after surgical removal.

**Self-Inflicted Lesions.** Local inflammatory lesions of the gingiva may be the result of trauma inflicted by repeated manipulation of the gingiva with the fingernails or small utensils. This mutilation may be simply a habit or one ramification of a psychologic disorder.

**Gingival Enlargement Associated with Orthodontic Therapy.** The placement of bands or direct bonded attachments on a tooth often leads to gingival enlargement. This is due in large part to poor hygiene measures during treatment. Sites where spaces have been closed or where teeth have been extracted also may develop a local excess of gingiva tissue. This tissue may be removed or recontoured during treatment. In most cases improved hygiene during the post-treatment retention period makes recontouring of the tissue the only necessary therapy.

## Mucosal Manifestations of Disease

### SYSTEMIC DISEASE

**Epidermolysis Bullosa.** An hereditary disease, epidermolysis bullosa is characterized by epithelial and mucosal bullae which arise following minor trauma. The bullae are usually followed by healing and scarring. Disfigurement of the oral structures may occur after numerous traumatic insults. Restorative dentistry and other oral manipulations by the dentist should be carried out with extreme care to eliminate all trauma.

**Erythema Multiforme.** Erythema multiforme is a disease of unknown etiology. Like the similar syndromes which affect various combinations of epithelial and mucosal tissue with erythematous macules or papules, it reoccurs periodically during the patient's lifetime. The oral lesions may become very painful and ulcerated, but they heal without scarring. Antibiotic therapy may be indicated to prevent subsequent bacterial infections.

**Histiocytosis X.** In the complex of diseases known as histiocytosis X mucosal ulcerations are generally accompanied by headache, malaise and fever. Radiolucencies of the skull, jaw, and long bones give a characteristic "punched-out" appearance to the bone. Teeth may be mobile and appear, on a radiograph, to be floating in the air. Treatment of the oral lesions is most appropriately palliative and pointed toward prevention of subsequent bacterial infections. The prognosis for this disease depends on the involvement of the reticuloendothelial system.

**Rubeola.** In the prodromal period the patient exhibits macules encompassed by inflamed margins on the buccal mucosa; these macules are termed Koplik's spots. The mucosal lesions are generally not evident when the epithelial lesions occur.

**Chickenpox.** The vesicular lesions associated with chickenpox may be found on either the epithelium or the oral mucosa. The vesicles rupture and heal in 7–10 days. There is no indication for treatment of the oral lesions.

*Mononucleosis.* Mononucleosis may be accompanied by malaise, fever, lymphadenopathy, and occasionally palatal petechiae. These petechiae are not pathognomonic, however, since they do not occur in all cases of mononucleosis.

### LOCAL MUCOSAL DISEASE

*Diphtheria.* Diphtheria is a virulent bacterial disease which may affect the oral mucosa in addition to the palatal and tonsillar areas. The fibrous membrane which covers the mucosal tissue is found in conjunction with malaise, fever, sore throat, nausea, and vomiting.

*Coxsackieviruses.* Diseases caused by coxsackieviruses are usually self-limiting, mildly acute, only moderately painful, and associated with fever, malaise, and sore throat. The ulcerative lesions of the mucosa usually resolve in less than 1 week and demand no treatment. Herpangina and acute lymphonodular laryngitis are the most common forms of this disease complex.

*Recurrent Aphthous Ulcer.* Of unknown etiology, recurrent aphthous ulcers are painful and usually last 7–10 days. There is no vesicular lesion associated with these ulcers. Symptomatic relief is sufficient treatment in the majority of cases.

*White Sponge Nevus.* The white sponge nevus, which is hereditary, is a manifestation of thickened epithelium of the oral mucosa. It cannot be wiped off the tissue and is asymptomatic. No treatment is necessary.

*Candidiasis.* Candidiasis usually affects debilitated children or those taking large doses of antibiotics. The white nodules can be wiped off the mucosa, although there is subsequent bleeding. Systemic or topical nystatin is recommended as treatment.

*Pentz–Jehgers Syndrome.* Pigmentation of the mucosa, perioral epithelium, and intestinal polyps characterize Jehgers syndrome. The oral pigmentation requires no treatment, and the epithelium pigmentation is often reduced at puberty. The intestinal polyps, on the other hand, may significantly influence the general health of the patient.

*Mucocele.* Mucoceles are elevated translucencies which usually occur on the mucosa following traumatic injury. Accessory salivary gland flow accumulates in the connective tissue and gives rise to the swellings. Complete excision of these lesions or marsupialization is the treatment of choice if recurrence is to be avoided.

## Hard Tissue Lesions Associated with Disease

### SYSTEMIC DISEASE

*Papillon–LeFèvre Syndrome.* The dermatologic signs of hyperkeratosis of the palms and soles of the feet are combined with periodontal pathosis in Papillon–LeFèvre syndrome, which is an autosomal recessive disease. Inflammation of the gingiva is followed by progressive bone loss around the incisors and molars. The periodontal pathology usually begins during the primary dentition, resolves after the loss of the primary teeth, and appears again before and during loss of the permanent dentition.

*Hypophosphatasia.* Like Papillon–LeFèvre syndrome, hypophosphatasia is an autosomal recessive disorder. It should be suspected when there is early loss of primary teeth. Severe bone loss, decreased alkaline phosphatase, hypocementogenesis, and increased excretion of phosphoethanolamine in the urine are characteristic of this disorder.

*Sickle Cell Anemia.* Sickle cell anemia is an autosomal recessive disorder which is being diagnosed more frequently in the black population. Radiographs of the skull exhibit the characteristic "hair-on-end" effect of the diploic spaces. The mandible demonstrates osteoporosis and thinning of the cortical bone. Management of subsequent periodontal lesions is best handled conservatively with great care to control infection.

*Thalassemia.* Thalassemia is an autosomal recessive disorder often seen in people of Mediterranean descent. Again the hair-on-end effect is observed in the diploic spaces of the skull. Osteoporosis and protrusion of the maxilla are commonly observed in these patients.

*Neutropenia.* As neutropenia progresses, the inflammation of the gingiva (see Gingival Manifestations of Disease) is followed by bone loss around the primary and permanent teeth. The bone loss often leads to loosening and premature loss of the teeth.

*Fibrous Dysplasia.* Fibrous dysplasia is a disease of unknown etiology which sometimes leads to alveolar enlargement and loss of permanent teeth. Root development may be arrested; in some cases resorption of the roots of the teeth is observed. Cystlike lesions which later appear to have the radiolucency of "ground glass" are often observed in conjunction with this disorder.

### LOCAL HARD TISSUE LESIONS

*Periodontitis.* Periodontitis destroys the underlying periodontal membrane and bony structures and undoubtedly proceeds from marginal gingivitis. Poor oral hygiene and the resultant inflammation have progressively greater effect on periodontal structures until bone loss and interosseous cratering occurs. Improved oral hygiene and surgical correction of the defects appears to be the treatment of choice.

*Central Giant Cell Reparative Granuloma.* A tissue-filled cystic cavity, central giant cell reparative granuloma is usually located in the mandible of persons under 20 years of age. The lesion appears radiolucent, is expansile, and is located within the bone. Tooth migration often accompanies enlargement of this lesion. The treatment of choice is curettage. Since these lesions are sometimes confused with those of hyperparathyroidism, serum calcium levels should be determined before treatment.

***Central Ossifying Fibroma.*** The central ossifying fibroma is also an expansile lesion which causes tooth migration. Upon radiographic examination it appears both radiolucent and radiopaque. Histologic section reveals a combination of connective tissue and bony trabeculae which give rise to the radiographic appearance. This lesion is best treated by curettage.

***Ewing's Tumor.*** A rare tumor which is found in the mandible of persons under 20 years of age, Ewing's tumor is accompanied by fever, pain, and swelling with erosion of the cortical plate in the area of the lesion. Although there is a poor prognosis for this lesion, radiation therapy appears to be the treatment of choice.

***Odontogenic Myxoma, Odontogenic Fibroma, and Adenoameloblastoma.*** Odontogenic myxoma, odontogenic fibroma, and adenoameloblastoma are commonly found in persons under 20 years of age. These radiolucent lesions, usually associated with erupting teeth, are expansile and asymptomatic. Although all appear to be cystlike cavities, histologic sectioning reveal quite different structures requiring different treatment. The odontogenic myxoma, which is best treated by curettage, reveals myxomatous tissue. At excision the odontogenic fibroma appears to be not a cystic cavity but a firm mass of tissue. When the adenoameloblastoma is excised, it reveals a well-defined composition of ductlike structures. Each of these lesions responds well to conservative treatment.

***Ameloblastic Odontoma.*** Commonly found in the maxilla of children under 15 years of age, ameloblastic odontoma is a combination of radiopacities and radiolucencies. This is accounted for by the ameloblastic epithelium, enamel, and dentin which make up this lesion. The treatment of choice is excision.

***Aneurysmal Bone Cyst.*** Although not true cysts, aneurysmal bone cysts appear in the mandibular anterior area of children under 20 years of age. Painless enlargement usually follows a history of trauma. The treatment of choice is curettage.

***Traumatic Bone Cyst.*** Most commonly found in the mandibular anterior area of males under 20 years of age, a traumatic bone cyst is a painless enlargement associated with vital teeth. When the lesion is entered for curettage, an empty cavity is usually revealed. Uneventful healing follows curettage.

***Osteopetrosis.*** Osteopetrosis is an hereditary disorder which is revealed before 30 years of age. There are two forms of the disease, one with an early childhood onset and one with a late childhood onset. Dense sclerotic bone is continually laid down, without the normal resorptive processes taking place. Because the enlargement of the bone is accompanied by a decrease in the quantity of vascular supply, there is an increased possibility of infection. No treatment is indicated.

## QUESTIONS

64. Odontogenic myxoma, odontogenic fibroma, and adenoameloblastoma are differentiated radiographically by their classic radiographic signs.
    1. In all cases.
    2. Only in some cases.
    3. Only the fibroma has a characteristic radiographic appearance.
    4. Never reliably.

65. Aphthous ulcers are found on the
    1. gingiva
    2. mucosa
    3. Both
    4. Neither

66. Immediate antibiotic coverage is indicated for periodontal abscesses in children due to the high incidence of subsequent cellulitis.
    1. The statement is true, and the reason is true.
    2. The statement is true, but the reason is false.
    3. The statement is false, and the reason is false.
    4. The statement is false, but the reason is true.

67. A mucocele may be
    a. incised
    b. excised
    c. marsupialized
    1. a and b
    2. b and c
    3. All of the above
    4. None of the above

68. A 2½-year-old child has an acute oral infection characterized by small reddish yellow vesicles in the buccal mucosa and on the hard palate. The temperature is 102° F, the mouth is sore, and the child will not eat or drink. The condition described is
    1. candidiasis
    2. infantile impetigo
    3. acute herpetic stomatitis
    4. acute streptococcal infection
    5. acute necrotizing ulcerative gingivitis

69. In a patient with a suspected case of leukemia and a badly infected primary tooth, the procedure of choice would be to
    1. administer antibiotics and refer the patient to a physician
    2. consult with a physician before determining the course of action
    3. obtain a blood count and admit the child to a hospital for extraction
    4. provide palliative treatment only
    5. extract the tooth under local anesthetic and refer the patient to a physician

70. If one single factor could be designated as contributing most to the development of simple gingivitis in children, it would be
    1. high fever
    2. poor oral hygiene
    3. pernicious oral habits
    4. physical nature of food ingested

71. With periodontitis there is an increase in sulcus depth due to the apical migration of the attachment epithelium.
    1. The pocket formed is a pseudopocket.
    2. The pocket formed is a true pocket.
    3. There is no pocketing with the periodontitis.
    4. The entity described is periodontosis, not periodontitis.

72. For a patient with generalized acute herpetic stomatitis, a dentist should
    1. begin series of treatments with diluted chickenpox vaccines
    2. gently debride the mouth, sustain oral hygiene, and treat the elevated temperature
    3. immediately distinguish from acute necrotizing ulcerative gingivitis with bacterial cultures
    4. promptly prescribe 300,000 units of penicillin orally.

# REFERENCES

1. ACKERMAN J, PROFFIT WB: The characteristics of malocclusion: A modern approach to classification and diagnosis. Am J Ortho 56:443–454, 1969
2. ANAISE JZ: The toothbrush in plaque removal. J Dent Child 42:186–189, 1975
3. ANDREASEN JO: Traumatic Injuries of the Teeth. St. Louis, CV Mosby, 1972
4. BAER PN, BENJAMIN SD: Periodontal Disease in Children and Adolescents. Philadelphia, JB Lippincott, 1974
5. BASHKAR SN (ed): Orban's Oral Histology and Embryology, St. Louis, 8th ed. CV Mosby, 1976
6. BASHKAR SN: Synopsis of Oral Pathology, 4th ed. St. Louis, CV Mosby, 1973
7. CHAMBERS D: Managing the anxieties of the young dental patient. J Dent Child 37:363–373, 1970
8. CRAIG W: Hand over mouth technique. J Dent Child 38:387–389, 1971
9. FINN SB: Clinical Pedodontics, 4th ed. Philadelphia, WB Saunders, 1973
10. FRANKL SN: Pulp therapy in pedodontics. In Siskin M (ed.) The Biology of the Human Pulp. St. Louis. CV Mosby, 1973, pp. 355–371
11. GESSELL A, ILG F: Infant and Child in the Culture of Today. New York, Harper and Brothers, 1943
12. GRABER TM: Orthodontics: Principles and Practice. 3rd ed, Philadelphia, WB Saunders, 1969
13. HICKS EP: Treatment planning for the distal shoe space maintainer. Dent Clin N Am 17:135–150, 1973
14. HYMES JL: Early childhood. Children 7:111, 1960
15. KENNEDY DB: Pediatric operative dentistry, Dental Practitioner Handbook #21, Bristol, John Wright and Sons, 1976
16. LAW DB, LEWIS TM, DAVIS JB: An Atlas of Pedodontics. Philadelphia, WB Saunders, 1969
17. LEVITAS TC: HOME—Hand over mouth exercise. J Dent Child 41:178–182, 1974
18. LEWIS J: The Effect of Duration and Technique of Toothbrushing on Oral Hygiene of Third Grade Students. Thesis, Chapel Hill N.C. University of North Carolina, 1973
19. MCDONALD RE: Dentistry for the Child and Adolescent. 2nd ed, St. Louis, CV Mosby, 1974
20. MEICHER AH, BEERTSEN W: The physiology of tooth eruption. In McNamera JA (ed): The Biology of Occlusal Development. Center for Human Growth and Development. Craniofacial Growth Series, 7:1–24, 1977.
21. NIZEL AE: Nutrition in Preventive Dentistry: Science and Practice. Philadelphia, WB Saunders, 1972
22. OWEN DG: The incidence and nature of space closure following the premature extraction of deciduous teeth: A literature survey. Am J Orthodont 59:37–49, 1971
23. PROFFIT WR, BENNETT C: Space maintenance, serial extraction and the general practitioner. J Am Dent Assoc 74:411–417, 1967
24. RUSHTON M: A new form of dental dysplasia: Shell teeth. Oral Surg., Oral Med., Oral Path 7:543–547, 1954
25. SANGNES G: Effectiveness of vertical and horizontal toothbrushing techniques in the removal of plaque: Comparison of brushing by six-year-old children and their parents. J Dent Child 41:119–123, 1974
26. SCHOUR I, MASSLER M: Studies in tooth development: The growth pattern of human teeth, Part I. J Am Dent Assn 27:1778–1873, 1940
27. SCOPP IW: Oral Medicine. St. Louis, CV Mosby, 1973
38. SHAFER WG, HINE MK, LEVY BM: A Textbook of Oral Pathology, 3rd ed. Philadelphia, WB Saunders, 1974
29. SILVERSTONE LM, DOGAN IL (ed): Proceedings of an International Symposium on the Acid–Etch Technique. St. Paul, North Central Pub., 1975
30. SPOUGE JD: Oral Pathology. St. Louis, CV Mosby, 1973
31. SWEENEY EA: Epidemiology of Oral Disease. In Sweeney EA (ed.) The Food That Stays: An Update on Nutrition, Diet, Sugar and Caries. New York, Medcom, 1977
32. TERHUNE JA: Predicting the readiness of elementary school children to learn an effective dental flossing technique. J Am Dent Assn 86:1332–1336, 1973
33. TINANOFF N, WEI SHY, PARKINS FM: Effect of a pumice prophylaxis on fluoride uptake of tooth enamel. J Am Dent Assn 88:384–389, 1974
34. GUSTAFSSON BE, QUENSEL CE, LONKE L, LUNDQUIST C, GRAHNEN H, BONOW BE, KRASSE B: The Vipeholm dental caries study: Effect of different levels of carbohydrate intakes on caries activity in 436 individuals observed for five years. Acta Odont Scand 11:232, 1954
35. WRIGHT EZ: Behavior Management in Dentistry for Children. Philadelphia, WB Saunders, 1975

# ANSWER KEY

| | | | |
|---|---|---|---|
| 1. 4 | 19. 4 | 37. 2 | 55. 1 |
| 2. 3 | 20. 2 | 38. 4 | 56. 1 |
| 3. 3 | 21. 3 | 39. 4 | 57. 4 |
| 4. 2 | 22. 1 | 40. 4 | 58. 4 |
| 5. 2 | 23. 3 | 41. 1 | 59. 4 |
| 6. 2 | 24. 3 | 42. 1 | 60. 1 |
| 7. 2 | 25. 4 | 43. 5 | 61. 5 |
| 8. 1 | 26. 4 | 44. 2 | 62. 1 |
| 9. 4 | 27. 1 | 45. 4 | 63. 2 |
| 10. 1 | 28. 7 | 46. 1 | 64. 4 |
| 11. 3 | 29. 4 | 47. 4 | 65. 2 |
| 12. 4 | 30. 4 | 48. 4 | 66. 3 |
| 13. 1 | 31. 2 | 49. 4 | 67. 2 |
| 14. 1 | 32. 3 | 50. 2 | 68. 3 |
| 15. 5 | 33. 1 | 51. 4 | 69. 2 |
| 16. 1 | 34. 3 | 52. 1 | 70. 2 |
| 17. 3 | 35. 4 | 53. 2 | 71. 2 |
| 18. 1 | 36. 2 | 54. 4 | 72. 2 |

# 8
# ORTHODONTICS

## Robert M. Little / Terry R. Wallen

## CRANIOFACIAL GROWTH AND DEVELOPMENT

### Definitions

**Growth:** an increase in size.

**Development:** the progress that any organism makes towards maturity. For example, the increase in height that a boy attains during puberty is considered growth; however, concomitant changes, such as the change of voice or the appearance of facial hair, may be considered development.

**Interstitial growth:** the growth of soft tissues. Interstitial growth involves expansive changes in the tissue components already present, i.e., cellular proliferation, enlargement of existing cells, or an increase in the material located between the cells. For example, a muscle cell may divide within the center of a mass of muscle and thus increase the total volume of that muscle.

**Appositional growth:** the essential mechanism for increasing bone size. It can only occur on inner or outer surfaces of the bone, since such hard tissues are not capable of expanding by growth within the center of the tissue.

**Endochondral bone growth:** lengthwise growth of long bones by deposition of bone at the epiphyseal junctions at their distal and proximal ends. This occurs by the proliferation of cartilage cells and the replacement of the older cartilage cells by new bone.

**Subperiosteal bone growth:** circumferential growth of long bones by subperiosteal surface addition. This type of growth may be considered appositional growth in that the overlying periosteal tissue produces cells which form layers of bone on the external surface of the shaft. Concomitant to this, there is resorption of the inner wall of the bone in the marrow cavity, which keeps the weight of the bone to a minimum without reducing its strength.

**Sutural bone growth:** appositional bone growth in which the bone is deposited upon the margins of adjoining bones.

**Endosteal bone growth:** appositional growth upon the various trabeculae within the body of the bone itself.

### Study of Craniofacial Growth

There are several methods of studying craniofacial growth (9).

**ANTHROPOMETRY.** The physical anthropologists started the metric study of the head of both living persons and specimens. Their techniques involve measurements between a series of selected landmarks which have been standardized and generally accepted.

**VITAL STAINING WITH ALIZARIN RED S.** Vital staining involves the injection into the living animal of dye which colors new bone that is growing at the time of injection. Bone that is not growing at the time of the injection remains unstained and comparatively white. Thus growth sites can be located. The use of several injections with a known period of time between them enables growth rates to be calculated.

Hunter (7) and Brash (2) pioneered the application of this technique in studying the growth sites of the craniofacial skeleton.

**RADIOISOTOPES.** The subject is injected with labeled salts (isotopes) which can be located within growing bones by means of Geiger counters or autoradiographic techniques. In the latter methods the bones or sections of them are placed against photographic emulsions which are exposed by emission of the radioactive salts.

**IMPLANT MARKERS.** Metallic markers inserted into a growing bone can provide a point, or points, from which to measure future growth relative to the markers' position as seen on radiographs (1).

**ROENTGENOGRAPHIC CEPHALOMETRY.** Historically cephalometric radiographs were developed as workers sought a method of applying the techniques of physical anthropologists to the use of radiographs in making serial measurements of the growing head. The first attempt to gain more information about skull morphology by means of radiograph was made by Paccini in 1922. The cephalostat, or cephalometer as it is known today, was developed simultaneously by Broadbent (3) in the United States and Hofrath (6) in Germany. Broadbent's cephalometric technique proved to be the most practical and even today is the most effective means of studying skull growth and dental position.

A technique of producing reproducible oriented head films (lateral, frontal, and oblique projections) is dependent upon a fixed source of x-rays, fixed head position, and fixed film position. All three factors must also be in a fixed relationship to each other. Studying the growth of children by means of oriented head films has many advantages. Both the cross-sectional and longitudinal methods of study may be employed. The same child may be studied over a long period of time by taking successive films. Bony landmarks may be accurately located and measured. Findings from head films may be correlated with other physical records of the same individual.

### Growth of the Cranial Bones

It was formerly believed that the cranium grew by surface apposition of bone upon its outer surface and resorption upon the inner surface. Little attention was focused upon the sutures as growth sites. The present concept of cranial growth, however, is that the tension produced by the enlarging brain tends to separate the bones of the cranial vault at their sutures, thereby stimulating sutural bone growth. As the brain enlarges and the various bones in the calvaria tend to separate, contact at the sutures is maintained by sutural growth at the free margins (4). Additionally, bone growth activity occurs on all periosteal and endosteal surfaces.

### Growth of the Facial Bones

Growth of the face (8) is rather generalized during the first 6 or 7 years of life. After that time localized areas of growth become predominant. Hence, by vital staining, it has been found that prior to 6 or 7 years of age there is a generalized staining of all bones of both the face and cranium. After this age generalized staining is no longer found; only the more active growth sites show evidence of the stain.

MAXILLARY GROWTH. Enlargement of the maxilla during the first 6 years of life occurs by generalized deposition of bone on all of its surfaces. Subsequent to this time there is still generalized bone deposition but at a much slower rate. During this latter period certain areas of the maxilla grow at a more rapid rate, which accounts for alterations in the proportions of the component parts of the bone itself and changes in the interrelationship of facial bones concomitant with the overall enlargement of the craniofacial complex. These active growth sites of the maxilla are

1. the maxillary tuberosity areas
2. the various sutures that join the maxilla to the rest of the facial skeleton
3. the alveolar process
4. surface apposition on the oral surface of the palatal shelves.

The maxillary sinus starts to develop sometime during the first several years of life and continues to enlarge through remodeling resorption until it reaches its adult size and configuration. In addition, other areas of the maxilla undergo remodeling resorption during the developmental process. This, together with the more rapid growth at some sites, accounts for the change in proportion which can be observed when the younger maxilla is compared with its adult form.

MANDIBULAR GROWTH. The mandible also increases in size from birth until 6–7 years of age by generalized deposition of all surfaces of the bone. Like that of the maxilla, the rate of growth is greater at several localized areas, which causes a change in mandibular proportions before and after 6–7 years of age. After 6–7 years of age local sites of growth continue to enlarge the total mandibular form, while a marked reduction occurs in the rate of generalized appositional growth. The localized active growth areas of the mandible which are prolific throughout its developmental process are

1. the posterior border of the ramus
2. the mandibular condyle and coronoid process
3. the alveolar process

Remodeling resorption occurs on the anterior border of the ramus and certain other areas of the mandible which also contributes to the change in proportions of the mandibular form from birth to maturation.

### Facial Growth in the Three Planes of Space

ANTEROPOSTERIOR GROWTH OF THE FACE. The upper face or maxilla grows by appositional bone growth as well as endosteal bone growth in the tuberosity region of the maxilla. Growth in this region produces a forward positioning of the maxilla relative to the cranial base. Growth occurs at the transverse palatal suture both on the palatine and the maxillary side of the suture (Fig. 8–1). This growth may be interpreted as an adjustment mechanism to keep the transverse palatal suture closed during the forward growth of the maxilla.

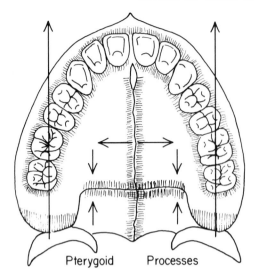

**FIG. 8-1.** Areas of appositional bone growth important during growth of the maxilla in both transverse and anteroposterior planes of space (**shading**). The pterygoid processes are relatively stable anteroposteriorly during growth of the face relative to the cranium.

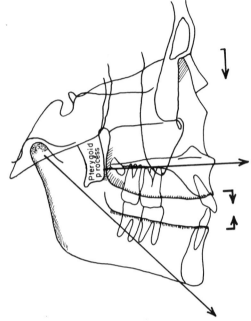

**FIG. 8-3.** Areas of active growth important for vertical and anteroposterior facial development (**shading**).

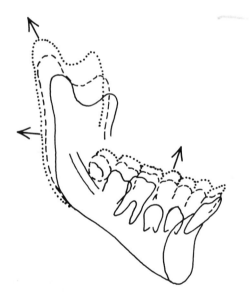

**FIG. 8-2.** Growth mechanism of the lower face or mandible, illustrating appositional growth at the posterior border of the ramus and alveolar margin, as well as endochondral growth of the condyle. Remodeling resorption occurs on the anterior border of the ramus.

The growth of the lower face or mandible in an anteroposterior direction is achieved by deposition of bone at the head of the condyle, which is an endochondral type of bone formation. It is covered by a cap of cartilage which continually proliferates and increases the length of the head and neck of the condyle throughout the growth of the mandible. Appositional growth on the posterior border of the ramus of the mandible also helps to increase the overall length of the mandible (Fig. 8–2).

**VERTICAL GROWTH OF THE FACE.** Growth of the frontonasal processes of the maxilla produces a downward positioning of these bones relative to the anterior cranial base. The height of the alveolar process of both the maxilla and mandible continues to increase concomitant with tooth eruption throughout the growth period from birth to maturation. The condylar growth of the mandible adds to the vertical height of the mandible as well as to the total increase of face height relative to the cranial base (Fig. 8–3).

**LATERAL GROWTH OF THE FACE.** The maxilla increases in width primarily through growth at the midsagittal suture. The lateral halves of the mandible diverge in a lateral direction, producing an increased interramus distance as the mandible enlarges in a posterior direction.

QUESTIONS

1. By what mechanism does the mandibular condyle grow?
   1. Subperiosteal surface addition
   2. Endosteal bone growth
   3. Appositional growth
   4. Endochondral borne formation

The mandibular condyle grows by endochondral bone formation. The head of the mandibular condyle is covered by a cap of cartilage which continually proliferates and increases the length of the head and neck of the condyle throughout the growth of the mandible.

2. By what mechanism does the mandible grow downward and forward as viewed on successive superimposed head films?
   1. Growth of the alveolar process
   2. Condylar growth
   3. Growth of the frontonasal process
   4. Sutural growth

The growth of the lower face or mandible in an anteroposterior direction is achieved by deposition of bone at the head of the condyle which is an endochondral type of bone formation. The condylar growth of the mandible also adds to the vertical height of the mandible as well as to the total increase of face height relative to the cranial base.

3. What are the active growth sites of the mandible?
   1. Posterior border of the ramus
   2. Condyle, coronoid process
   3. Alveolar process
   4. All of the above.

The localized active growth areas of the mandible which are prolific throughout its developmental process are the posterior border of the ramus and the summit of the ramus, which consists of the mandibular condyle and coronoid process. Concomitant with tooth eruption the alveolar process increases in height throughout the entire growth period.

4. According to current concepts of mandibular growth, what is the mechanism of action of the following mandibular expansion appliance?
   1. Arch expansion by dental tipping
   2. Arch expansion by widening of the body of the mandible
   3. A combination of 1 and 2
   4. Skeletal expansion of the midsymphysis suture

In contrast to sutural growth which contributes to lateral growth of the maxilla, the mandible increases in width as the ramus grows vertically and posteriorly thereby increasing intercondylar width. There is no mechanism to allow the mandible to expand skeletally in response to the appliance illustrated above, and therefore any changes would be dental in origin.

5. What are the active growth sites of the maxilla?
   1. Maxillary tuberosity areas
   2. Frontonasal process
   3. Midpalatal and transpalatal suture
   4. All of the above

The localized active growth sites of the maxilla are the maxillary tuberosity areas, and the various sutures that connect the maxilla to the rest of the craniofacial complex. Concomitant with the eruption of teeth there is an increase in height of the alveolar process throughout the entire developmental process.

6. How does the maxilla grow in width?
   1. Appositional bone growth
   2. Endochondral bone growth
   3. Endosteal bone growth
   4. Sutural growth

The maxilla increases in width primarily through growth at the mid-sagittal suture. Growth also occurs on the transverse palatal suture, both on the palatine as well as the maxillary side of the suture.

7. In assessing overall facial growth, what are important considerations in treatment planning?
   1. Amount of growth to be expected
   2. Direction of growth expected
   3. General physical development
   4. All of the above

It is important to identify the amount of growth, the direction of growth, and the timing of growth, particularly when planning treatment for the Class II division I malocclusion.

8. What are the typical facial profile changes that occur during the transition from childhood to adulthood?

   1. The profile remains essentially constant.
   2. As the face enlarges, there is a general accentuation of lips relative to nose and chin structures.
   3. Flattening of the profile typically occurs with maturation.
   4. The face elongates, narrows, and thins with time.

There is a general trend toward decreasing lip convexity concomitant with nose and chin development and overall vertical growth of the face resulting in a flatter facial profile.

## ORTHODONTIC TOOTH MOVEMENT

### Biology of Tooth Movement

THE PERIODONTAL LIGAMENT.    The periodontal ligament is composed primarily of connective tissue fibers made of collagen. Bundles of fibers connect the cementum of teeth to the bone of the alveolus and the gingiva. Between the fibers is a meshwork of blood and lymph vessels, as well as fibroblasts. The periodontal fibers which are attached to, and continued in, the alveolus are known as Sharpey's fibers. Between the cementum and the alveolus, bundles of fibers are intermeshed at the center of the periodontal membrane where they form the intermediate plexus. The intermediate plexus is believed to be an adjustment mechanism, allowing rearrangement of the periodontal fibers during tooth movement (16).

RESPONSE TO ORTHODONTIC FORCES.    When a force is applied to the crown of a tooth, there are two reactions at the level of the root. On the side to which the force is applied, tension is created in the periodontal ligament. Apically on the same side there is a zone of pressure in the opposite direction. On the opposite side pressure is present gingivally; tension, apically.

In tension areas new bone and cementum are laid down, whereas in pressure areas bone is resorbed. A light force compresses the periodontal membrane, stimulating the formation of osteoclasts (bone removers) and bone resorption in the areas of pressure. Periodontal fibers are stretched in the areas under tension, partly unraveling in the intermediate zone, and osteoblasts (bone builders) form in the periodontal membrane. If the force greatly exceeds physiologic limits, the periodontal membrane is crushed on the pressure side, blood vessels are occluded, and necrosis occurs. With necrosis and stasis of fluids, activity at the pressure site is minimal. Further up the root, away from the actual pressure site, blood supply is increased and osteoclasts (bone removers) proliferate. The osteoclasts infiltrate the alveolar wall behind the necrotic pressure site to remove the bone and dead cells. This phenomenon is known as undermining resorption. If heavy forces are continuous and active over a distance beyond the thickness of the periodontal membrane, chances of root resorption are increased appreciably (12).

### General Principles of Tooth Movement

#### TYPES OF TOOTH MOVEMENT

*Tipping.* Tipping is an alteration in the axial inclination of a tooth. It may be due to the movement of the crown or of the root. The application of an orthodontic force in terms of direction, magnitude, and duration alters the degree of crown versus root movement. Tipping movements are primarily directed in a labiolingual or a mesiodistal direction.

*Torque.* An alteration in root angulation with the objective being to maintain crown position is called torque. Torque changes are primarily directed at moving incisor roots labially or lingually or moving molar roots buccally or lingually. The major difference from simple tipping is that force must be applied at two different points on the crown.

*Translation.* The two basic types of tooth translation are horizontal and vertical. The objective of a horizontal translation is to move a tooth while maintaining the axial inclination of that tooth. The objective of a vertical translation is to produce either extrusion or intrusion of a particular tooth or segment of teeth.

*Combinations.* In actual practice torque tipping and translation forces are usually applied simultaneously in orthodontics.

#### TYPES OF ANCHORAGE.
Depending on how orthodontic forces are applied, different teeth have different resistance values to tooth movement. The term anchorage refers to the nature and degree of resistance to displacement offered by a tooth, group of teeth, or anatomic unit when used for the purpose of effecting tooth movement. There are a number of different types of anchorage (13).

**Cervical anchorage:** anchorage in which the back of the neck is used for resistance by means of a cervical headgear.

**Extraoral anchorage:** anchorage in which the resistance unit is outside the oral cavity, such as cranial, occipital, or cervical anchorage (headgear).

**Intermaxillary anchorage:** anchorage in which the units in one jaw are used to effect tooth movement in the other jaw.

**Intramaxillary anchorage:** anchorage in which the resistance units are all situated within the same jaw.

**Intraoral anchorage:** anchorage in which the resistance units are all located within the oral cavity.

**Multiple anchorage (reinforced anchorage):** anchorage in which more than one type of resistance unit is utilized.

**Occipital anchorage:** anchorage in which the top and back of the head are used for resistance by means of a headgear.

**Reciprocal anchorage:** anchorage in which the movement of one or more dental units is balanced against the movement of one or more opposing dental units.

**Simple anchorage:** dental anchorage in which the resistance to the movement of one or more dental units comes solely from the resistance of the anchorage unit to tipping movement.

**Stationary anchorage:** dental anchorage in which the resistance to the movement of one or more dental units comes from the resistance of the anchorage unit to bodily movement.

#### QUESTIONS

9. What is the response of alveolar bone to orthodontic forces?
   1. Tooth movement stimulates jaw growth, thereby allowing arch expansion.
   2. Bone is deposited at pressure sites and resorbed at tension sites.
   3. Bone is deposited at tension sites and resorbed at pressure sites.
   4. Alveolar bone does not respond to orthodontic forces unless the individual is growing.

Forces applied to a tooth are transmitted to the supporting bone via the periodontal ligament. Pressure and tension are produced resulting in bone resorption at pressure sites and bone deposition at tension sites.

10. Changes in the pressure side of the alveolar crest when orthodontic forces exceed physiologic limits are called
    1. direct resorption
    2. undermining resorption

3. osteoblastic activity
4. All of the above

Undermining resorption is a type of bone resorption which occurs when forces are heavy enough to produce a cell-free zone in the compressed periodontal membrane.

11. What are some of the potential negative tissue responses to heavy forces?
    1. Root resorption
    2. Excessive tooth mobility
    3. Discomfort
    4. All of the above

Orthodontic forces vary from a few grams to several pounds. Fixed orthodontic appliances are capable of moving teeth rapidly over great distances and therefore careful control of such variables as direction, magnitude, and continuity is of paramount importance to minimize negative tissue responses.

12. An example of simple anchorage is
    1. diastema closure by elastic traction, tipping the crowns together
    2. extraoral force
    3. diastema closure by bodily movement of incisors
    4. intraarch elastics

Simple anchorage applies to the situation where resistance of the anchorage unit to tipping is utilized to move another tooth or teeth.

13. An example of extraoral anchorage is
    1. chin cup
    2. cervical headgear
    3. occipital headgear
    4. All of the above

Extraoral anchorage makes use of cranial, occipital, cervical, or mandibular areas to act as resistance units for tooth movement. Extraoral anchorage is often employed in the correction of maxillary and mandibular protrusions.

14. Which of the following is not an example of intermaxillary anchorage?
    1. Criss-cross elastics to correct crossbites
    2. Class II elastics between maxillary incisors and mandibular molars
    3. Baker anchorage
    4. Retraction of maxillary incisors by tipping them lingually, using maxillary molars as anchorage

The case of retracting maxillary incisors using the molars as an anchorage unit is a form of reciprocal anchorage.

15. Given an orthodontic force of 30 grams applied in a lingual direction to the crown of a maxillary central incisor (illustrated below), the areas of bone resorption or osteoclastic activity are
    1. A and B
    2. D and E
    3. A and E
    4. A, B, D, and E

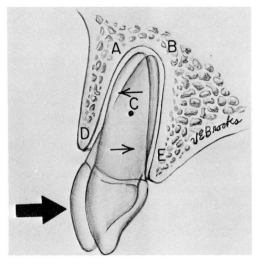

16. The areas of bone deposition or osteoblastic activity in the above illustration are
    1. A and B
    2. B and D
    3. A and E
    4. A, B, D, and E

The above illustration is an example of a simple tipping which takes place when force is applied to the crown so that the tooth is free to tip. A force applied in this way causes the tooth to pivot about a point (labeled C) resulting in areas of pressure or osteoclastic activity, (areas labeled A and E), and areas of tension or osteoblastic activity (areas labeled B and D).

17. The type of anchorage being used in the illustration below is
    1. simple anchorage
    2. reciprocal anchorage
    3. intraoral anchorage
    4. intermaxillary anchorage
    5. All of the above

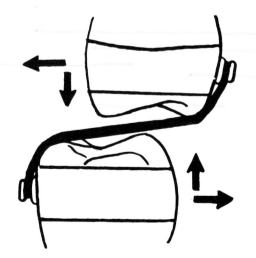

The use of criss-cross elastics to correct a molar cross-bite is an example of all of the above concepts of orthodontic anchorage.

## CLASSIFICATION OF MALOCCLUSION

### Anteroposterior Classification

#### DENTAL RELATIONSHIPS (CLINICAL AND CAST DATA)

*Angle's Classification of Malocclusion.* There are so many varieties of tooth malpositions that description and discussion of malocclusion are quite complicated. To simplify the study of these myriad types of dental abnormalities, it is obviously desirable to group them according to their similarities. The most commonly used categorization of malocclusion was introduced by Angle in 1889. Although many malocclusions do not fit neatly into Angle's system, it does give the practitioner a starting point in analyzing and describing a case.

The basis of Angle's classification was his hypothesis that the maxillary first molar is the "key to occlusion"—he felt that Nature rarely erred in its placement. The way the upper and lower molars occlude in an anterior–posterior direction was the basis of the system. The Angle classification does not describe normal or ideal occlusion, only malocclusion; it does not describe vertical or lateral discrepancies, only mesiodistal. Angle assumed that all permanent teeth are present and that the patient is biting in a position of normal maximum occlusal contact or centric occlusion. The Angle classification does not describe the deciduous or mixed dentition (it is commonly used to classify the preadult dentition even though Angle did not describe this use), nor does it describe the discrepancies between centric relation and centric occlusion.

All types of malocclusion are grouped into three classes based on the position of the maxillary to the mandibular first permanent molars.

*Class I (Neutroclusion).* Class I malocclusion is characterized by a normal mesiodistal relationship of the jaws and dental arches. The mesiobuccal cusp of the upper first molar occludes in the mesiobuccal groove of the lower first molar. Class I cases are generally dental dysplasias; these patients have normal muscle function and usually well-balanced faces. Certainly a small percentage of patients with Class I molar position has protrusive or retrusive upper and lower jaws and lips, but most Class I types are essentially dental malalignments, i.e., crowding or spacing within a normal jaw and face (Fig. 8–4). Approximately 50%–55% of the U.S. child and adolescent population have a Class I molar position; however, this figure includes those with normal or ideal occlusion as well as Class I malocclusion. There is considerable racial variation in categorizing malocclusion. For example, the percentage of whites in this category is estimated at 50%–55% while the figure for blacks is 60%–75% (11, 12).

*Class II (Distoclusion).* Class II malocclusion is characterized by the lower first molar being positioned more than one-half cusp distal from the normal location. The mesiobuccal cusp of the maxillary first molar articulates more than one-half cusp mesial to the buccal groove of the lower first molar. Approximately 30%–35% of the U.S. population are in this category. The percentage of blacks in this category is considerably lower, being below 20% (11, 12).

This major class is divided into two subgroups labeled division 1 and division 2. In Class II division 1 types (Fig. 8–5) the following is usually noted:

**FIG. 8–4.** Typical Class I malocclusion. A. Facial profile. B. Anterior view. C. Lateral view.

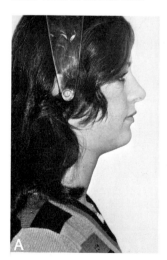
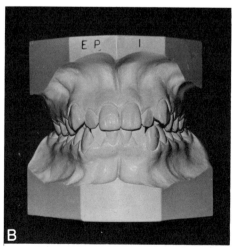
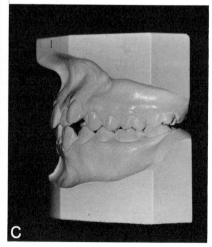

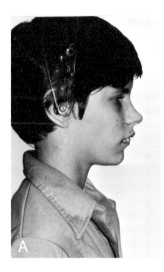
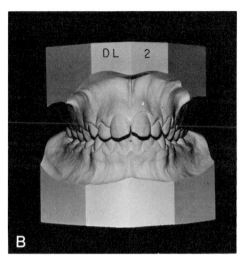
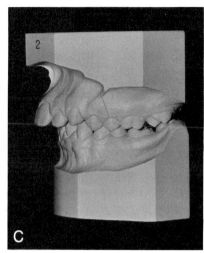

**FIG. 8–5.** Typical Class II division I malocclusion. A. Facial profile. B. Anterior view. C. Lateral view.

1. Upper anteriors protrude ahead of lower anteriors.
2. The lower incisors often overerupt, causing a deep overbite
3. The palate is often narrow and V shaped.
4. The Curve of Spee is usually quite steep.
5. The face is usually in poor balance, with protruding upper lip and/or the appearance of a recessive lower jaw and chin.

In Class II division 2 types (Fig. 8–6) the molars are also in Class II position, but the upper anteriors are not usually protrusive. The more common picture is as follows:

**FIG. 8–6.** Typical Class II division 2 malocclusion. A. Facial profile. B. Anterior view. C. Lateral view.

1. Upright or retruded upper central incisors with labially tipped upper lateral incisors which may even overlap the central incisors.
2. The overbite is deep; the palate is normal to wide.
3. The facial profile is usually quite acceptable, often with a rather prominent chin.

*Class III (Mesioclusion).* Class III malocclusion is characterized by the mesiobuccal cusp of the maxillary first molar occluding more than one-half cusp distal to the buccal groove of the mandibular first molar (Fig. 8–7). Approximately 10%–15% of the U.S. population are in this category, with the percentage being slightly higher for blacks than it is for whites (11, 12). In this major class the following usually occurs:

1. The classic Class III case has mandibular incisors in total crossbite and labial to the maxillary incisors.

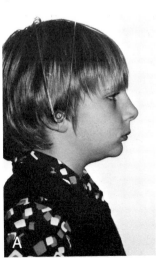
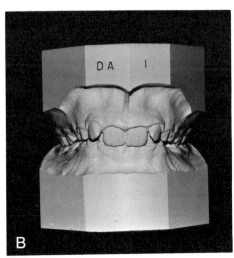
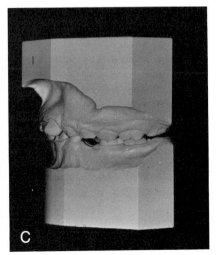

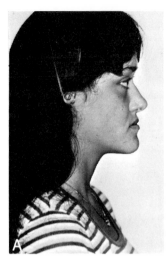
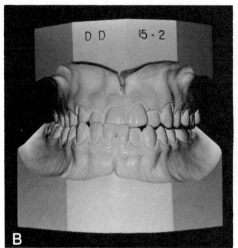
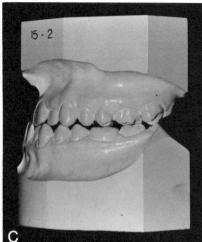

**FIG. 8–7.** Typical Class III malocclusion. A. Facial profile. B. Anterior view. C. Lateral view.

However, a Class III molar relationship can exist without anterior crossbite.
2. In most cases the lower incisors are inclined lingually despite the crossbite.
3. Facial balance is usually poor with a rather prominent mandible or retrusive maxilla.

*Subdivisions.* Angle noted that occasionally a patient had a Class I molar relation on one side and a Class II on the other (Fig. 8–8). This asymmetric pattern could occasionally be seen with a Class III molar position on one side and Class I on the other. Asymmetric cases of these types were labeled subdivisions which

Angle felt usually demonstrated the normal characteristics of the Class II or Class III side. The following are possible subdivision varieties.

Class II division 1 subdivision (Class II one side, Class I other side with division 1 anterior pattern)
Class II division 2 subdivision (Class II one side, Class I other side with division 2 anterior pattern)
Class II subdivision (Class III one side, Class I other side)

*Overjet.* Measuring parallel to the occlusal plane, the most common measure of maxillary to mandibular incisor protrusion is the millimeter displacement of upper incisors relative to mandibular incisors. The measurement is (+) if the maxillary teeth are forward of the mandibular and (−) if the lower teeth are forward. It is estimated that 80%–85% of children and adoles-

**FIG. 8–8.** Class II division I subdivision malocclusion. A. Class II side. B. Anterior view. C. Class I side.

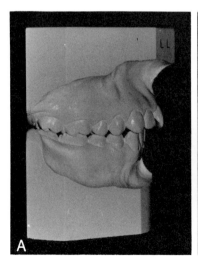
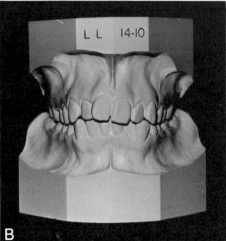
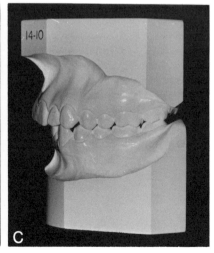

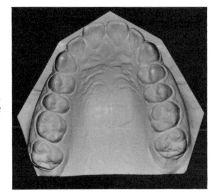
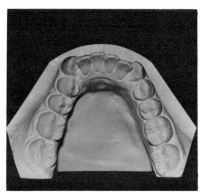

**FIG. 8-9.** Trimming the rear of the casts perpendicular to the midpalatal raphe allows assessment of buccal segment anteroposterior asymmetry. Note the more anterior position of the maxillary and mandibular left segments.

cents have a positive overjet from 0–5 mm. Approximately 15%–20% have more extreme maxillary incisor overjet, while negative overjet occurs in 1%–2.5% of U.S. children and adolescents, with the percentage for blacks being somewhat higher, 3%–5% (11,12).

*Centric Relation vs. Centric Occlusion.* Any anteroposterior difference between centric relation and centricocclusion must be noted when describing overjet and Angle class, since evaluation of such a discrepancy is an integral part of a thorough diagnosis.

*Asymmetry.* Casts trimmed so that the posterior surfaces are perpendicular to the maxillary midpalatal raphe allow evaluation of symmetry. Viewed from the occlusal, anteroposterior asymmetry can be noted (Fig. 8–9).

#### SKELETAL–FACIAL–DENTAL RELATIONSHIPS

*Cephalometry.* Cephalometric radiography is a standardized technique of studying the skull by means of oriented head radiographs. The apparatus orients the patients at a given target-to-film distance (5 ft) with the film and patient midsaggital plane perpendicular to the central beam (Fig. 8–10). The design of the head holder allows for fairly accurate positioning of the head so that serial radiographs of the same patient can be compared. Most cephalometric analyses are made from tracings of the cephalogram rather than directly from the film (Fig. 8–11).

*Anteroposterior Analysis of Maxilla and Mandible Position.* Pinpointing whether growth of the maxilla and mandible has been insufficient or excessive is the first step in the assessment of a cephalometric radiograph. For example, a Class II case could result from 1) excess forward growth of the upper jaw (protrusive maxilla), 2) lack of adequate forward growth of the

**FIG. 8-10.** Cephalometric apparatus.

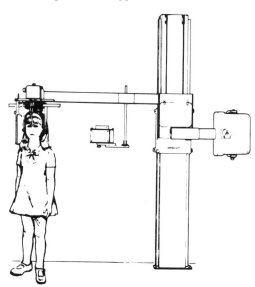

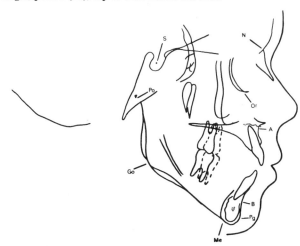

**FIG. 8-11.** Cephalometric tracing and common landmarks. Midsagittal landmarks: sella (**S**), center of hypophyseal fossa; (**N**), junction of frontal and nasal bones; A point (**A**), innermost point of maxillary alveolus; B point (**B**), innermost point of mandibular anterior alveolus; pogonion (**P_g**), most anterior chin point; menton (**Me**), lowest point on the symphysis. Bilateral landmarks: orbitale (**Or**), lowest point of the orbits; gonion (**Go**), middle of mandibular angle; porion (**Po**), top of head holder ear rods.

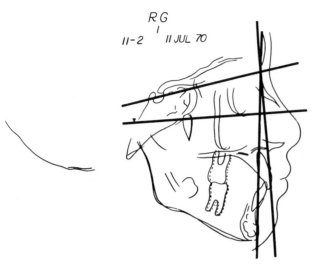

**FIG. 8–12.** Cephalometric tracing and common reference planes.

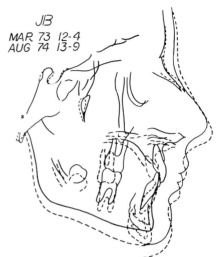

**FIG. 8–13.** Serial cephalometric superimposition.

lower jaw (retrusive mandible), or 3) a combination of these factors. A Class III case could result from a protrusive mandible, retrusive maxilla, or a combination of these factors.

Numerous methods have been proposed to measure the anteroposterior position of the maxilla and mandible. The cephalometric plane sella–nasion (S–N) represents a relatively stable anatomic structure known as the anterior cranial base. Angular measurements such as S–N–A and S–N–B when compared to known cephalometric norms, can identify areas that deviate from normal. The Frankfort Horizontal line, a line from porion to orbitale, can be used to measure linear or angular dimensions in the same manner. A great variety of linear, angular, and archial methods have been proposed in the literature to assess maxilla to mandible, maxilla to cranium, mandible to cranium, chin dimension, and facial profile (Fig. 8–12) (13).

All of these measurements are designed to assess the patient at one moment in time. Treatment and growth effects can be further assessed by superimposition of serial tracings (Fig. 8–13).

***Anteroposterior Analysis of the Dentition.*** Clinical and dental cast assessment of incisor and molar anteroposterior position should be compared with the cephalometric tracing to note centric relation–occlusion errors in either dental cast preparation or mandible position during exposure of the head film. The cephalometric radiograph offers the opportunity to examine the relative spatial position of the most prominent maxillary and mandibular incisors. Examination of various incisor angular and linear relationships to their

respective bones or to cranial landmarks and planes can help to identify any deviation from normal standards. Serial evaluation of the dentition by superimposition of subsequent tracings orienting on the maxilla for maxillary teeth and on the mandible for mandibular teeth provides further insights to growth, eruption, treatment effects, and posttreatment change (Fig. 8–14).

***Anteroposterior Analysis of the Facial Profile.*** A thorough assessment of the profile is a necessary step in formulating a comprehensive diagnosis. Any possible treatment decision must be weighed against the potential improvement or deleterious effect on the profile. A clinical or cephalometric appraisal of the profile should, at the very least, answer the following questions:

1. Is the soft tissue chin relative to the rest of the profile prognathic (prominent), mesognathic (normal or straight profile), or retrognathic (recessive)?
2. Do the lips appear convex, straight, or concave in relation to the nose and chin?
3. Are the upper and lower lips thick, normal, or thin? Do they appear short to the extent that incisor teeth could not be covered even if the teeth were less prominent? At rest, are the lips competent or incompetent (do they touch or not)?
4. Does the nose appear unusually prominent or small relative to the patient's developmental age? How do the parents and siblings compare?
5. Is there evidence of facial muscle strain or flaccidity? Does the muscle activity during swallowing appear to be related to the malocclusion?
6. Does the face appear unusually long or short?
7. Does the profile assessment consider racial, ethnic,

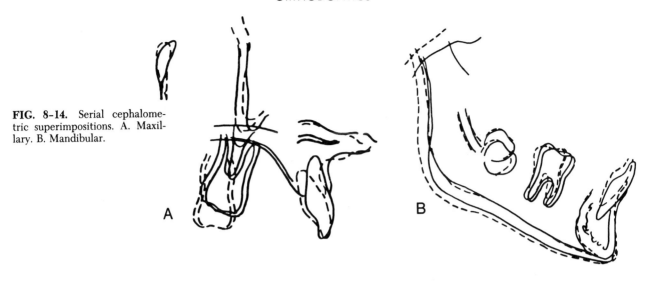

**FIG. 8-14.** Serial cephalometric superimpositions. A. Maxillary. B. Mandibular.

and familial characteristics? Would it be appropriate to try and influence the facial profile pattern?

## Vertical Classification

### DENTAL RELATIONSHIPS (CLINICAL AND CAST DATA)

***Vertical Analysis of the Anterior Dentition.*** Overbite is a vertical measure of the overlap of the upper incisors to the lower incisors. One method of expressing overbite is the number of millimeters of overlap that can be measured on casts when the ruler is held perpendicular to the occlusal plane (plane bisecting the first molar and incisor overbite). This value is (+) if there is overlap and (−) if there is no overlap of the incisors. Percent overlap is an alternative description method. Frequently the term "deep overbite" is used to describe a marked amount of overlap, such as when the lower incisors touch either the palate or lingual surfaces of the upper incisors. "Open bite" describes any case in which the lower incisors are not in contact with the palate or upper dentition; an open bite can range from minimal space to an extreme opening often associated with a tongue thrust or digit-sucking habit (Fig. 8–15).

In the U.S. population ages 6–17 it is estimated that approximately 5%–6% have an open bite, while 45%–50% have a 0–3 mm overbite, which is considered normal. There is considerable racial variation. Black children show a trend toward more open bites, 16% for blacks compared to 4% for whites. Conversely, there is a much higher incidence of extreme overbite in white children, 8%–12% for white and 1% for black children (11, 12).

***Vertical Analysis of the Posterior Dentition.*** When any opposing posterior teeth are not in contact

when the patient is in centric occlusion, open bite describes the condition, usually with the number of millimeters specified. In centric occlusion each tooth is either in occlusion or displays an open bite.

### SKELETAL–FACIAL–DENTAL RELATIONSHIPS

***Vertical Analysis of Skeletal Position.*** Several cephalometric analyses have been proposed to assess the proportionality between and the relative cant of skeletal–dental planes, including the S–N, Frankfort, palatal, occlusal, and mandibular planes. Proportions between upper and lower face can be measured in the anterior face, for example, between nasion, the palate, and menton or in the posterior face between sella, articulare, and gonion. Ratios illustrate areas of deviation from the norm. Study of the cant of various planes locates morphologic deviation and further locates the area of disproportion. Deviation from the norm of any one or several planes can signal a poorer prognosis for correction (Fig 8–16).

***Vertical Analysis of Dental Position.*** The millimeter overlap (overbite) of the incisors or lack of overlap (open bite) can be measured from the cephalometric tracing and compared to clinical and cast data. Incisor overbite or open bite should also be compared to the cant of planes and vertical skeletal proportions. In general the more skeletal in nature the deviation, the poorer the prognosis for long-term success in correction.

***Vertical Analysis of Facial Profile.*** The clinician treating malocclusion must consider vertical facial balance by assessing the proportionality between forehead, nose, lips, and chin. Lip length must be considered both at rest and during function since lip coverage of the dentition is an important aspect of planning the

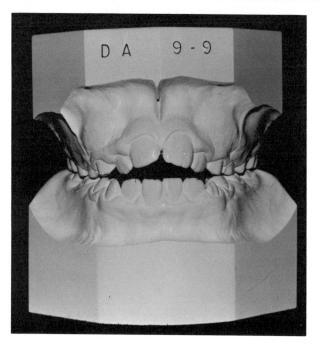

**FIG. 8-15.** Anterior open bite malocclusion associated with a thumb-sucking habit.

final vertical position of incisors. In certain instances the clinician cannot improve on what exists but can at least design appropriate therapy to prevent further detrimental vertical facial changes (Fig. 8–17).

## Transverse Classification

**DENTAL RELATIONSHIPS (CLINICAL AND CAST DATA)**
*Midlines.* Observing the upper and lower dental midlines of the casts alone does not relate the dentition to the face. The patient must be carefully examined to assess both upper and lower dental midlines relative to an estimated midsagittal facial vertical line. Although viewing the casts from the occlusal direction may allow identification of midline deviation relative to the palatal raphe and incisive papilla, assessment relative to the nose and lips is also necessary. To plan proper treatment for a midline correction, the number of millimeters from the facial vertical plane should be measured for both the upper and lower midlines, not just the total number of millimeters that the two midlines deviate from each other. Any lateral shift of the mandible from centric relation to centric occlusion must be noted as well.

*Asymmetry.* Viewing the casts from the occlusal direction, asymmetry involving one or several teeth can be measured by determining the number of millimeters that each tooth is located from the midpalatal raphe. If the posterior surfaces of the casts are trimmed perpendicular to this line, the lower cast can be viewed from the occlusal direction and deviation from normal arch form noted (Fig. 8–18). Posterior crossbites, buccolingual malposition of maxillary to mandibular teeth, should be noted in both centric relation and centric occlusion.

**SKELETAL–FACIAL–DENTAL RELATIONSHIPS.** Most modern cephalometric head holders can be rotated 90° so that the patient can face the film. Tracing the posterior–anterior radiograph allows transverse assessment of skeletal and dental midline asymmetry. Even though facial asymmetry should be evaluated clinically as a routine part of the patient evaluation, extreme deviation should be confirmed and measured with the posterior–anterior radiograph (Fig. 8–19).

## Perimeter Classification

**TRADITIONAL ARCH LENGTH ANALYSIS TECHNIQUES.** Nance proposed measuring arch length available on diagnostic casts as the distance of an even arc from the mesial of the first molar on one side to the same point on the opposite side (10). Arch length required for tooth alignment is the sum of the sizes of all erupted permanent teeth mesial to the first molars plus the sizes of unerupted teeth estimated from periapical radiographs. Any excess when comparing space available to space required is labeled leeway space (5, 9, 15).

Numerous other authors have advocated prediction formulas to compute the size of unerupted teeth. Unfortunately there is a fairly poor correlation between the size of erupted and unerupted teeth. To overcome this weakness at least partially Moyers suggests use of a probability chart which can be used to predict size at various levels of statistical confidence (98).

**ARCH PERIMETER CALCULATED BY SEGMENTS**
*Anterior Arch Perimeter (Central and Lateral Incisors).* Space available in the anterior arch can be determined by measuring each side from the midline to a point which represents the distal of the lateral incisor (Fig. 8–20A). Space required can be determined by measuring the mesiodistal dimension of each incisor from the diagnostic casts (Fig. 8–20B). Net anterior arch perimeter is the difference on each side between space available and space required.

*Intermediate Arch Perimeter (Cuspids and Bicuspids).* In the intermediate arch space available in each quadrant can be determined by measuring from the distal of the lateral incisors to the anatomic contact point of the first permanent molars (Fig. 8–21). To determine the space required the mesiodistal dimension of each erupted cuspid and bicuspid is measured. Unerupted tooth dimensions can be obtained from long cone periapical radiographs compensating for distor-

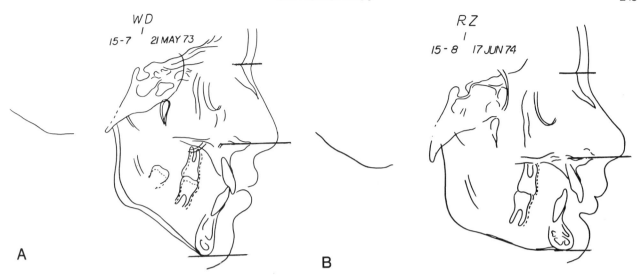

**FIG. 8–16.** Cephalometric tracings demonstrating facial proportions. A. Greater than normal anterior lower face height. B. Decreased anterior lower face dimension.

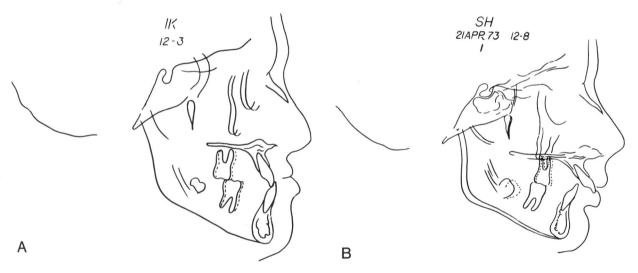

**FIG. 8–17.** Cephalometric tracings of cases which demonstrate poor vertical as well as anteroposterior facial balance. A. Class III malocclusion with increased lower face height. B. Class II division I malocclusion with decreased lower face height.

tion and enlargement. The net intermediate arch perimeter is computed in each quadrant; it is the difference between space available and space required.

From panoramic radiographs, the sequence of eruption in each intermediate quadrant can be assessed (Fig. 8–22). Is impaction likely? Is the sequence favorable?

**Posterior Arch Perimeter (Second and Third Molars).** From periapical and panoramic radio-graphs, the angular position of unerupted second and third molars can be subjectively evaluated. Can they erupt? Will they impact? These radiographs, can also be utilized for a subjective assessment of the proximity of first, second, and third molars. Are they tightly positioned? Do they have adequate space to erupt normally?

***Summary.*** The clinician should determine if the patient has definitely excessive arch length (+ 2 mm or more), definitely deficient arch length (− 2 mm or more), or is a borderline arch length situation (± 2mm). By this method each section of the developing dental arches can be viewed separately, specific areas of defi-

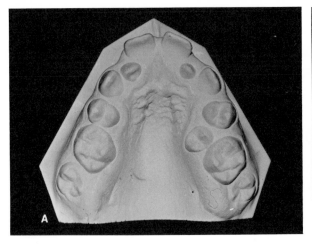
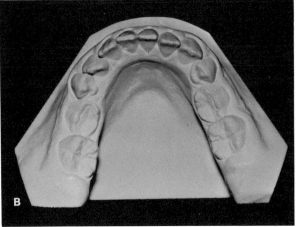

**FIG. 8–18.** Casts demonstrating marked transverse asymmetry. A. Pronounced maxillary arch construction, greater on the patient's left. B. Mandibular left buccal quadrant lingual deviation.

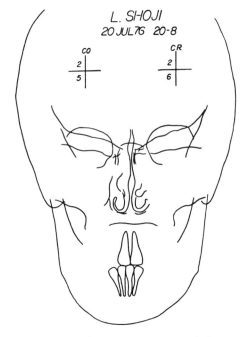

**FIG. 8–19.** Tracing of a posteroanterior cephalometric radiograph demonstrating mandibular asymmetry toward the patient's right.

ciency or excess identified, and an appropriate plan of treatment designed.

### QUESTIONS

18. Serious and difficult open bite cases are often characterized by which of the following cephalometric findings?
    1. Shortened face height
    2. Parallel relationship of anterior cranial base, palatal, occlusal and mandibular planes
    3. Palatal plane tipped upward in the anterior in conjunction with a steep mandibular plane
    4. Class II skeletal and dental pattern

Open bites with the poorest prognosis are not limited to a single Angle Class but do typically have a disproportionate vertical face problem. Often the lower face is lengthened, the palatal plane and mandibular plane are more obtuse and the incisors appear to have a longer than normal alveolar base while maxillary molars often are positioned higher relative to the palate.

19. Which of the following cannot be assessed with cephalometric radiographs?
    1. Mandibular retrusion
    2. Mandibular lateral asymmetry
    3. Vertical facial disproportion
    4. Incisor position and angulation
    5. Adequacy of dental arch perimeter

Arch length is best assessed by evaluation of dental casts and intraoral radiographs.

20. A 7-year-old patient demonstrates unilateral buccal crossbite in centric occlusion, deviation of the mandibular midline, bilateral construction of the maxillary arch, and a lateral deviation from centric relation to centric occlusion. What is the most likely treatment for this case?
    1. Unilateral cross-elastics to widen the constructed side
    2. Bilateral arch wire expansion
    3. Bilateral palatal expansion
    4. Reassess the malocclusion in the permanent dentition.

Since most unilateral crossbites in centric occlusion in association with a functional shift are actually bilateral in centric relation, bilateral palatal expansion is the usual treatment of choice.

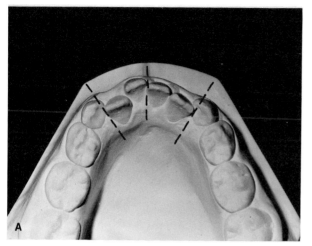

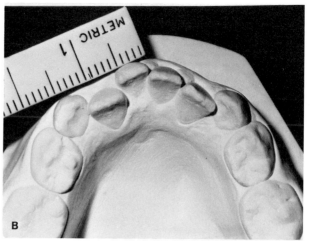

**FIG. 8–20.** A. Measurement of anterior space available. B. Anterior space required is the sum of each incisor width.

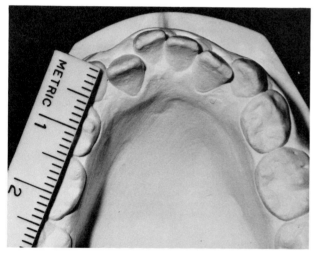

**FIG. 8–21.** Intermediate segment measured from the distal of the lateral incisor to the mesial of the first permanent molar.

21. A mixed dentition patient with anterior crossbite of all incisors in centric occlusion and Class I molar relationship can be positioned in centric relation so that the incisors are in an edge-to-edge relationship. If the crossbite is correctable through maxillary incisor advancement and centric relation and centric occlusion are then coincident, what will be the molar classification?

1. Class I
2. Class II
3. Class III
4. Not predictable

A Class II molar relation could be the molar relationship following correction of this "pseudo Class III" case. Cor-

rection of the centric shift which is described can result in considerable distal positioning of the lower molar.

22. A patient presents with a history of cleft palate and anterior crossbite. What is the most likely skeletal cephalometric finding?

1. Maxillary protrusion
2. Maxillary retrusion
3. Normal maxillary position
4. Mandibular protrusion
5. Maxillary retrusion and mandibular protrusion

23. How does the evaluation of posterior arch length influence the management of intermediate segment deficiency?

1. Molar spacing or crowding can be ignored in the child and adolescent patient.
2. Posterior crowding could eventually cause anterior crowding.
3. Evaluation of the posterior segment may help determine bicuspid removal.
4. Since mesial drift improves molar positioning, the posterior segment should be observed but not treated in the mixed dentition.

The extent of posterior crowding, specifically the eruption position of developing second molars, could influence extraction decisions. For example, a case with a good facial profile and mild to moderate mandibular arch length deficiency might better be treated by second bicuspid removal than the more typical first bicuspid extraction.

24. What is the incidence of anterior open bite among children and adolescents?

1. Under 1%
2. 5%
3. 10%
4. 25%

Although black children have a higher incidence of open bite and a much lower incidence of deep overbite, 5% open bite is usually considered the figure for the U.S. population.

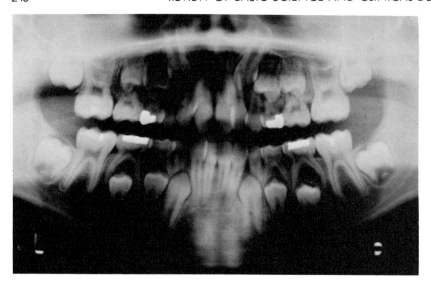

**FIG. 8-22.** Eruption sequence of cuspids in the upper arch somewhat delayed relative to bicuspids, but advanced in the lower arch.

25. In an early mixed dentition case with insufficient space in the anterior segment for erupting permanent lateral incisors, what treatment is indicated?
    1. No treatment—allow the incisors to erupt in a crowded state and treat the case in the permanent dentition
    2. Disc the proximal surfaces of the permanent incisors to reduce the space required.
    3. Disc the deciduous cuspids.
    4. Extract the deciduous cuspids.

Discing of the mesial surfaces of deciduous cuspids will often allow self-alignment of permanent incisors but in cases of marked space deficiency extraction of deciduous cuspids may be required.

26. What is the rationale for selective early removal of deciduous teeth in cases involving deficient arch length?
    1. To promote permanent tooth alignment by creating space
    2. To hasten eruption of underlying permanent teeth
    3. To reduce subsequent orthodontic treatment time
    4. To begin the several steps leading to selected bicuspid extractions
    5. All of the above

Selective and sequential removal of deciduous teeth, sometimes termed "serial extraction," is utilized to gain alignment of erupting permanent teeth and often is carried to the removal of certain bicuspid teeth in cases of marked space inadequacy. Although controversial, proponents claim reduced active treatment time and improved long-term results.

## REFERENCES

1. BJORK A: Facial growth in man, studied with the aid of metallic implants. Acta Odont Scand 13:9–34, 1955

2. BRASH JC: The Growth of the Jaws and Palate. London, Dental Board of the United Kingdom, 1924
3. BROADBENT B: A new x-ray technique and its application to orthodontia. Angle Orthod 1:45–66, 1931
4. ENLOW D: The Human Face. New York, Evanston, and London, Harper and Row, 1968, pp 194–226
5. GRABER T (ed): Orthodontics, Principles and Practice, 2nd ed. Philadelphia, WB Saunders, 1957, pp 489–528
6. HOFRATH H: Die Bedeuntung der Rötgenfern und abstandsaufrahme fur die Diagnostik der Kieferanomdien. Fortschr Orthodonik 1:232, 1931
7. HUNTER J: The natural history of the human teeth. A practical treatise on the disease of the teeth. Essays and observations. London, 1771, 128 pages, 16 plates, 4°.
    * Dordraci, 1773, xxii, 213 pp, 16 pl, 4°, Pietro Boddaert
    * Te Dordrecht, 1773–80, xxii, 214 u. xii, 66 pp, 16 pl;
    * London, 1778 (reprint of 1st edition?), 128 pp, 16 l., 16 pl; Pt. 2, 128 pp, 4°; index at end of Pt. 2
8. MOORE A: Personal communication, 1978
9. MOYERS R (ed): Handbook of Orthodontics, 2nd ed. Chicago, Year Book Medical, 1963
10. NANCE H: The limitations of orthodontic treatment. Am J Orthodontics and Oral Surgery 33:177–223, 1947
11. National Center for Health Statistics: An assessment of the occlusion of the teeth of children 6–11 years, United States. Vital and Health Statistics. Series 11, No. 130, DHEW Publ No. (HRA) 74–1612. Health Resources Administration, Washington DC, US Government Printing Office, 1973
12. National Center for Health Statistics: An assessment of the occlusion of the teeth of children 12–17 years, United States. Vital and Health Statistics. Series 11, No. 162, DHEW Publ No. (HRA) 77–1644. Health Resources Administration, Washington DC, US Government Printing Office, 1977
13. Orthodontic Glossary. Council on Orthodontic Education, St Louis, American Association of Orthodontists, 1972
14. REITAN K: Biomechanical principles and reactions. In Graber T (ed): Current Orthodontic Concepts and Techniques, Vol 1. Philadelphia, WB Saunders, 1969, pp 56–159
15. SALZMANN J: Orthodontics in Daily Practice. Philadelphia, JB Lippincott, 1974, pp 197–210
16. SICHER H (ed): Oral Anatomy, 3rd ed. St. Louis, CV Mosby, 1960, pp 247–249
17. THUROW R (ed): Edgewise Orthodontics, 3rd ed. St. Louis, CV Mosby, 1972

# SUGGESTED READING

ACKERMAN J, PROFFIT W: The characteristics of malocclusion: a modern approach to classification and diagnosis. Am J Orthod 56:443–454, 1969

BROADBENT B SR, BROADBENT B JR, GOLDEN W (eds): Bolton Standards of Dentofacial Developmental Growth. St. Louis, CV Mosby, 1975

ENLOW D (ed): The Human Face. New York, Harper & Row, 1968

GIANELLY A, GOLDMAN H (eds): Biologic Basis of Orthodontics. Philadelphia, Lea & Febiger, 1971

GRABER T (ed): Orthodontics, Principles and Practice, 3rd ed. Philadelphia, WB Saunders, 1957

MOORREES C (ed): The Dentition of the Growing Child. Cambridge, Harvard University Press, 1959

NANCE H: The limitations of orthodontic treatment: mixed dentition diagnosis and treatment. Am J Orthod Oral Surg 33:4, 177–223, 1947

PROFFIT W: Myofunctional therapy for tongue-thrusting: background and recommendations. J Am Dent Assoc 90:403–411, 1975

RIOLO M, MOYERS R, MCNAMARA J, HUNTER W (eds): An Atlas of Craniofacial Growth: Cephalometric Standards from the University School Growth Study, The University of Michigan. Ann Arbor, University of Michigan, 1974

SASSOUNI V, FORREST E (eds): Orthodontics in Dental Practice. St. Louis, CV Mosby, 1971

SICHER H (ed): Oral Anatomy, 3rd ed. St. Louis, CV Mosby, 1960

THUROW R (ed): Atlas of Orthodontic Principles. St. Louis, VC Mosby, 1977

## ANSWER KEY

| | | | |
|---|---|---|---|
| 1. 4 | 8. 3 | 15. 3 | 21. 2 |
| 2. 2 | 9. 3 | 16. 2 | 22. 2 |
| 3. 4 | 10. 2 | 17. 5 | 23. 3 |
| 4. 1 | 11. 4 | 18. 3 | 24. 2 |
| 5. 4 | 12. 1 | 19. 5 | 25. 3 |
| 6. 4 | 13. 4 | 20. 3 | 26. 5 |
| 7. 4 | 14. 4 | | |

# 9
# ENDODONTICS

## James L. Gutmann

Endodontics is that branch of dentistry that deals with diagnosis and treatment of oral conditions which result from pathoses of the dental pulp. Its study encompasses basic science, i.e., the biology of the normal pulp and supporting structures, and clinical science, i.e. the etiology, diagnosis, prevention, and treatment of diseases and injuries of the pulp and periradicular tissues.

## PULPAL BIOLOGY

The dental pulp is a loose connective tissue system comprised of 1) cells, 2) ground substance, 3) fibers, 4) vessels, and 5) nerves. Each component plays an integral part in the dental pulp functions, which are formative, nutritive, sensory, and defensive (reparative).

### Cells of the Dental Pulp

The basic cells of the pulp are *fibroblasts*. They occupy the body of the pulp and are active in collagen synthesis. The *odontoblast*, which is a highly differentiated cell, produces dentin. Odontoblasts are lined up along the periphery of the pulp at the predentin border and extend their processes into the dentinal tubules. Injury to the dentin of the tooth may cause disruption of the odontoblastic layer, resulting in a reparative response or ultimate cell death.

The bulk of the remaining cell types in the pulp are primarily defensive in nature. *Histiocytes* or *wandering rest cells* which can change into macrophages are found closely aligned with the blood vessels. *Undifferentiated mesenchymal cells* form a reservoir of cells which are capable of differentiating into fibroblasts, odontoblasts, or dentinoclasts. This capability allows the pulp to respond in various ways to a multitude of stimuli. Following injury, polymorphonuclear leukocytes, lymphocytes, plasma cells, or eosinophils may also be found in the pulp tissue.

### Ground Substance of the Pulp

The ground substance of the pulp is composed of protein associated with glycoproteins and acid muco-polysaccharides (hyaluronic acid and chondroitin sulfate). The metabolism of the cells and fibers in the pulp is mediated through the ground substance. Its integrity influences the spread of infection, metabolic changes in pulpal cells, and the effects of other metabolic substances on the pulp.

### Fibers of the Pulp

Pulp tissue is composed primarily of *collagen* fibers, although *reticular* or fine *argyrophilic fibers* are present in small quantities. Collagen deposition throughout the pulp may be diffuse (apical segment) or of the bundle type (coronal segment). The apical portion of the pulp is usually more fibrous than the coronal portion.

### Vessels of the Pulp

Many blood vessels, either arteries or arterioles, enter the pulp at its apical termination and course coronally, increasing and branching into capillaries subjacent to the odontoblastic layer. The odontoblastic layer is in close contact with the blood stream, which ensures continuous and adequate nutrition to the functioning odontoblasts. Many thin-walled veins, larger and more centrally located than the arterioles, drain the capillary plexus; at the apex they decrease in number. Lymphatic capillaries, originating as blind sacs among the odontoblasts, accompany the veins in their course through the pulp.

### Nerves of the Pulp

Nerve trunks enter the pulp at its apical segment with the afferent blood vessels either as accompanying individual units or as intimately associated nerve sheaths. The pulpal nerve proceeds coronally with the blood vessels until it enters the coronal pulp. At this point the pulpal nerve divides into cuspal nerves which, still proceeding coronally, form a massive plexus (plexus of Raschkow) and either terminate in the pulp proper or among the odontoblasts. Although approximately 90% of the nerves are *myelinated*, once among the odontoblasts they are unmyelinated. Occasionally the nerves pass into the predentin and dentin. The majority of sensory receptors on the dental nerves are free nerve endings or slight modifications suggestive of synaptic nerve endings in other tissues.

## Pulpal Functions

The primary function of dental pulp, being of mesenchymal origin, is the production of dentin. This is accomplished by odontoblasts, which also furnish the dentin with nourishment through their odontoblastic processes. The nerves of the pulp are responsible for the sensitivity of the pulp and dentin along with the initiation of reflexes for the control of the circulation in the pulp.

When exposed to irritation, whether mechanical, thermal, chemical, or bacterial, the pulp can produce an effective defense reaction. The defense reaction may be the formation of new dentin (reparative) if the irritation is mild or an inflammatory reaction if the irritation is more severe.

## Pulpal Response to Aging

Changes due to aging are commonly seen in the pulp. They may include

1. Decrease in cellular components
2. Dentinal sclerosis
3. Decrease in the number and quality of blood vessels and nerves
4. Reduction in size and volume of the pulp owing to continued (secondary) dentin deposition and to reparative dentin formation
5. Increase in number and thickness of collagen fibers
6. Increase of pulp stones and dystrophic mineralizations

### QUESTIONS

1. Which of the following pulpal cell types is a reservoir of multipotential cells capable of responding in an effective defensive manner following irritation?
   1. Polymorphonuclear leukocytes
   2. Odontoblasts
   3. Lymphocytes
   4. Undifferentiated mesenchymal cells
   5. Histiocytes

2. A common change seen in the pulpal tissue during the aging process is
   1. an increase in the cellular components
   2. the development of new capillary buds in the apical portion of the pulp
   3. an increase in the number and thickness of collagen fibers
   4. a decrease in pulp response to thermal changes
   5. the loss of dystrophic mineralization

3. Which of the following structures are integral components of normal pulp tissue?

   a. Osteoclasts
   b. Odontoblasts
   c. Myelinated nerves
   d. Pulp stones
   e. Collagen fibers

   1. a, b, and c
   2. a, b, d, and e
   3. b and c
   4. a, c, and e
   5. b, c, and e

## MICROBIOLOGY OF ENDODONTICS

Endodontic therapy is essentially a débridement procedure to remove microorganisms and their end products, debris, and potential substrate from the root canal prior to obturation. Because microorganisms have been implicated in pulpal and periapical disease, it is necessary to know and understand 1) the types of microorganisms found in root canals, 2) the potential pathways of microbial access to the pulp, 3) microbial virulence factors, 4) host resistance factors, 5) immunologic considerations, 6) clinical detection of microorganisms, and 7) clinical management of the infectious state.

### Types of Microorganisms Found in Root Canals

The most commonly isolated microorganisms found in root canals are the *streptococci*, primarily the *α-hemolytic streptoccus*, which is a gram-positive facultative anaerobe. Other gram-positive microorganisms frequently isolated include the *enterococci, diphtheroids, lactobacilli,* and *staphylococci.* Isolated gram-negative cocci primarily include species of the genera *Neisseria* or *Veillonella.* Yeasts such as *Candida* have also been isolated. Although the isolation of strict anaerobic bacteria from root canals is a difficult procedure, there is increasing evidence that species of *Peptostreptococcus,* a gram-positive anaerobic cocci, and *Bacteroides* and *Fusobacterium,* both gram-negative anaerobic rods, may also be present in significant concentrations.

### Pathways of Microbial Ingress

Microorganisms and their by-products may reach the pulp and periapical tissues through several pathways:

1. Direct extension through an open cavity or carious lesion (most common route)
2. Penetration of dentinal tubules exposed by cavity preparations or adjacent carious lesions
3. Hematogenous anachoresis, that is, localization of blood-borne bacteria (bacteremia) in a traumatized or inflamed pulp

4. Apical extension of periodontal disease where bacterial invasion may occur through patent dentinal tubules, lateral or accessory canals, or the apical foramen
5. Extension of a periapical infection from adjacent, infected teeth.

## Microbial Virulence Factors

Microorganisms produce specific substances capable of causing tissue damage. The nature of these substances alone and in combination may determine the virulence of the organism. Some common microbial virulence factors produced by root canal microorganisms include:

1. Coagulase and collagenase
2. Endotoxins
3. Enzymes and kinases
4. Ground substance spreading factors, i.e., hyaluronidase
5. Proteases and gelatinases
6. Deoxyribonuclease
7. Various microbial breakdown products, i.e., indole, skatole, amines, antigens

Although microorganisms possess these virulence factors, the ultimate pathogenicity of a specific organism depends on the host–parasite relationship which involves various host resistance factors.

## Host Resistance Factors

The response of the host to the presence of microorganisms and their virulence factors may be beneficial or detrimental. Specific cell types and substances released by these cells may modify or alter microbial elements and their secretions. Common host resistance factors include:

1. Polymorphonuclear leukocytes }phagocytitic action
2. Macrophages
3. Lysosomal enzymes
4. Substances released as a result of immunologic reactions, i.e., histamine, lymphotoxin
5. Fibrinolysin and collaginase
6. Proteolytic enzymes

## Immunologic Considerations

Bacterial degradation products, along with specific virulence factors, may act as antigens by stimulating what histologically appears as an inflammatory response, but actually may be an immunologic response. This response may take place in pulpal and periapical tissue where a rich supply of cell mediators (plasma cells, lymphocytes, polymorphonuclear leukocytes) are found. Although immune as well as inflammatory reactions can be destructive in the pathogenesis of disease, they may be beneficial in healing as well.

## Clinical Detection of Microorganisms

The presence of microorganisms from root canal exudate, or fluid from a sinus tract or fluctuant lesion, can be detected through 1) Gram-stains, 2) phase microscopy, and 3) culture tests. *Gram staining* provides some indication as to the flora involved in a particular situation, i.e., gram-negative or gram-positive organisms, but it is not specific in the diagnosis of any endodontic symptom or disease. *Phase microscopy* is used primarily for the visualization of living, unstained microorganisms.

The *culture test* is used to determine the presence or absence of microorganisms in the root canal. Commonly employed culture media include thioglycollate broth, glucose ascites medium, and trypticase soybroth with 0.1% agar. The innoculated paper point is placed in the culture medium, which is then incubated at 37°C for 48–96 hours to allow sufficient time for any microorganisms present to grow.

Although the use of the microbial culture to determine when to obturate a root canal has been severely criticized, it may be useful as an adjunctive diagnostic tool.

RATIONALE FOR CULTURING.   Those who favor culture tests point out that there is some evidence for greater root canal success with a negative culture prior to obturation. Clinical management of infection is enhanced through antibiotic sensitivity testing. The culture test may be used to assess roughly the effectiveness of the biomechanical cleansing of the root canal system.

RATIONALE AGAINST CULTURING.   There are several reasons why culturing is considered inadvisable. Contamination during the culture procedure causes false-positive results. The difficulty of properly sampling, detecting, and growing any microorganisms present can cause a false-negative result. There is no positive correlation between root canal microorganisms and any specific disease state. Microbial virulence, population, or host resistance cannot be determined by the culture test. Microorganisms can remain undetected in lateral or accessory canals, dentinal tubules, and cemental lacunae. Previous clinical studies of success and failure relative to culture results are inconclusive. Culture reversals often occur between the culture appointment and the obturation appointment.

## Clinical Management of Infection

*Antibiotics* are used in endodontic therapy as 1) premedication when the systemic condition of the patient is compromised and 2) adjuncts to help eliminate the acute infectious state, i.e., acute cellulitis, osteomyelitis, and periapical abscess. The drug of choice is *penicillin,* followed by *erythromycin.* Guidelines for dosage and administration follow those of accepted therapy.

Between appointments *intracanal medicaments* are effective in reducing bacterial populations within the root canal. Commonly used medicaments include 1) formocresol, 2) camphorated *p*-monochlorophenol, and 3) Cresatin. Less than 1 drop of the medicament is placed in the coronal part of the canal on a sterile cotton pledget. Medicaments are either bacteriostatic or bacteriocidal, and their mode of action is through vaporization as opposed to direct contact. They are severe tissue irritants, however, and if used injudiciously can cause pain and retard healing. The use of intracanal medicaments does not preclude thorough biomechanical cleansing of the root canal system.

### QUESTIONS

4. The most common route for microorganisms and their toxic by-products to reach the pulp tissue is
   1. hematogenious anachoresis
   2. direct extension through an open cavity or carious lesion
   3. through exposed dentinal tubules following cavity preparation
   4. from the extension of periapical infection from adjacent, infected teeth
   5. through the pulpal lymphatic system

5. Although microorganisms possess specific virulence factors, the ultimate pathogenicity of a specific organism depends on
   1. ground substance spreading factors
   2. the ability of the organism to alter its metabolic activity
   3. the host–parasite relationship
   4. antigen–antibody complex formation
   5. proteolytic enzymes

6. During endodontic therapy, appropriate clinical management of infection may include
   a. thorough biomechanical cleansing of the root canal
   b. using intracanal medicaments
   c. incision and drainage if fluctuant swelling is present
   d. antibiotic administration
   e. tooth extraction
   1. a, c, and d
   2. c and d
   3. a, b, and d

4. d
5. All of the above

7. Strict anaerobes commonly isolated from root canals include
   1. *Veillonella*
   2. α-hemolytic streptococci
   3. *Bacteroides*
   4. *Candida*
   5. lactobacilli

8. (A) method(s) used both to detect and identify the microorganisms present in root canals is(are)
   a. Gram staining
   b. blood tests
   c. phase microscopy
   d. culture for 48–96 hours and plating of positive findings
   e. antibiotic sensitivity tests
   1. a, b, and c
   2. a, d, and e
   3. c, d, and e
   4. d
   5. a and d

9. In a culture procedure it is common practice to use an enriched culture medium and to incubate it at 37 °C for 48–96 hours because thorough incubation under the right conditions permits organism identification, appropriate antibiotic administration, and successful root canal therapy.
   1. Both statement and reason are correct and related.
   2. Both statement and reason are correct but not related.
   3. The statement is correct but the reason is not.
   4. The statement is not correct, but the reason is.
   5. Neither statement nor reason is correct.

10. Effective root canal sterilization relies solely on the use of intracanal medicaments in the canal between appointments because long periods of medicament and root wall contact ensure total bacterial death and tissue neutralization.
   1. Both statement and reason are correct and related.
   2. Both statement and reason are correct but not related.
   3. The statement is correct but the reason is not.
   4. The statement is not correct, but the reason is an accurate statement.
   5. Neither statement nor reason is correct.

## DIAGNOSIS

Diagnosis requires a logical, systematic approach to the gathering and interpretation of the subjective patient history and the available clinical data. The proper integration of this information allows the practitioner to formulate a clinically accurate diagnosis of the pulpal and/or periapical status.

From an endodontic standpoint the primary focus in

diagnosis is to determine *if a tooth is causing the patient discomfort and, if so, to determine if the pulpal tissue is reversibly or irreversibly affected.* If a tooth is not the source of discomfort, further patient interrogation and differential diagnostic testing may be necessary to elucidate the problem.

## Medical History

It is mandatory to review a patient's medical history prior to questioning the patient about the immediate problem since various systemic or local disturbances may mimic those of pulpal or periapical disease. In addition, a proper regimen of premedication or alteration in the planned usage of drugs may be necessary in the medically compromised patient, i.e., the patient with rheumatic heart disease, allergies, or coronary problems.

## Dental and Pain History

A good dental history often leads to a tentative diagnosis of the patient's problem. The patient should be interrogated with both general and leading questions, followed by very pointed questions. Specific and essential questions which should be asked of the patient include

1. Have you been experiencing pain?
2. Can you identify the source of the pain?
3. Have there been previous episodes of pain?
4. Is the pain severe? How long does it last?
5. Is the pain spontaneous?
6. Does it hurt to bite or chew?
7. Do thermal changes stimulate pain?
8. Has there been any swelling?

Factors in the patient dental history that indicate the presence of irreversible pulpal disease are

1. The increased presence of pain
2. Pain localized to a single tooth
3. A history of previous intermittent or continuous pain
4. The presence of severe pain of long duration
5. Spontaneous pain
6. Pain when biting or chewing
7. Pain of long duration following thermal stimulation
8. The presence or history of swelling

## CLINICAL TESTS

ORAL-VISUAL EXAMINATION.    Examination of the patient should begin with a complete visual inspection of the patient's face, head, and neck to note any changes in symmetry, tissue texture, or color. The oral cavity should then be inspected with special attention

to *sinus tracts,* the presence of any *swelling, discoloration* (tooth and tissue), *caries,* obvious *fractures* of tooth structure, and the *integrity of any restorations.*

PALPATION TEST.    Palpation is commonly employed with the oral–visual examination to determine if any swellings are present over root apices or if there is lymphadenopathy in the submental, submandibular, or cervical lymph nodes. The degree of tooth mobility should also be ascertained. Tenderness to palpation may be indicative of irreversible pulp disease which has communicated with the surrounding tissues.

PERCUSSION TEST.    Percussion testing is performed by tapping with a mirror handle the tooth/teeth in question along with adjacent or contralateral teeth. Sensitivity to percussion indicates that there is an inflammatory process at the apex of the tooth, which may indicate irreversible pulpal disease.

PERIODONTAL PROBING.    Evaluation of the surrounding periodontal tissues is often necessary to differentiate between pulpal and periodontal disease, as well as to establish the integrity of the supporting structures.

RADIOGRAPHIC EXAMINATION.    Radiographs provide a tremendous amount of information relative to accurate diagnosis. Periapical radiographs, along with bite-wing radiographs in the posterior, are a necessity for good endodontic diagnosis. Occasionally a panorex or occlusal radiograph is also necessary as a differential diagnostic tool.

Radiographic changes which might be indicative of degenerative pulpal changes include

1. Deep carious lesions
2. Deep restorations
3. Pulp cappings and pulpotomies
4. Pulp stones, canal calcifications
5. Resorptive defects
6. Radiolucent/radiopaque lesions
7. Thickened or obliterated periodontal ligament space
8. Root fractures
9. Periodontal disease with bone loss.

ELECTRIC PULP TEST.    The electric pulp tester is used to determine whether a pulp is responsive or nonresponsive to an electric current passed through the tooth. It does not measure pulpal vitality, which is determined by the presence or absence of a vascular supply. Pulp tests are always performed on the tooth in question and adjacent contralateral teeth. Wide variances in response between teeth may be indicative of a degenerative pulp.

It is important to note that a test of this nature can be greatly influenced by patient factors such as the mental or emotional status, pain threshold, drug influence, age, and tooth status.

False-negative responses to electric pulp testing may be due to

1. The presence of diffuse pulpal calcifications
2. Large amounts of reparative dentin
3. An incompletely formed apex
4. Poor contact of tooth and electrode
5. Recently traumatized teeth
6. Operator error

The total absence of response to electric pulp testing, provided there is little or no chance for a false-negative response, strongly suggests pulp necrosis.

False-positive responses to electric pulp testing may be due to

1. A multicanaled tooth with varying degrees of vitality
2. Transference of current between teeth via approximating restorations
3. Transference of current via fluid to the gingiva
4. Placement of an electrode in contact with the gingiva
5. Pulp tissue undergoing degenerative changes
6. Totally necrotic pulp tissue in a fluid state
7. Operator error

**THERMAL TESTS.** Thermal tests can be valuable in differentiating between a reversible and irreversible pulpitis. When tested, the patient may have a hypersensitive response, a normal response, no response, or an abnormal response. The response is hypersensitive if, upon application of cold (ice, ethylchloride) or heat (heated temporary stopping), the patient responds immediately to a sharp sensation which subsides rapidly upon removal of the stimulus. Upon application of cold or heat the normal response is a mild to moderate discomfort which disappears almost immediately upon removal of the stimulus. The absence of a response to any thermal testing as compared to adjacent or contralateral teeth strongly suggests pulpal necrosis. A prolonged hypersensitive response (pain that lingers after the stimulus is removed) is an abnormal response which strongly suggests irreversible pulpal disease.

**TEST CAVITY.** The test cavity is utilized when the results of other tests prove inconclusive. Without the use of an anesthetic, a small hole is drilled into a tooth to the dentinoenamel junction. If the patient feels a sharp pain, the pulp is presumed to be vital. Immediate restoration of the small opening is recommended. If no pain is felt upon access, the pulp chamber should be opened and endodontic therapy instituted.

**ANESTHETIC TEST.** In situations where pain is diffuse or vague where the pain seems to move from one location to another, i.e., maxillary arch to mandibular arch and vice versa (referred pain), block anesthesia or selective infiltration can be utilized. For example, if block anesthesia is used in the mandible and the pain subsides with the onset of numbness, it can be surmised that a mandibular tooth is the source of the pain. Likewise, when subperiosteal infiltration of anesthesia is used over the maxillary teeth, starting from the most distal tooth, the pain will subside when the anesthesia reaches the source of pain. Pulpal pain, even if referred, is invariably unilateral and stems from only one of two branches of the trigeminal nerve supplying sensory innervation to the jaws. Referred pain may also originate from or radiate to other areas of the head and neck, i.e., ear, temple.

**TRANSILLUMINATION.** The transillumination test employs a high intensity light source (fiberoptic) that is passed through the teeth in a dimly lit room. It is useful in identifying necrotic teeth (dark opaque appearance) or fractured teeth.

### Cracked Tooth Syndrome

The diagnosis of the cracked tooth syndrome can be a very difficult task. Patient symptoms may be vague or may encompass the total spectrum of symptomatology. Clinical examination may reveal an incipient fracture line on a marginal ridge or an actual separation of the tooth into two or more segments. Teeth suspected of being cracked can be evaluated by having the patient bite forcefully on an object (orangewood stick, cotton-tipped applicator) that has been placed on a specific cusp, ridge, or inclined plane. Noting the occlusion when the pain occurs aids in the location of the cracked tooth.

### Endodontic Diagnostic Scheme

A logical, rational diagnostic scheme can be utilized efficiently and effectively to manage a patient who has dental pain. After giving a medical history and answering selected questions concerning dental and pain history, the patient will state either that the pain is definitely localized to one tooth or that it is diffuse and its source cannot be accurately identified. If the pain is localized to a tooth, the information obtained from the visual examination, palpation, percussion test, periodontal probing, and radiographs, along with the patient's history, will usually result in a definite diagnosis. The same diagnostic procedures are carried out when the pain is diffuse or nonlocalized, but if a diagnosis cannot be made at this point, further comparison testing such as electric pulp tests and thermal tests may be necessary. If all testing still proves inconclusive and the dentist is suspicious of a single tooth, a test cavity may be used. The anesthetic test is appropriate if the possibility of referred pain exists. The transillumination test and evaluation for a cracked tooth are the final diagnostic procedures.

An inconclusive diagnosis at this point may indicate the need to consider that the pain is from a nondental origin. Pain in the oral region that is not of dental origin may be caused by an ear infection, coronary insufficiency, sinus infection, emotional problems, migraine headache, temporomandibular joint dysfunction, malignancies, and occlusal dysfunction.

## QUESTIONS

11. A 24-year-old male presents with continuous diffuse pain in the maxillary left canine region. Upon visual examination the tissue in the mucobuccal vestibule appears inflamed and slightly swollen. Palpation reveals a tenderness over the apex of the lateral incisor and the canine. Both teeth are slightly percussion sensitive. Radiographically no pathology is noted. Further evaluation and/or treatment should consist of
    1. initiating root canal therapy on both teeth because irreversible pulpal disease is present
    2. further diagnostic testing, specifically thermal or electric pulp testing
    3. a test cavity on each of the two teeth
    4. evaluation of pain of nondental origin
    5. dismissing the patient until the pain localizes

12. A patient presents with an occasional vague pain in the lower left first molar. The pain began 2 weeks ago and is present upon chewing. Hot and cold stimuli do not bring on discomfort. Radiographically there is bone loss evident in the immediate bifurcation of the tooth. Further diagnostic testing may consist of
    a. limited periodontal probing around the tooth in question
    b. periodontal probing and radiographic evaluation of the entire dentition
    c. evaluation of occlusal discrepancies
    d. evaluation for the presence of a cracked tooth
    e. electric pulp testing

    1. a, d, and e
    2. a, b, and e
    3. b, c, d, and e
    4. b, d, and e
    5. a and e

13. A 14-year-old patient presents with severe pain in tooth #7 and relates a history of trauma in that region. A visual examination reveals a large carious lesion on the distal surface of #7. Tooth #7 is tender to percussion. Radiographically a periapical lesion is present at the apex of #8. The initial consideration should be
    1. immediate initiation of root canal therapy on tooth #8
    2. excavation of tooth #7, placement of an indirect pulp cap, and initiation of root canal therapy on #8

    3. thermal and electric pulp tests of #6, #7, #8, and #9
    4. immediate initiation of root canal therapy on #7 and #8
    5. excavation and pulpectomy on #7

14. An 8-year-old patient presents with mild discomfort in teeth #9 and #10. The teeth were traumatized the day before in a fall from a bicycle. Both teeth are slightly percussion sensitive and the crowns are intact. Electric pulp tests indicate that neither tooth is responsive to electric stimulation. Treatment of choice is
    1. pulpectomy on both #9 and #10
    2. pulpotomy on #9 and #10
    3. thermal testing
    4. observation of the patient over the next few weeks
    5. referral to a pedodontist

15. A 40-year-old female patient presents with vague pain that radiates from the lower right mandible into the right ear and sometimes is located in the upper right maxillary teeth. The pain is spontaneous, may last for 1–2 hours and has been present for 3 weeks. The patient relates that she cannot identify any specific stimulus that brings on the pain. Oral examination reveals large but intact restorations throughout the mouth. Radiographically #29, #30, and #31 all have deep restorations with bases and #2 and #3 have full crown coverage. No periapical pathology is present. The next step in the diagnosis and/or treatment of this patient should consist of
    1. referral to an ear, nose, and throat physician
    2. anesthetic testing when the patient is experiencing pain
    3. dismissal of the patient until the pain localizes
    4. excavation of the mandibular teeth in an attempt to identify a pulpal exposure
    5. test cavities in the maxillary teeth

16. An excited patient comes into your office complaining of continuous tooth pain. She relates that she cannot chew or drink cold liquids and has had little if any sleep in the past 48 hours. The first question you should ask to determine the specificity of the patient's problem is,
    1. Has there been any swelling?
    2. Is the pain spontaneous?
    3. How long does the pain last?
    4. Can you identify the source of the pain?
    5. Is the pain severe?

17. A 34-year-old black female presents for a routine oral examination. She only has the six mandibular anterior teeth remaining in her mouth. There is no evidence of decay or tooth destruction, although slight periodontal disease is present. She is totally asymptomatic. Radiographically there are periapical radiolucencies present on the two lower central incisors. Electric pulp testing indicates all teeth are responsive in a similar fashion. Treatment of choice is
    1. test cavities on the lower central incisors
    2. transillumination to identify dark, potentially necrotic, pulp chambers

3. initiate root canal therapy on two teeth
4. extract and replace these teeth when fabricating a lower partial denture
5. No treatment is necessary

18. An elderly male patient presents with a vague diffuse pain in the lower mandibular anterior teeth. The pain comes and goes and has been present for 3 months. Although the medical history is noncontributory, the patient has not had a physical exam in 5 years. You are unable to elicit any positive findings through diagnostic testing. Your next consideration should be to
    1. prescribe an analgesic and dismiss the patient
    2. set up another appointment to reevaluate the situation in 2 weeks
    3. refer the patient to a physician for full examination and consultation prior to any further dental treatment
    4. extract the teeth and replace them with a denture
    5. investigate possible pain referral from the posterior mandibular teeth

19. A 13-year-old female presents with intermittent pain in tooth #31 that began 2 weeks ago. The pain comes and goes, sometimes is severe, and lasts more than 2 hours. The tooth hurts slightly on biting, and she has noticed a tenderness in the vestibule next to the tooth. A radiograph shows a large restoration with a deep base and the presence of immature root development. Your diagnosis and treatment consists of
    1. reversible pulpal disease; excavation and placement of a sedative dressing
    2. irreversible pulpal disease; pulp extirpation and initiation of root canal therapy
    3. reversible pulpal disease; occlusal adjustment and observation
    4. irreversible pulpal disease; open for drainage
    5. irreversible pulpal disease; pulpotomy and apexification procedures

20. A 36-year-old male presents with severe pain to biting on tooth #18. In the past 2 days the pain has increased to the point where it constantly hurts and the patient cannot and does not want to eat. Clinically a recently placed mesial–occlusal–distal inlay is present in #18 and a mesial–occlusal–distal onlay is present in #19. Radiographically no pathology is noted. The patient refuses to let you touch the tooth until an anesthetic is administered. Possible diagnosis(es) and etiology(ies) may be
    a. reversible pulpal disease; hyperocclusion
    b. reversible pulpal disease; restorative procedures
    c. irreversible pulpal disease; marginal leakage
    d. irreversible pulpal disease; vertical fractures
    e. irreversible pulpal disease; restorative procedures
    1. a
    2. a and b
    3. c and d
    4. c and e
    5. d and e

21. A 12-year-old patient arrives at your office complaining of pain in tooth #7. Yesterday he was hit in the mouth during basketball practice. The tooth is slightly mobile but not tender to percussion. Thermal changes do not affect the tooth, and the electric pulp tester registers a response at 8. Diagnosis and treatment consist of
    1. irreversible pulpal disease; pulpectomy
    2. necrotic pulp; open and debride
    3. reversible pulpal disease; reduce occlusion and place a sedative dressing
    4. acute abscess formation; open and drain
    5. An accurate diagnosis cannot be made at this point; treat palliatively and observe.

22. A 22-year-old male presents with continuous mild to moderate pain in the area of tooth #3. You ascertain the following information: history of rheumatic fever and hay fever, pain of 2 days duration, no caries or restorations, no abnormal visual or radiographic findings, a weakly positive percussion test, and a normal response to thermal and electric pulp tests. The most probable diagnosis is
    1. irreversible pulpal disease in #3
    2. reversible pulpal disease in #3
    3. sinusitis
    4. referred pain
    5. fracture

23. A 50-year-old male presents with pain in the area of tooth #30. The pain has been present off and on for 3 months with increasing severity that is now bothering his sleeping. There are no medical problems. On radiographic examination there are no apparent lesions; however, a deep distal–occlusal amalgam is present. Palpation is negative and percussion evokes a positive response. The electric pulp test gives a reading of 4. The treatment of choice is to
    1. perform pulpotomy or pulpectomy
    2. wait for further symptoms or remission
    3. prescribe analgesics and adjust the occlusion
    4. remove the amalgam and replace with a zinc–oxide–eugenol temporary
    5. refer the patient to a periodontist

## TREATMENT PLANNING

Endodontic therapy has a high rate of success and patient acceptance. Successful therapy is based upon a thorough evaluation and integration of patient factors, clinician factors, and the oral environment of each individual patient. Patient factors to be considered in determining the advisability of endodontic treatment include 1) patient motivation and understanding, 2) economic status of the patient as related to the *whole* treatment plan, and 3) health considerations. Clinician factors to be considered in endodontic treatment planning include 1) the ability of the clinician to perform the treatment, 2) the availability of the proper armamentarium, and 3) time.

## Indications for Endodontic Therapy

There are only *two* definite indications for endodontic therapy. One is the presence of irreversible pulpal disease. The other involves prophylactic pulpal therapy which may be needed for other disciplines, i.e., restorative dentistry, prosthetics, periodontics.

## Contraindications to Endodontic Therapy

True contraindications to endodontic therapy are few in themselves. Only in light of the total treatment plan do many of the following contraindications come into play:

1. Severe, untreatable periodontal disease
2. Condition of the remaining dentition
3. Nonrestorable teeth
4. Extensive resorption
5. Vertical root fractures
6. Malpositioning of teeth
7. Limited accessibility
8. Nonstrategic tooth
9. Aberrant root morphology
10. Unfavorable crown:root ratio
11. Predictable failures
12. Proximity to vital structures
13. Health; elective procedure

## Endodontic–Periodontic Treatment Planning

Due to the intimate relationship of the pulp and periodontal tissues (through dentinal tubules, accessory and lateral canals, the apical foramen), pathologic interactions may occur via toxic products and/or inflammatory extensions, or through incomplete crown–root fractures which result in concomitant pulpal–periodontal disease. Of prime importance in planning and carrying out treatment of pulpal–periodontal disease is the recognition of the effects the tissues may have upon each other, the possible etiology, the likely route of communication, and the duration of the disease process. Pulpal and periodontal lesions of short duration often heal following appropriate therapy. Periodontal lesions of short duration which are caused by pulpal infection often heal subsequent to endodontic therapy while those of longer duration may respond with additional adjunctive periodontal therapy. Periodontal lesions of long duration, even if endodontic therapy is indicated, will require surgical procedures to correct the periodontal situation."

## Endodontic–Restorative Treatment Planning

Many teeth requiring endodontic therapy have had their structural integrity severely compromised. Of-

tentimes a post-core restoration is required to prevent further crown and/or root fracture and to restore the tooth adequately. Following the placement of a post-core, full coverage is recommended.

If teeth which are relatively intact require endodontic therapy, their role in the patient's overall functioning occlusion must be evaluated. Intact anterior teeth with only a lingual endodontic access opening require simply a well-placed composite or silicate, whereas a lower premolar with a two surface amalgam might call only onlay coverage.

Factors which must be considered in evaluating the restoration of endodontically treated teeth include

1. Amount and quality of remaining tooth structure
2. Position of the tooth in the arch
3. Periodontal status of the tooth
4. Use of the tooth as an abutment for prosthetic purposes
5. Cervical circumference of the tooth
6. History of previous tooth fracture
7. Patient economics
8. Endodontic prognosis for the tooth

## Endodontic–Orthodontic Treatment Planning

Teeth requiring endodontic therapy can and should be treated prior to any anticipated orthodontic intervention. Even if endodontic treatment is required during or after orthodontic therapy, however, the teeth heal uneventfully. Endodontic therapy can also be employed to stop root resorption that may be orthodontically induced.

Orthodontic therapy may also be considered for the extrusion of teeth that have been fractured in the coronal one-third of the root below the osseous crest. This technique, known as the vertical extrusion technique, evaluates the remaining root segment above the alveolar bone and gingival epithelial level, allowing for its appropriate restoration.

## Endodontic–Prosthodontic Treatment Planning

Endodontically treated teeth serve well as abutments for fixed, partial, and removable dentures; overdenture techniques requiring the retention of roots alone; or as anchors for bar and stud attachments, telescopic crowns, and removable prostheses. In planning the prosthetic restoration, care must be taken to evaluate the amount of bone support along with the proper force distribution allotted to the treated tooth.

## Endodontic–Pedodontic Treatment Planning

Pulpal management in the child and adolescent should take into consideration *pulp therapy* as a means to preserve arch integrity and to protect the erupting tooth.

**PRIMARY TEETH.**  A formocresol pulpotomy is often performed in primary teeth when the pulp tissue has been invaded by caries. A zinc oxide-eugenol base is placed in the chamber and the tooth is restored with a stainless steel crown."

### PERMANENT TEETH

*Indirect Pulp Cap.*  An indirect pulp cap in a permanent tooth is indicated when a large carious lesion is present and complete caries removal may result in a pulpal exposure. Clinically, the pulp must be vital and radiographically there should be no signs of apical pathology. The patient should be in good health and have no history of pain from the tooth in question. Any abnormal diagnostic tests or history of irreversible pulpal disease would be a contraindication to an indirect pulp cap.

*Direct Pulp Cap.*  A direct pulp cap is indicated when a small (¼–½mm) aseptic, mechanical exposure has occurred in a tooth which has a clinically normal pulp. Any abnormal diagnostic tests or history of irreversible pulpal disease would contraindicate the use of a direct pulp cap.

*Pulpotomy.*  A *pulpotomy* in a child's permanent tooth is a temporary procedure indicated for mechanical, carious, and traumatic exposures, especially when root development is incomplete. Following apical closure, endodontic therapy may be necessary should calcification of the canals become evident during recall evaluation. If the canals remain patent, endodontic therapy may be required when a post-core is necessary for adequate restorative procedures.

### QUESTIONS

24. Contraindications to endodontic therapy may include
    - a. untreatable periodontal disease
    - b. the presence of a wide-open apex
    - c. vertical root fracture
    - d. nonstrategic tooth
    - e. incipient internal resorption
    1. a, b, and c
    2. b, c, and e
    3. a, c, and d
    4. b, d, and e
    5. All of the above

25. When endodontically treated teeth are evaluated for an appropriate restoration, the factors which must be considered are
    - a. periodontal status of the tooth
    - b. amount and quality of remaining tooth structure
    - c. position of the tooth in the arch
    - d. endodontic prognosis for the tooth
    - e. patient economics

    1. a and b
    2. a, b, and c
    3. a, d, and e
    4. d and e
    5. All of the above

26. Due to clinical success and patient acceptability, endodontic therapy has been advocated as the treatment of choice in cases of
    - a. periodontal lesions of short duration due to pulpal infection
    - b. teeth planned for overdentures
    - c. teeth having complete coronal fractures
    - d. teeth misaligned and planned for full crown coverage
    - e. teeth with reversible pulpal disease
    1. b, d, and e
    2. b, c, and d
    3. c, d, and e
    4. a, b, c, and d
    5. a, c, d, and e

27. You have just completed root canal therapy on a patient whose lower left second molar had a pulpal–periodontal disease. Prognosis for the endodontic therapy is good, but the periodontal prognosis is guarded. The tooth is missing the two buccal cusps and the distal marginal ridge due to caries. You want to begin restoration of the tooth next week. Your treatment of choice is
    1. full cast crown
    2. post-core with full porcelain to gold crown with margins above the gingival crest
    3. pin amalgam core with full cast crown
    4. amalgam build-up and reevaluation of periodontal status at a later date
    5. reverse three-quarter crown with margins below the gingival crest

28, Effective management of pulpal–periodontal disease process is accomplished by
    - a. early recognition of a combined disease process
    - b. accurate identification of the etiologic agent
    - c. determination of the duration of the disease process
    - d. identification of the microorganism responsible for the disease process
    - e. initial periodontal surgical intervention
    1. a, b, and d
    2. b, d, and e
    3. a, b, and e
    4. a, b, and c
    5. All of the above

29. During the preparation of tooth #31 to receive a MO amalgam you find that you have inadvertently created a mechanical exposure of the mesiobuccal pulp horn. The tooth had been properly isolated with a rubber dam and all the decay has been removed. The patient is 13 years old and has no history of symptoms with this tooth. The radiograph reveals no apparent pathology although the root apices are not fully formed. Treatment of choice consists of

*(Continued)*

1. an indirect pulp cap with calcium hydroxide followed by an amalgam restoration
2. an indirect pulp cap with zinc oxide–eugenol followed by an amalgam restoration
3. a direct pulp cap with calcium hydroxide followed by an amalgam restoration
4. a direct pulp cap with zinc oxide–eugenol followed by an amalgam restoration
5. a pulpotomy with calcium hydroxide placed over the vital stumps to allow for continued rooth growth.

## ENDODONTIC TREATMENT

### Dentin Protection

Dentin must be protected in deep excavations or in cases of exposed tubules following fracture. Materials advocated for this purpose are calcium hydroxide and/or zinc oxide–eugenol.

### Pulpal Protection

Pulp can be protected by either an indirect pulp cap or a direct one. The object of the indirect pulp cap is to preserve pulpal vitality under deep lesions in which the pulp might be exposed if all the caries is excavated. The infected surface layer of dentin is removed without penetrating the underlying leathery dentin. The cavity is washed with warm water and dried; then a dressing of calcium hydroxide is placed over the leathery dentin, followed by a zinc oxide–eugenol temporary restoration. Partial remineralization and sclerosis of the underlying dentin usually occurs after a period of several weeks.

A direct pulp cap is used to protect a slightly exposed (¼–½ mm) pulp. Calcium hydroxide is placed over the exposed site to allow the pulp to recover and maintain its normal vitality and function. A layer of zinc oxide–eugenol is then placed over the capping material, and the tooth is restored in a normal fashion.

### Pulpotomy

A pulpotomy is the removal of the coronal portion of the pulp. The course of treatment is determined by the extent of root development. If the root apex is undeveloped, the radicular pulp stumps are capped with calcium hydroxide to allow for continued radicular growth. If the apical segment is completed, full pulpectomy and root canal therapy should follow.

### Pulpectomy

Pulpectomy, which is the removal of the entire pulp, is usually accomplished with a barbed broach or small root canal file. Care must be exercised to remove the pulp throughout the total length of the canal because any remaining shredded segments of pulp can be a source of postoperative discomfort.

### Root Canal Therapy

Actual treatment of the root canal system is divided into three phases: 1) access opening, 2) biomechanical preparation, and 3) obturation.

ACCESS OPENING.    Access to the root canal system is the initial phase of root canal therapy. It is necessary to establish a straight line access to the apical foramen to ensure complete débridement and proper preparation of the canal.

The procedure for access openings begins with a periapical radiograph to determine the size, shape, and location of the pulp chamber and root canals. Then the tooth is isolated with a rubber dam. Once an opening has been made into the pulp chamber, all cutting and refining of the access should be performed as the bur is removed from the chamber. The passive type of preparation allows the size and shape of the chamber to dictate the ultimate access extent and outline. Finally, all unsupported tooth structure should be reduced to prevent fracture during root canal procedures.

As a general rule the access outlines for all anteriors can be oval or triangular; those for the premolars are usually oval; and those for molars are trapezoidal (mandibular) or triangular (maxillary).

In developing the access opening on anterior teeth, especially mandibular anterior teeth care must be taken to remove enough of the lingual shoulder to identify a possible second canal. In the lower molar a trapezoidal opening is recommended for identification of any second canal in the distal root. In the maxillary molars an effort should be made to clear out all overhanging dentin on a line drawn between the mesiobuccal canal and the palatal canal. A fourth canal frequently occurs anywhere from 1–4 mm palatal to the mesiobuccal orifice.

Most errors in access opening fall into the following categories:

1. Root or chamber perforation
2. Gouging of the pulpal floor
3. Failure to unroof the chamber
4. A proximal access opening
5. Overconservation of tooth structure
6. An inverted access (greatest width toward the pulpal floor)

BIOMECHANICAL PREPARATION.    There are two major objectives of biomechanical preparation of the root canal: 1) removal of the canal contents and

2) preparation of the apex and dentinal walls to receive and retain a filling material. In order to achieve both of these objectives, instruments such as broaches, files, and reamers are necessary.

*Broaches* are primarily designed to remove the bulk tissue contents of the canal. *Files* are used with a push–pull action with emphasis on the withdrawal motion. *Reamers* are used in a clockwise rotational fashion to remove dentinal shavings or old canal filings. The actual physical action involved when any particular instrument is used determines the final shape of the canal preparation.

Keeping in mind that all canals have individual characteristics regarding curvative, taper, length, width, presence of obstructions, or degree of calcifications, objectives in canal preparation include 1) instrumentation maintained within the canal, 2) maintenance of original canal shape, 3) development of a sound apical seat, and 4) creation of a tapered funnel.

Ideally the apical point where the canal preparation is to end is the dentinocemental junction, which most investigators have identified as being located approximately 0.5 mm from the radiographic apex of the tooth. In practicality the establishment of a *working length* 0.5–1.0 mm from the radiographic apex is clinically acceptable. It is at this point that a sound apical seat must be developed to allow for adequate obturation procedures.

Once the working length has been established, the preparation of the root canal can be accomplished. In order to establish a continuously tapering funnel, special attention must be paid to preparing the apical segment, the body of the canal, and the coronal orifice. The *apical segment* is prepared to preserve the integrity of the natural apical constriction. It is necessary to maintain near parallel walls in the apical 2–3 mm of the preparation to provide tugback of retention of a master cone. The *body of the canal* is developed into a rapidly tapering funnel to allow for placement of the master cone without premature binding and to allow for adequate depth of placement for the appropriate root canal spreaders or pluggers. The *coronal orifice* is also enlarged and tapered to permit a straight line access for obturation of the apical and body portions of the canal.

Preparation of any root canal in the manner described also allows for efficient and effective post space preparation.

Suggested aids or guidelines which may be used in canal preparation include

1. Root canal preparation is always prepared in a wet environment. Common irrigants used during preparation may include sodium hypochlorite (0.5%–5.0%) hydrogen peroxide (3%), normal saline (0.9%), sterile water, or chelating agents (ethylene diamine tetraacetic acid). Their prime purpose is to provide

a medium whereby dentinal filings and tissue debris can be easily removed from the canal. Secondarily, they may act as lubricants, tissue dissolvents or softeners, and/or antimicrobial agents.
2. Examine and discard fatigued instruments.
3. Use precurved instruments for initial canal entry.
4. File sequentially (avoid skipping sizes).
5. Use clean instruments to reenter the canal.
6. Maintain a patent canal with a small instrument by clearing the apical segment every one or two sizes that the canal is increased.
7. Avoid forcing debris past the apical foramen.
8. Do not force an instrument if binding occurs.

**CANAL OBTURATION.** The basic objective of canal obturation is to fill the prepared root canal space in all dimensions. The most commonly used materials for this purpose are *gutta-percha* and *silver cones*. Indications for using gutta-percha as a root canal filling material include

1. Irregular internal anatomy or noncircular shape of prepared canal
2. Anticipated lateral or accessory canals
3. Large canals amenable to condensation techniques
4. Lack of apical constricture and possibility of material overextension
5. Internal resorption
6. Anticipated periapical surgery

Although the routine use of silver cones is not indicated, they may be used where

1. Condensation techniques cannot be performed.
2. Severe canal dilaceration exists.
3. The tooth is extremely long and condensation techniques would be difficult.

A *root canal sealer* is commonly employed in conjunction with gutta-percha and silver cones. These sealers are basically some type of zinc oxide–eugenol cement modified by certain additives. The sealer is intended to fill the discrepancies between the fit of the filling material and the dentin walls and to facilitate placement of the filling material by acting as a lubricant.

Before the root canal can be obturated certain criteria must be met. The tooth must be asymptomatic. The canal must be properly prepared to allow the operator to seal the root canal system satisfactorily, and it should be clean and dry at the time of filling.

Common techniques employed to obturate the root canal system with gutta-percha include 1) the lateral condensation technique, 2) the vertical condensation technique (with or without heat), and 3) the chloropercha technique or diffusion techniques.

Each technique allows for many variations and subtle changes which enables the operator to meet the individual needs of each tooth.

In the *lateral condensation technique* a master gutta-percha cone is placed to the prepared apical seat. Resistance to displacement of the cone from this position, in a coronal direction, is referred to as tugback or retention. Once adequately fit, the cone is removed, the canal walls are coated with sealer, and the master cone is seated in place. A root canal spreader is inserted, and the master cone is condensed in a lateral fashion to make room for the placement of a smaller accessory cone. This procedure is repeated until the canal is adequately obturated. The excess gutta-percha is removed with a heated instrument, and a temporary or permanent restoration is placed.

The *vertical condensation technique* involves the vertical movement of a gutta-perha cone (whole or segmented) which has been fit to within 1.5 mm of the prepared apical seat. Movement is accomplished by using root canal pluggers to force the material (cold or heat softened) apically to the prepared seat.

The *chloropercha technique* consists of flooding the prepared canal with chloropercha rosin and then seating a previously fitted master cone to the desired apical position. Lateral or vertical condensation may follow.

## Miscellaneous Procedures

The scope of root canal therapy also includes apexification procedures, management of internal and external resorptive defects, intracanal procedures on primary teeth, retreatment procedures, and bleaching procedures.

*Apexification* procedures are necessary when pulpal vitality has been lost prior to the completion of root growth. Biomechanical procedures are carried out, and the tooth is packed with calcium hydroxide paste in an attempt to induce hard tissue formation at the apex of the tooth. The calcium hydroxide is replaced every 4–8 weeks. Once an adequate calcific stop is formed at the apex, normal obturation procedures are carried out.

*Resorptive* defects are also treated with calcium hydroxide, especially in cases of external resorption. Internal resorption only requires removal of the pulpal tissue and root canal procedures.

*Primary teeth* are amenable to full root canal therapy when the nature of the case warrants. Biomechanical cleansing is followed by obturation with a resorbable paste of zinc oxide–eugenol or root canal sealer placed under pressure.

*Retreatment* procedures can also be performed in an effective manner. Removal of gutta-percha can be accomplished by using heated instruments or softening with chloroform or xylene. Often silver cones can be removed with an endodontic spoon excavator or he-

mostat. Once the old filling has been removed, normal cleansing and obturation follows.

*Bleaching* of endodontically treated teeth is a relatively effective treatment modality provided the discoloration is not due to penetration of metallic salts or silver-containing medicaments, sealers, or restorative materials. Bleaching is accomplished by using hydrogen peroxide 30% alone or in combination with sodium perborate. The chemicals can be heat forced into the dentinal tubules or mixed into a paste and placed in the tooth for varying degrees of time (walking bleach). The bleaching of intrinsic stains in vital teeth is also considered acceptable therapy, but the prognosis for total stain elimination is guarded. Success depends upon the etiology of the stain, i.e., systemic medication, fluorosis.

## Endodontic Surgery

Endodontic surgery is a term used to cover surgical fistulation, periradicular surgery, resectional surgery, and replantation procedures.

SURGICAL FISTULATION.   Surgical fistulation, via soft tissue or hard tissue, creates a route to evacuate pus and toxins from an acutely inflamed area. *Incision and drainage* is indicated when a localized, fluctuant intraoral swelling from an acute abscess is present. Local anesthesia is achieved via block or infiltration, and an incision is made directly below the most convex aspect of the swelling, which allows for a rapid evacuation of frank pus. To achieve a maximum effect, a drain may be placed (rubber dams, Penrose, iodoform gauze, etc.) to keep the incision patent for 24–48 hours. Saline rinses may be prescribed.

*Trephination* is indicated when the acute process has not broken through the cortical plate of bone. After local anesthesia is achieved, a small incision is made in the mucosa at a point opposite the anticipated area of entry into the bone. A round bur on slow speed is used to perforate the cortical bone into the area of acute inflammation. A drain may or may not be needed, and saline rinses are prescribed.

Prior to or following surgical fistulation, antibiotics may or may not be prescribed, depending upon the

1. Patient's medical history
2. Patient symptomatology, i.e., amount and location of swelling, presence of a temperature, physical impairment
3. Amount of drainage obtained from the surgical procedure

PERIRADICULAR SURGERY.   Periradicular surgery implies both periapical surgery and corrective surgical measures. Basic procedures employed in periradicular surgery include 1) apicocurettage, 2) apicoectomy, 3) retrofilling, and 4) repair of root defects.

**RESECTIONAL SURGERY.** Resectional surgery refers to root amputation, hemisection, or bicuspidization procedures. Often these procedures are carried out because of concomitant pulpal–periodontal lesions or because it is impossible to perform adequate endodontic therapy.

**REPLANTATION PROCEDURES.** Replantation procedures, in the context of endodontic surgical procedures, refer to the internal removal of teeth which are absolutely inoperable *in situ* and their replantation after treatment.

**INDICATIONS FOR ENDODONTIC SURGERY.** Indications for endodontic surgical intervention are relatively few. Most teeth respond favorably to adequate nonsurgical therapy. In straightforward cases of inadequate root canal therapy retreatment, if possible, is the treatment of choice.

Endodontic surgery should be performed, however, if there is a strong possibility of failure via nonsurgical treatment, if earlier treatment failed to achieve complete root closure (apexification) and symptoms are present, and if nonsurgical treatment failed and retreatment would not achieve a better result or is impossible. Surgery is also necessary if a biopsy is needed.

**CONTRAINDICATIONS TO ENDODONTIC SURGERY.** Endodontic surgical intervention is contraindicated if the proposed surgery is an elective procedure and the patient's health prohibits it. Anatomic inaccessibility is another contraindication. In addition, endodontic surgery should not be used as a panacea for poor nonsurgical therapy.

**TECHNIQUES**
*Flaps.* Tissue flaps in endodontic surgery are either *full thickness* or *partial thickness* flaps. The design of these flaps is either *semilunar, full vertical* with releasing incision(s), or *envelope* flaps (modified to meet the needs of the individual case).

There are certain guidelines which should be followed in designing and handling any flap:

1. The base of the flap should be the widest point of the flap.
2. Incisions over bony defects should be avoided.
3. There should be no sharp corners in the flap design.
4. The flap should be designed for the unexpected and for maximum visibility.
5. The flap must be handled with care during retraction and manipulative procedures.

*Retrofilling Technique.* Whenever there is any chance that the apical seal is faulty, a reverse filling must be placed. In most instances a silver amalgam is placed in the root apex. An alloy either with or without zinc may be used, depending on the ability of the operator to dry the field in which the retrofilling is to be placed.

**POSTOPERATIVE CARE.** Postoperative care following the surgical procedure should include the intermittent placement of an ice pack extraorally over the treated area, administration of an appropriate analgesic, and instructions to the patient on how to maintain the area for the following 3–5 days prior to suture removal.

## Clinical Asepsis and Sterilization Procedures

Endodontic procedures should be carried out in an aseptic environment, and primary sterilization is required for all instruments used in clinical procedures. Instruments can be acceptably sterilized by dry heat at 320°F for 1 hour, or they can be sterilized along with paper products in an autoclave at 250°F for 20–30 min. Although glass bead or salt sterilizers are available for chairside sterilization (450°F for 5–10 sec.), they should not be used as a method for primary sterilization.

## Evaluation of Root Canal Therapy

Upon completion of root canal therapy, the patient is usually seen on a recall basis every 6 months to a year for a period of 2 years. Factors which should be checked in the evaluation of root canal therapy include

1. The presence or absence of pain and swelling
2. Disappearance of a sinus tract
3. Loss of function
4. Evidence of tissue destruction
5. Roentgenographic evidence of an eliminated or arrested area of rarefaction after a posttreatment interval of 6 months to 2 years

If symptoms persist or if there is no evidence of satisfactory healing, the case should be considered for retreatment or possible surgical intervention.

QUESTIONS

30. A new patient comes to you for total dental care. During treatment planning you find a radiolucency associated with the apex of tooth #12. Endodontic therapy was performed on the tooth 1 year ago, and the patient has had no symptoms or problems with the tooth since then. You are unable to locate previous x-rays. Your treatment would be to

    1. perform endodontic surgery as the persistent radiolucency indicates a failure

(Continued)

2. wait and observe, checking for clinical signs or symptoms of pathology, or changes in the radiolucency, at recall visits
3. retreat the endodontic fill and observe for 6 months
4. adjust the occlusion because continual trauma to the tooth may cause the lesion to persist

31. The primary purpose of the endodontic access opening is to
   1. remove the coronal pulpal tissue
   2. allow for removal of the canal contents
   3. allow for the preparation of the dentinal walls
   4. establish a straight line access to the apical foramen
   5. allow the enlargement of the coronal orifice

32. A 10-year-old boy comes to your office with a coronal fracture of #8. The accident happened about 1 hour ago, and there is a large pulp exposure. On x-ray you see the apex of #8 is still not closed. Treatment would consist of
   1. direct pulp cap with calcium hydroxide
   2. pulpectomy and later gutta-percha fill
   3. pulpotomy with $Ca(OH)_2$
   4. pulpectomy and fill with $Ca(OH)_2$
   5. smoothing edges and placing zinc oxide–eugenol over the exposure

33. Objectives in root canal preparation include
   a. establishment of a sound apical seat
   b. complete obturation of the apical one-third of the canal
   c. creation of a tapered funnel
   d. preparation of the canal in a wet environment
   e. establishment of a working length 0.5–0.75 mm from the radiographic apex
   1. a, c, and e
   2. a, d, and e
   3. a, c, d, and e
   4. a, b, c, and d
   5. All of the above

34. During the excavation of a very deep lesion on tooth #30 on an 8-year-old patient, you initially find large amounts of mushy, decayed tooth structure over a leathery, demineralized dentin. The tooth is asymptomatic and has given all signs that it is vital. Treatment contemplated should include
   1. total excavation; if no exposure is present, apply a base and restore
   2. total excavation; if a pulp exposure is present, do a direct pulp cap
   3. total excavation; if a pulp exposure is present, perform a pulpotomy
   4. application of a cavity sealer over the leathery dentin, followed by restoration with amalgam
   5. application of calcium hydroxide and/or zinc oxide–eugenol over the leathery dentin and restoration with amalgam

35. A 21-year-old female presents with slight discomfort on tooth #7. She complains that it is tender to biting and occasionally gives her an ache near the apex. A radiograph reveals a previous root canal filling (silver cone) which extends 1 mm past the apex. Around the silver cone is a $3 \times 5$ mm periapical lesion. The crown of the tooth is partially broken down, and you can see the coronal end of the silver cone. Treatment of choice is
   1. periapical surgery, retrofilling and restoration of the tooth with a synthetic material
   2. extraction of the tooth and replacement with a three unit fixed partial denture
   3. trephination of the lesion and prescription of antibiotics
   4. retreatment, removing the silver point, and preparation of the tooth for a post-core restoration
   5. periapical curretage and simple cutting off of the extended silver point

36. In preparing the root canal of tooth #9 you have achieved the following sizes: #50 file to the apex, a #70 file in the body of the canal, and #90 file in the coronal aspect of the canal. Upon seating your master cone with sealer and placing a spreader down the canal you find that it is difficult to get any apical depth with the spreader or to place more than one or two accessory cones in the prepared canal. Reflecting upon the situation you identify the potential reason(s) for your problem as
   a. too much hardened sealer in the canal
   b. too large a spreader
   c. failure to flare the body of the root canal adequately
   d. too large accessory cones
   e. failure to flare the occlusal access opening adequately
   1. a, b, and d
   2. a, c, and e
   3. b, c, and d
   4. b, c, and e
   5. All of the above

37. A patient presents with localized, fluctuant swelling associated with tooth #28. The patient complains of extreme pain on biting. You open the tooth and establish good drainage. You should also consider
   1. prescribing saline rinses
   2. relieving occlusion
   3. closing the tooth
   4. incising and draining soft tissue
   5. All of the above

## PULPAL AND PERIAPICAL PATHOSIS

### Pulpal Inflammation

In order to understand pulpal and periapical pathosis, and their sequelae, an understanding of pulpal inflammation is necessary. When there is a cellular injury to the pulp (caries, chemical or thermal injury, trauma), intracellular products (histamine and histaminelike substances) which have a direct effect on the microcirculation in the immediate area are released. Initial vascular contraction is followed by vessel dilation, endothelial cell damage, and tissue edema. The first cells to appear are the *polymorphonuclear leukocytes* (PMNs) which escape the vessel walls through diapedesis. An accumulation of PMNs and *monocytes* in the affected area is histologically termed *acute inflammation*. If the source of irritation is removed or reduced, the potential for healing is enhanced.

If irritation continues, PMNs can break down, releasing proteolytic enzymes. The resultant dead tissues and PMNs constitute pus, termed a *microabscess*, in the pulp. If this process continues, lymphocytes, *macrophages,* and *plasma cells* are drawn into the area and essentially constitute a histologic picture of *chronic inflammation*.

Acute and chronic inflammatory processes can exist concomitantly in the pulp and, along with the potential presence of antibodies and antigen–antibody complex formation, can cause the following sequence of events:

1. Increase in tissue pressure
2. Collapse of venous circulation
3. Localized tissue anoxia and localized necrosis
4. Increase in toxic product release from necrotic tissue
5. Further spread of the inflammatory process
6. Total pulpal necrosis from a continued local spread of inflammation

From a clinical standpoint there is no correlation between severity of symptoms and the extent of pulpal disease. The critical decision for the clinician is whether or not to treat the tooth endodontically or to provide palliative treatment, i.e., whether reversible or irreversible pulpal disease is present (see Diagnosis).

## Periapical Pathoses

Periapical pathoses result from inflammatory responses of the periapical connective tissue of pulpal irritants. They may be symptomatic or asymptomatic, depending on the nature, duration, and extent of the pulpal inflammatory process (Table 9–1).

Based on histologic criteria, the classification of periapical pathoses has little clinical relevancy. Often the pathologic status of the periapical tissues is in a state of flux between various histologic entities. As in irreversible pulpal disease, appropriate treatment must be rendered to eliminate the etiologic agent before healing and repair can take place.

Periapical pathology of nondental origin may occur and mimic, radiographically, pulpally induced pathosis. Common examples include osteomyelitis, central giant cell granuloma, malignancies, and periapical osseous dysplasia. Appropriate pulpal and laboratory tests are necessary to confirm a true diagnosis.

## Management of Endodontic Emergencies

Endodontic emergencies fall into three categories: 1) initial emergency situation, 2) intratreatment emergencies, and 3) post fill emergencies.

**INITIAL EMERGENCY SITUATION.** The initial emergency situation requires identification of the offending tooth, determination of the pathologic process present, and appropriate treatment. In the case of *reversible pulpitis* the etiologic agent must be removed and palliative treatment given. *Irreversible pulpitis* is treated with initial pulpotomy or pulpectomy followed by root canal therapy.

**Table 9-1.  Periapical Pathoses**

| CONDITION | HISTOLOGY | CLINICAL SIGNS | RADIOGRAPHIC APPEARANCE | PULP STATUS |
|---|---|---|---|---|
| Acute apical periodontitis | Concomitant with acute inflammation | Tender to percussion; pain | Normal to slight thickening of the periodontal membrane | Vital or nonvital |
| Acute apical abscess | Acute inflammation; suppuration | Tender to percussion; pain | Normal to slight thickening of the periodontal membrane to an area of rarefaction | Nonvital |
| Phoenix abscess (recrudescence) | Acute inflammation superimposed on chronic inflammation | Tender to percussion; pain | Well defined area of rarefaction | Nonvital |
| Chronic apical periodontitis | Concomitant with minimal chronic inflammation | Asymptomatic; sinus tract maybe present | Diffuse area of bone rarefaction with or without demarcation | Nonvital |
| Apical granuloma | Granulomatous tissue; capsule fibrous | Asymptomatic | Well defined area of rarefaction | Nonvital |
| Apical cyst | Central, fluid-filled cavity; epithelium lining; peripheral fibrous encapsulation | Asymptomatic | Well defined area of rarefaction | Nonvital |

When acute apical pathology is present an attempt is made to achieve drainage through the root canal. If this is unsuccessful or if a fluctuant swelling is also present, incision and drainage is performed. If there is no evidence of a fluctuant swelling and no drainage obtained through the root canal, trephination may be necessary.

**INTRATREATMENT EMERGENCIES.** Intratreatment emergencies are primarily due to overinstrumentation, remnants of pulp tissue in the canal, the necrotic debris forced into the periapical tissues, or overmedication. When a patient presents with intratreatment discomfort every attempt should be made to identify the etiology of this pain and to treat accordingly. If overinstrumentation is suspected, the tooth should be opened to establish drainage and a new working length should be established. Following copious irrigation the canal is dried and the access opening is sealed. If remnants of pulpal tissue are discovered in the canal, the canals must be reinstrumented, irrigated and closed. If it is felt that debris has been forced past and apex, the tooth is opened for drainage, the canal is irrigated, and the access opening is sealed. The presence of excessive medication requries a thorough irrigation of the canal, placement of a sterile cotton pledget without medication, and the sealing of the access opening.

Although there are no automatic indications to leave a tooth open for drainage, it may be necessary to do so in some cases to achieve maximum drainage. The patient should be advised to rinse the area frequently, especially after meals, to maintain the patency of the canal.

**POSTFILL EMERGENCIES.** Postfill emergencies usually fall into two categories, abscess formation and tenderness to biting or touch without abscess. If there is an *abscess*, the filling material must be removed; any fluctuant swelling is incised and drained. If there is no swelling, trephination may be considered. When *no abscess* is present, occlusion is reduced and analgesics prescribed. The patient is recalled for observation and possible retreatment.

### QUESTIONS

38. Yesterday you did a pulpotomy on an emergency patient with pain on tooth #30 caused by irreversible inflammation of a vital pulp. Today the patient has called with moderate–severe pain. You should
    1. prescribe antibiotics
    2. prescribe antibiotics and analgesics
    3. inform the patient it will probably go away
    4. have patient return and perform complete pulpectomy
    5. have patient return, open the tooth, and leave it open

39. From a histologic standpoint a Phoenix abscess or recrudescence would consist of

    a. PMNs
    b. macrophages
    c. plasma cells
    d. lymphocytes
    e. circumferential areas of bone resorption
    1. a, c, and e
    2. b, c, and d
    3. a and e
    4. c, d, and e
    5. All of the above

40. You have completed all the biomechanical preparation of the root canal of tooth #8. The patient returns in 24 hours with severe pain to biting on #8. You open the tooth and upon x-ray you find that your final file size (#55) is right at the radiographic apex. Treatment of choice is to
    1. enlarge the canal one or two sizes, irrigate, and close the tooth
    2. trephinate at the apex
    3. enlarge the canal two or three sizes to remove any pulpal remnants
    4. decrease your working length, open, irrigate, and close the tooth, reduce the occlusion, and prescribe analgesics
    5. open the tooth for drainage and leave open

## SUGGESTED READING

Accepted Dental Therapeutics, 37th ed. Chicago, American Dental Association, 1977

ARENS DE, RICH JJ, HEALEY HJ: A practical method of bleaching tetracycline-stained teeth. Oral Surg 34:812, 1972

BAILEY RW, CHRISTEN AG: Bleaching of vital teeth stained with endemic dental fluorosis. Oral Surg 26:871, 1968

BENCE R: Handbook of Clinical Endodontics. St. Louis, CV Mosby, 1976

BENDER IB, SELTZER S: Roentgenographic and direct observation of experimental lesions of bone. J Am Dent Assoc 62:153, 1961

BENDER IB, SELTZER S: The effect of periodontal disease on the pulp. Oral Surg 33:458, 1972

BHASKAR SN: Periapical lesions—types, incidence, and clinical features. Oral Surg 21:657, 1966

COHEN S, BURNS R (eds): Pathways of the Pulp. St. Louis, CV Mosby, 1976

FRANK AL: Endodontic endosseous implants and treatment of the wide open apex. Dent Clin North Am 11:675, 1967

GREEN D: Morphology of the pulp cavity of permanent teeth. Oral Surg 8:743, 1955

GROSSMAN LI: Endodontic Practice. Philadelphia, Lea & Febiger, 1974

GUTMANN JL: Preparation of endodontically treated teeth to receive a post-core restoration. J Prosthet Dent 38:413, 1977

HARTY FJ: Endodontics in Clinical Practice. Bristol, John Wright & Sons, 1976

HEITHERSAY GS: Combined endodontic-orthodontic treatment of transverse root fractures in the region of the alveolar crest. Oral Surg 36:404, 1973

INGLE JI, BEVERIDGE EE: Endodontics, 2nd ed. Philadelphia, Lea & Febiger, 1976

KRAKOW AA, BERK H: Efficient endodontic procedures with the use of a pressure syringe. Dent Clin North Am 9:387, 1965

KRAKOW AA, BERK H, GRØN P: Therapeutic induction of root formation in the exposed incompletely formed tooth with vital pulp. Oral Surg 43:755, 1977

MASSLER M: Preventive endodontics: vital pulp therapy. Dent Clin North Am 11:663, 1967

MASSLER M: Therapy conducive to healing of the human pulp. Oral Surg 34:122, 1972

NAIDORF IJ: Clinical microbiology in endodontics. Dental Clin North Am 18:329, 1974

NATKIN E: Treatment of endodontic emergencies. Dental Clin North Am 18:243, 1974

NUTTING EB, POE GS: Chemical bleaching of discolored endodontically treated teeth. Dental Clin North Am 11:655, 1967

PULVER WH, TAUBMAN MA, SMITH DJ: Immune components in normal and inflamed human dental pulp. Arch Oral Biol 22:103, 1977

ROBINSON HBG, BOLING LR: The anachoretic effects in pulpitis. I. Bacteriologic studies. Am Dent Assoc 28:268, 1941

SCHILDER H: Filling root canals in three dimensions. Dental Clin North Am 11:723, 1967

SCHILDER H: Cleaning and shaping the root canal. Dental Clin North Am 18:269, 1974

SELTZER S: Endodontology: Biologic Considerations in Endodontic Procedures. New York, McGraw-Hill, 1971

SELTZER S, BENDER IB: The Dental Pulp, 2nd ed. Philadelphia, Lea & Febiger, 1976

SHEETS CE: Dowel and core foundations. J Prosthet Dent 23:58, 1970

SHOJI Y: Systematic Endodontics. Chicago, Buch- und Zeitschriften-Verlag "Die Quintessenz," 1973

SIMON JH, GLICK DH, FRANK AL: The relationship of endodontic-periodontic lesions. J Perio 43:202, 1972

SISKIN M (ed): The Biology of the Human Dental Pulp. St. Louis, CV Mosby, 1973

STEWART GG: Evaluation of endodontic results. Dental Clin North Am 11:711, 1967

TEN CATE AR: The epithelial cell rests of malassez and the genesis of the dental cyst. Oral Surg 34:957, 1972

WALTON RE: Endodontic radiographic techniques. Dental Radiogr Photogr 46:51, 1973

WEINE FS: Endodontic Therapy, 2nd ed. St. Louis, CV Mosby, 1976

## ANSWER KEY

| | | | |
|---|---|---|---|
| 1. 4 | 11. 2 | 21. 5 | 31. 4 |
| 2. 3 | 12. 3 | 22. 3 | 32. 3 |
| 3. 5 | 13. 5 | 23. 1 | 33. 1 |
| 4. 2 | 14. 4 | 24. 3 | 34. 5 |
| 5. 3 | 15. 2 | 25. 5 | 35. 4 |
| 6. 5 | 16. 4 | 26. 4 | 36. 3 |
| 7. 3 | 17. 5 | 27. 4 | 37. 5 |
| 8. 4 | 18. 3 | 28. 4 | 38. 4 |
| 9. 3 | 19. 5 | 29. 3 | 39. 5 |
| 10. 5 | 20. 5 | 30. 2 | 40. 4 |

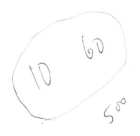

# 10
# PERIODONTICS

### Carole N. Hildebrand / Leslie M. Salkin

## DIAGNOSIS

### Medical and Dental History

The initial interview of a patient is a most important one. At this time the therapist should elicit the patient's chief complaint, if there is one, the medical history, and dental history. The patient should be afforded the opportunity to describe the present problem in his or her own words. The patient's description can be most helpful. Some preliminary observations of the patient's physical and mental state may provide valuable added information. Examination of areas of pain, swelling, or bleeding, along with any necessary radiographs, should follow so that a course of action to alleviate immediate distress can be planned.

The medical history should be taken before any work is begun because it helps the dentist determine if the patient's oral condition is a result of a systemic problem. Systemic disease may alter the patient's resistance to oral disease or modify the patient's response to therapy. A thorough medical history also alerts the therapist to any disease entities that may call for special precautions (valve damage from rheumatic fever, allergies, bleeding problems, cardiac history, etc.).

A thorough dental history should be obtained from all patients. It should include the frequency of previous dental visits, the type of treatment rendered, the type and frequency of toothbrushing, the other types of oral hygiene aids used, any areas of chronic pain in teeth or supporting structures, and the situations which initiate the pain. In addition, information about oral habits (grinding and clenching) and muscle soreness should be obtained.

When data are gathered for history (medical or dental), a standard written questionnaire may be helpful in providing an outline for interviewing the patient to assure that all necessary topics are covered.*

---

* For further reading applicable to the material covered in the foregoing section, see the following entries in the Suggested Reading at the end of this chapter: Glickman, 1972, pp 482–483; Goldman, pp 298–301; Grant, pp 300–301; Prichard, pp 77–78; Schluger, pp 263–275

1. Which of the following statements about medical and dental history is *not* accurate?
   1. At the initial interview, the therapist should elicit the chief complaint, medical history, and dental history.
   2. The patient should be allowed to describe the chief complaint in his or her own words.
   3. A thorough dental history should be obtained from all patients.
   4. Use of a standard written questionnaire may be a helpful outline for gathering both the medical and dental history.
   5. The medical history, although often useful, is still considered optional information for the dental patient.

2. Which of the following statements about the medical history is *most* accurate?
   1. No dental work should begin until the history is taken and evaluated.
   2. The medical history may provide insight into the etiology of an existing dental problem.
   3. Systemic disease may alter the response to therapy.
   4. A medical history may alert the therapist to any disease status that requires special treatment of the patient.
   5. All of the above are accurate statements.

### Radiography

The radiograph is a valuable tool for diagnosis of periodontal diseases. Radiographic examination should comprise a complete periapical survey, including four posterior bite-wing films. Although a panoramic film can be a valuable addition to this survey, by itself it is totally inadequate.

A good deal of important information for diagnosis is provided by a proper radiographic series. The position of the septal bone (in two dimensions) is visualized readily. Also crown:root ratios, and any thickening of lamina dura and periodontal ligament space, are documented on radiographs. This information provides insight into the causes of mobility and the type of treatment that may be necessary. Certain etiologic factors (subgingival calculus and faulty restorations) may also be visualized on radiographs.

It is important to remember, however, that the role of the radiograph is to corroborate clinical findings. Combined with the clinical data which result from probing, as well as visual and digital examination of the periodontal tissues, radiographs provide information which is necessary for an accurate diagnosis. By themselves they are not diagnostically definitive.

Although radiographs are critical to establishing an accurate diagnosis, they have many limitations. Since soft tissue is not depicted on radiographs, one cannot see pockets and cannot evaluate the hard and soft tissue relationship. Even though the level of bone change in disease may be seen, the true morphology of intraosseous defects is not depicted accurately because bony defects are three dimensional entities and the radiographic image is only two dimensional. Also the buccal, labial, and lingual bony aspects cannot be seen because of the radiopacity of the teeth. The only accurate way to visualize these defects is by surgical exploration. Generally bone loss is less severe in a radiographic image than in actuality.

There are no radiographic changes associated with gingivitis. Any change associated with periodontal bone loss immediately rules out a diagnosis of gingivitis. The loss of bone is associated with periodontitis.

Several radiographic changes are characteristic of periodontitis. There is often a fuzziness or break in the crestal lamina dura as a result of the reduction in calcified tissue caused by the spread of inflammation into the bone. The loss of alveolar bone height in the interdental septum is indicative of periodontitis. This may be accompanied by a loss of trabeculation and widening of the medullary spaces.

Aside from the initial full series of radiographs required for proper diagnosis, a periodic radiographic survey should be undertaken posttreatment. The frequency depends upon the complexity and problems associated with each individual case.*

## QUESTIONS

3. The role of radiographs as a tool for diagnosis may be best described by which one of the following statements?
   1. Periapical radiographs by themselves serve as a definitive tool for diagnosing periodontal disease.
   2. Although the radiograph is a valuable diagnostic tool, it may be used only to corroborate clinical findings and by itself is not definitive diagnostically.

* For further reading applicable to the material covered in the foregoing section, see the following numbered entries in the Suggested Reading at the end of this chapter: Glickman, 1972, pp 483–484, pp 499–518; Goldman, pp 319–321; Grant, pp 306–609; Prichard, pp 103–108, pp 142–144; Schluger, pp 265–266, pp 288–291, pp 544–717

   3. Although it is best to have clinical findings available, accurate diagnosis of periodontal disease can be made with radiographs alone.
   4. Only bite-wing radiographs are needed for the diagnosis of periodontal disease.
   5. When bite-wings, a full periapical series, and a panograph are available, it is possible to make a definitive diagnosis of periodontal disease from radiographs alone without any clinical data.

4. Which of the following statements best describes the diagnostic information provided by a proper radiographic series?
   1. Radiographs provide a two dimensional visualization of the position of the septal bone.
   2. Radiographs provide information about the crown: root ratios.
   3. Radiographs provide information about the thickness of the periodontal ligament space.
   4. Radiographs may reveal such etiologic factors as subgingival calculus and faulty restorations.
   5. All of the above

5. Which of the following statements can *not* be considered a limitation of radiographic examination?
   1. A proper radiographic series is very costly and time-consuming.
   2. A proper radiographic series does not provide any information about the presence or absence of soft tissue pockets.
   3. A proper radiographic series does not accurately depict the morphology of intraosseous defects.
   4. Radiographs do not depict the buccal and lingual bony aspects because of the inherent radiopacity of the teeth.
   5. The radiographic image of bone loss is generally less severe than the degree of loss that actually exists.

6. Which of the following statements best describes the proper interval for a post-periodontal treatment radiographic survey?
   1. A full series of radiographs should be taken every 6 months.
   2. A bite-wing survey should be performed every 6 months, and a panoramic film should be taken.
   3. A full radiographic series along with a panoramic film should be taken every year.
   4. A bite-wing series and panoramic film should be taken every year.
   5. The frequency of posttreatment radiographic surveys depends upon the complexity and problems of each individual case.

7. The radiographic changes associated with gingivitis may best be described by which of the following statements?
   1. There is often a fuzziness or break in the crestal lamina dura.
   2. There is often an increase in the width of the periodontal ligament space.
   3. There is often loss of alveolar bone height in the interdental septum.
   4. There are no radiographic changes associated with gingivitis.

(Continued)

5. There is often a loss of trabeculation and widening of the medullary spaces.

## Clinical Findings

Well over 90% of periodontal diseases are classified as inflammatory. Clinical examination must include changes in color, size, shape, contour, consistency, surface texture, position of gingival margin, presence of bleeding and/or exudate, presence of pain, and depth and type of pockets.

**COLOR.** The color of the normal gingiva (marginal, attached, and interproximal) is described as a coral pink. Any deviations from this are considered clinical signs of inflammation. Varying shades of red, reddish blue, or blue indicate the presence of inflammation. These changes may occur only within the interdental papilla (localized) or spread to the marginal and attached gingiva (diffuse). Depending upon the number of areas of the mouth affected, color change may be characterized as localized or generalized.

Often in dark-skinned individuals the gingiva contains patches of brown pigmentation. This color change is considered a normal variation, not a sign of disease.

**SIZE, SHAPE, AND CONTOUR.** The normal parabolic contour and knife-edged margins of the gingiva may be changed by alterations in tooth position, enlargement of the gingiva due to the inflammatory process, or hyperplasia caused by a drug such as diphenylhydantoin (Dilantin) or an inherited condition such as idiopathic gingival hyperplasia. Changes in contour may also result from cleft formation or recession as a result of inflammation, trauma, or both.

**CONSISTENCY.** Normal gingiva is firm and resilient, but inflammation causes the tissue to become boggy and swollen. It takes on a soft and spongy character as a result of inflammatory exudate and connective tissue destruction. The numerous attempts of the body to heal areas of chronic inflammation result in an increase in connective tissue fibers and cells, which along with the edema of inflammation yields a fibroedematous tissue consistency.

**SURFACE TEXTURE.** The normal gingival surface is keratinized or parakeratinized to protect it from the forces of mastication, toothbrushing, etc. The attached gingiva may or may not be stippled (similar to the surface of an orange peel). If stippling is present originally, its loss is considered one of the first signs of gingivitis. If stippling is not present at the patient's initial visit, however, the clinician cannot determine whether this is a normal finding or whether it indicates gingivitis.

**POSITION OF THE GINGIVAL MARGIN.** Enlargement of the gingiva due to inflammation or hyperplasia may cause a coronal positioning of the gingival margin. On the other hand, areas of recession or clefts cause an apical placement of the gingival margin, exposing the cementoenamel junction and root surfaces.

**BLEEDING AND SUPPURATION.** With gingivitis, the wall of the pocket exhibits numerous microulcerations. Disturbance of these ulcerated surfaces by gentle probing, toothbrushing, or at times mastication causes bleeding. In addition, gentle pressure or probing often reveals an exudate in the pockets. This is the result of phagocytosis of broken down tissue products and debris.

**PAIN.** Chronic periodontal disease usually is not associated with pain. If pain is reported, the clinician must suspect other complications such as an acute gingival problem (acute necrotizing ulcerative gingivitis or herpes), a concomitant endodontic involvement, or a periodontal abscess.

**POCKETS.** The only accurate way to determine the presence or absence of a pocket is with a pocket probe. The level of the attachment (the position of the base of the pocket) is of greater significance than the depth of the pocket. If the bottom of the pocket is at or near the cementoenamel junction, it can be assumed that the pocket is not a result of migration of the epithelial attachment, but instead is due to gingival enlargement in a coronal direction because of inflammation of the gingiva. If the margin of the gingiva is at its normal position and there are probable pockets down the root surfaces, it is then assumed that the pocket has formed by the apical migration of the epithelial attachment. This may be corroborated by examination of radiographs for evidence of the bone loss which accompanies such a migration of the epithelial attachment.

A pocket formed by a coronal shift of the gingival margin, without migration of the epithelial attachment, is referred to as a pseudopocket. A pocket associated with apical migration of the epithelial attachment and loss of bone is called a true periodontal pocket and is indicative of periodontitis. The treatment of true pockets is far more complex than the treatment of pseudopockets.[*]

[*] For further reading applicable to the material covered in the foregoing section, see the following numbered entries in the Suggested Reading at the end of this chapter: Glickman, 1972, pp 494–498; Goldman, pp 303–313; Grant, pp 309–321; Prichard, pp 77–98; Schluger, pp 275–279, pp 291–293

8. The normal color of gingiva (marginal, attached, and interproximal) may best be described by which one of the following statements?
   1. Normal gingival color is described as coral pink.
   2. Normal gingival color is described as bright red.
   3. Normal gingival color is described as reddish blue.
   4. Normal gingival color is described as reddish pink.
   5. Normal gingival color may vary from coral pink to varying shades of red or reddish blue.

9. Which of the following statements about the clinical findings of normal gingiva is *not* true?
   1. Depending upon the number of areas of the mouth affected, color change may be characterized as localized or generalized.
   2. Often in dark-skinned individuals the gingiva contains patches of brown pigmentation and these patches are considered a normal finding.
   3. Gingival contour is normally described as having a parabolic form with blunted margins.
   4. When color changes associated with gingival inflammation have occurred in the interdental papilla and have spread to the marginal and attached gingiva, these changes are described as diffuse.
   5. Changes in gingival contour may be the result of cleft formation or recession.

10. Which of the following statements about the gingiva is not true?
    1. Normal gingiva is firm and resilient.
    2. Normal gingival surface is either keratinized or parakeratinized.
    3. Gingival enlargement may cause a coronal positioning of the gingival margin.
    4. Bleeding of the gingiva during toothbrushing usually is not considered an abnormal finding.
    5. Fibroedematous gingival consistency indicates the presence of an increase in connective tissue fibers and cells along with the edema of inflammation.

11. Which of the following signs and symptoms is not usually associated with chronic gingival inflammation?
    1. Suppuration
    2. Bleeding
    3. Color change
    4. Pain
    5. Spongy, swollen gingiva

12. The only accurate way to determine the presence or absence of a pocket is by
    1. radiographic examination
    2. occlusal examination
    3. pocket probing
    4. visual examination for gingival enlargement
    5. visual examination for color change

13. A true periodontal pocket is best defined by which one of the following statements?
    1. A true periodontal pocket is one formed by a coronal shift of the gingival margin, without migration of the epithelial attachment.
    2. A true periodontal pocket is one which is over 5 mm in depth.
    3. A true periodontal pocket is one which is over 7 mm in depth.
    4. A true periodontal pocket is one which is associated with apical migration of the epithelial attachment and loss of bone.
    5. A true periodontal pocket is one which is associated with loss of bone without any migration of the epithelial attachment.

14. Which one of the following statements best describes the significance of pocket probing in the diagnosis of periodontitis?
    1. The level of the epithelial attachment (position of the base of the pocket) is of greater significance than the depth of the pocket.
    2. The greater the pocket depth probings, the more severe the periodontal disease.
    3. The position of the gingival margin determines whether a diagnosis of periodontitis can be made.
    4. Bleeding elicited by gentle probing is indicative of periodontitis.
    5. When suppuration of the pocket is evident during pocket probing, a diagnosis of periodontitis is automatic.

15. Which one of the following statements best describes the value of stippling as a diagnostic aid in gingival inflammation?
    1. The presence of stippling always indicates a total lack of gingival inflammation.
    2. The absence of stippling is always indicative of gingival inflammation.
    3. The absence of stippling is never a diagnostic sign of gingival inflammation.
    4. The lack of stippling may not be considered a sign of inflammation unless stippling is known to have been present previously.
    5. In order for gingiva to be truly healthy, stippling must always be present.

## Occlusal Analysis

If occlusal forces delivered to the periodontium exceed physiologic limits, the result is a breakdown of these tissues (cementum, bone, and periodontal ligament). Excessive forces may cause thrombosis, necrosis and hyalinization in the periodontal ligament, along with cemental tears and resorption of supporting bone. The necrosis related to occlusal trauma is not associated with inflammation; there are no leukocytes, lymphocytes, or plasma cells. Radiographically there may be widening of the periodontal ligament spaces and loss of clarity of the lamina dura. Clinically the patient should be examined for and/or questioned about clenching, bruxism, speech problems, pain, soreness in the temporomandibular joint, tooth position, any deviant swallowing pattern, chewing patterns, overbite and overjet, Angle classification, and aesthetics. Careful examination of initial contact in retruded centric should be made. The discrepancy in millimeters between maximum intercuspation and retruded centric should be recorded, and all teeth exhibiting fremitus or frank mobility, balancing side contacts, or interferences should be noted.

Movements during bruxism or clenching, which are called parafunctional, can be extremely destructive. Occlusal prematurities may set off parafunctional movements with resultant destruction of the attachment apparatus. Destruction manifests itself clinically as tooth mobility, excessive tooth wear, muscle spasms, or temporomandibular joint disorders either singly or in various combinations.

Most people have prematurities in retruded contact, but do not display any signs or symptoms of them. Therefore, most individuals have a good adaptive capacity and suffer no pathologic effects. For this reason it is not proper therapy to undertake occlusal correction on a prophylactic basis.

Since excessive occlusal forces have never been shown to be associated with the formation of periodontal pockets, it can be stated that trauma to the periodontal tissues from such forces does not cause pocket formation. Many investigators, however, do believe that excessive forces may alter the pathway of inflammation in the presence of periodontal disease and cause angular as opposed to horizontal bone loss.

When excessive occlusal forces cause destruction of sound periodontium, it is termed primary occlusal trauma. Elimination of these forces should bring about a resolution of the destruction to the periodontium. However, bone loss due to periodontal disease may so erode support for the teeth that the normal forces of chewing and swallowing become destructive to the weakened periodontium and other supporting structures. This situation is referred to as secondary occlusal trauma.*

#### QUESTIONS

16. Occlusal analysis would not usually include examination for which one of the following parameters?
    1. The presence of parafunctional movements
    2. Soreness in the temporomandibular joint
    3. The presence of gingival inflammation
    4. The initial contact in retruded centric position
    5. Overbite, overjet and Angle classification

17. Which one of the following statements best describes the role of excessive occlusal forces in the etiology of periodontal disease?

* For further reading applicable to the material covered in the foregoing section, see the following numbered entries in the Suggested Reading at the end of this chapter: Glickman, 1972, pp 329–342; Goldman, pp 315–317; Grant, p 313, pp 570–589; Prichard, pp 98–100, pp 131–134, pp 718–823; Schluger, pp 299–307

1. Excessive occlusal forces cause the formation of periodontal pockets.
2. Excessive occlusal forces may alter the pathway of inflammation causing an alteration in the morphology of periodontal pockets.
3. Excessive occlusal forces cause a more rapid horizontal bone loss.
4. Excessive occlusal forces cause the formation of "pseudo-pockets."
5. Excessive occlusal forces increase the severity of gingival inflammation.

18. Parafunctional movements during bruxism or clenching have been described as potentially very destructive. This destruction may manifest itself by
    1. tooth mobility
    2. excessive wear of teeth
    3. muscle spasms
    4. temporomandibular joint discomfort
    5. All of the above

19. When conducting an occlusal analysis, the therapist should elicit information from the patient about all the following clinical signs except
    1. clenching or bruxism
    2. soreness in the temporomandibular joint
    3. bleeding of the gums when chewing or brushing
    4. speech problems
    5. looseness of any teeth

### Differential Diagnosis

There are several extensive classifications of periodontal diseases. The more complex and subdivided, the more confusing these classifications tend to become. Current terminology aims at simplification in an effort to avoid ambiguity.

The two major disease entities in periodontics are gingivitis and periodontitis.

**GINGIVITIS.** Gingivitis is defined as an inflammatory lesion that is confined to the gingiva. The primary etiologic agents of this disease entity are plaque products. There are also certain ulcerative conditions which affect the gingiva as well as certain conditions that render the gingiva more susceptible to the initiation of the inflammatory lesion.

*Plaque Associated Gingivitis.* The most common of the periodontal diseases is gingivitis associated with plaque. It has been shown conclusively that, if plaque is left on the teeth, an inflammation of the gingiva results. Thorough removal of the plaque mat once a day brings about resolution of the inflammatory lesion.

*Ulcerative Gingivitis.* Several ulcerative conditions affect the gingival tissue.

*Acute Necrotizing Ulcerative Gingivitis.* Acute necrotizing ulcerative gingivitis (ANUG), also called trench mouth and Vincent's infection, has a sudden onset. It is most common in young adults and often is associated with periods of psychologic stress such as final examinations, divorce, a new job, etc.

Clinically there are ulcerated soft tissue craters in the tips of the papillae, and often the marginal gingiva is ulcerated as well. The lesions are usually quite painful; they may be localized to one or two teeth or generalized throughout the mouth. They may be covered by a gray pseudomembrane that, when removed, reveals a raw ulcerated surface. Microscopic smears from these lesions show bacteria that are predominantly spirochetes and fusiform bacilli. Recent electron-microscopic observations have revealed four distinct surface layers: 1) bacterial zone, 2) neutrophile-rich zone, 3) necrotic zone, and 4) a zone of spirochetal infiltration. ANUG has been reported to be associated sometimes with an increase in body temperature. However, many investigators feel that a temperature elevation concomitant with ANUG is indicative of another disease entity (herpes) or a superimposed systemic infection.

*Primary Herpes.* Rarely seen in adults, primary herpes lasts 7–14 days and often involves the buccal mucosa and lips as well as the gingiva. Vesicles erupt which tend to rupture and leave a painful ulcerated surface. The characteristic ulcerated papillae associated with ANUG are not seen with herpes. There is often a temperature elevation and the patient may feel sick.

*Recurrent Aphthous Ulcers.* Recurrent aphthous is characterized by the formation of discrete ulcers that often coalesce to form larger ulcerative areas. These ulcers persist for 1–2 weeks and may be precipitated by the manipulation of the oral tissues during dental treatment.

*Chemical Burns.* Localized ulcerative areas may be seen on the gingiva, buccal mucosa, and vestibule as a result of holding some caustic agent (aspirin, etc.) in a particular area of the mouth. Chemical burns are associated frequently with a patient's effort at a home remedy for a toothache.

*Desquamative Gingivitis.* Desquamative gingivitis appears as a diffuse involvement of the gingiva and may be extremely painful. The epithelium tends to desquamate in patches, leaving an exposed underlying connective tissue base. It is thought to be a disease of the connective tissue and not the epithelium. The etiology is not known.

*Predisposing Factor.* There are several predisposing conditions which modify the host's response to plaque: 1) hormonal factors, 2) gingival enlargement, 3) systemic disease, and 4) nutrition.

*Hormonal.* It is believed that certain hormonal imbalances associated with puberty and pregnancy may alter the tissue response to plaque products and cause an exaggerated inflammatory response in the gingiva.

*Gingival Enlargement.* Sodium diphenylhydantoin (an anticonvulsant drug) often results in a hyperplastic enlargement of the gingiva which makes plaque control more difficult. Enlargement of the gingiva has also been reported where a familial pattern was revealed without any apparent etiology (idiopathic gingival hyperplasia).

*Systemic Disease.* Systemic disease may cause a generalized reduction in body resistance to disease. Blood dyscrasias such as leukemia may present a very similar clinical picture in the mouth to that of ANUG, for example, but gingival disease resulting from a systemic condition will not respond to local treatment.

*Nutrition.* Frank nutritional deficiencies may cause an exaggerated response to plaque. For example, vitamin C deficiency is believed to cause a disturbance in collagen formation which weakens the connective tissue and makes it more susceptible to plaque.

**PERIODONTITIS.** Periodontitis is distinguished from gingivitis by the presence of true periodontal pockets with concomitant bone loss. Clinical signs of inflammation are not pathognomonic of periodontitis, and the amount of clinical inflammation has no relationship to the degree of pocket depth or bone loss.

Mobility of teeth may be a result of excessive and/or traumatic occlusal forces. It is believed by many clinicians that traumatic occlusal forces may alter the pathways of inflammation into the bone and periodontal ligament. In the presence of periodontal disease these altered pathways may cause an angular type of bone loss which is more severe and more difficult to treat than a horizontal type bone loss.

In advanced periodontal disease pocket depths are often greater in the interproximal than on the facial, buccal, palatal, or lingual surfaces. This bone loss pattern, which is the reverse of normal, is referred to as reverse architecture. Proper therapy dictates that this condition be corrected and the likelihood that it can be corrected greatly affects the prognosis. Also advanced bone loss may cause the teeth to shift and flare, complicating occlusal relationships and treatment of the occlusion.

Although few clinicians believe that periodontitis is one disease entity, it is difficult to subclassify periodontitis because of the lack of clear-cut criteria. It is stated in texts that periodontitis begins as gingivitis, but that all gingivitis does not progress to periodontitis. Absolute scientific proof of this progression is still lacking, however. Probably all clinicians who treat periodontal disease are painfully aware that all cases of periodontitis do not respond satisfactorily to accepted modes of therapy. There are marked differences in amounts of gingival inflammation, presence of plaque and other local factors, progression, types and amount of bone loss, and age of individuals affected.

*Juvenile vs. Adult Periodontitis.* One subclassification that is, more or less, accepted today is that of juvenile periodontitis as opposed to *adult* types of periodontitis. Juvenile periodontitis appears to be a more widely accepted term than periodontosis to describe a rapidly advancing and severe periodontal condition in adolescents. Periodontosis has been described as a degenerative lesion. The initial breakdown, which is believed to start in the supporting structures (bone, cementum, and periodontal ligament), is due to a noninflammatory degenerative response which later has an advanced inflammatory component superimposed upon it. A major problem with this theory is that there are no histologic data showing a degenerative lesion. Instead, histology of periodontosis always reveals a very advanced inflammatory component. Since the degenerative phase has never been demonstrated, this theory must be viewed as speculative. The only hard data available show that some young individuals display a rapidly advancing periodontal disease that is not evident in most of the population.

There is evidence that the type of organisms associated with juvenile and adult periodontitis may be different. The flora of young individuals with this rapidly progressive disease appear to be associated with gram-negative rods (*Bacteroides aucraceus* or *capnocytophigus*) which are not present in the more slowly progressive adult type of periodontitis.

*Periodontal Abscess.* If a periodontal pocket becomes occluded, there is the possibility of a rapid build-up of bacterial products and pus, causing an acute inflammation with pain and swelling. The affected tooth or teeth may be very sensitive to pressure. This is one of the few instances that periodontitis is associated with pain. The periodontal abscess should be differentiated from pulpal disease by electric and thermal pulp testing. If the pain is caused by a periodontal abscess, both of these tests will reveal no change since the pulp is normal and vital.*

### QUESTIONS

20. Acute necrotizing ulcerating gingivitis (ANUG) is best described by which one of the following statements?
    1. ANUG is characterized by a sudden onset and is often associated with periods of psychologic stress.
    2. ANUG is rarely seen in the adult population.
    3. ANUG is characterized by the presence of discrete ulcers on the lips, cheeks, or gingiva that persist for up to 2 weeks.
    4. ANUG is often precipitated by the manipulation of the oral tissues during dental treatment.

---

* For further reading applicable to the material covered in the foregoing section, see the following numbered entries in the Suggested Reading at the end of this chapter: Glickman, 1972, pp 416–431; Goldman, pp 362–363; Grant, p 322; Prichard, pp 115–140; Schluger, pp 65–71

5. ANUG is often associated with patches of desquamative tissue that have an extremely painful exposed connective tissue surface.

21. Predisposing factors have been described as those conditions which modify the host's response to plaque. Which of the following factors may not be considered a predisposing factor?
    1. Hormonal imbalance
    2. Gingival enlargement
    3. Temporomanidibular joint disorders
    4. Blood dyscrasias
    5. Inadequate nutrition

22. Which of the following signs or symptoms best differentiates periodontitis from gingivitis?
    1. The presence of pocket depths in excess of 3 mm
    2. The severity of gingival inflammation
    3. The presence of pocket depths where the epithelial attachment has migrated apically, past the cementoenamel junction, with radiographic evidence of bone loss
    4. Radiographic evidence of a widening of the periodontal ligament space
    5. The presence of gingival recession

23. Juvenile periodontitis (periodontosis) is best described by which one of the following statements?
    1. Juvenile periodontitis is a rapidly advancing, severe periodontitis in individuals of adolescent age.
    2. A diagnosis of juvenile periodontitis is a condition that always clearly manifests signs and symptoms of a degenerative process.
    3. Juvenile periodontitis is not associated with the presence or absence of bacterial organisms.
    4. Juvenile periodontitis never reveals any signs of supperation or bleeding.
    5. Juvenile periodontitis is best described as a rapidly advancing ulcerative condition affecting the periodontium of younger individuals.

24. Which of the following statements most accurately describes the plaque flora of individuals afflicted with juvenile periodontitis?
    1. The plaque formed in cases of juvenile periodontitis has been shown to calcify far more rapidly.
    2. The plaque formed in cases of juvenile periodontitis is believed to be identical to the plaque formed with cases of adult periodontitis.
    3. There is some evidence that the plaque formed in cases of juvenile periodontitis is associated with a flora that is different from that associated with adult periodontitis.
    4. There is little or no plaque formed in cases of juvenile periodontitis.
    5. The plaque formation associated with juvenile periodontitis is far more tenacious and more difficult to remove with standard home care procedures.

25. Which of the following statements best describes the clinical appearance of desquamative gingivitis?
    1. Desquamative gingivitis is a diffuse involvement of the gingiva where the epithelium tends to desqua-

mate in patches, leaving an exposed underlying connective tissue base.

2. Desquamative gingivitis is characterized by the formation of discrete ulcers that tend to last up to 2 weeks.

3. Desquamative gingivitis reveals the formation of vesicles which tend to rupture and leave a painful ulcerated surface.

4. Desquamative gingivitis is characterized by ulcerated soft tissue craters in the tips of the papillae.

5. Desquamative gingivitis reveals no clinically evident changes; however, patients generally report a painful burning sensation in the gums.

26. When there is an elevated temperature associated with a suspected ANUG which one of the following statements best describes the possible clinical significance of this finding?

1. With an elevation in temperature, the disease entity is in a very advanced state and antibiotic therapy should be instituted immediately.

2. When there is a temperature elevation with ANUG, another disease entity (Herpes) or a superimposed systemic infection should be suspected.

3. A temperature elevation is pathognomonic of ANUG.

4. When there is an elevation in temperature, treatment of ANUG should be postponed.

5. When there is an elevation in temperature in ANUG, local debridement should begin immediately.

27. Which one of the following statements is not a correct sign or symptom of a periodontal abscess?

1. There is a localized swelling of the gingiva.

2. There is an abnormal response to electric and thermal pulp testing.

3. Pain in the area of the abscess

4. Tooth or teeth very sensitive to pressure

5. Heavy deposits of subgingival calculus in the affected area

## ETIOLOGY

### Plaque

Dental plaque is a soft, amorphous, granular deposit which accumulates on tooth surfaces, dental restorations, and dental calculus. It is so adherent that it can be removed only by mechanical cleansing, and it is the principal etiologic factor in periodontal disease as well as caries. There is a high correlation between poor oral hygiene, the presence of plaque, and the prevalence and severity of periodontal disease. In humans, when oral hygiene procedures are discontinued, plaque accumulation leads to a gingivitis in 10–21 days.

Plaque is neither food nor food residue. It is a complex, metabolically interconnected, highly organized bacterial system that consists of dense masses of a large variety of microorganisms embedded in an intermicrobial matrix. It is this organization of the matrix and its firm adherence to the tooth which distinguishes plaque from materia alba. Although materia alba is also composed of bacteria, exfoliated epithelial cells, and food debris, it lacks the organization of plaque and can be removed with a water spray.

The first step in plaque formation on a clean tooth surface is usually the attachment of a monolayer of microorganisms to an acquired salivary pellicle. With the attachment of additional bacteria and the proliferation of those already attached, measurable amounts of plaque may form in as little as 6 hours. In 2–5 days colonies have fused to form a continuous deposit over the teeth, primarily in areas protected against friction from food, tongue, lips, and cheeks. The gingival third of the tooth, the gingival margin, and the gingival sulcus therefore are prime locations for bacterial plaque accumulation.

The rate of formation and location of plaque vary among individuals, on different teeth in the same mouth, and on different areas of individual teeth. Plaque formation is not directly related to food consumption because plaque tends to form more rapidly during sleep when no food is ingested.

Plaque consists of 20% solids and 80% water. Of the solid components 70% is bacteria. Plaque matrix is composed of an organic component and an inorganic component. The organic matrix consists of a polysaccharide–protein complex of which the principal components are carbohydrates and proteins (30%) and lipids (15%). They represent extracellular products of plaque bacteria, their cytoplasmic and cell membrane remnants, ingested foodstuff, and derivatives of salivary glycoproteins. The carbohydrates present in greatest amount in the matrix are dextran (9.5% of the total plaque solid) and levan (4% of the plaque solid), both bacteria-produced polysaccharides. Bound to the organic matrix are the inorganic plaque components. The major components are calcium and phosphorus; there are small amounts of magnesium, potassium, and sodium.

As plaque develops, three distinct phases of floral transition can be observed. In phase 1 (1–24 hours) discrete colonies composed of 80%–90% gram-positive cocci and short rods appear. In phase 2 (2–4 days) rods and filamentous microorganisms appear, and the number of cocci is reduced. In phase 3 (6–10 days) vibrios and spirochetes appear, and there is a relative increase in the size of the gram-negative anaerobic population.[*]

---

[*] For further reading applicable to the material covered in the foregoing section, see the following numbered entries in the Suggested Reading at the end of this chapter: Glickman, 1972, pp. 291–301; Goldman, pp. 181–184; Grant, pp. 109–113; Schluger, pp. 142–157.

QUESTIONS

28. Appearing almost immediately after the cleansing of a tooth, the film of salivary origin which coats the surface is called
   1. plaque
   2. materia alba
   3. pellicle
   4. levans
   5. lipoproteins

29. The predominant microorganisms in the first 24 hours of plaque formation are
   1. vibrios
   2. filaments
   3. spirochetes and vibrios
   4. rods and cocci
   5. cocci and filaments

30. Plaque microorganisms are organized into a matrix which is composed of
   a. dextrans
   b. lipoproteins
   c. monosaccharides
   d. levans
   1. a
   2. b
   3. a and c
   4. a and d
   5. b and d

31. Plaque is differentiated from materia alba by which of the following characteristics?
   a. Plaque consists of an organized matrix while materia alba is not organized.
   b. Plaque adheres firmly to the tooth surface while materia alba is easily dislodged.
   c. Plaque can be removed with a water spray while material alba must be mechanically removed.
   d. Plaque cannot be differentiated from materia alba because they are the same entity.
   1. a
   2. c
   3. d
   4. a and c
   5. a and b

## Contributing Factors

Although the primary etiologic agent in periodontal disease is dental plaque, there are contributing factors, both extrinsic and intrinsic, which influence the initiation and/or maintenance of disease by either enhancing plaque formation or retention, or by modifying the host resistance to the disease.

### EXTRINSIC FACTORS

*Calculus.* Calculus, classified by location on the tooth as supragingival (salivary) or subgingival (serumal), is dental plaque which has undergone mineraliza-tion. Soft plaque is hardened by precipitation of mineral salts beginning from 4 hours to the 14th day of plaque formation.

Like plaque, calculus is composed of an organic component and an inorganic one. The inorganic portion, which makes up 70%–90% of the calculus, consists of calcium phosphate (76%), calcium carbonate (3%), and magnesium phosphate with trace amounts of other metals.

It is difficult to separate the effects of calculus from those of plaque because calculus is always covered with a nonmineralized layer of plaque. Since gingivitis can occur in the absence of calculus, it is felt that plaque is more important than calculus in the etiology of periodontal disease. Calculus is considered a significant contributing factor, however, because it provides a fixed nidus for the continued accumulation of irritating surface plaque and holds the plaque against the gingiva.

*Other Extrinsic Factors.* There is a long list of extrinsic contributing factors in addition to calculus. The most common are faulty dental restorations, dental caries, poor tooth position, etc. In general these contributing factors in some way enhance plaque retention; therefore, in the process of therapy it becomes important to modify these factors to make plaque removal as easy as possible.

### INTRINSIC FACTORS

*Heredity.* The association of hereditary factors with commonly observed forms of inflammatory periodontal disease has not been clearly established, although clinicians indicate there may be a significant relationship.

*Systemic Influences.* While various systemic conditions such as hormonal imbalance during puberty, pregnancy, and menopause and systemic disorders such as diabetes and blood dycrasias predispose to the development of inflammatory disease and aggravate previously existing disease, in the absence of the bacterial component none of these conditions has the capacity to induce inflammatory periodontal disease.

*Other Intrinsic Factors.* Intrinsic factors in general, such as drugs, nutrition, oral habits, etc., tend to affect periodontal disease by altering host resistance. In other words, these factors cause an exaggerated response to the local factors (plaque), and the severity of the disease appears more advanced than one would normally expect.[*]

---

[*] For further reading applicable to the material covered in the foregoing section, see the following numbered entries in the Suggested Reading at the end of this chapter: Glickman 1972, pp 302–305; Goldman pp 89–90, 128–129, 182; Grant, pp 144–151; Schluger pp 92–100.

32. The importance of an overhanging margin on a crown as an etiologic agent in periodontal disease is primarily related to which of the following factors?
    1. It serves to retain plaque.
    2. It serves as a mechanical irritant.
    3. It causes poor food deflection.
    4. It tears the gingival fibers.
    5. It leaves an unaesthetic result.

33. Which of the following statements is true of dental calculus?
    1. It is composed entirely of inorganic materials.
    2. It is the primary etiologic agent in periodontal disease.
    3. It is classified according to the degree of the inflammatory response it creates.
    4. It is dental plaque which has become mineralized.
    5. It is precipitated saliva.

34. In regard to pregnancy gingivitis, which of the following statements is correct?
    1. The hormonal imbalance creates the inflammatory changes in the tissues.
    2. Bacterial plaque creates a greater than usual inflammatory response.
    3. It can be modified by hormonal therapy to bring the body back to a state of equilibrium.
    4. It occurs in women with a hereditary predisposition to hormonal imbalance.
    5. Bacterial plaque accumulation is accelerated by the hormonal changes in pregnancy.

## Occlusion

Occlusion plays an important role in the function of the periodontium; however, it must be emphasized that occlusal problems which exceed the host's adaptive capabilities and create pathologic alterations in the supporting structures do not lead to inflammatory periodontal disease. In other words, the pathologic features in occlusal disease are basically different from those in inflammation. Occlusion is believed by many clinicians to be significant in inflammatory periodontal disease when both disease processes are concurrently present. Experimentally induced occlusal trauma of teeth kept free of plaque failed to bring about periodontitis, but similarly traumatized teeth in the same animal, allowed to accumulate plaque, exhibited periodontitis with rapid bone destruction.

TRAUMA FROM OCCLUSION.  To remain structurally and metabolically sound the periodontal ligament and alveolar bone require the mechanical stimulation of occlusal forces, although an inherent margin of safety common to all tissues permits some variation in force. When the occlusal force is insufficient, however, the periodontium atrophies; when occlusal forces exceed the adaptive capacity of the tissues, the tissues are injured. This injury is referred to as trauma from occlusion.

### Stages of Occlusal Traumatism

*Stage 1: Injury.*  The severity, location, and pattern of tissue damage depend upon the severity, frequency, and direction of the injurious forces. Slightly excessive pressure stimulates increased osteoclastic resorption of the alveolar bone, resulting in a widening of the periodontal ligament space and a reduction in the size of numerous blood vessels. Slightly excessive tension causes elongation of the periodontal ligament fibers, apposition of alveolar bone, and enlarged blood vessels. As pressure increases from moderate to severe, changes in the periodontal ligament progress from compression of the fibers and thrombosis of blood vessels to hyalination and then necrosis of the periodontal ligament and bone. With severe pressure bone is resorbed by cells from viable periodontal ligament adjacent to the necrotic area and from the marrow spaces, a process called undermining or rear resorption. On the tension side, as forces increase from slightly excessive to severe, there is increased widening of the periodontal ligament, thrombosis, hemorrhage, tearing of the periodontal ligament, and resorption of alveolar bone.

*Stage 2: Repair.*  In the repair process the damaged tissues are removed by phagocytes and all the body's natural repair potential; new connective tissue cells and fibers, bone, and cementum are formed in an attempt to restore the injured periodontium. When bone is resorbed by excessive occlusal forces, nature attempts to reinforce the thinned bone trabeculae with new bone. This attempt to compensate for lost bone is called buttressing bone formation.

*Stage 3: Adaptive Remodeling of the Periodontium.*  If repair cannot keep pace with the destruction caused by the occlusion, the body adapts by remodeling the periodontium in an effort to create a structural relationship in which the forces are no longer injurious to the tissues. To cushion the impact of the offending forces the periodontal ligament is widened and the adjacent bone is resorbed, causing mobility. The results are a thickened periodontal ligament, funnel-shaped at the crest, and angular defects in the bone.

***Primary Occlusal Traumatism.***  Maldirected or excessive occlusal force exerted on a tooth with normal bone support is primary traumatism. In primary occlusal trauma, forces must be so excessive and/or misdirected as to lead to 1) tooth wear, 2) widened periodontal ligament space (upon radiographic examination), or 3) mobility in a mouth free from inflammation.

***Secondary Occlusal Traumatism.***  If bone loss and weakening of the supporting tissues due to prior periodontal disease is complicated by occlusal trauma which has led to periodontal damage, the traumatism is termed secondary occlusal trauma. Since the periodontium has already been weakened by bone loss, the alveolar surface available for the insertion of periodontal fibers is reduced. This decreased support so weakens the periodontium that normal occlusal forces cannot be withstood and therefore become traumatic, resulting in damage and mobility.

Excessive occlusal forces caused by clenching and bruxing habits can lead to trauma from occlusion of both a primary and secondary nature. The origin of these parafunctional habits is not entirely understood; in addition to the importance of occlusal discrepancies in triggering the habits, there is considerable influence of psychologic factors. Even when the occlusal prematurities and interferences are eliminated by selective grinding, it is frequently necessary for the patient to wear an occlusal guard (night guard, bite plane) to stabilize and to protect the teeth during parafunctional habits.

**INADEQUATE OCCLUSAL FUNCTION.** Degeneration of the periodontium caused by insufficient stimulation is manifested by thinning of the periodontal ligament, atrophy of the fibers, osteoporosis of the alveolar bone, and reduction in bone height. Hypofunction results from an open bite relationship, absence of functional antagonists, or unilateral chewing habits.*

### QUESTIONS

35. Trauma from occlusion leads to alteration in the
    a. periodontal ligament
    b. cementum
    c. alveolar bone
    d. epithelial attachment
    1. a
    2. c
    3. a and b
    4. a, c, and d
    5. a, b, and c

36. The stages of trauma from occlusion include
    a. injury to the periodontium
    b. change in the morphology of the periodontium
    c. stimulation of the periodontium
    d. repair of the periodontium
    1. a and b
    2. a and c
    3. a, b, and c
    4. a, b, and d
    5. a, c, and d

* For further reading applicable to the material covered in the foregoing section, see the following numbered entries in the Suggested Reading at the end of this chapter: Glickman, 1972, pp 328–335; Goldman, pp 419–464; Grant, pp. 583–588; Schluger, p 87.

37. Histologic changes found in trauma from occlusion include
    a. inflammation in the periodontal ligament
    b. hemorrhage and thrombosis of blood vessels in the periodontal ligament
    c. apical migration of the epithelial attachment
    d. replacement of collagenous fibers in the periodontal ligament with elastic tissue fibers.
    1. a
    2. b
    3. a and c
    4. b and d
    5. a, b, and d

38. Primary occlusal traumatism can be differentiated from secondary traumatism by which of the following?
    1. Excessive occlusal forces in primary traumatism lead to mobility, but in secondary traumatism they lead to tooth wear.
    2. Primary traumatism is more likely to occur in a patient with advanced periodontal disease than secondary traumatism.
    3. Primary traumatism can lead to insufficient stimulation of the periodontal ligament, whereas in secondary traumatism there is excessive stimulation of the periodontal ligament.
    4. Primary traumatism occurs in teeth with decreased bone support, whereas secondary traumatism occurs in teeth with normal bone support.
    5. Misdirected or excessive occlusal forces on a tooth with normal bone support may lead to primary traumatism, and normal occlusal forces on a tooth which cannot withstand them because of decreased support may lead to secondary traumatism.

## TREATMENT PLANNING

All data gathered from the examination must be analyzed so that an orderly plan of action, based on the diagnosis and prognosis, can be formulated to treat the disease entity. This is the treatment plan for resolving the patient's periodontal problems and restoring the oral cavity to periodontal health. The periodontal treatment is divided into three broad categories: 1) initial therapy, 2) surgical therapy, and 3) maintenance.

### Initial Therapy

Initial therapy involves those steps or therapeutic modalities aimed at elimination of all etiologic factors. Initial therapy may include all or some of the following:

1. Alleviation of all emergency problems, chief complaint, rampant caries, iatrogenic restorations, and extraction of teeth which cannot be saved

2. Plaque control program
3. Scaling and root planing
4. Occlusal adjustment: selective grinding, orthodontic tooth movement, temporary splinting, and reevaluation

Probably the most important aspects of initial therapy are the plaque control program and scaling and root planing because they are concerned with the elimination of the primary bacterial etiologic agents and débridement necessary to eliminate inflammation.

## Surgical Phase

When the etiologic agents have been removed or controlled, the more definitive surgical phase may be undertaken. The surgical phase is aimed at correcting the damage to the periodontal structures from the disease process. It is designed to eliminate pockets and to establish an adequate zone of attached gingiva.

Upon completion of all necessary surgery and final check of the occlusion, any necessary refinements should be undertaken. When treatment is complete, a posttreatment examination should be performed to establish a baseline for maintenance.

## Maintenance

Maintenance is as important as active therapy, and a definite schedule should be established. Since the patient is always challenged by plaque formation, constant maintenance and evaluation is necessary so that the therapist can determine if the patient is remaining stable or falling into various stages of relapse.*

QUESTIONS

39. Which of the following statements best describes the treatment plan?
    1. The treatment plan is the result of the analysis of all the data gathered during the examination.
    2. The treatment plan is the orderly plan of action based on diagnosis and prognosis of the particular disease.
    3. The treatment plan is the orderly plan of action for resolving the patient's problems.
    4. The periodontal treatment plan is usually divided into the broad categories of 1) initial therapy, 2) surgical therapy, and 3) maintenance.
    5. All of the above.

* For further reading applicable to the material covered in the foregoing section, see the following numbered entries in the Suggested Reading at the end of this chapter: Glickman, 1972 pp 531–534; Goldman, pp 354–371; Grant, pp 328–331; Pritchard, pp 362–381; Schluger, pp 322–331.

40. The major role of initial therapy is the
    1. alleviation of all emergency problems
    2. elimination or control of all etiologic factors
    3. establishment of a functional physiologic occlusion by means of selective grinding and orthodontic therapy where indicated
    4. removal of calculus
    5. None of the above

41. Which of the following statements concerning treatment planning is not accurate?
    1. Initial therapy is that phase of treatment where etiologic factors are removed or controlled.
    2. The surgical phase of the treatment plan is aimed at correction of the damage to the periodontal structures resulting from periodontal disease.
    3. The maintenance phase of the treatment plan is as important or more important than the active phase of the treatment plan.
    4. Periodontally treated patients should be kept in the maintenance phase for up to 6 months after treatment.
    5. One of the most important aspects of the treatment plan is the removal of plaque and plaque control program.

42. Initial therapy does not include
    1. alleviation of all emergencies, rampant caries, chief complaint, iatrogenic restorations
    2. scaling and root planing
    3. bone grafting
    4. occlusal adjustment
    5. temporary stabilization

## PROGNOSIS

Prognosis is the prediction of the chances for success of a given treatment. Its accuracy depends heavily upon proper diagnosis and a good deal of clinical experience. The ability of the practitioner to recognize and eliminate or control the factors causing periodontal disease, as well as to correct any resultant damage, and the particular patient's ability to maintain a meticulous oral cleanliness determine whether a prognosis is good, guarded, or hopeless. After the prognosis has been determined, a more rational and realistic treatment plan may be formulated. Several factors influence the prognosis.

### Periodontal Pockets

The type of periodontal pocket is very significant. Pseudopockets (gingival pockets) are not an indication of bone loss. The true periodontal pocket with migration of the epthelial attachment is indicative of periodontitis, which is far more difficult to treat than gingivitis. If pocket depth cannot be reduced to 2–3 mm, the control of the bacterial environment is greatly impeded.

## Bone Loss

Since bone loss essentially is not reversible, the amount of bone loss is most significant. If too much bone is lost, the stability of the dentition is in question (secondary occlusal trauma). The pattern of bone loss is also important. Horizontal bone loss may be easier to treat than angular defects and craters. Treatment of a condition with angular defects and reverse architecture of a physiologic osseous contour may require the removal of too much supporting bone to be successful. Loss of bone in the furcation presents a serious problem. Generally mandibular bifurcations can be treated more successfully than maxillary trifurcations. A distal maxillary molar furcation involvement has a very poor prognosis because access is very poor for cleansing; a maxillary first bicuspid has a very poor prognosis when the furcation is involved because access is very poor for maintenance.

## Tooth Mobility

Tooth mobility may be caused by inflammation, trauma from occlusion, or excessive loss of periodontal tissues. If it is due to inflammation, resolution should reduce the mobility. Destruction due to traumatic forces, without inflammatory periodontal disease, is reversible if the trauma is eliminated (primary occlusal trauma). If excessive bone loss has resulted in secondary occlusal trauma, destruction is not reversible. Treatment may involve complex restorative dentistry which is difficult to execute and maintain.

## Tooth Morphology

The anatomy of the roots (length and width) have a great deal to do with how much bone loss is too much. The wider and broader the roots, the greater is the surface that is available for attachment of periodontal ligament fibers.

## Duration of Disease

If periodontal disease has been present for a long time and has not progressed rapidly, the prognosis is much more favorable than it is if there is evidence of an active, rapidly progressive disease state. In general the greater the loss and the younger the individual, the poorer the prognosis.

## Etiology

The most significant etiologic factor in periodontal disease is poor oral hygiene; however, there are people with significant disease despite good plaque control.

Where there is much disease but little plaque, the prognosis is far less favorable.

## Prosthetic Conditions

Missing teeth, tilted teeth, badly broken-down teeth, and teeth with weakened periodontal support may require complex prostheses. These are difficult treatments to execute and to maintain. Loss of key abutments may require partial dentures which in themselves are a compromise from a fixed prosthesis.

## Patient Motivation and Dexterity

A patient must be motivated not only to maintain good oral health but also to develop the skill needed to do so. Only then will the patient give the time and energy necessary to maintain an adequate level of oral hygiene. The patient must also possess a certain level of dexterity, for even the best intentioned patient will not be able to maintain an adequate level of plaque control without the ability to handle the various hygiene aids.

## Prognosis for Dentition

The therapist must also view the dentition as a whole to determine the overall prognosis as opposed to the individual tooth prognosis. For instance, a clinician might decide that a particular tooth could be retained but so much supporting bone from adjacent teeth would have to be removed that there would be a negative effect on the overall prognosis. In this case the tooth in question would be sacrificed because an individual tooth prognosis is superseded by the prognosis for the overall dentition.*

QUESTIONS

43. Which of the following statements concerning the prognosis of periodontal therapy is not accurate?
    1. Prognosis depends heavily upon proper diagnosis and the therapist's clinical experience.
    2. Prognosis is concerned with the ability of the practitioner to recognize and eliminate or control the factors causing periodontal disease.
    3. The ability to correct the resultant damage of periodontal disease does not relate to prognosis.
    4. The ability to achieve goals of a specific treatment plan determines whether a prognosis is good, guarded, or hopeless.
    5. The individual patient's ability to maintain an adequate level of plaque control has great bearing upon the prognosis.

* For further reading applicable to the material covered in the foregoing section, see the following numbered entries in the Suggested Reading at the end of this chapter: Glickman, 1972, pp 523–530; Goldman, pp 345–353; Grant, pp 324–327; Prichard, pp 254–300; Schluger, pp 333–341.

44. Which of the following statements regarding periodontal prognosis is true?
    1. The presence of a pseudopocket makes the prognosis far more guarded than the presence of a true periodontal pocket.
    2. The pattern of bone loss does not affect the prognosis, while the amount of bone loss definitely does.
    3. A distal maxillary molar furcation involvement has a poor prognosis because access for cleaning is poor.
    4. Generally the wider and broader the roots, of the tooth, the poorer the prognosis.
    5. A younger person with severity of disease equivalent to that of an older person has a better prognosis than the latter.

45. Which of the following statements concerning prognosis is true?
    1. A long-standing periodontal disease that progresses slowly has a poorer prognosis than a disease state that progresses more rapidly but is of shorter duration.
    2. If the cause of periodontal disease is directly and clearly related to plaque, then the prognosis is much more favorable than it is in cases where the etiologic agent is not obvious.
    3. Patient motivation and normal dexterity plays only a minor role in the prognosis.
    4. The overall prognosis is a less important consideration than the individual tooth prognosis.
    5. The greater the need for a prosthesis following periodontal therapy, the better the prognosis.

## THERAPY

### Background

The effectiveness of periodontal therapy is made possible by the remarkable healing capacity of the periodontal tissue. Periodontal therapy is aimed at accomplishing the following objectives:

1. Control of etiology
2. Elimination of inflammation
3. Creation of physiologic occlusion
4. Elimination of mobility
5. Establishment of physiologic gingival and osseous contour
6. Establishment of adequate zones of attached gingiva
7. Motivation of the patient to perform necessary plaque control techniques

As the objectives suggest, periodontal treatment consists principally of local procedures to eliminate etiologic agents and/or to alter hard and soft tissues so that local factors can be controlled. When systemic therapy is employed, it is usually as an adjunct to local measures and for specific purposes, such as the control of systemic complications from acute infections, chemotherapy, and the control of systemic diseases which aggravate the patient's periodontal condition or necessitate special precautions during treatment.[*]

### QUESTIONS

46. Select from the following the objectives of periodontal therapy.
    a. Elimination of inflammation
    b. Extension for prevention
    c. Establishment of adequate zones of attached gingiva
    d. Motivation of the patient to perform plaque control

    1. a and b
    2. a and c
    3. b, c, and d
    4. a, c, and d
    5. All of the above

### Armamentarium

Periodontal instruments are classified according to the purposes they serve:

1. Periodontal probes and pocket marking forceps for location, measurement, and marking of pockets and for determining their shape on individual tooth surfaces
2. Explorers for location of deposits on the teeth
3. Heavy scalers for removal of supragingival calculus
4. Fine scalers for removal of subgingival calculus
5. Hoe scalers for removal of subgingival calculus and planing root surfaces
6. Curettes for removal of the inner surface of the pocket wall and the epithelial attachment and for smoothing root surfaces
7. Ultrasonic instruments for scaling and cleansing tooth surfaces with tenacious deposits and curetting the gingival wall of periodontal pockets
8. Surgical periodontal instruments
9. Cleansing and polishing instruments (rubber cups, bristle brushes, dental tape) for cleansing and polishing tooth surfaces[†]

### QUESTION

47. Select from the following the instruments which are correctly matched with their function in periodontal therapy.
    a. Ultrasonic instruments for sounding pocket depths
    b. Curettes for the cleansing of root surfaces

(Continued)

[*] For further reading applicable to the material covered in the foregoing section, see the following numbered entry in the Suggested Reading at the end of this chapter: Glickman, 1972, p 536.
[†] For further reading applicable to the material covered in the foregoing section, see the following numbered entry in the Suggested Reading at the end of this chapter: Glickman, 1979, p 548

    c. Fine scalers for the removal of subgingival calculus

    d. Explorers for the location of deposits on the teeth

1. a and b
2. a and c
3. c and d
4. a, b, and d
5. All of the above

## Root Planing and Curettage

**THEORY AND RATIONALE.**   Scaling, root planing, and curettage techniques are the basic, most commonly employed procedures for the treatment of gingival disease. Scaling removes calculus, plaque, and other deposits; planing the root smooths it and removes cementum; and curetting the inner surface of the gingival wall of periodontal pockets removes diseased soft tissue.

In the process of scaling and root planing, the operator often performs an inadvertent curettage; therefore the terms scaling, root planing, and curettage frequently are linked together. One must be careful to note the context in which the word curettage is used because curettage is also performed intentionally. Both the closed technique (subgingival curettage) and the open technique (flap curettage), which are used when the curettage is intentional, are considered surgical procedures. In the following discussion of scaling and root planing it should be assumed that inadvertent curettage accompanied the technique. Specific mention of curettage indicates one of the two intentional types.

The purpose of removing deposits from the teeth and removing the epithelial lining is to resolve the inflammation, thereby bringing about soft tissue shrinkage and/or reattachment. As much as 2 mm of shrinkage and/or reattachment may occur with root planing and curettage.

Root planing is a part of every treatment of gingivitis and periodontitis. It may eradicate some of the shallower pockets through the resolution of inflammation. When deep pockets are accompanied by edematous gingiva, they may be reduced or eliminated entirely by root planing. When gingiva are largely fibrotic, however, total pocket reduction cannot be accomplished by root planing.

Root planing may be performed alone, as a presurgical procedure, or as a final step procedure, depending upon such factors as the extent of the disease, physical status of the patient, healing response, the patient's plaque control ability, etc. Root planing alone, or followed by an intentional curettage, often comprises the principal therapeutic modality when shallow pockets (4–5 mm deep) are present in edematous tissue or when there are extremely deep infrabony defects (especially three-walled) which cannot be removed by osteoplasty or ostectomy.

Presurgical root planing is intended to resolve edema and exudation so that the soft tissues will shrink, normal color will return, and bleeding will diminish. After all these things have occurred, the therapist can determine areas that must be corrected by surgery and those that may be resolved by conservative means. Morphologic features in the gingiva and mucosa are more clearly delineated after inflammation has been resolved. Other advantages of presurgical root planing are that surgery may be performed in a relatively clean field devoid of calculus and plaque, gingiva is firm to the scalpel and is of good texture to be beveled or split as required, and bleeding from surgery is definitely less than it would be in an inflamed gingiva. Also with this type of tissue preparation exuberant granulation tissue is rarely present postoperatively. Finally, the interval required for recovery provides an insight into the patient's management of etiologic agents and healing response.

Immediately after root planing and/or curettage, a blood clot fills the gingival sulcus. This is followed by a rapid proliferation of granulation tissue with a decrease in the number of small blood vessels as the tissue matures. Restoration and epithelialization of the sulcus generally require 2–7 days, and the restoration of the epithelial attachment occurs in animals in as early as 5 days. Immature collagen fibers appear within 21 days posttreatment. Healthy gingival fibers inadvertently severed from the tooth by scaling, root planing, and curettage, and tears in the sulcular epithelium and epithelial attachment, are repaired in the healing process.

### TECHNIQUES

*Root Planing.*   First the area is isolated and anesthetized; either topical or infiltration and block anesthesia are used according to the needs. Then the calculus is removed both supragingivally and subgingivally and the tooth surface is planed.

*Curettage.*   After the area has been isolated and anesthetized with infiltration or block anesthesia, the pocket lining and epithelial attachment are removed. The curette is inserted to engage the inner lining of the pocket wall and carried along the soft tissue to the crest of the gingiva. Supporting the pocket wall by gentle finger pressure on the external surface, the operator then places the curette under the cut edge of the epithelial attachment so as to undermine it. The epithelial attachment is separated away with a scooping motion of the curette to the tooth surface. Curettage removes the degenerated tissue, proliferating epithelial buds, and granulation tissue which form the inner aspect of the pocket wall; it also creates a cut, bleeding connective tissue surface. The bleeding reduces the height of the gingiva, reduces pocket depth, and facilitates healing by removing tissue debris.*

QUESTIONS

48. Root planing and curettage are performed to achieve which of the following gingival tissue changes?
1. Remission of inflammation and reduction of fibrotic tissue
2. Remission of inflammation and soft tissue shrinkage
3. Resolution of inflammation and conversion from fibrotic to edematous tissue
4. Eradication of deep pockets and conversion from fibrotic to edematous tissue
5. Reduction of 7-mm pockets to 3-mm pockets and reattachment of edematous tissue

49. Which of the following statements are true of root planing?
1. Root planing is frequently a presurgical technique when shallow pockets are present.
2. Root planing is used entirely as a presurgical technique.
3. Root planing with or without a curettage may reduce edematous 4-mm pockets to normal sulci.
4. 1 and 3
5. None of the above

50. Root planing is performed as a presurgical technique to achieve which of the following alterations?
a. To reduce bleeding during surgery
b. To provide an insight into the patient's healing response
c. To provide a better tissue consistency for incision
d. To resolve edema and exudation
1. a and c
2. a and d
3. a, c, and d
4. b, c, and d
5. All of the above

51. In some circumstances root planing will resolve the periodontal problem. Root planing can be expected to
a. reduce shallow edematous pockets to normal sulci
b. reduce shallow fibrotic pockets to normal sulci
c. cause shrinkage and/or reattachment of a three-walled infrabony defect
d. increase the zone of attached gingiva in edematous tissue
1. a and c
2. a and d
3. b and c
4. b and d
5. None of the above

* For further reading applicable to the material covered in the foregoing section, see the following numbered entries in the Suggested Reading at the end of this chapter: Glickman, 1972, pp 623–630; Goldman, pp 393–399, pp 599–608; Grant, pp 364–383, pp 436–442; Schluger, pp 376–382

52. When performing root planing, which of the following steps must be taken?
1. Isolate and anesthetize the area with block anesthesia and plane the tooth
2. Anesthetize the area with infiltration or block anesthesia, remove the calculus, plane the tooth
3. Isolate and anesthetize the area with block anesthesia, remove the calculus, remove the pocket lining and epithelial attachment
4. Anesthetize the area with infiltration or block anesthesia, plane the tooth, remove the pocket lining and epithelial attachment
5. Remove the calculus, plane the root, remove the epithelial attachment

53. Which of the following statements apply to curettage?
1. The epithelial attachment is separated and planed with a scaler.
2. The epithelial attachment is undermined and scooped away with a curette.
3. The inner lining of the pocket wall is planed smooth with a scooping motion.
4. The inner lining of the pocket wall is cut and removed with a scalpel.
5. The inner lining of the pocket wall is removed with a rotary motion of the curette.

## Surgery

Objectives of periodontal therapy include the elimination of pockets, the establishment of physiologic gingival and osseous contour, and the development of an adequate zone of attached gingiva. Periodontal surgery constitutes the major modality in the attainment of these therapeutic objectives. Periodontal surgical techniques may be divided conveniently into three broad categories: 1) gingival, 2) mucogingival, and 3) osseous.

GINGIVAL SURGERY
*Rationale for Gingival Surgery.* The main procedures of gingival surgery are gingivectomy and gingivoplasty. Gingivectomy involves the excision of the soft tissue wall of the pocket, while gingivoplasty involves the recontouring of the gingiva that has lost its physiologic gingival form. Gingivectomy and gingivoplasty are most often performed together, although they may be considered separately for teaching purposes. The two names reflect only the two different objectives of the same procedure.

There are certain basic prerequisites for gingivectomy/gingivoplasty. First, the zone of attached gingiva must be wide enough that excision of part of it will still leave a functionally adequate zone. Second, the underlying alveolar crest must be normal in form. If bone loss has occurred, the loss must be horizontal in nature so that there is a relatively regular crestal bone form at the new lower level. Third, there should be no infrabony defects or pockets.

If these prerequisites are met, gingivectomy/gingivoplasty may be used to

1. Eliminate supraalveolar pockets and pseudopockets
2. Remove fibrous or edematous enlargements of the gingiva
3. Transform rolled or blunted margins to ideal (knife-edge) form
4. Create more aesthetic form in cases in which the anatomic crown has not been fully exposed or in which there is asymmetry due to varying rates of marginal recession
5. Expose additional clinical crown to gain added retention for restorative purposes

*Techniques for Gingival Surgery.* The pockets on each surface are explored to determine their depth and morphology. Each pocket is marked in several areas so as to outline its course on each surface. The gingiva is resected apical to the points marking the course of the pockets between the base of the pocket and the crest of bone. The incision should be beveled at approximately 45° to the tooth surface, should pass completely through the soft tissue to tooth, and should recreate the normal festooned pattern of the gingiva as much as possible.

After the pocket wall is excised, the granulation tissue is removed with curettes and the roots examined to make sure débridement has been thorough. Areas with remaining calculus and rough cementum should be rescaled and planed.

### MUCOGINGIVAL SURGERY

*Rationale for Mucogingival Surgery.* Mucogingival surgery is performed for several purposes. One purpose is to relocate frena and muscle attachments which encroach upon the margin of the gingiva, causing the marginal tissue to pull away from the tooth surface.

Another purpose is to widen the zone of attached gingiva or create a new zone of attached gingiva, which must be accomplished when periodontal pockets extend close to or beyond the mucogingival junction or when the existing zone of attached gingiva is deemed inadequate for function. (The width of attached gingiva varies in different individuals and on different teeth. No minimum width has been established as a standard necessary for gingival health; even as little as 1 mm may create no problem in a patient with excellent plaque control. It does appear, however, that teeth which are to be covered with crowns placed subgingivally require more attached gingiva than teeth without crowns.)

It may also be necessary to perform mucogingival surgery in order to deepen the oral vestibule or to cover denuded root surfaces.

*Techniques for Mucogingival Surgery.* A number of methods are available to manage the various types of mucogingival problems.

*Apically Repositioned Flap.* A flap is raised; roots are scaled and planed, and osseous deformities may be corrected. Then the flap is repositioned at a more apical level and sutured to place.

*Replaced Flap (Flap Curettage, Flap for New Attachment).* After a flap is raised, chronically inflamed tissue is removed, and roots are scaled and curetted. Then the flap is placed back in its original position and sutured. This technique is used in areas where aesthetics are a major concern and the use of an apically repositioned flap would result in recession that would be cosmetically objectionable. The goal is to achieve connective tissue reattachment/new attachment to root surfaces.

*Laterally Repositioned Flap (Sliding Flap, Pedicle Flap.* A flap at least one and one-half times as wide as the defect is prepared from a donor site, reflected by sharp or blunt dissection, and placed over the prepared denuded root surface. Many variations of this procedure have been reported (oblique rotated flap, double papillae flap, etc.). All these types of flaps, when placed submarginally on an adjacent area, increase the zone of attached gingiva.

*Free Gingival Graft.* Attached gingiva, approximately 1 mm in thickness, is dissected free from a donor site (with a fairly wide zone of attached gingiva, frequently the palate) and placed onto a prepared tissue bed of either periosteum or bone and sutured in place.

*Frenectomy (Frenotomy, Frenum Repositioning).* Excision of the heavy fibrous frenum down to the periosteum is performed to relieve frenum pull on the marginal gingiva.

### OSSEOUS SURGERY

*Rationale for Osseous Surgery.* Osseous surgical techniques are performed either to reshape or to restore bone to an idealized form on the assumption that periodontal pockets will recur unless gingiva and bone have the same contour. To gain access to the alveolar bone, a flap is reflected.

*Types of Surgical Flaps.* Flaps may be classified as full thickness and partial thickness flaps. Full thickness flaps are reflected when the thickness of bone over the radicular root surfaces is adequate, and partial thickness flaps are reflected to protect facial and/or lingual surfaces when bone is thin.

The periodontal flap is incised (with a reverse beveled incision) and the outline is scalloped to follow the contour of the teeth. Depending upon the operator's need to preserve attached gingiva, the incision can be made in the sulcus (preserving the most attached gingiva) or submarginally when there is a wide zone present.

Once the flap has been raised, the pocket tissue removed, and the granulation tissue entirely cleaned away, the architecture of the osseous tissue is revealed.

*Types of Osseous Change.* Horizontal bone loss is the most common pattern of bone loss in periodontal disease. The bone is reduced in height, and the bone margin is horizontal or slightly angulated. Interdental septa and the facial and lingual plates are affected, but not necessarily to an equal degree around the same tooth.

Osseous craters are concavities in the crest of the interdental bone usually confined within facial and lingual walls. They occur less frequently between the tooth surface and facial and lingual bony plate.

Infrabony defects are hollowed-out troughs in the bone alongside one or more denuded root surfaces enclosed within one, two, three, or four bony walls. The base of the defect is located apical to the surrounding bone.

Bulbous bone contours are bony enlargements caused by exostoses, adaptation to function, or buttressing bone formation.

Hemisepta is the portion of an interdental septum remaining after the mesial or distal portion has been destroyed by disease.

Inconsistent margins are angular or V-shaped defects produced by resorption of the facial or lingual alveolar plate or by abrupt differences between the height of the facial or lingual margins and the height of the interdental septa.

Ledges are plateaulike bone margins caused by resorption of thickened bony plates.

Locations of special concern in the bone destruction occurring in periodontal disease are the furcations. Bifurcation and trifurcation involvement are stages of progressive periodontal disease and have the same causes. The bone destructive pattern may be horizontal, or it may produce angular osseous defects associated with infrabony pockets. Furcation involvements are a problem to manage because of the extreme difficulty in maintaining the areas; caries, idiopathic resorption, and abscess formation may develop along an endodontic, periodontic, or combined pathway.

It sometimes becomes necessary in molar teeth with deep furcation involvements to hemisect and/or to resect roots. The rationale for performing such procedures is either to create a separation that can be cleaned more readily or to remove an especially bad root which tends to jeopardize the longevity of other roots on the same tooth or roots of adjacent teeth.

*Techniques for Osseous Surgery.* The procedures in osseous surgery fit into categories: (1) bone resectioning and reshaping to correct osseous defects and create physiologic osseous contours, and (2) implant procedures to stimulate bone growth and restore tissue destroyed by disease.

*Bone Reshaping and Resection Procedures.* Bone reshaping and resection techniques are commonly referred to as osteoplasty, bone reshaping without removing tooth-supporting bone, and ostectomy, the bone reshaping which involves some portions of tooth-supporting bone.

*Bone Stimulative Procedures.* Implant procedures to stimulate bone growth in infrabony defects is being utilized by some practitioners. Success is considered unpredictable, however, so these procedures are usually reserved for the very few cases in which the support of key teeth would be compromised by osseous resection.

Osseous defects which seem to respond best to implantation procedures are the three-walled infrabony type. This is not surprising since three-walled defects are more likely than any other type of osseous deformity to be filled by natural repair if the operator simply removes the granulation and debrides the root.

Bone grafts may be autogenous, homogenous, or heterogeneous. Autogenous grafts obviously produce the best results because they do not provoke immune reactions leading to rejection. In successful cases the bone graft serves as a source of osteoblasts and activates connective tissue cells which develop into osteoblasts. The bone graft itself ultimately is resorbed and replaced by new bone.

Grafts may consist of cancellous or cortical bone, or a combination. Cancellous bone is preferable because the marrow spaces and the greater vascularity and cellularity are presumed to permit easier incorporation in the healing process.

Some of the grafting procedures utilized are bone swaging, osseous coagulum (cortical and cancellous bone), tuberosity grafts, hip marrow grafts, and grafts from fresh extraction sites (cancellous).*

### QUESTIONS

54. Gingivectomy can be performed under which of the following conditions?
    a. To eliminate pockets when the alveolar crest is normal or bone loss is horizontal
    b. When an adequate zone of attached gingiva is present
    c. To eliminate three-walled infrabony defects
    d. When gingival margins are rolled

    1. a and b
    2. a and c
    3. a, b, and c
    4. a, b, and d
    5. All of the above

*For further reading applicable to the material covered in the foregoing section, see the following numbered entries in the Suggested Reading at the end of this chapter: Glickman 1972, pp 228–235, pp 635–653, pp 712–714, pp 672–682, p 768; Goldman, pp 616–636, pp 638–757; Grant, pp 446–449, p 473, pp 530–546; Schluger, pp 444–445, p 523, pp 568–569

55. Mucogingival surgery is performed for which of the following purposes?
    a. To deepen the vestibule
    b. To cover denuded root surfaces
    c. To decrease the zone of attached gingiva
    d. To relocate frena and high muscle attachment
    1. a and b
    2. a and c
    3. a, b, and c
    4. a, b, and d
    5. All of the above

56. Select from the following those procedures which are considered mucogingival surgery.
    a. Apically repositioned flap
    b. Free gingival graft
    c. Gingivectomy
    d. Curettage.
    1. a and b
    2. a and c
    3. a, b, and c
    4. a, c, and d
    5. All of the above

57. Select from the following the osseous changes which can occur in periodontal disease.
    a. Osseous craters
    b. Osseous bulges
    c. Hemisepta
    d. Infrabony defects
    1. a and b
    2. a and c
    3. a, b, and c
    4. a, c, and d
    5. All of the above

58. Which of the following statements is true of osseous surgery?
    1. Reshaping of the bone is referred to as ostectomy or osteoplasty.
    2. Implantation of bone is referred to as ostectomy or osteoplasty.
    3. Implantation procedures are utilized with increasingly greater frequency since the surgical results are reasonably predictable.
    4. Reshaping of bone should not be performed when supporting bone will have to be removed to eliminate the defect.
    5. Bone swaging and osseous coagulum are ostectomy procedures.

## Splinting

There are several different methods of splinting teeth. Major classification is based on the length of time the splint is to be used. Minor classifications are based on whether the technique of splinting involves removal of coronal tooth structure or leaves teeth unaltered.

I. Temporary stabilization
   A. Extracoronal splints not requiring cavity preparation
      1. Removable (acrylic; cast continuous clasps)
      2. Fixed (wire/acrylic; soldered orthodontic bands)
   B. Intracoronal splints requiring cavity preparation (wire/acrylic; wire/amalgam; composite; combination)
II. Provisional stabilization
   A. Acrylic splints
   B. Gold-band and acrylic splints
III. Permanent or long-term stabilization
   A. Removable
   B. Fixed
   C. Combination

When teeth are seriously loosened by periodontal disturbances, stabilization by splinting is extremely valuable before, during, and after corrective therapy. The prime objective of stabilization by splinting is to rest the affected structures by redistributing functional and parafunctional forces and especially by reducing those forces that act in a horizontal direction.

If there is reason to believe that the mobility is temporary, any form of stabilization should be conservative; the teeth should not be altered by removal of tooth structure. However, if mobility is due to a permanent loss of support, the overall projected treatment plan must take long-term stabilization by permanent splinting into consideration; a form of stabilization that is less conservative of tooth structure may be justified. Removable acrylic splints, normally used for temporary stabilization, can be used by patients (especially those with clenching and bruxing habits) on a rather permanent basis.*

For the majority of patients, splinting should be considered only after the preliminary phase of periodontal therapy has been completed, that is, after all local factors contributing to inflammation have been eliminated and occlusal adjustment selective grinding has been performed. The method of splinting should neither impede normal functions nor frustrate the oral hygiene and physiotherapeutic efforts of the patient.

QUESTION

59. Select from the following statements about splinting those which are true.
    a. Splinting of a permanent nature is the treatment of choice for mobile teeth.
    b. Splinting should be performed as the first treatment procedure in mobile teeth.
    c. Splinting is usually performed after the local factors causing inflammation have been eliminated.

*For further reading applicable to the material covered in the foregoing section, see the following numbered entries in the Suggested Reading at the end of this chapter: Goldman, p 465; Schluger, pp 408–409

d. Splinting with a removable acrylic splint can sometimes be used on a permanent basis.

1. a and b
2. a and c
3. c and d
4. b and d
5. a, b, and d

## Occlusal Correction

More has been written, but perhaps less is known, about the precise role of occlusion in periodontal disease than about most aspects of periodontics. There is probably no other phase of dentistry as confused by divergence of terminology and definitions as the field of occlusion.

RATIONALE. Occlusal correction is the establishment of a functional relationship favorable to the periodontium by one of the following procedures: 1) reshaping the teeth by grinding, 2) reshaping the teeth by restorations, and 3) repositioning the teeth with orthodontic tooth movement. Occlusal correction is based upon the premise that tissue damage and excessive tooth mobility caused by unfavorable occlusal forces undergo repair naturally when injurious forces are corrected.

Occlusal correction or adjustment from the periodontal frame of reference is performed via selective grinding. The occlusion is adjusted when patients show evidence of occlusal trauma 1) which is manifested as periodontal injury (mobility of the anterior teeth), muscle dysfunction, and temporomandibular joint disorders or 2) which results from occlusal prematurities and bruxing. Occlusal adjustment is not recommended as a preventive therapy for the correction of what appear to be abnormal occlusal relationships in patients without signs of trauma from occlusion.

TECHNIQUE. There are three times in the course of periodontal treatment when occlusal interventions may be undertaken: 1) preliminary grinding, 2) definitive grinding, and 3) check grinding.

Preliminary grinding is a necessity early in the treatment when the patient complains of pain or discomfort or when normal function is prevented by excessive mobility.

Definitive grinding is usually performed after resolution of inflammation. Whether it is performed after initial therapy or after periodontal surgery is usually determined by the degree of mobility of the teeth. In instances where mobility is considerable, the adjustment should be performed prior to surgery and refined after final healing. In instances when mobility is less significant the occlusal adjustment can be done after surgery. In such cases definitive and check grinding can be done simultaneously.

Check grinding is generally performed after all other therapy has been completed. Usually a month is allowed to elapse after surgery; then the mouth is checked for trauma that may have resulted from slight shifting of the teeth.

There are many different philosophies and techniques of occlusal adjustment, but no matter which concept is being followed, the first step is the elimination of gross prematurities and the adjustment of centric relation–centric occlusion discrepancies. In those techniques involving adjustment of lateral and protrusive moments, the elimination of balancing interferences is the second step; correction of protrusive interferences is the final step.*

QUESTIONS

60. Occlusal correction is performed in which of the following circumstances?
    a. When patients exhibit migration of anterior teeth
    b. When patients' radiographs exhibit thickening of the periodontal ligament space
    c. When patients have abnormal occlusal relationships which may lead to future damage
    d. When patients have temporomandibular joint disorders

    1. a and b
    2. b and c
    3. a, b, and c
    4. a, b, and d
    5. All of the above

61. Occlusal correction can be accomplished by which of the following types of procedures?
    a. Repositioning the teeth with orthodontic tooth movement
    b. Repositioning the teeth with periodontal surgical procedures
    c. Reshaping the teeth with restorations
    d. Reshaping the teeth by grinding

    1. a and b
    2. a and c
    3. a, b, and c
    4. a, c, and d
    5. All of the above

## Maintenance

Preservation of the periodontal health of the treated patient requires as positive a program as the elimination of periodontal disease. After treatment is completed, patients are placed on a program of periodic recall visits which are the foundation of a meaningful long-term prevention/maintenance program. The interval between visits is varied according to the patient's needs, although a 3–4 month interval is a common one

*For further reading applicable to the material covered in the foregoing section, see the following numbered entries in the Suggested Reading at the end of this chapter: Glickman 1972, pp 852–856; Goldman, p 563, p 632

for patients who have required periodontal therapy. Transfer of the patient from active treatment status to a maintenance program is a definitive step in total patient care which requires time and effort on the part of the dentist and staff. Patients must be made to understand the purpose of the maintenance program.

Recall visits should include examination for dental caries and lesions of the oral mucosa. A complete series of intraoral radiographs should be taken periodically at recall visits and compared with previous ones for preservation of bone height, repair of osseous defects, signs of trauma from occlusion, periapical pathology, and caries. Periodontal care at the recall visit is concerned with two primary areas: gingival health and occlusion.

Since gingival health is maintained by proper plaque control, methods of plaque control must be reviewed at recall visits until the patient demonstrates the necessary proficiency, even if it requires additional instruction sessions. Combined with plaque control, periodic scaling, root planing, and curettage are the most effective means of minimizing the recurrence of gingivitis and periodontal pockets.

The occlusion changes as the natural dentition and dental restorations wear with function. Patients must be checked for the earliest signs of trauma from occlusion, and the occlusion should be adjusted when necessary. Periodic evaluation is especially important in patients whose periodontal treatment included correction of the occlusion by means of extensive dental restorations or occlusal adjustment.*

QUESTIONS

62. Select from the following statements the one which is true of periodontal maintenance.
   1. Periodontal maintenance therapy is an active part of treatment which is concerned with pocket elimination.
   2. Periodontal maintenance appointments occur at 6-month intervals.
   3. Periodontal maintenance visits should include a full series of radiographs at each appointment.
   4. Periodontal maintenance is necessary only in patients who have demonstrated poor plaque control.
   5. Periodontal maintenance is a definitive phase of therapy, and the recall intervals vary according to patient needs.

63. Recurrence of periodontal disease is minimized in which of the following circumstances?
   1. Recurrence is minimized when the patient demonstrates proper plaque control.
   2. Recurrence is minimized when periodic radiographs are taken at recall appointments.

* For further reading applicable to the material covered in the foregoing section, see the following numbered entries in the Suggested Reading at the end of this chapter: Glickman, 1972, p 984; Goldman, pp 1014–1032

3. Recurrence is minimized when the occlusion is adjusted at recall appointments.
4. Recurrence cannot be minimized since people are either susceptible or not susceptible to periodontal disease.
5. Recurrence is not a concern in patients who have received periodontal therapy.

## Specific Disease Therapy

ACUTE PROBLEMS. Periodontal diseases are generally considered to be chronic. There are, nevertheless, a few acute inflammatory periodontal diseases.

*Acute Periodontal Abscess.* The classic signs of acute inflammation, i.e., swelling, redness, and pain, are not always present with the acute periodontal abscess; the signs may be masked and subtle. Adenopathy, extrusion of the tooth involved, loosening, and tenderness to even slight percussion are most common. A slight elevation of the patient's temperature is an occasional finding.

The first objective in treating the acute abscess is to establish drainage. As with many acute pyogenic infections, the release of pressure through the evacuation of pus has a salutary effect on the lesion. Pain is relieved, swelling is resolved, the extended tooth returns to its normal position, mobility is reduced, the pericementitis no longer gives acute pain on occlusion, and in general the patient begins to feel better.

Drainage may be established in one of two ways: 1) by finding the orifice of the occluded pocket and gently distending the aperture so that instruments can be used to evacuate the pus or 2) by traditional incision and drainage. In both approaches the complete evacuation of the contents of the pocket is highly desirable to end the acute phase, both to relieve pain and to end the rapid bone loss due to the acute inflammatory infiltrate.

After the acute phase has subsided, there remains a chronic inflammatory lesion which must be treated. These lesions often occur in a three-walled infrabony defect, since such a site is more prone to occlusion of the aperture and to subsequent acute flare-up than one with a wide aperture and few, if any, confining bony walls. This feature provides an occasional favorable morphologic arrangement for a reversal of bone and connective-tissue attachment loss, which responds well to early pocket therapy with a natural reconstitution of lost bone and reattachment.

The administration of antibiotics is standard supportive treatment of the periodontal abscess, especially when an elevated temperature and/or lymphadenopathy are present.

*Pericoronitis.* Inflammation of the gingiva in relation to the crown of an incompletely erupted tooth, which occurs most frequently in the mandibular third molar, is called pericoronitis. It may be acute, subacute, or chronic. Since the space between the crown of the tooth and the overlying gingival flap (operculum) is an ideal area for the accumulation of food debris and bacterial growth, acute inflammatory involvement is always a possibility. The clinical picture is that of a markedly red, swollen, suppurating lesion that is exquisitely tender, with radiating pains to the ear, throat, and floor of the mouth.

Treatment consists of flushing the area of debris by injecting warm saline under the operculum as well as administering antibiotics if the patient has a fever and/or lymphadenopathy. Once the acute phase has subsided, further treatment may consist of excision of the operculum with a distal wedge flap or gingivectomy.

*Acute Necrotizing Ulcerative Gingivitis* **(ANUG).** As the characteristics of ANUG have been discussed earlier in this chapter, they need not be repeated here.

Treatment of ANUG is usually managed in a series of appointments because of the extreme discomfort experienced by the patient even without tissue manipulation. At the first visit, superficial deposits are removed with either a hand instrument (scaler or curette) or frequently an ultrasonic scaler. If the patient has a fever or lymphadenopathy, antibiotics are prescribed. Frequently peroxide mouth rinses are recommended. The cycle is repeated at subsequent appointments until all the deposits are removed, temperature is normal, and the patient's reparative processes are underway. Residual deformities often occur and appropriate treatment is undertaken to eliminate the defects.

***Acute Herpetic Gingivostomatitis.*** Acute herpetic gingivostomatitis is an infection of the oral cavity caused by the herpes simplex virus. Secondary bacterial infection frequently complicates the clinical picture. Although it most frequently occurs in infants, it can be found in adolescents and adults.

The condition appears as a diffuse, erythematous, shiny involvement of the gingiva and the adjacent oral mucosa with varying degrees of edema and gingival bleeding. In its initial stage it is characterized by the presence of discrete spherical gray vesicles which may occur on the gingiva, mucosa, soft palate, pharynx. After 24 hours the vesicles rupture and form painful small ulcers with a red, elevated, halolike margin and a depressed yellowish or grayish white central portion. Only palliative treatment is recommended, and the use of antibiotics if fever is present. The duration of involvement is 7–10 days, followed by uneventful healing.

## ATROPHY AND HYPERTROPHY

***Periodontal Atrophy.*** Atrophy is a decrease in the size of an organ or part because of the loss of its cellular elements after it has attained mature size. There are two forms of periodontal atrophy: gingival recession and disuse atrophy.

Gingival recession involves a noninflammatory loss of periodontal tissue with concurrent apical movement of the soft tissue attachment to the tooth but without pocket formation. The etiology may be traumatic, resulting from vigorous long-term use of a hard-bristled toothbrush, for example; it may result from excessive occlusal force; or it may occur spontaneously with aging.

Disuse atrophy is a condition in which functional forces have been removed from the tooth; there is a loss of alveolar bone and the principal fibers of the periodontal ligament without gingival recession. The alveolar bone proper persists, but the supporting bone trabeculae become thin and finally disappear as the marrow spaces increase in size.

***Hypertrophy.*** Hyperplastic lesions occur primarily in the gingiva. Gingival hyperplasia is an overgrowth of tissue due to an increase in the number of its elements, and it serves no functional purpose. Gingival hyperplasia is generally subclassified on the basis of its etiology. It may result from chronic irritation, from the endocrine imbalance of adolescence or pregnancy, or from long-term use of certain drugs such as diphenylhydantoin (Dilantin). It may be hereditary, as in cases of familial fibromatosis.*

## QUESTIONS

64. Treatment of ANUG consists of which of the following procedures?

    a. Removal of deposits, usually in a series of appointments
    b. Peroxide injected into the ulcerated lesion
    c. Antibiotics when a fever is present
    d. Antibiotics when a lymphadenopathy is present

  1. a and b
  2. a and c
  3. a, b and c
  4. a, c, and d
  5. All of the above

65. Select from the following situations those in which gingival hyperplasia may occur.

    a. Diphenylhydantoin
    b. Familial fibromatosis
    c. Pregnancy
    d. Chronic irritation

  1. a and b
  2. a and c
  3. a, b, and c
  4. a, c, and d
  5. All of the above

* For further reading applicable to the material covered in the foregoing section, see the following numbered entries in the Suggested Reading at the end of this chapter: Glickman, 1972, p 126, pp 129–138, p 143, p 242; Goldman, p 144, pp 167–177; Schluger, p 68, pp 240–243

## PREVENTION

### Theory

Oral hygiene can be considered both a therapeutic and prophylactic modality. In order to achieve and maintain good dental health there must be a regular disruption of bacterial colonization on the surface of the teeth. This is difficult to accomplish because these bacterial colonizations (plaque) are transparent, are sticky, and cover a myriad of difficult-to-reach tooth surfaces. The products of these colonies, if left undisturbed, cause the onset of tissue inflammation. However, the plaque mat can be reduced to levels compatible with gingival health if daily meticulous oral hygiene is practiced.

The therapist can only work toward establishing a healthy environment that can be maintained with proper hygiene; the maintenance itself must be the responsibility of the patient. If a patient will not put forth the necessary efforts for controlling plaque formation, then the disease process will surely return. In fact, patient neglect is one of the principal reasons for the wide distribution of chronic inflammatory periodontal disease. Unfortunately the only effective means of control of periodontal disease is by means of a difficult and demanding regimen of mechanical removal on a daily basis. There are many techniques for plaque control, but no single one has been proven best or universally applicable to all patients.

Motivating the patient to perform the necessary procedures regularly is a most difficult aspect of periodontal therapy. The therapist must deal with the patient's psychologic makeup, intelligence, and manual dexterity. The patient must be educated about etiology, proper method for controlling its agents, and ways to recognize early warning signs of disease. Plaque disclosants and phase contrast microscopy often prove to be invaluable aids in the education process. However, these efforts to educate the patient are of little value if the patient does not perform the necessary procedures. Therefore, along with information, the therapist must give the patient a desire to do these procedures. The therapist's skills in relating to patients become most important, since these skills may be the difference between success and failure.°

### QUESTIONS

66. Which of the following statements about plaque control is not accurate?
    1. There must be a regular disruption of bacterial colonization on the surface of the teeth.

° For further reading applicable to the material covered in the foregoing section, see the following numbered entries in the Suggested Reading at the end of this chapter: Glickman, 1972, pp 443–444; Goldman, pp 291–295; Grant, pp 385–386; Prichard, p 778; Schluger, pp 344–349

2. Plaque removal is difficult because it is transparent, sticky, and covers very hard to reach surfaces.
3. Plaque products, left undisturbed, will cause inflammation of the periodontal tissues.
4. Current theory is that plaque causes gingivitis which left untreated will become periodontitis.
5. Adequate plaque control can readily be obtained without patient cooperation and individual effort.

67. Which of the following statements about patient motivation for oral hygiene is not accurate?
    1. Motivating and educating the patient about etiology and proper removal of the etiologic factors is usually a straightforward and simple procedure.
    2. Motivating the patient toward proper oral hygiene is most difficult because it is concerned with the patient's psychologic make-up, intelligence, and manual dexterity.
    3. The use of such aids as plaque disclosants and phase contrast microscopy are often valuable tools in efforts to educate and motivate a patient.
    4. The passing on of information is of little value if the patient does not perform the necessary procedures.
    5. The therapist must instill in a patient, not only knowledge about oral hygiene, but also the desire to perform the necessary hygiene procedures.

68. Which of the following statements about prevention of periodontal disease is not true?
    1. Patient neglect is only a minor reason for the wide distribution of chronic inflammatory periodontal disease.
    2. The therapist is greatly limited in the treatment of periodontal disease because it is necessary to rely upon the patient to remove the primary etiologic agent (plaque).
    3. Plaque removal, which is a major portion of any preventive program, is most difficult to perform.
    4. There are many techniques to achieve the proper level of plaque control, but no single one has been proven best.
    5. Plaque products bring about the onset of inflammation which, when left uncontrolled, progresses to more advanced periodontal disease.

69. Which of the following statements best describes the therapist's role in the prevention of periodontal disease?
    1. The therapist is the primary force in prevention of periodontal disease, although a strong supportive role is allocated to the patient.
    2. If the patient will not put forth the necessary effort for plaque control, then the therapist must assume the responsibility.
    3. The therapist can only work toward establishing an environment that can be maintained with proper hygiene; proper oral hygiene can only be achieved by the patient.
    4. Since plaque control is a difficult task for the patient to accomplish adequately, this responsibility rests with the therapist.

5. Poor plaque control can be compensated for by careful control of nutrition.

70. Which of the following statements best describes the place of adequate oral hygiene in control of periodontal disease?
    1. Oral hygiene is usually considered a prophylactic modality.
    2. Oral hygiene is usually considered a therapeutic modality.
    3. Oral hygiene is considered both a therapeutic and prophylactic modality.
    4. Periodontal health is maintained in a different manner posttreatment than pretreatment.
    5. Meticulous oral hygiene on a daily basis is not compatible with general health because of potential damage to the soft tissues.

71. The only orally effective means of control of periodontal disease is by
    1. daily rinses with warm salt water
    2. daily use of commercial mouth rinses
    3. a daily regimen of plaque control via mechanical removal
    4. a weekly regimen of plaque control via mechanical removal
    5. yearly professional removal of plaque and calculus

## Brushing

There have been numerous techniques of toothbrushing reported in the literature (e.g., Roll, Stillman's, Charter's, Fones', Bass). The proponents of each method give myriads of reasons to explain why their method is best. However, there are no conclusive studies to show that one method is superior to any other. It appears that thoroughness on the part of the patient is far more important than technique. The patient must be able to detect plaque and take the time necessary to remove it.

The most popular methods of brushing taught today are probably the Bass, Roll, Scruds, and Charter. The most popular toothbrush is the soft nylon because it is believed that a soft nylon brush can be inserted into areas critical for plaque removal without irritating or damaging the gingiva.

At one time a great deal of effort was devoted to the study of hand versus power toothbrushes. It appears that there is no difference between the two.*

### QUESTIONS

72. The most effective method of toothbrushing is
    1. Roll
    2. Stillman's

* For further reading applicable to the material covered in the foregoing section, see the following numbered entries in the Suggested Reading at the end of this chapter: Glickman, 1972, pp 444–460; Goldman, pp 429–432; Grant, pp 391–405; Prichard, pp 782–783; Schluger, pp 350–353

3. Charter's
4. Fones'
5. No one method has been shown to be best.

73. Which of the following is the most important aspect of toothbrushing?
    1. The design of the brush head
    2. The method of toothbrushing
    3. Thoroughness on the part of the patient
    4. The frequency
    5. The use of toothpaste containing fluoride

74. Which of the following statements best describes the popularity of the soft nylon toothbrush?
    1. Soft nylon brushes are the most readily available.
    2. Soft nylon brushes are cheaper.
    3. Soft nylon brushes last longer.
    4. Soft nylon brushes are not irritating to the gingiva.
    5. Soft nylon brushes do not scratch dental restorations.

## Flossing

The interproximal areas of the teeth are the most difficult from which to remove plaque, and not surprisingly, the incidence of periodontitis is greatest in these areas. Since these areas cannot be reached effectively by any of the standard toothbrushing techniques, other methods must be utilized.

The most common method of interproximal plaque removal is the use of dental floss. It is the best way to clean these areas when the interdental space is filled by the interdental papilla. There has been a good deal of controversy concerning unwaxed floss versus waxed floss, but whether one is better than the other is still unestablished. No matter which type of dental floss is utilized, it is important to remember that its purpose is primarily to remove plaque from the teeth. There are some aides to facilitate flossing such as various floss holders for reaching posterior areas and plastic needles for threading through splints and under pontics.†

### QUESTION

75. Which of the following statements about dental flossing is not accurate?
    1. It is not proper for individuals without periodontal disease to use dental flossing.
    2. The most efficient method of interproximal plaque removal is the use of dental floss.
    3. Unwaxed dental floss has not been shown definitely superior to waxed floss.
    4. The primary purpose of dental floss is the removal of plaque from the interproximal tooth surfaces.
    5. Dental floss can be used on areas of splints and bandages with the aid of plastic needles.

† For further reading applicable to the material covered in the foregoing section, see the following numbered entries in the Suggested Reading at the end of this chapter: Glickman, 1972, p 461; Goldman, p 432; Grant, pp 387–389; Prichard, pp 783–784; Schluger, pp 350–353

## Adjunctive Procedures

Often the interdental spaces of a patient who has undergone periodontal therapy are no longer filled with tissues. Instead this area is an open space. In such a case other methods of interproximal cleaning may be used quite effectively, for example, toothpicks, rubber tips, Perio-aids, Proxabrushes, and Stimudents.

The use of water-irrigating devices to remove loose particles is often helpful. However, it must be remembered that these devices do not remove bacterial plaque unless it is first loosened from the tooth surfaces by brushing and flossing. There have been many tests performed on mouthwashes containing a wide variety of chemotherapeutic agents; none has been found that is both effective and safe for regular use.

Even with all the brushing methods and oral hygiene aids available, it can be said that the patient's thoroughness in removing plaque every 24 hours is the most critical factor upon which effective oral hygiene and ultimately success or failure of periodontal treatment rests.*

### QUESTIONS

76. Patients who have undergone periodontal therapy may no longer have interdental spaces filled with tissue. These areas can now be cleaned by means other than dental floss. Which of the following is a floss substitute?
    1. Proxabrushes
    2. Perio-aids
    3. Rubber tips
    4. Stimudents
    5. All of the above

77. Which of the following statements most accurately reflects the use of adjunctive home care procedures?
    1. The most effective adjunctive interproximal cleaner has been proven to be the rubber tip.
    2. There are many effective mouthwashes available for clinical use
    3. The water-irrigating devices available today, when used properly, make adequate substitutes for the use of floss.
    4. Water-irrigating devices should usually be utilized prior to dental flossing.
    5. No matter which adjuncts are used, the most important feature for oral hygiene is patient thoroughness.

## PATHOGENESIS

### Inflammatory Periodontal Disease

Pathogenesis is the course of events in the disease process. It is assumed that the pathogenesis of chronic

* For further reading applicable to the material covered in the foregoing section, see the following numbered entries in the Suggested Reading at the end of this chapter: Glickman, 1972, pp 462–467; Goldman, pp 434–437; Grant, pp 389–391, p 392, pp 405–508; Prichard, p 782; Schluger, pp 356–363

inflammatory periodontal disease begins with an inflammatory process in the gingival tissue which is initiated by the products of plaque. If there is no migration of the epithelial attachment or loss of alveolar bone, this inflammation is referred to as gingivitis. It appears that, although it is unproven, in many cases of gingivitis the inflammatory process spreads with a resultant loss of attachment of epithelium and connective tissue to the tooth and loss of bone. This is periodontitis, which is assumed to be an extension of gingivitis and not a distinct disease entity. In other words, the difference between gingivitis and periodontitis is the degree of destruction associated with the inflammatory lesion.

Classifications such as initial, early, established, and advanced have been created to describe the series of events leading from the earliest inflammatory signs to the more advanced signs of chronic inflammation associated with a great degree of tissue destruction and loss of attachment to the teeth.†

The junctional epithelium is a point of weakness. It is here that the primary entry of bacterial products probably occurs. Inflammation begins in the connective tissue just below the junction and spreads to the deeper tissues. It is believed that this spread of inflammatory products follows the connective tissue immediately surrounding the blood vessels. As collagen fibers are destroyed, the attachment of gingival fibers to the root is destroyed; the epithelial attachment begins to migrate apically. At the same time, inflammation reaches the crest of the alveolar bone and bone resorption begins.

The various stages of inflammation are associated with the presence of leukocytes, lymphocytes, plasma cells, macrophages, altered fibroblasts, extravascular serum proteins, and exudate from the gingival sulcus. Collagen fiber destruction, alterations in the junctional epithelium with rete peg formation, destruction of perivascular collagen, and loss of alveolar bone and periodontal ligament are also associated with inflammation. As the lesion advances, there is a shift in population of inflammatory cells. In the earliest lesion neutrophils make up the largest percentage of inflammatory cells; in the more established lesion there are more lymphocytes; and in the advanced stages, more plasma cells.

The inflammatory process is protective, but it has a destructive component which causes the breakdown associated with periodontal disease. Much of the current research in periodontics is directed at finding the actual products associated with this breakdown. Evidence indicates that plaque substances activate various host defense mechanisms. There seems to be a strong relationship between immunopathology and the in-

† The periodontal lesion does not usually reveal a straight line progression, however; many patients reveal periods of active disease and periods of remission.

flammatory destruction associated with periodontal diseases.*

QUESTIONS

78. A basic assumption concerning the pathogenesis of chronic inflammatory periodontal diseases is that
    1. the onset of gingival inflammation is closely linked to heredity
    2. the onset of gingival inflammation follows the radiographic signs of alveolar bone loss
    3. chronic inflammatory periodontal disease is initiated by the products of plaque
    4. the products of plaque play only a minor role until periodontal disease has been initiated, usually by occlusal trauma
    5. before migration of the epithelial attachment, plaque products are not capable of causing any damage to the gingiva

79. The relationship of periodontitis and gingivitis is best described by which of the following statements?
    1. Gingivitis is the result of inflammation initiated by plaque products while periodontitis is the result of inflammation initiated by trauma from occlusion.
    2. Gingivitis is always associated with bone loss while periodontitis usually is not.
    3. There is no relationship between gingivitis and periodontitis.
    4. Gingivitis is a disease of the epithelium while periodontitis is a disease of the connective tissue.
    5. The difference between gingivitis and periodontitis is the degree of destruction associated with the chronic inflammatory lesion.

80. Which of the following statements concerning the spread of inflammation in the periodontal disease is least accurate?
    1. The junctional epithelium is a weak barrier to plaque products and the onset of inflammation.
    2. Inflammation usually begins in the connective tissue just below the junctional epithelium.
    3. Inflammation is believed to spread to the deeper tissues by following along the collagen fibers of the gingival fiber apparatus.
    4. Inflammation is believed to spread to the deeper tissues by following the connective tissue immediately surrounding the blood vessels.
    5. The spread of inflammation results in a destruction of the gingival fiber and apical migration of the epithelial attachment.

81. Which one of the following statements accurately reflects the population shift of inflammatory cells as the inflammatory lesion advances?
    1. There is a shift from neutrophils in the earliest lesion, to mast cells in the established lesion, and to macrophages in the more advanced lesion

    2. There is a shift from neutrophils in the earliest lesion, to plasma cells in the established lesion, and to lymphocytes in the more advanced lesion.
    3. There is a shift from plasma cells in the earliest lesion, to lymphocytes in the established lesion, and to neutrophils in the more advanced lesion
    4. There is a shift from neutrophils in the earliest lesion, to lymphocytes in the established lesion, and to plasma cells in the advanced lesion
    5. The population of inflammatory cells remains constant.

82. Which of the following statements about inflammatory periodontal disease is most accurate?
    1. The periodontal lesion does not usually reveal a straight line progression; many patients reveal periods of active disease and periods of remission.
    2. The inflammatory process is protective, but has a destructive component.
    3. Plaque substances seem to activate various host defense mechanisms.
    4. There is a strong relationship between immunopathology and the inflammatory destruction associated with periodontal disease.
    5. All of the above are accurate statements.

## Other Periodontal Diseases

Except for the ulcerative and traumatic lesions of the gingiva, the pathogenesis of other gingival disease entities, such as enlargements and nutritional diseases, is the same as in plaque-induced disease. These disease entities alter resistance to the products of plaque, but the same inflammatory lesion results. The ulcerative and traumatic lesions, on the other hand, have a different etiology and pathogenesis. The ulcerative gingival lesions are not caused by plaque; they are surface ulcerations of the gingiva. They may be caused by bacteria, viruses, systemic disease, chemical burns, etc.

Excessive occlusal forces damage the attachment apparatus. Associated with this damage is a sterile necrosis without loss of horizontal bone height or soft tissue attachment to the tooth. In the absence of underlying inflammatory periodontal disease, this condition is believed to be totally reversible with elimination of the excess forces.†

QUESTIONS

83. Which of the statements about excessive occlusal forces is not accurate?
    1. Excessive occlusal forces may damage the attachment apparatus.
    (*Continued*)

* For further reading applicable to the material covered in the foregoing section, see the following numbered entries in the Suggested Reading at the end of this chapter: Glickman, 1972, pp 81–82, pp 211–213; Goldman, pp 101–138; Grant, pp 193–204, pp 206–230; Prichard, pp 1–50, pp 67–68; Schluger, pp 196–231.

† For further reading applicable to the material covered in the foregoing section, see the following numbered entries in the Suggested Reading at the end of this chapter: Glickman, 1972, p 95, p 98, p 101, pp 129–131, p 140, pp 152–153, pp 190–193, pp 213–217; Goldman, pp 198–203; Grant, p 225, pp 245–247, pp 266–270, pp 272–273; Prichard, p 3, pp 135–213; Schluger, p 241, pp 243–244, pp 255–256

2. Damage associated with excessive occlusal forces results in a sterile necrosis.
3. The damage associated with excessive occlusal forces does not cause a loss of horizontal bone height.
4. The damage associated with excessive occlusal forces does not cause any alteration in the soft tissue attachment to the tooth.
5. The damage associated with excessive occlusal forces is not reversible even when the excessive forces are eliminated.

84. Which of the following statements concerning ulcerative lesions of the gingiva is correct?
    1. These lesions have the same pathogenesis as chronic inflammatory gingival disease.
    2. These lesions are primarily caused by plaque products.
    3. These lesions alter the resistance of the tissues to the plaque products.
    4. These lesions have a different etiology, but the same pathogenesis as chronic inflammatory gingival disease.
    5. These lesions have a different etiology and pathogenesis from chronic inflammatory gingival disease.

## EPIDEMIOLOGY

Epidemiology is concerned with the study of the disease state of large populations. In order to conduct studies effectively in large populations indices which reduce clinical observations to numerical values have been developed. Some of the more common periodontal indices are the PMA, PI, PDI, etc. Much of the data gathered can be misleading, however. For instance, periodontal disease incidence is very high but much of it can be cured. Therefore, knowing the occurrence without the severity would not be very helpful.

Epidemiology studies of periodontal disease have shown a strong relationship between plaque, home care, and gingivitis. Poor oral hygiene seems to be the most important factor in the prevalence and severity of gingivitis. This does not hold true, however, for periodontitis, since there does not seem to be a correlation between the severity of the signs of inflammation and the amount of destruction associated with periodontitis.[*]

### QUESTIONS

85. Which of the following statements concerning epidemiology is not accurate?
    1. Epidemiology is concerned with the study of the disease state of large populations.

[*] For further reading applicable to the material covered in the foregoing section, see the following numbered entries in the Suggested Reading at the end of this chapter: Glickman, 1972, pp 275–286; Goldman, pp 57–64; Grant, pp 156–160; Schluger, pp 74–82

2. In order to conduct epidemiologic studies effectively, the development of indices has been necessary.
3. Indices are the reduction of clinical observations to numerical values.
4. PMA, PI, PDI are designations for commonly used periodontal indices.
5. The fact that periodontal disease incidence is very high can be readily interpreted to mean that the need for active treatment is very high.

86. Which of the following statements concerning the results of epidemiologic studies of periodontal disease is true?
    1. There is only a weak relationship between plaque, home care, and gingivitis.
    2. Poor oral hygiene does not seem to be a major factor in the prevalence and severity of gingivitis.
    3. There is a strong relationship between plaque, home care, and gingivitis.
    4. There is a strong relationship between plaque and destruction associated with periodontitis.
    5. There is a strong correlation between severity of the signs of inflammation and the amount of destruction associated with periodontitis.

### SUGGESTED READING

1. BAER PN, BENJAMIN SD: Manual of Periodontal Disease in Children and Adolescents. Philadelphia, JB Lippincott, 1973
2. CARANZA FA: Glickman's Clinical Periodontology: Prevention, Diagnosis and Treatment of Periodontal Disease in the Practice of General Dentistry, 5th ed. Philadelphia, WB Saunders, 1978
3. GLICKMAN I: Clinical Periodontology, 4th ed. Philadelphia, WB Saunders, 1972
4. GLICKMAN I, SPEIRS DM, MERGENHAGEN SE, et al: Periodontal Disease: Immunological Factors, No. 1. New York, Mss Information Corporation, 1973
5. GLICKMAN, I, SMULOW JB: Periodontal Disease: Clinical Radiographic and Histopathologic Features. Philadelphia, WB Saunders, 1974
6. GOLDMAN HM, COHEN DW: Periodontal Therapy, 5th ed. St. Louis, CV Mosby, 1973
7. GOLDMAN HM, COHEN DW: Introduction to Periodontia, 5th ed. St. Louis, CV Mosby, 1972
8. GRANT DA, STERN IB, EVERETT FG: Orban's Periodontics, 4th ed. St. Louis, CV Mosby, 1972
9. HURT WC: Periodontics in General Practice. Springfield, Il, CC Thomas, 1976
10. MELCHER AR, BOWEN WH: Biology of the Periodontium. New York, Academic Press, 1969
11. PRICHARD JF: Advanced Periodontal Disease, 2nd ed. Philadelphia, WB Saunders, 1972
12. PRICHARD JF: The Diagnosis and Treatment of Periodontal Disease. Philadelphia, WB Saunders, 1978
13. RAMFJORD SP, ASH MM, JR: Periodontology and Periodontics. Philadelphia, WB Saunders, 1978
14. SCHLUGER S, YUODELIS RA, PAGE RC: Periodontal Disease: Basic Phenomena, Clinical Management and Occlusal and Restorative Interrelationships. Philadelphia, Lea & Febiger, 1977
15. WARD HL: A Periodontal Point of View: A Practical Expression of Current Problems Integrating Basic Science with Clinical Data. Springfield, Il, CC Thomas, 1973

16. WARD HL, SIMRING M: Manual of Clinical Periodontics. St. Louis, CV Mosby, 1973
17. WENTZ FM: Principles and Practice of Periodontics with an Atlas of Treatment. Springfield, Il, CC Thomas, 1977

## ANSWER KEY

| | | | |
|---|---|---|---|
| 1. 5 | 9. 3 | 17. 2 | 25. 1 |
| 2. 5 | 10. 4 | 18. 5 | 26. 2 |
| 3. 2 | 11. 4 | 19. 3 | 27. 2 |
| 4. 5 | 12. 3 | 20. 1 | 28. 3 |
| 5. 1 | 13. 4 | 21. 3 | 29. 4 |
| 6. 5 | 14. 1 | 22. 3 | 30. 4 |
| 7. 4 | 15. 4 | 23. 1 | 31. 5 |
| 8. 1 | 16. 3 | 24. 3 | 32. 1 |

| | | | |
|---|---|---|---|
| 33. 4 | 47. 3 | 61. 4 | 74. 4 |
| 34. 2 | 48. 2 | 62. 5 | 75. 1 |
| 35. 5 | 49. 3 | 63. 1 | 76. 5 |
| 36. 4 | 50. 5 | 64. 4 | 77. 5 |
| 37. 2 | 51. 1 | 65. 5 | 78. 3 |
| 38. 5 | 52. 2 | 66. 5 | 79. 5 |
| 39. 5 | 53. 2 | 67. 1 | 80. 3 |
| 40. 2 | 54. 4 | 68. 1 | 81. 4 |
| 41. 4 | 55. 4 | 69. 3 | 82. 5 |
| 42. 3 | 56. 1 | 70. 3 | 83. 5 |
| 43. 3 | 57. 4 | 71. 3 | 84. 5 |
| 44. 3 | 58. 1 | 72. 5 | 85. 5 |
| 45. 2 | 59. 3 | 73. 3 | 86. 3 |
| 46. 4 | 60. 4 | | |

# 11

# ORAL PATHOLOGY

## Kenneth P. Hopkins

When the dental student sits down to begin a review of oral pathology in preparation for the National Board Examinations, he or she is usually confronted with pages of class notes, "hand-outs," copies of old tests ("T–R"), and a thick textbook describing, in sometimes laborious detail, over 200 disease entities which may directly or indirectly affect the oral cavity. It probably has been some time since the formal undergraduate course in oral pathology. The confusing classification of odontogenic tumors, once memorized verbatim, has become only a list of "-omas," few of which have actually been encountered in the oral diagnosis clinic. Judgment day, however, is now at hand and one is still faced with the Gargantuan task of sifting, sorting, and organizing the material so that the review time may be spent most efficiently. The purpose of this chapter is to help the student with this task.

The oral pathology/radiology National Board Examination consists of approximately 100 questions, including over 30 questions on radiology. Nearly two-thirds of the questions on radiology are related to technical principles, radiation hygiene, and anatomy. These particular subjects are discussed in Chapter 13, Dental Radiology, but certain radiographic interpretive recognition points as they relate to oral pathologic entities are included here.

## DENTAL CARIES

Ironically dental students tend to neglect the review of dental caries, yet a significant number of National Board Examination questions deal with the etiology and interactions of the various modifying factors in the carious process. There are also a few references to the clinical and histopathologic aspects of dental caries.

### Etiologic Theories of Caries Formation

The acidogenic theory, which is the most widely accepted, states that acids produced by microorganisms first demineralize the inorganic portion of enamel. This is followed by the dissolution of the organic portion by certain proteolytic organisms. First proposed by Miller in 1890 (41), this theory still explains most carious lesions and emphasizes the roles of plaque, cariogenic diets, and acid in the carious process.

The proteolytic theory explains penetrating and recurrent decay as essentially the reverse of the process described in the acidogenic theory, stating that proteolysis precedes inorganic demineralization. In this theory organic defects such as lamellae in the enamel are significant in the initiation of a carious lesion.

The proteolysis–chelation theory is most recent, but least supported by experimental evidence (49). It attempts to resolve the question of caries initiation by stating that proteolysis and demineralization of enamel take place simultaneously and that neither plaque nor an acid pH are essential to the process.

### Contributing Factors in Caries

Microorganisms, probably the most important contributing factors, apparently must be present for caries to develop. Animal experimentation has shown streptococci, specifically *Streptococcus mutans*, to be most suspect as the initiator of dental caries (7, 22, 44). These are often referred to as "cariogenic streptococci." Lactobacilli seem to increase in number in active carious lesions, but do not initiate the lesion (21).

Plaque, primarily composed of microorganisms and extracellular matrix (dextran), acts to hold or localize acid (lactic acid) in close contact with the enamel surface.

Carbohydrates, especially sucrose, are considered cariogenic because they become the main source of acid for demineralization when microorganisms have acted upon them (47).

Xerostomia is often associated with an increase in caries activity. This reduction in salivary flow may occur with aging, as a component of Sjögren's syndrome, after radiation therapy, etc.

### Histopathology of Caries

The greatest degree of lateral spreading in a carious lesion is at the dentinoenamel junction, probably due to

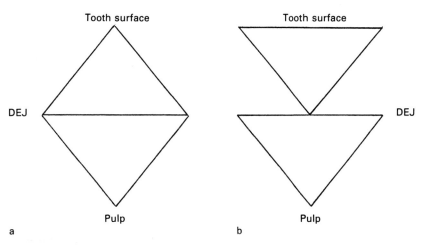

**FIG. 11-1.** Caries attack patterns from outer tooth surface, through enamel, dentinoenamel junction (**DEJ**), and dentin towards the pulp chamber for pit and fissure caries (**a**) and smooth surface caries (**b**).

the increased amount of organic material in this region. Caries tends to progress towards the pulp in certain conical "attack patterns." In enamel, the pattern follows the arrangement of the enamel rods. In smooth surface caries of enamel, the base of the cone is at the tooth surface, and its apex is at the dentinoenamel junction; in pit and fissure caries, the reverse is true. The attack pattern in dentin, however, is constant, with the base of the cone being at the dentinoenamel junction and the apex nearest the pulp (Fig. 11-1).

## Clinical Aspects of Caries

Acute caries, characterized by pain and rapid progression, tends to occur more often in children whose dentinal tubules are more open and nonsclerotic. The decayed dentin is of a soft, "cheesy" consistency and is more yellow in color than that of chronic caries. Little pain is associated with chronic caries, which is seen more in adults. The production of sclerotic and secondary dentin tends to slow the advance of the process towards the pulp. Usually the cavity is more open and larger, which leads to the compression of the carious dentin into a tough, leathery mass which in some cases may actually become hard or eburnated.

## Preventive Measures

Currently the use of fluorides, both systemically ingested and topically applied to the teeth, is the most effective anticariogenic strategy. The mechanisms whereby fluoride reduces caries are many and complex. The most important one is the incorporation of the fluoride into the enamel crystal structure (fluoroapatite) rendering the enamel more resistant to acid dissolution (54). Evidence is also available that demonstrates a significant caries reduction with properly applied occlusal sealants (6, 12, 23). The use of antibiotics such as penicillin to reduce caries incidence does not seem to be

particularly effective and carries the risk of causing hypersensitivity reactions in the patient, as well as developing penicillin-resistant strains of microorganisms.

QUESTIONS

1. The major portion of dental plaque consists of
   1. mucin
   2. levan
   3. dextran
   4. microorganisms
   5. calcium phosphate

2. The routine use of oral penicillin as an anticariogenic agent in humans is not now recommended because
   1. it is not a particularly effective anticariogenic agent
   2. there is the possibility of developing penicillin-resistant pathogenic microorganisms
   3. the patient may become hypersensitive to the drug
   4. All of the above

3. The lateral spread of dental caries is facilitated most by the
   1. dentinoenamel junction
   2. sclerotic dentin
   3. striae of Retzius
   4. enamel spindles
   5. enamel lamellae

4. Current evidence indicates that the most important contributing factor in the etiology of dental caries is
   1. the pH of the saliva
   2. poor oral hygiene
   3. salivary amylase activity
   4. malformation of tooth structure
   5. the activity of certain oral microorganisms

5. Acute caries progresses rapidly to pulpal involvement because
   1. the dentinal tubules of younger people are wider and more open
   2. advanced dentinal sclerosis in the teeth of younger persons is more readily demineralized
   3. little or no pain accompanies acute caries to indicate the rapidity of the process

*(Continued)*

4. cementum is usually involved and thus the decay has a shorter distance in which to reach the pulp

6. The most widely accepted theory for the etiology of dental caries is the
   1. zonation theory
   2. proteolytic theory
   3. proteolysis–chelation theory
   4. lactobacillus theory
   5. acidogenic theory

7. Caries which is initiated via a lamella or organic defect in enamel and progresses rapidly through this defect to the dentin, producing extensive undermining of enamel with little involvement of the enamel is most correctly named
   1. acute caries
   2. chronic caries
   3. penetrating caries
   4. rampant caries

8. Experimental evidence is accumulating which reveals that the organism primarily responsible for the initiation of most dental caries is
   1. *Staphylococcus*
   2. *Lactobacillus*
   3. *Mycobacterium*
   4. *Streptococcus*
   5. *Actinomyces*

9. The effectiveness of ingested fluoride in caries prevention is related to the
   1. prevention of carbohydrate degradation
   2. inhibition of microorganisms
   3. reduction of acid solubility of enamel
   4. lowering of plaque pH
   5. None of the above

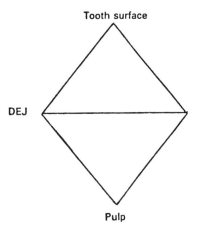

10. The caries attack pattern diagramatically represented here is the form commonly seen in
    1. interproximal smooth surface caries
    2. pit and fissure caries
    3. penetrating caries
    4. cervical, labial smooth surface caries

# PULP PATHOLOGY

The pulp, being essentially like connective tissue elsewhere in the body, responds to injury by the process of inflammation. The basics of this process are discussed in the section on general pathology and should be reviewed along with the following discussion of the specific pulpal diseases. Usually several questions on the National Board Examination are allotted to this subject.

## Inflammation of the Pulp (Pulpitis)

**ETIOLOGY.** Most commonly, the pulp becomes inflamed and/or infected via a carious lesion. Though there may be no clinical or microscopic exposure of the pulp which permits actual bacterial invasion, toxic products of an advancing carious lesion can enter the pulp through dentinal tubules and result in an inflammatory response. Microorganisms may also enter the pulp by the blood stream (43), a process known as anachoresis ("a safe refuge"). Physical injuries to the teeth, such as extreme temperature and trauma, can lead to pulpal inflammation. Chemical injuries also produce pulpal irritation and inflammation. Silicate cements, resins, and medicaments used in restorative procedures (particularly when placed in deep cavity preparations without an intermediate base) may cause sufficient irritation to result in pulpal inflammation (48).

**CLASSIFICATION.** Inflammation of the pulp may be acute or chronic, depending on the etiology and speed of pulpal involvement. The amount of total pulpal tissue affected by an inflammatory process determines whether the inflammation is referred to as partial or total. The presence or absence of pulp exposure, as well as the size of any area exposed, may also be used to classify a pulpitis as being either open or closed. Combinations of these terms may be applied to the description of a pulpal inflammation.

It is important to remember that the pulp may become inflamed without being infected (37). The presence or absence of microorganisms strongly determines whether or not a pulp will survive an injury.

The initial inflammation is most commonly localized to the site of injury, but if it is not treated, it subsequently extends to involve the entire pulp. This process may take years in some cases of chronic pulpitis, however. Some pulpal inflammations are asymptomatic, but pain is usually manifested in some degree and has certain characteristic features. The pain may be severe and out of proportion to the small (sometimes microscopic) amount of tissue involved. Localization of pulpal pain is poor since proprioceptive nerves are not involved until the inflammation reaches the periapical regions. Pulpal pain may be referred away from the actual site of involvement, even to the opposing jaw, but not across the midline.

The relationships between the symptoms, microscopic findings and treatments of pulpitis are presented as an overview in Table 11-1.

**POINTS TO REMEMBER.**   There are several key points to remember regarding pulpal inflammation:

1. Acute inflammation is characterized by vascular dilatation and a polymorphonuclear cellular exudate.
2. A pulpal abscess is a localized degeneration of pulpal tissue, breakdown of leukocytes, and bacteria.
3. Chronic pulpitis is characterized by lymphocytes and plasma cells along with increased fibrosis and decreased cellularity of the pulpal tissue.
4. Tooth vitality cannot be determined radiographically.

## Other Pulpal Entities

**INTERNAL ROOT RESORPTION.**   An idiopathic hyperplasia of the pulp at the expense of the surrounding dentin, internal root resorption leaves the dentinal walls of the pulp chamber and/or root canal irregularly scalloped by the activity of clastic, multinucleated giant cells (63). The tooth is usually asymptomatic and may appear clinically normal, although it may have a somewhat pinkish hue (pink tooth of Mummery). A radiograph reveals a focally enlarged radiolucency in the coronal and/or radicular pulp. Treatment consists of endodontic intervention to halt the process.

**TYPES OF DENTIN.**   The formation of the various types of dentin, whether physiologic or in response to injury, is an important function of the pulp. Secondary dentin, which is more physiologic in nature than patho-

**Table 11-1.   Correlation of Clinical Symptoms, Probable Microscopic Findings°, and Treatment Rationale in the Various Forms of Pulpitis**

| TYPE | USUAL CLINICAL SYMPTOMS | EXPECTED MICROSCOPIC FINDINGS | TREATMENT |
|---|---|---|---|
| Focal reversible pulpitis (hyperemia) | Sensitivity to thermal or chemical changes; disappearance of pain with removal of stimulus; response to lower level of current on pulp tester; usually a deep carious lesion, large, unbased restoration, or defective margins on tooth | Dilatation and congestion of vessels, edema; possible white cell exudation; reaction localized beneath the area of injury; possibly evidence of reparative dentin | Removal of irritant before more severe damage occurs |
| Acute pulpitis (usually irreversible) | Occurrence in tooth with a large carious lesion or defective restoration; pain, elicited by thermal or chemical changes, which persists after removal of stimulus; severe and continuous pain, especially when lying down; reaction to a low level on pulp tester; pain possibly spontaneous | Extensive, acute inflammation (edema, polys); possibly pulpal abscess | Endodontic therapy, extraction, or possible pulpotomy |
| Acute suppurative pulpitis | Severe, continuous pain; patient complaint that tooth feels "high" | Liquefactive and suppurative necrosis of entire pulp | Opening of chamber to establish drainage, endodontic therapy, or extraction |
| Chronic pulpitis | Mild, dull ache (intermittent); little reaction to thermal change; higher setting on pulp tester required for response; possibly no symptoms; patient complaint that tooth "hurts on going to bed" | Fibroblastic and endothelial proliferation; increased collagen (fibrosis); monocytes, lymphocytes, and plasma cells, calcification | Same as for acute pulpitis |
| Chronic hyperplastic pulpitis (pulp polyp) | Exuberant, exophytic mass of pulp tissue proliferating from a large, open carious exposure in tooth of a child or young adult with large apical foramen; relatively painless lesion which bleeds easily | Basically granulation tissue and chronic inflammatory cells, with an epithelialized surface | Pulpotomy, endodontic therapy, or extraction |

° There is NO clinical sign or symptom which designates with certainty the histopathologic status of the pulp.

logic, is less calcified and has fewer and more irregular tubules than primary dentin. Both the primary and secondary dentin are formed rather diffusely around the entire coronal and radicular pulp by odontoblasts. Reparative dentin, however, is a localized deposit of highly irregular dentin in an area of pulpal irritation or injury by the activity of reserve mesenchymal cells from deeper pulpal tissue. This dentin is rather poorly calcified and has few or no tubules. The term osteodentin is sometimes used to describe the more irregular forms of this type of dentin.

### QUESTIONS

11. Chronic pulpitis is characterized microscopically by
    1. increased fibrosis
    2. decreased cellularity
    3. presence of lymphocytes and plasma cells
    4. All of the above

12. Which of the following has the greatest significance in determining whether or not a pulp will survive an episode of injury?
    1. An open pulpitis
    2. A closed pulpitis
    3. A large apical foramen
    4. Presence or absence of reparative dentin
    5. Presence or absence of microorganisms

13. Blood-borne seeding of bacteria into an area of previously damaged or irritated pulp with a resultant inflammation is known as
    1. bacterial endocarditis
    2. Koplik's spots
    3. chronic hyperplastic pulpitis
    4. anachoretic pulpitis
    5. ulcerative pulpitis

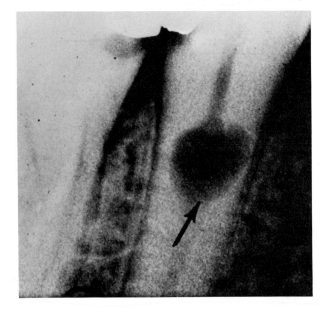

14. The bicuspid is vital and asymptomatic. The most probable diagnosis of the area indicated by the arrow is
    1. lateral periodontal cyst
    2. pulp stone (denticle)
    3. acute pulpal abscess
    4. idiopathic internal resorption
    5. fixation artifact

15. A microscopic comparison of reparative dentin and secondary dentin shows that reparative dentin
    1. has fewer tubules than secondary dentin
    2. is more calcified than secondary dentin
    3. is more evenly distributed about the pulp chamber than is secondary dentin
    4. has more organization of tubules than secondary dentin

16. The development of a pulp polyp is usually related to the combination of which of the following circumstances or features?
    a. A patient younger than 20 years of age
    b. Acute pulpitis (closed type)
    c. Exuberant fibroendothelial proliferation
    d. An open carious exposure
    e. Large apical foramina of the involved tooth
    1. a, b, c, and e
    2. c, d, and e
    3. a, b, and d
    4. a, c, d, and e
    5. All of the above

17. Pulpal pain as a response to injury or disease is probably the result of
    1. increased pressure on nerve endings
    2. irritation of nerve endings by toxic products of inflammation
    3. crowding of odontoblasts by reparative dentin
    4. the presence of active pulp stones
    5. Both 1 and 2

18. Although the clinical and microscopic features cannot always be correlated, the tooth characterized by a severe throbbing pain which is worse when lying down, by extreme sensitivity to hot or cold, and by a painful response to a very low setting on the electric pulp tester most likely possesses which of the following types of inflammation?
    1. Chronic inflammation
    2. Subacute inflammation
    3. Acute inflammation
    4. Hyperplastic pulpitis

## PERIAPICAL PATHOLOGY

The National Board Dental Examination on oral pathology includes several basic questions on periapical diseases with additional questions on radiographic interpretive recognition, some of which include photoreproductions of actual radiographs. Familiarity with the pathogenesis, usual radiographic appearances, treatment, and pertinent histologic components of the following periapical lesions is advisable:

Apical periodontal entities
1. Pericementitis
2. Dental granuloma
3. Radicular cyst
4. Acute and chronic dentoalveolar abscesses
5. External resorption
6. Apical scar

Apical alveolar bone lesions
1. Condensing osteitis
2. Chronic diffuse sclerosing osteomyelitis
3. Garré's osteitis

When a pulp dies, the necrotic debris and toxins from within the confines of the chamber and canals spill out of the apical foramen, injuring the tissues of the periodontal ligament and initiating an inflammatory response (pericementitis). If the inflammation is severe enough, granulation tissue begins to proliferate at the apex of the root (at the expense of the surrounding alveolar bone) and a localized periapical lesion is formed known as a periapical granuloma.

## Periapical Granuloma (Dental Granuloma)

**CLINICAL AND RADIOGRAPHIC FEATURES.** The involved tooth may be asymptomatic or slightly tender to percussion; it responds poorly to pulp testing or is completely nonvital. Often there is a gross carious lesion, a deep restoration, or a history of previous trauma to the tooth. The earliest radiographic evidence is a slight thickening of the periodontal ligament at the apex (49). Later a well-circumscribed radiolucency of varying size is produced.

**MICROSCOPIC FINDINGS.** Basically microscopic examination of a periapical granuloma reveals fibroendothelial proliferation (or granulation tissue) with a rather diffuse infiltration of chronic and some acute inflammatory cells (lymphocytes, plasma cells, and polymorphonuclear neutrophils). Also present may be some phagocytic cells with ingested lipids (foam cells) as well as cholesterol spaces or slits, and epithelial rests of Malassez.

**TREATMENT.** Removal of the cause is the basis for treatment of the periapical granuloma. This consists of extraction of the tooth with curettage of the granulation tissue mass from the socket or endodontic therapy with or without accompanying apicoectomy.

If not treated, some unknown component of the inflammatory process in the periapical granuloma may act upon the rests of Malassez, resulting in a proliferation of these epithelial cells which leads to central cystic degeneration of the epithelial cell nest and the formation of a periapical cyst (56).

## Periapical Cyst (Apical Periodontal or Radicular Cyst)

This lesion is a true cyst (lined by epithelium) and is a common sequela to the periapical granuloma.

**CLINICAL AND RADIOGRAPHIC FEATURES.** The tooth associated with a periapical cyst is in almost every case nonvital and asymptomatic unless the area is secondarily acutely inflamed. The cyst develops slowly over a long period of time. Like the periapical granuloma, the periapical cyst may show gross evidence of probable pulpal destruction such as a large carious lesion, a deep restoration, etc. The radiograph reveals a well-outlined periapical radiolucency similar to that of the granuloma. There is no accurate method to distinguish a cyst from a granuloma radiographically (18).

**MICROSCOPIC FINDINGS AND TREATMENT.** Histologic examination of the cyst reveals tissue similar to that of the granuloma, but the cyst contains a lumen area lined totally or in part by stratified squamous or respiratory epithelium. The lumen may contain amorphous material, cholesterol, and inflammatory cells.

The treatment modalities for the periapical granuloma and cyst are basically the same, since it is usually impossible to determine clinically which one is present. Treatment consists of extraction or endodontic therapy with enucleation of the cyst. There is some controversy as to whether endodontic therapy should be followed by an apicoectomy in the case of a suspected periapical cyst.

Failure to remove or destroy the cyst completely may result in its persistence or recurrence after the tooth has been extracted. This persistent lesion is known as a residual cyst. Should this occur, it must then be removed in a second procedure.

## Periapical Abscess (Dentoalveolar Abscess)

The extension of pulpal infection into the apical periodontal ligament may give rise to a periapical abscess. This lesion may precede or accompany a granuloma or periapical cyst. It most often arises when caries exposes the pulp and produces a pulpitis that spreads rapidly to the periapical area. It may, on the other hand, represent an acute flare-up (Phoenix abscess) in a previously chronic lesion such as a granuloma or apical cyst.

**CLINICAL AND RADIOGRAPHIC FEATURES.** With an acute periapical abscess the involved tooth is extremely painful and sensitive to percussion (feels "high"). The patient may be systemically ill with fever and malaise, and some redness or swelling of the soft tissue may be apparent over the apical area of the root. An acute dentoalveolar abscess may form so rapidly following pulp destruction that no radiographic evidence or bone destruction is present. An abscess arising in a previously existing granuloma or cyst is indistinguishable from the radiographic representation of those entities.

**MICROSCOPIC FEATURES AND TREATMENT.** A periapical abscess consists primarily of a localized accumulation of viable and nonviable polymorphonuclear neutrophils (PMN'S), amorphous proteinaceous material, debris, etc. surrounded by a zone of fibroendothelial proliferation and the other components of the entity (granuloma or cyst) in which it may have arisen. The treatment of the abscess is, of course, to remove the cause, the infected tooth. If the pressure of the abscess is relieved, either by spontaneous pointing or incision, and the offending tooth is not removed, the acute process subsides to a state of chronicity which is usually asymptomatic. The resulting lesion may be called a chronic alveolar abscess and requires the same treatment as a granuloma or cyst.

The periapical, intrabony area occupied by a granuloma, cyst, etc., normally organizes and reossifies following treatment or removal of the cause. Occasionally reossification fails to take place and the area progressively fibroses, leaving a sterile, connective tissue scar which results in a persisting radiolucency on routine radiographs. This lesion, known as an apical scar, generally occurs following endodontic therapy. The associated tooth is asymptomatic, and the lesion does not enlarge. Consequently this entity requires no treatment, just periodic observation.

## Other Periapical Entities

Although periapical lesions usually result in some destruction of the surrounding bone, there are situations in which the resistance of the host and the virulence of the inflammatory process reach a sort of balance and bone is actually produced rather than being resorbed. There are three entities in which this reaction occurs: 1) chronic focal sclerosing osteomyelitis, 2) chronic diffuse sclerosing osteomyelitis, and 3) proliferative periostitis.

**CHRONIC FOCAL SCLEROSING OSTEOMYELITIS.** The most frequent of these types is chronic focal sclerosing osteomyelitis, more commonly referred to as condensing osteitis. It usually occurs about the apices of mandibular molars in patients under the age of 20. Apical infection evokes a sclerotic reaction in the immediate surrounding alveolar bone. There are generally no clinical signs or symptoms; the condition is revealed on radiographic examination as an area of increased density. Treatment consists of removing the cause by extraction or endodontic therapy of the involved tooth. Following treatment, however, the sclerosed area may persist for years.

**CHRONIC DIFFUSE SCLEROSING OSTEOMYELITIS.** As the name implies, chronic diffuse sclerosing osteomyelitis is characterized by more widespread reaction than the chronic focal type. It is actually a form of chronic osteomyelitis in which the bone is able to tolerate, but not overcome, the infection. In contrast to the focal type previously described, this condition predominantly affects older individuals and is found more often in the edentulous mandible. The true nature of this lesion is very controversial. Symptoms may be largely absent, but exacerbations to acute osteomyelitis may occur. Radiographically the condition is characterized by patchy areas of sclerotic medullary bone. Treatment is usually conservative and palliative since the lesion is too extensive to remove all infected bone surgically and antibiotics seem to have a limited effect.

**PROLIFERATIVE PERIOSTITIS (GARRÉ'S OSTEITIS).** The third type of proliferative osteomyelitis, proliferative periostitis, most often occurs in the lower jaw of young patients in response to the presence of a molar with periapical infection. In this case, however, the reaction takes place at the periosteum adjacent to the area. Clinically a localized overgrowth of cortical bone produces an expansion on the surface of the mandible. Removal of the infective focus leads to a gradual return of the normal contour of the bone, though it is often a slow process.

## Points to Remember

Some final miscellaneous points to remember about periapical lesions are

1. The periapical granuloma may very likely be a sterile lesion, particularly if the cause of the original pulpal injury was trauma.
2. Both the mental foramen and the incisive canal may be superimposed over the apices of teeth on a radiograph, giving a false impression of a periapical lesion.
3. Although the rests of Malassez are the most common sources of epithelium in a periapical granuloma, others include a) oral epithelium growing in a fistulous tract, b) respiratory epithelium of the maxillary sinus, and c) oral epithelium from a periodontal pocket.

QUESTIONS

19. Which of the following is normally characterized by pain?
    1. Periapical dental granuloma
    2. Radicular cyst
    3. Periapical scar
    4. Pulp polyp
    5. Acute periapical abscess

20. The most constant microscopic feature in the periapical cyst is
    1. cholesterol slits
    2. foam cells
    3. epithelium
    4. polymorphonuclear leukocytes
    5. multinucleated giant cells

21. Which of the following would most likely be associated with a nonvital tooth?
    1. Internal resorption
    2. Hyperplastic pulpitis
    3. Radicular cyst
    4. Active formation of a pulp stone
    5. Periapical cementoma

22. Destruction and/or proliferation of bone may occur in osteomyelitis. Proliferation is prominent in which of the following types of this disease?
    a. Acute suppurative
    b. Chronic suppurative
    c. Garré's osteitis
    d. Chronic diffuse sclerosing
    e. Condensing osteitis

    1. a, c, and d
    2. b, c, and d
    3. c, d, and e
    4. c and d

23. The most common cyst of the oral regions is the
    1. dermoid inclusion cyst
    2. dentigerous cyst
    3. incisive canal cyst
    4. primordial cyst
    5. periapical cyst

24. A tooth which is extremely sensitive to percussion, shows some elevation in the socket so as to feel "high" in occlusion, shows no changes at the apex on radiographs, and exhibits swelling and redness in the overlying soft tissue, most likely has a
    1. periapical scar
    2. periapical abscess
    3. periapical granuloma
    4. radicular cyst

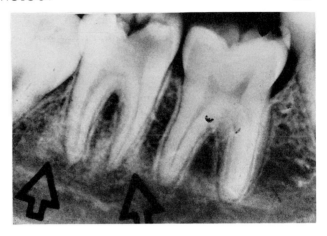

25. The increased radiopaqueness about the apices indicated by arrows (above) is probably due to
    1. hypercementosis
    2. periapical cemental dysplasia
    3. sequestration in osteomyelitis
    4. condensing osteitis

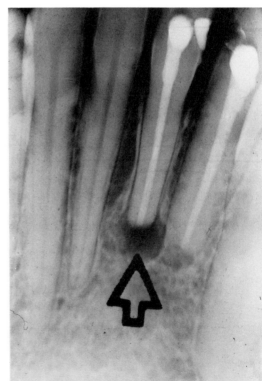

26. The radiograph shown was taken 1 year after endodontic therapy on the two incisors. The radiolucency (arrow) has neither decreased nor increased in size since the pretreatment radiograph. The patient has been asymptomatic since the root canals were completed. Diagnosis and present course of action should be

*(Continued)*

1. cementoma, no treatment
2. apical scar, no treatment
3. radicular cyst, apicoectomy
4. periapical granuloma, apicoectomy

## NEOPLASMS

Approximately eight basic questions plus two interpretive recognition questions on the National Board Examination are concerned with neoplasms, including both benign and malignant types, as well as mere tumorlike proliferations or hyerplasias.

### Odontogenic Tumors

**AMELOBLASTOMA.**    The ameloblastoma is an important neoplasm which is classified as an ectodermal odontogenic tumor. It is found most often in the mandibular molar–ramus area where it may appear as a multilocular, "soap bubble" radiolucency on the radiograph. Although there are many histologic variations of the ameloblastoma, the tumor is treated by a relatively radical surgical excision to prevent recurrence (25).

**CRANIOPHARYNGIOMA (RATHKE'S POUCH TUMOR).** Although not truly odontogenic, the craniopharyngioma is of interest to the dentist and pathologist in that histologically it resembles the ameloblastoma. It arises from remnants of the embryonic invagination of ectodermal cells from the oral cavity to the anterior pituitary region (Rathke's pouch).

**CEMENTOMA (CEMENTAL DYSPLASIA).**    The most significant feature of the cementoma is the production in its early stages of multiple, well-circumscribed apical radiolucencies in the lower incisor regions, which may resemble apical cysts or granulomas. The associated teeth, however, are vital, and no treatment is indicated (18). In later stages of the cementoma, the radiolucencies become radiopaque as the tissue calcifies. This entity seems to occur more often in middle-aged black females.

**MYXOMA.**    A multilocular or honeycombed radiolucency of the mandible is the typical radiographic appearance of the myxoma, which is an uncommon neoplasm. The tumor itself is difficult to remove during surgery because of its jellylike consistency. Microscopically much faintly staining ground substance, containing a few small, spindle-shaped cells, is seen.

**ODONTOMAS.**    Usually seen in association with an impacted tooth, odontomas are predominantly radiopaque lesions which occur in two forms. The compound odontoma is composed of numerous toothlike structures and is found more commonly in the anterior portion of the jaws. The complex odontoma, in contrast, represents an unorganized mass of enamel, dentin, cementum, and small amounts of soft tissue: it occurs more often in the posterior jaws (11).

**ADENOMATOID ODONTOGENIC TUMOR (ADENOAMELOBLASTOMA).**    The adenomatoid odontogenic tumor produces an expansion of bone; it occurs most often in the anterior maxilla of young individuals (25). Its name is derived from the histologic pattern in which gland or ductlike structures are noted. The lesion is well encapsulated, thus easily removed, and has an excellent prognosis (42).

### Benign Tumors and Tumorlike Proliferations

**HAMARTOMA.**    The term hamartoma is used to describe a developmental overgrowth of tissue which is native to a certain area. For example, many consider hemangiomas to be hamartomatous lesions rather than true neoplasms.

**FIBROMA.**    The most common benign tumor of the oral region is the fibroma (49). Originating from connective tissue, it is composed primarily of dense fibrous tissue and is lined on its surface by normal stratified squamous epithelium. It is indistinguishable clinically and microscopically from the nonneoplastic irritation fibroma which is merely a reactive fibrous hyperplasia responding to some local stimulus. Clinically the fibroma is most often smooth, firm, raised, of normal color, and has a broad or sessile base. The lesion is treated by surgical excision.

**PAPILLOMA.**    Much less common in the oral cavity than the fibroma, the papilloma is a true epithelial neoplasm which usually appears as a rough, white, often pedunculated lesion. The oral papilloma has little or no malignant potential (28). Like the fibroma, it is treated by simple excision.

**HEMANGIOMA.**    The majority of hemangiomas occur about the head and neck regions and also may be found centrally in the jaws. Some are considered true vascular neoplasms, while others may be simply hamartomas. Microscopically the hemangioma is composed of numerous vascular spaces in a stroma of normal connective tissue.

**GRANULAR CELL MYOBLASTOMA.**    Although the name implies muscle tissue origin, the granular cell myoblastoma is currently thought to arise from nerve sheaths (18). A decided predilection for the tongue has been shown by this tumor, which produces a swelling covered by apparently normal mucosa. Microscopically, however, it appears that the tumor cells, which contain fine, eosinophilic granular cytoplasm, induce the overlying surface epithelium to undergo pseudoepitheliomatous hyperplasia.

**RHABDOMYOMA.** The rhabdomyoma (adult or extracardiac type) is a benign neoplasm of skeletal muscle, and is extremely rare in the oral cavity. It presents as a painless, well-circumscribed nodule or mass, sometimes occurring on the soft palate causing difficulty in swallowing (65). Adequate local excision is the preferred treatment.

**SCHWANNOMA (NEURILEMOMA).** Another tumor having a predilection for the tongue is the schwannoma. The neoplastic cells arise in the sheath of Schwann and their nuclei are arranged into palisades forming the characteristic Antoni type A pattern with numerous Verocay bodies. The tumor is encapsulated and has a good prognosis, although rare malignant transformation does occur.

**NEUROFIBROMA.** The neurofibroma may occur as a solitary lesion. If there are multiple nodules of the skin and bones, the condition is known as neurofibromatosis or Recklinghausen's disease of the skin. In the multiple form skin pigmentations (café au lait spots) are often present. Sarcomatous transformation is a strong possibility when multiple lesions are present, but solitary lesions may be simply excised, with no problem of recurrence.

**PYOGENIC GRANULOMA.** The pyogenic granuloma is a nonneoplastic proliferative response of connective tissue to a nonspecific infection or irritation. The lesion may occur in both intraoral and extraoral locations. The most common intraoral site is the gingiva, an area frequently subjected to minor irritations. Pregnancy tumor is a term sometimes applied to the tumor when it occurs on the gingiva of a pregnant patient. Basically the mass is an exuberant proliferation of granulation tissue lined on the surface by mucosal epithelium which may be ulcerated.

**GIANT CELL GRANULOMA.** The giant cell granuloma is also an overzealous proliferative response of vascular connective tissue which occurs both peripherally and centrally. Multinucleated giant cells characterize the microscopic appearance. The peripheral lesions always occur on the alveolar ridges, and a history of trauma, such as a recent extraction, often precedes its development. When the central type is encountered, blood calcium levels should be assayed to rule out hyperparathyroidism, because similar bone lesions occur in this endocrine dysfunction (1).

**ANEURYSMAL BONE CYST.** Another possible overactive repair response is the aneurysmal bone cyst, an expansive, cystic bone lesion primarily seen in young persons. Again, a history of trauma is often obtained. Radiographically the lesion is a multilocular or honeycombed radiolucency. Microscopic examination reveals a highly vascular lesion with young fibroblasts and giant cells.

**EXOSTOSES.** Exostoses are dense, bony expansions, technically including the tori, which are usually present as distinct radiopacities upon radiographic examination. Clinically the torus palatinus and torus mandibularis are distinguished from exostoses, although they are the same type of bone tissue as seen in multiple exostoses which occur on the buccal aspects of the alveolar ridges.

## Hyperplasias and Premalignant Lesions

**LEUKOPLAKIA.** Most correctly defined as a white lesion which will not wipe off and cannot be diagnosed as any other white lesion (such as lichen planus, leukoedema, etc.), leukoplakia is considered by most authorities to be a possible premalignant condition (62). The lesion should be biopsied and closely followed as patients with the condition show a significantly higher risk for developing squamous carcinoma.

**ERYTHROPLAKIA.** Appearing clinically as smooth to slightly elevated and finely granular, or velvety red areas, erythroplakia carries a serious premalignant potential. It may even represent carcinoma in situ or invasive carcinoma (50).

**SOLAR CHEILITIS.** A common degenerative or aging condition of the lips, solar cheilitis results in wrinkling and poor definition of the vermilion border. The condition is characterized microscopically by an increase in elastic fibers in the connective tissue.

**BOWEN'S DISEASE.** Usually seen on the skin of older individuals, Bowen's disease appears as a brownish lesion which harbors carcinoma in situ when examined microscopically. The condition is often associated with a coexisting internal malignancy (49).

## Malignant Tumors

**SQUAMOUS CELL CARCINOMA (EPIDERMOID CARCINOMA).** Squamous cell carcinoma is the most prevalent oral malignancy (32, 59), often appearing clinically as a painless ulcer or erosion. It may, however, be manifested in many other guises, such as an erythematous, velvety area; a roughened mucosal texture; etc. In fact, any change from normal tissue appearance may be cancer. Histologically squamous cell carcinoma features invading nests and sheets of epithelial cells demonstrating hyperchromatic nuclei, numerous and abnormal mitoses, pleomorphic nuclei, and keratin pearls.

**BASAL CELL CARCINOMA.** Basal cell carcinoma is a locally malignant (nonmetastasizing) erosive lesion of the skin, usually occurring in older persons having a light complexion and with a history of habitual exposure to sunlight, wind, etc. On the face this lesion generally occurs above an imaginary line from the corner of the mouth to the tragus of the ear. This form of carcinoma apparently does not arise primarily in the mouth (14).

**METASTATIC LESIONS.** Cancer from other regions of the body may seed to the oral cavity. Such an occurrence most commonly arises from cancer of the breast, lung, and prostate. The process most often manifests in the mandibular molar–premolar area, producing an irregular radiolucent or radiopaque lesion on x-ray. Clinically it may produce vague pain, loosening of teeth, and/or paresthesia or numbness.

**TREATMENT OF ORAL MALIGNANCIES.** Most primary oral malignant lesions are treated by surgery and/or radiation. Chemotherapy is reserved for widespread malignancies such as leukemia, myeloma, the lymphomas, etc.

### Salivary Gland Tumors

In the benign category the most common salivary gland tumor is the pleomorphic adenoma, also referred to as a benign mixed tumor. The latter is a misnomer since the tumor is not truly mixed, but is entirely of ductal epithelium origin. *Warthin's tumor* (also papillary cystadenoma lymphomatosum) is another benign salivary gland tumor of importance and occurs primarily in the parotid gland of older adult males (38).

Malignant salivary gland tumors are of several types, but one of the most important is the mucoepidermoid carcinoma, so-named because it is composed of both mucus-secreting cells and sheets of epidermoid or squamous epithelial cells. This tumor may arise in both major and minor glands and is characterized by varying degrees of malignancy. The adenoid cystic carcinoma is the most common malignancy of the palatal region (18); it originates in the abundant accessory or minor salivary glands found there.

In general both benign and malignant varieties of salivary gland tumors have a strong tendency to recur due to an infiltration of the connective tissue capsules by neoplastic cells. Malignant forms are generally fixed to underlying tissues and may cause pain and/or paralysis, particularly when the parotid gland is involved. Benign tumors are usually freely moveable, slow-growing, and asymptomatic. These are important points to remember in clinically distinguishing a benign from a malignant salivary gland tumor.

Surgery, the usual treatment modality for these tumors, in the parotid area may result in injury to or severance of the auriculotemporal nerve, leading to gustatory sweating (46) or Frey's syndrome.

QUESTIONS

27. The radiopacities about the apices of these vital incisors most likely represent

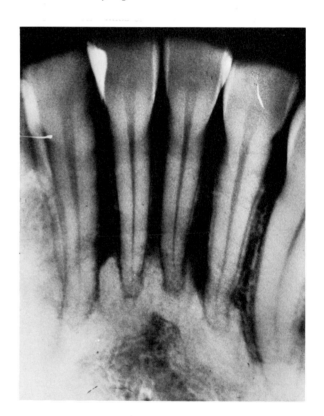

1. Garré's osteitis
2. condensing osteitis
3. mature cementomas
4. hypercementosis

28. A hamartoma is best defined as
    1. an overzealous repair process
    2. a true tumor, in that it has no apparent etiology
    3. an overproduction of tissue normal to a particular area
    4. a degenerative process of connective tissue

29. The malignant tumor of salivary glands which is seen most often in the posterior palatal area is the
    1. papillary cystadenoma lymphomatosum
    2. mucoepidermoid carcinoma
    3. malignant mixed tumor
    4. adenoid cystic carcinoma

30. The great tendency for recurrence in benign salivary gland tumors is largely due to
    1. the presence of tumor cells in the capsule
    2. an inherent tendency of the patient to develop tumors
    3. the presence of many minor salivary glands in the oral cavity
    4. the inductive effect in the connective tissue

31. Which of the following clinical lesions is most likely to harbor dysplastic changes, carcinoma in situ, or even early invasive cancer?
    1. Lichen planus
    2. Erythroplakia
    3. Leukoplakia
    4. Stomatitis nicotina

32. Entities to be considered in the differential diagnosis of a white oral lesion suspected of being leukoplakia should not include
    1. leukoedema
    2. lichen planus
    3. lupus erythematosus
    4. silver nitrate burn
    5. Stevens–Johnson syndrome

33. Facial nerve paralysis is a rather common finding associated with
    1. pleomorphic adenoma of the parotid
    2. epidermoid carcinoma of the parotid
    3. Warthin's tumor
    4. benign lymphoepithelial lesion

34. Pseudoepitheliomatous hyperplasia seen microscopically in a granular cell myoblastoma is considered
    1. an integral part of the tumor
    2. a sign of early malignant change
    3. a response of the epithelium to the tumor cells
    4. true invasion of the epithelium

35. A multilocular radiolucency on a radiograph from the mandibular molar area is pathognomonic for
    1. ameloblastoma
    2. Pindborg's tumor

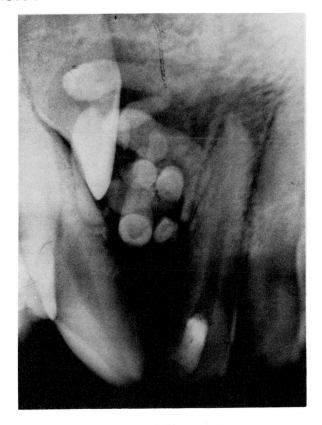

    3. dentigerous cyst
    4. ameloblastic fibroma
    5. None of the above

36. The photo is a reproduction of a periapical radiograph taken on a 26-year-old female. What is the diagnosis of the radiopaque mass?
    1. Complex odontoma
    2. Adenomatoid odontogenic tumor
    3. Fibrous dysplasia
    4. Ossifying fibroma
    5. Compound odontoma

37. The photomicrograph shown on the next page is from an excisional biopsy of a rough, white lesion of the lower lip. The lesion is covered by a hyperkeratotic stratified squamous epithelium producing fingerlike projections, each possessing cores of connective tissue. The lesion is a
    1. lipoma
    2. fibroma
    3. mucocele
    4. papilloma
    5. hemangioma

(See figure on p. 306.)

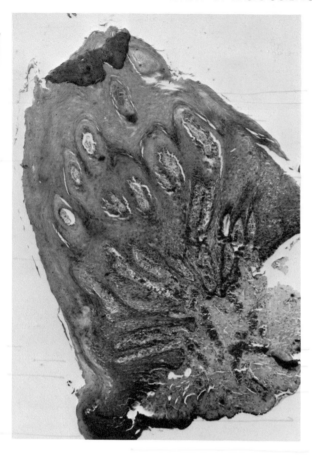

## ANOMALIES

Developmental anomalies of the teeth, jaws, and soft tissues are referred to in several questions of the National Board Examination.

### Soft Tissue and Jaw Anomalies

**CLEFT PALATE AND LIP.** Clefts occur in varying degrees, ranging from a simple bifid uvula to a complete palatal cleft including bilateral lip involvement (5). Heredity appears to be one of the most important etiologic factors (55), though many drugs (teratogens) have been implicated when maternally ingested during the formative stages of the embryo (49).

**DOWN'S SYNDROME (MONGOLISM).** The pathologic basis of Down's syndrome is a chromosomal aberration known as trisomy 21. The oral manifestations include prognathism, macroglossia, microdontia, delayed eruption and relative caries immunity (49, 55). These patients also have a high incidence of leukemia.

**PEUTZ–JEHGERS SYNDROME (HEREDITARY INTESTINAL POLYPOSIS).** Melanin pigment distributed as macules on the lips and buccal mucosa is the distinguishing oral manifestation of Peutz–Jehgers syndrome. Of primary concern, however, are the multiple intestinal polyps. Found primarily in the small intestine, these polyps have a low malignant potential, but they may be the precipitating factor in an abdominal emergency.

**FORDYCE'S GRANULES (SPOTS).** Representing ectopically situated sebaceous glands, Fordyce's granules are commonly found bilaterally on the buccal mucosa as well as labial mucosa. Clinically they appear as yellow, flat, or slightly raised spots which may coalesce into patches.

**WHITE SPONGE NEVUS (CANNON'S DISEASE).** White sponge nevus is a hereditary condition in which there is a thickening of the mucous membranes which gives the mucosa a folded, spongy appearance (67) with a characteristic grayish white or parboiled hue. The lesion microscopically exhibits marked acanthosis with parakeratosis and spongiosis. The condition may be indistinguishable from the nonhereditary leukoedema.

**HEREDITARY BENIGN INTRAEPITHELIAL DYSKERATOSIS (WITKOP'S DISEASE).** In addition to oral features similar to those of white sponge nevus, manifestations of hereditary benign intraepithelial dyskeratosis include foamy or gelatinous corneal lesions which show a seasonal incidence, increasing in severity in the spring (49). Microscopic examination reveals a thickened, spongiotic epithelium with numerous round, pearllike cells undergoing keratinization (67) constituting the so-called dyskeratosis. The condition, however, carries no premalignant potential.

### Anomalies of the Teeth

**DENTINOGENESIS IMPERFECTA.** Affecting both deciduous and permanent teeth, dentinogenesis imperfecta is a hereditary condition in which the teeth are characterized by a brownish, opalescent color; short, conical roots; and small or obliterated pulp chambers. The dentin, microscopically, is highly irregular, and the dentinoenamel junction is flat and smooth rather than normally scalloped. The condition may also be associated with the more generalized connective tissue defect known as osteogenesis imperfecta.

**AMELOGENESIS IMPERFECTA.** Amelogenesis imperfecta is another hereditary condition affecting both deciduous and permanent teeth. The enamel formed is of both poor quality (hypocalcification) and quantity (hypoplasia). Varying degrees of the defect are noted. Dentin is unaffected.

**VARIABLE TEETH.** Variable teeth is a term sometimes applied to those teeth which are most commonly affected by anomalies. These are the maxillary lateral incisors, all third molars, and bicuspids.

**ENAMEL HYPOPLASIA.** Disturbances during amelogenesis may result in enamel hypoplasia. The disturbance may be local, involving only a single tooth and resulting in a Turner's tooth. A systemic disturbance during enamel formation such as produced from a prolonged high fever, however, may affect the enamel of any or all of the teeth undergoing amelogenesis at that time (18). The result is several teeth with enamel pits or defects (environmental hypoplasia). A hereditary interference in amelogenesis affects all teeth, both deciduous and permanent as is seen in amelogenesis imperfecta.

**DENS IN DENTE.** Dens in dente is caused by an invagination of the enamel organ of a developing tooth into the dental papilla (pulp), resulting in a deep, enamel-lined pit. The lingual surface of the maxillary lateral incisor is the most common site for this anomaly (57).

**INTRINSIC STAINS OF THE TEETH.** Several systemic conditions occurring during the time of tooth formation may lead to intrinsic staining of the teeth. These include erythroblastosis, which gives the teeth a green, brown, or bluish hue; porphyria, which results in a red or brownish cast of the teeth; and tetracycline therapy, which causes the teeth to have a yellow or brownish gray color.

It should be noted that endemic fluorosis, or mottled enamel, is not due to intrinsic staining.

**ECTODERMAL DYSPLASIA.** Ectodermal dysplasia is a hereditary condition characterized by hypotrichosis (sparse hair), anhidrosis (abnormal deficiency of sweat), and hypodontia or rarely anodontia (2).

**CONCRESCENCE.** Concrescence is the union of the roots of teeth by confluent cementum. The condition is not truly developmental since it occurs after the teeth are formed. Its primary significance lies in the difficulty of extracting such teeth.

**FUSION.** Fusion occurs when two adjacent developing teeth (usually single-rooted incisors) join by a union of dentin. The result is a tooth having a large or double crown and two distinct root canals.

**CLEIDOCRANIAL DYSOSTOSIS.** Often hereditary in nature, cleidocranial dysostosis is characterized by abnormalities of the cranium, clavicles, jaws, and teeth (40). More specifically, the important oral features are a high, narrow, arched palate; prolonged retention of deciduous teeth with delayed eruption of permanent teeth; and impacted supernumerary teeth.

**DILACERATION.** Dilaceration (to tear apart) is a term used to denote a rather sharp, angular deviation of the root/roots of a tooth from the long axis. The condition is probably the result of trauma during development of the root (55).

**GARDNER'S SYNDROME.** The dentist is concerned with Gardner's syndrome primarily because of the oral manifestations of multiple, impacted supernumerary teeth. Other findings are polyposis of the intestine, osteomas, sebaceous cysts, and desmoid tumors (18).

**ENDEMIC FLUOROSIS.** More commonly referred to as mottled enamel, endemic fluorosis is a form of enamel hypoplasia resulting from the ingestion of excessive amounts of fluoride in the drinking water. The enamel becomes extrinsically stained, but is highly resistant to carious attack.

**TAURODONTISM (BULL TEETH).** Taurodontism is the term applied to teeth characterized by large coronal pulp chambers and short roots. When present, both deciduous and permanent teeth are affected (24).

QUESTIONS

38. Although rare, most instances of true, total anodontia are seen in males and are associated with which of the following conditions?
    1. Congenital syphilis
    2. Hereditary ectodermal dysplasia
    3. Peutz–Jehgers syndrome
    4. Osteogenesis imperfecta

39. Damage of a developing permanent tooth germ by periapical infection in the overlying deciduous tooth could result in defective enamel when the permanent tooth erupts. Such a case would be referred to as
    1. amelogenesis imperfecta
    2. a Turner's tooth
    3. Hutchinson's tooth
    4. a paramolar

40. A large, double-crowned maxillary central incisor having a single root and canal is probably the result of
    1. fusion
    2. dentinal dysplasia
    3. dens in dente
    4. taurodontism
    5. None of the above.

41. Which of the following conditions affect both deciduous and permanent dentitions?
    a. Amelogenesis imperfecta
    b. Dentinogenesis imperfecta
    c. Congenital syphilis
    d. Erythroblastosis fetalis
    1. a and c
    2. b and d
    3. c and d
    4. a and b
    5. b and c

42. Teeth which exhibit a brownish gray discoloration and fluoresce a bright yellow under ultraviolet light have probably been affected by
    1. dentinogenesis imperfecta
    2. tetracycline staining
    3. erythroblastosis fetalis
    4. porphyria
    5. enamel hypoplasia

43. A young patient of yours has multiple areas of pigmentation on the lips and buccal mucosa. His mother states that he frequently complains of the colic. You should suspect
    1. Pierre Robin syndrome
    2. Peutz–Jehgers syndrome
    3. Melkersson–Rosenthal syndrome
    4. Gardner's syndrome

44. A pit on the labial surface of a central incisor which is a result of inadequate enamel matrix formation is known as (a) _____, while the localized failure of complete mineralization in the presence of normal enamel matrix is termed (b) _____.
    1. (a) agenesis; (b) hypoplasia
    2. (a) dysplasia; (b) metaplasia
    3. (a) hypocalcification; (b) hypogenesis
    4. (a) hypoplasia; (b) hypocalcification

45. A patient 18 years of age has several sebaceous cysts on the scalp and back of the neck, as well as an apparent osteoma on the right mandible. Radiographs indicate the presence of multiple impacted supernumerary teeth in both jaws. These findings suggest
    1. cleidocranial dysostosis
    2. Gardner's syndrome
    3. ectodermal dysplasia
    4. dentinogenesis imperfecta
    5. osteogenesis imperfecta

## SOFT TISSUE PATHOLOGY

The questions allotted to the area of soft tissue pathology on the National Board Examination cover some basic general pathology material on infections and inflammations, such as abscess, cellulitis, etc. The questions deal primarily, however, with bacterial, viral, and mycotic diseases, manifestations of blood diseases, metabolic disturbances, and the dermatoses.

## Infections

**BACTERIAL INFECTIONS.** Virulent forms of streptococci may initiate a diffuse, spreading type of inflammation referred to as a cellulitis. The enzyme hyaluronidase produced by these organisms is partly responsible for the extensive spreading through tissue spaces. Ludwig's angina is a serious form of cellulitis of the floor of the mouth, usually initiated by an infected mandibular molar.

An abscess in contrast, is a more localized, purulent area of infection. Although the dentist is more concerned with alveolar abscesses associated with teeth, an abscess of the lung may result from aspiration of infected material during operative procedures in the mouth.

Of increasing importance to the dentist and staff are the several oral manifestations of syphilis. These include the chancre of primary syphilis, the mucous patch of the secondary stage, and the gumma and glossitis associated with the uncommon tertiary stage. Differential diagnosis is important, as the chancre may mimic herpetic lesions of the lips as well as oral cancer. The dentist should also be aware that serologic tests for syphilis may not be positive in the early primary stage. Equally deceptive is the mucous patch of the secondary stage because it may resemble an area of leukoplakia. Though seldom seen now because of early diagnosis and treatment, the tertiary manifestations of syphilis are significant. Syphilitic glossitis may predispose to carcinoma of the tongue, and the gumma, which occurs primarily on the tongue and hard palate, may destroy large areas of tissue.

Oral lesions of tuberculosis usually represent manifestations of a more widespread systemic involvement and may be mistaken clinically for carcinoma, especially when they occur on the tongue.

Noma is a serious oral infection usually associated with a fusospirochetal involvement of the soft tissues. The patient is most often a malnourished, debilitated individual (55).

**VIRAL INFECTIONS.** The rather common herpes simplex infection occurs in both primary and secondary (recurrent) forms. The primary infection, if severe, produces fever, lymphadenopathy, vesicles and ulcers (single or clustered) on the lips, gingivae, tongue, and palate (52). Recurrent herpes usually occurs extraorally on the lips, or if intraorally, on the keratinized, tightly bound mucosa.

Herpes zoster is a neurotropic viral infection which follows the distribution of a sensory nerve such as the trigeminal nerve. The lesions are painful and strikingly unilateral when involving the face or oral cavity.

Herpangina is a coxsackievirus-induced eruption of the soft palate and pharyngeal regions, primarily occurring in young children. The lesions may be confused with primary herpetic stomatitis (19).

Measles may produce oral manifestations. In rubeola the characteristic whitish areas known as Koplik's spots usually precede the skin eruptions by several days. In rubella palatal petechiae may be the only oral features.

Hand, foot, and mouth disease, caused by another strain of coxsackievirus, produces papular or vesicular eruptions in the areas indicated by its name. A common patient complaint is a "sore mouth." As in most viral diseases, the course is self-limiting.

**MYCOTIC DISEASES.** The most common oral mycotic or fungal disease is candidiasis (or moniliasis) which may occur in both acute and chronic forms. The incidence of this opportunistic overgrowth of *Candida albicans* has increased, possibly due to overzealous prescribing of antibiotics by both dentists and physicians resulting in opportunistic overgrowth (49). The very young and very old are particularly susceptible to this infection (34). Painful cracking and fissuring at the corners of the mouth (perlèche or angular cheilosis) often includes candidiasis as part of the etiology.

Another important fungal disease is actinomycosis. The dentist is primarily concerned with the cervicofacial type in which the causative organism is introduced into the deeper tissues via trauma such as a fracture or extraction. The result is a chronic suppurative infection characterized by multiple lumpy abscesses which may open and discharge a purulent material containing fine, yellowish granules. These so-called "sulfur granules" represent colonies of microorganisms.

### Blood Dyscrasias

**ANEMIAS.** Sickle cell anemia may result in certain radiographic changes on the bones of the skull and jaws. The skull may exhibit the "hair on end" pattern of cortical bone, while radiographs of the jaws reveal loss of normal trabeculation and large, irregular marrow spaces.

Iron deficiency anemia produces a hypochromic, microcytic red cell population. Clinically the most striking oral feature is a smooth, red, and painful tongue. This form of anemia is also an important feature of the Plummer–Vinson syndrome which predisposes to oral carcinoma.

Pernicious anemia is fundamentally produced by the deficiency of an intrinsic factor normally present in gastric secretions. This inability to utilize dietary vitamin $B_{12}$ may result in the oral manifestation of a painful, burning glossitis.

**OTHER BLOOD DISORDERS.** Leukemia, particularly the acute forms, may be characterized by lymphadenopathy, anemia, thrombocytopenia, hypertrophied gingivae, spontaneous bleeding from the gingivae, oral ulcers (39), and elevated leukocyte counts. Leukemic gingivitis may be confused and misdiagnosed as necrotizing ulcerative gingivitis.

Agranulocytosis, being of varied etiology, seems to be most commonly caused by the ingestion of certain drugs, resulting in decreased white cell production (granulocytes). The condition is frequently seen in members of the health professions due to their easy access to and imprudent use of drugs in general (49). The characteristic oral manifestations consist of gingival and mucosal ulcerations.

Thrombocytopenic purpura is characterized by spontaneous purpuric, petechial, or hemorrhagic lesions of the skin and oral mucosa. A deficient production of platelets is responsible.

### Metabolic Disturbances

**VITAMIN DEFICIENCIES.** The oral effects of vitamin C deficiency are seen primarily in the gingival and periodontal tissues as swollen, erythematous, or ulcerated areas. The B complex deficiency is usually manifested in oral soft tissues, particularly the tongue and lips. Patients often complain of a "burning tongue" (glossodynia).

**ENDOCRINE DISTURBANCES.** Hyperthyroidism in a child causes early exfoliation of the deciduous teeth and subsequent early eruption of the permanent teeth. Hypothyroidism produces cretinism in children and myxedema in adults, both of which feature a swollen, edematous tongue.

Acromegaly is the result of excessive growth hormone (hyperpituitarism) in an adult. Enlargement of the mandible is a striking oral feature. Hyperpituitarism occurring during childhood is the cause of gigantism.

In Addison's disease the underlying mechanism is a chronic insufficiency of the adrenal cortical hormones; this insufficiency produces a complex array of systemic symptoms. The most outstanding feature in the oral regions is the diffuse brownish pigmentation of the lips, buccal mucosa, gingivae, and tongue. This pigmentation should not be confused with that of Peutz–Jehgers syndrome.

### Dermatoses

**LICHEN PLANUS.** Lichen planus is basically a keratotic lesion and thus may resemble leukoplakia. Oral lesions, which may occur in the absence of skin involvement, are usually bilaterally situated with a characteristic lacey or filigree pattern of crisscrossing lines, with most patients having buccal mucosa involvement (53). Microscopic examination of the lesion reveals a band-like, subepithelial infiltrate of lymphocytes and degeneration of the basal layer of epithelium.

**PEMPHIGUS VULGARIS.** There are several varieties of pemphigus, but pemphigus vulgaris is the one of urgent concern to the dentist. The appearance of oral bullae may be the first symptom of this serious dermatologic disease (17). Microscopically the bulla is shown to be formed by epithelial cell acantholysis and suprabasalar cleavage. Two additional key words or terms are associated with pemphigus. The first, Nikolsky's sign, denotes the diagnostic test in which rubbing friction on an epithelial or mucosal surface raises the characteristic bulla. The second term of importance is the Tzanck cell, the microscopic acantholytic epithelial cell from the bulla fluid which in some instances may be harvested in a cytology smear preparation.

**PSORIASIS.** Although oral manifestations of psoriasis are rare, skin lesions do occur about the face and scalp as red, scaly, or violaceous areas. These lesions are pruritic, and scratching produces multiple pinpoint bleeding spots. This characteristic constitutes the diagnostic aid known as Auspitz's sign. It is also interesting to note that a significant percentage of psoriatic patients develop arthritis.

**LUPUS ERYTHEMATOSUS.** One of the so-called collagen or autoimmune diseases, lupus erythematosus occurs in a disseminated form and in a less widespread form referred to as chronic discoid lupus. The dentist is probably more often involved in treating patients with the latter. Intraoral lesions of lupus may appear as leukoplakia. The dentist should also be aware of the unique butterfly rash type of skin involvement on the nose and cheeks.

**SCLERODERMA.** Scleroderma, another slowly progressive collagen disease, is not common, but it is important to the dental practitioner because it results in a hardening or fixation of the oral mucosa to the underlying bone and muscle. The skin likewise becomes tight and bound down. Other oral features include difficulty in opening the mouth, immobility of the tongue, and a generalized widening of the periodontal ligaments visible on radiographs.

**EHLERS–DANLOS SYNDROME.** Ehlers–Danlos syndrome is an uncommon, but interesting, hereditary disorder of the connective tissue which is possibly related to osteogenesis and dentinogenesis imperfecta (31). In contrast to the tightness of the skin and joints seen in scleroderma, there is hyperelasticity of the skin and joints, as well as fragility of vessels, easy bruising, and defective healing. The underlying process is an increase

in elastic fibers (26) with a decrease in collagen fibers. The oral aspects include a fragile mucosa which is difficult to suture, easily bleeding gingivae, hypermobility of the temporomandibular joint, and microscopically, a defective dentinoenamel junction, similar to that seen in dentinogenesis imperfecta (lack of scalloping).

**ERYTHEMA MULTIFORME.** One of the most perplexing dermatoses is erythema multiforme, a disease of unknown etiology with an explosive onset primarily affecting young adult males. As the name implies, many manifestations may occur, although the disease usually appears as skin and mucosal erythematous macules, bullae, and ulcerations. The lesions, both intra- and extraoral may exhibit the target or iris effect caused by central resolution. The disease occurs in minor and major forms. In the most severe type, referred to as Stevens–Johnson syndrome, extensive lesions involve the skin, mucosa, ocular areas, and genitalia.

QUESTIONS

46. A 26-year-old male reports to your office complaining of an open sore on the buccal mucosa. The lesion is ulcerated, about 1 cm in diameter, and is covered by a grayish white exudate. The patient had a negative tuberculin test, but the blood examination revealed a positive VDRL test. This lesion is most likely to be
    1. an aphthous ulcer
    2. leukoplakia
    3. a mucous patch
    4. lupus vulgaris
    5. actinomycosis

47. Which of the following oral lesions may show a striking unilateral distribution?
    1. Herpes zoster
    2. Lichen planus
    3. Acute necrotizing ulcerative gingivitis
    4. Primary herpetic gingivostomatitis
    5. Erythema multiforme

48. The oral lesions which precede the cutaneous eruption of measles (rubeola) are known as
    1. Koplik's spots
    2. Fordyce's spots
    3. Aphthae
    4. Lipshütz bodies

49. Atrophy of the epithelium of the upper portion of the digestive tract; hypochromic, microcytic anemia; and dysphagia are symptoms characteristic of
    1. Behçet's syndrome
    2. Sjögren's syndrome
    3. Plummer–Vinson syndrome
    4. Stevens–Johnson syndrome

50. Oral manifestations of sickle cell anemia would be evident predominantly in the

1. gingival tissues as a hyperplasia
2. tongue as a burning sensation
3. lamina dura as a decreased radiopacity
4. medullary bone of the jaws as large marrow spaces
5. buccal mucosa as petechial hemorrhages

51. A smooth, red tongue may be seen as a striking oral manifestation in
    1. iron deficiency anemia
    2. riboflavin deficiency
    3. nicotinic acid deficiency
    4. vitamin B$_{12}$ deficiency
    5. All of the above

52. Pericoronitis, in most cases, is classified as a(n)
    1. abscess
    2. periodontal disease
    3. granulomatous process
    4. cellulitis

53. Difficulty in suturing, fragility of soft tissues, and poor wound healing are oral manifestations in patients with
    1. Frey's syndrome
    2. Ehlers–Danlos syndrome
    3. neuropolyendocrine syndrome
    4. Albers–Schönberg disease

54. A generalized widening of the periodontal ligaments is a finding associated with
    1. chronic discoid lupus erythematosus
    2. Paget's disease
    3. monostotic fibrous dysplasia
    4. scleroderma

55. What stage of syphilis would produce lesions which might be most easily confused with leukoplakia?
    1. Primary
    2. Secondary
    3. Tertiary
    4. Syphilis does not produce lesions which might be confused with leukoplakia.

56. Keratotic lesions of the oral mucosa include leukoplakia, lichen planus, and lupus erythematosus. Although of different etiologies, one common feature is that they are
    1. white in color
    2. related to local irritation
    3. premalignant
    4. painful
    5. associated with vitamin A deficiency

57. A 13-year-old boy with generalized gingival swelling and acute inflammation did not respond to conservative periodontal therapy and was referred to a physician for a blood work-up. Subsequent findings included a peripheral white cell count of 63,000, 95% of which were identified as immature lymphocytes. The patient was also severely anemic and numerous petechiae could be seen on the skin and mucous membranes. The most likely diagnosis is
    1. acute myelogenous leukemia
    2. infectious mononucleosis
    3. pancytopenia
    4. acute lymphocytic leukemia
    5. chronic granulocytic leukemia

58. Due to easy access and indiscriminate usage of drugs, medical, dental, and paramedical personnel are frequently affected by
    1. leukocytosis
    2. chronic lymphocytic leukemia
    3. pernicious anemia
    4. agranulocytosis
    5. achlorhydria

59. A coxsackie virus is implicated in the etiology of
    a. herpes zoster
    b. herpangina
    c. rubeola
    d. hand, foot, and mouth disease
    1. a and b
    2. b and c
    3. c and d
    4. b and d
    5. a and d

60. Enlargement of the mandible in an adult resulting in prognathism and spacing of the teeth would be most characteristic of
    1. hyperparathyroidism
    2. Addison's disease
    3. hyperthyroidism
    4. hyperpituitarism

61. Below is a photomicrograph of a tissue section taken from a large bulla on the soft palate of a 49-year-old woman. Nikolsky's sign was positive. These findings are most suggestive of
    1. lupus erythematosus
    2. pemphigus vulgaris
    3. erythema multiforme
    4. scleroderma

(See figure on p. 312.)

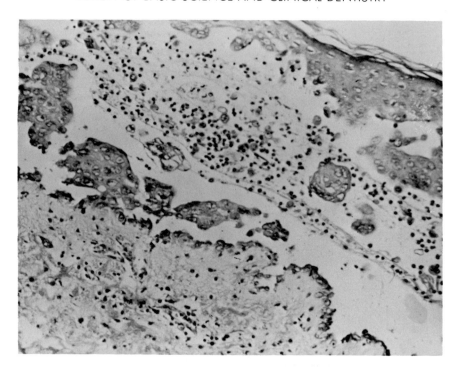

## OTHER ENTITIES

According to the general outline of the oral pathology section of the National Board Dental Examination, approximately 14 questions are allotted to this miscellaneous category, with the most emphasis being placed on diseases of bone. It is also advisable to master eponyms (Tables 11–2, 11–3, and 11–4) and synonyms for all entities.

### Bone Diseases

In reviewing for the examination, the dental student would be wise to spend a little extra time studying bone diseases as questions in other areas occasionally overlap this category.

#### HEREDITARY BONE DISEASES

*Osteogenesis Imperfecta.* Since osteogenesis imperfecta is basically due to a connective tissue defect, other tissues arising from mesenchyme and its derivatives may be affected, including dentin of teeth (dentinogenesis imperfecta), the sclera of the eye (blue sclera due to thinness), and of course, bone (10). Involved bones are extremely fragile, fracture easily, and heal imperfectly, leading to multiple deformities.

*Osteopetrosis.* Another genetic disease featuring bones which are easily fractured is osteopetrosis, also called marble bone disease and Albers–Schönberg disease. In contrast to osteogenesis imperfecta, however, the basic defect in this disease may be a failure of the osteoclasts to resorb and remove bone normally, resulting in bones which are dense, brittle, and extremely radiopaque. The gradual obliteration of the marrow spaces by this dense bone produces a myelophthisic anemia, along with leukopenia and thrombocytopenia. Oral manifestations and complications include features related to the denseness of the bone locally, as well as the systemic effects mentioned. Those most commonly exhibited are retarded eruption of teeth (15), fracture of the jaw, slow wound healing, and increased susceptibility to infection.

*Cherubism.* A condition considered by some pathologists in the past to be a familial type of fibrous dysplasia (55, 58), cherubism produces bilateral, asymptomatic, cystlike radiolucent lesions in the bone at the angles of the mandible in young children. Microscopically these lesions consist of a proliferative connective tissue containing large numbers of giant cells.

*Hypophosphatasia.* Hypophosphatasia is a hereditary condition characterized by a basic deficiency of the enzyme alkaline phosphatase. The major oral aspect is the loosening and premature loss of the deciduous incisors. Absence of cementum on the root surfaces may account for the early exfoliation (4).

*Caffey–Silverman Syndrome.* Caffey–Silverman syndrome (infantile cortical hyperostosis) is characterized by unusual cortical thickening in certain bones of

**Table 11-2. Important Syndromes in Oral Pathology**

| SYNDROME | MAJOR COMPONENTS | SIGNIFICANCE |
|---|---|---|
| Albright's | Polyostotic fibrous dysplasia, café au lait spots, precocious puberty in females | Involvement of mandible or maxilla by fibrous dysplasia, early eruption of teeth |
| Behçet's | Oral, genital, and occular ulcerations; mostly in young adult males | Oral lesions resembling aphthous ulcerations |
| Caffey–Silverman (infantile cortical hyperostosis) | Cortical thickening of certain bones in children, most often the mandible and clavicles | Possible confusion with cherubism |
| Ehlers–Danlos | Hereditary disorder of connective tissue; hyperelasticity of skin and fragile oral tissues (so-called "rubber man") | Difficulty in suturing, poor wound healing |
| Frey's (auriculo-temporal) | Flushing and sweating on involved side of face when eating (gustatory sweating) | Possible outcome of parotid surgery |
| Gardner's | Multiple impacted supernumerary teeth, polyposis of large intestine, osteomas, sebaceous cysts, desmoid tumors | Diagnosis via dental x-rays, dentigerous cysts |
| Heerfordt's (uveo-parotid fever) | A form of sarcoidosis; firm, painless, bilateral enlargement of parotids, uveitis, low-grade fever, 7th nerve paralysis | Salivary gland enlargement |
| Melkersson–Rosenthall | Fissured tongue, facial paralysis, cheilitis granulomatosa | Use as a differential diagnosis in swellings of the lip |
| Peutz–Jehgers | Pigmentations on lips, face, and oral mucosa; intestinal polyps (small gut) | Differential diagnosis of pigmented lesions |
| Pierre Robin | Microstomia, cleft palate, glossoptosis | Breathing difficulty |
| Plummer–Vinson | Iron deficiency anemia, atrophic oral and gastric mucosa, dysphagia | Predisposition to oral cancer |
| Reiter's | Nonspecific urethritis; arthritis; conjunctivitis; mucocutaneous lesions; usually seen in young males | Differential diagnosis in oral ulceration, possible resemblance to geographic tongue |
| Sjögren's | Dryness of eyes, mouth; primarily in middle-aged women; accompanied by rheumatoid arthritis; possibly an autoimmune reaction | Swelling of major salivary glands, xerostomia, biopsy of labial tissue possibly helpful in the diagnosis |
| Stevens–Johnson | Major form of erythema multiforme; explosive onset; lesions of mouth, lips, conjunctivae, skin, and genitals; self-limiting | Resemblance to recurrent herpes and other vesicular diseases, as well as Vincent's infections and allergic reactions |

**Table 11-3. Important Diseases with Eponyms**

| NAME | SYNONYMS | FEATURES |
|---|---|---|
| Albers–Schönberg | Osteopetrosis, marble bone disease | Generalized sclerosis of all bones, anemia, fractures, lack of osteoclastic activity |
| Bowen's | Carcinoma in situ | Premalignant lesion of the skin |
| Cannon's | White sponge nevus | Hereditary; gray white, thickened mucosa; generalized |
| Darier's | Keratosis follicularis | Genodermatosis with eruption of foul-smelling skin papules and "cobblestone" oral lesions, unique epithelial clefts with *corps ronds* and *corps grains* |
| Hand–Schüller–Christian | Histiocytosis X | Intermediate form of this disease process affecting young children, punched-out lesions on radiograph |
| Rendu–Osler–Weber | Hereditary hemorrhagic telangiectasia | Congenital angiomatous areas on skin and mucosa, spontaneous hemorrhage, more prominent at puberty |
| Sutton's | Major aphthae or periadenitis mucosa necrotica recurrens | Large, deep, painful aphthous ulcers which persist and heal with scarring |
| von Recklinghausen's (of skin) | Neurofibromatosis | Multiple neurofibromas, café au lait spots, possible malignant transformation |
| Witkop's | Hereditary benign intraepithelial dyskeratosis | Similar to white sponge nevus; microscopic resemblance to dyskeratosis, but completely benign |

**Table 11-4. Tumors with Eponyms**

| NAME | SYNONYM | FEATURES |
|---|---|---|
| Burkitt's | African jaw lymphoma | Rapidly growing tumor mass of the jaws in children, type of malignant lymphoma; possibly viral in origin |
| Ewing's | Endothelial myeloma | Very uncommon malignant neoplasm of bone occurring predominantly in children; pain and swelling may mimic an inflammatory disease |
| Pindborg's | Calcifying epithelial odontogenic tumor | Odontogenic tumor, most often in the mandible, often associated with an impacted tooth; may be a mixed radiolucent and radiopaque lesion |
| Warthin's | Papillary cystadenoma lymphomatosum | Benign salivary gland tumor seen primarily in older men, arising from ductal epithelium and lymphoid elements in the parotid and/or submaxillary glands |

infants. The clavicles and mandible are most often affected. In the mandible, a bilateral but asymmetric deformity of the angle–ramus area is produced, which should not be confused with cherubism. In addition, soft tissue swelling and fever may occur (27).

### METABOLIC DISTURBANCES INVOLVING BONE
*Rickets and Osteomalacia.* In growing children a deficiency of calcium and/or vitamin D produces the condition referred to as rickets. The oral findings of note are retarded eruption rates of the teeth, elongated pulpal horns, and abnormal alveolar bone patterns.

The adult counterpart of rickets is osteomalacia, in which improper mineralization of osteoid matrix leads to softening of the bones. A poorly defined lamina dura and abnormal trabecular bone patterns may be seen radiographically in such patients.

*Hyperparathyroidism.* Hyperparathyroidism (osteitis fibrosa cystica) is usually the result of a secreting primary adenoma of the parathyroids. The excessive serum parathyroid hormone thus released systematically causes calcium withdrawal from the bones, including the jaws as evidenced by 1) multiple "cystic" giant cell lesions, 2) loss of lamina dura, and 3) generalized rarefaction.

*Histiocytosis X.* Histiocytosis X is a complex disease process involving the reticuloendothelial histiocyte. The disease varies in its distribution and severity, ranging from the localized form, eosinophilic granuloma, to the diffuse Hand–Schüller–Christian disease and highly fatal Letterer–Siwe disease of infants. Oral lesions generally present as single or multiple radiolucent lesions of the jaws which in some instances mimic dental disease such as a periapical granuloma. For ex-

ample in the localized eosinophilic granuloma a tooth may appear on the radiograph to be "floating in air" or in a large radiolucency. Hand–Schüller–Christian disease, which occurs in younger age groups than eosinophilic granuloma, is characterized by multiple "punched-out" radiolucencies, particularly of the skull.

### PROLIFERATIVE OR NEOPLASTIC BONE DISEASE
*Paget's Disease.* Paget's disease also known as osteitis deformans, is a slowly progressive disease of older individuals in which there is a haphazard resorption and apposition of bone. The skull and maxilla enlarge. Radiographically the affected bones reveal the "cotton wool" effect. The microscopic manifestation of the abnormal resorption and apposition is a characteristic mosaic pattern of resting and reversal lines in rather dense bone. A most important laboratory finding is a markedly elevated serum alkaline phosphatase which is indicative of the hyperactive bone. A serious complication of the disease is the development of osteosarcoma in a significant percentage of the patients (66).

*Multiple Myeloma.* Multiple myeloma is another disease of older adults, particularly males between the ages of 40–70. This neoplastic process originates in the bone marrow from plasma cells, and the proliferation of these cells produces multiple osteolytic lesions of the bones, including the jaws, where the mandible is the most frequent site. Pain, swelling, and mobility of the teeth, as well as pathologic fracture, are not uncommon oral features. Radiographic examination reveals multiple, rather sharply punched-out radiolucencies in the skull, vertebrae, jaws, etc. Laboratory findings are extremely important in the diagnosis of multiple myeloma. These include 1) hyperglobulinemia from excessive globulins produced by the neoplastic cells, 2) reversal of the serum albumin–globulin ratio, 3) Bence–Jones protein in the urine, and 4) a myelophthisic (16) or replacement type anemia. Microscopic examination of tissue from the osteolytic areas exhibits sheets of cells resembling plasma cells. This disease carries a poor prognosis; treatment is primarily of a palliative nature.

*Fibrous Dysplasia.* Fibrous dysplasia, characterized by a painless, slow-growing jaw expansion producing facial deformity, is an idiopathic proliferative reaction of bone occurring primarily during the active periods of bone growth in young patients. The lesions may be single (monostotic) or involve multiple sites (polyostotic). Albright's syndrome, which is a form of the polyostotic type, includes skin pigmentations (café au lait spots) and precocious puberty in females (49). Radiographs of affected bones show an ill-defined mixed radiolucent/radiopaque area described as having a "ground glass" appearance (61).

*Osteosarcoma.* Osteosarcoma of the jaws occurs an average decade later than osteosarcoma of the extremities (30). Symmetric widening of the periodontal ligament about a tooth radiographically, accompanied by pain and loosening of the tooth may be suggestive (20). Advanced osteosarcoma of the jaw is characterized by a painful, enlarging mass.

## Nerve Diseases

Approximately three questions on the National Board Dental Examination concern the oral manifestations of nerve diseases.

**TRIGEMINAL NEURALGIA (TIC DOULOUREUX).** Trigeminal neuralgia is characterized by a paroxysmal disturbance of the fifth cranial nerve (usually the second division) in which severe transient pain is elicited by stimulation of a trigger zone. The condition most often affects older people and occurs on the right side of the face in the majority of cases (13).

**BELL'S PALSY.** A rapidly developing, unilateral paralysis of the seventh nerve is referred to as Bell's palsy. The motor paralysis leads to drooping of the corner of the mouth, slurring of speech, and inability to close the eyelid on the affected side. Fortunately the condition is usually temporary, lasting for about a month.

**MYASTHENIA GRAVIS.** Myasthenia gravis, a defect in the neuromuscular transmission process, is characterized by a progressive weakness of the skeletal muscles. The muscles of mastication may be involved early, as manifested by drooping of the jaw and difficulty in chewing. Tongue involvement is exhibited by slurring of speech.

**FREY'S SYNDROME (AURICULOTEMPORAL SYNDROME).** Surgery or injury to the auriculotemporal nerve and subsequent aberrant nerve regeneration is the etiology of Frey's syndrome (Table 11–2). As a result, sweat glands in the affected area are cross-enervated and become activated upon psychic, salivary, or gustatory activity (gustatory sweating).

**CAUSALGIA.** Causalgia is a term applied to severe pain which arises as a result of injury to a peripheral nerve such as may occur during a difficult tooth extraction.

## Temporomandibular Joint Disease

Only two or three questions in the oral pathology section of the National Board Examination deal directly with temporomandibular joint disease. These are usually related to developmental problems of the joint and inflammation, although other entities have sometimes been used as distractors in the examination questions.

**DEVELOPMENTAL DISTURBANCES.** Hypodevelopment of the temporomandibular joint may be congenital or acquired. Some etiologic factors are traumatic birth injury, external trauma in childhood, infections (otitis media), and radiation injury. Distinguishing features of such hypodevelopment include facial asymmetry and mandibular midline shift during opening or closing. The older the patient at the time of the growth disturbance, the less severe the facial deformity. Ankylosis of the joint, which may also be the result of injury or infection during early growth periods, can lead to hypodevelopment.

Hyperplasia of the temporomandibular joint area is much less common than hypoplasia and leads to a unilateral enlargement of the mandible in most cases. The etiology of the hyperplasia may be a mild chronic inflammation or neoplasm.

**TRAUMATIC DISTURBANCES OF THE TEMPOROMANDIBULAR JOINT.** A complete dislocation of the temporomandibular joint is referred to as luxation. Usually bilateral, the problem may be precipitated by sudden trauma, yawning, laughing, or excessive opening during dental procedures. Clinically there is a sudden locking and immobilization of the jaw with possible prolonged spasmodic muscle contraction. Treatment consists of relaxing the muscles and applying inferior and posterior pressure to guide the head of the condyle back into position.

Subluxation has been used to describe an incomplete or partial dislocation (51). The patient can generally return the jaw to its proper position.

**INFLAMMATORY CONDITIONS OF THE TEMPOROMAN-DIBULAR JOINT.** Inflammation of the temporomandibular joint or arthritis may be of several types, depending upon the etiology. Arthritis due to a specific bacterial infection may stem from a direct extension of an infection in the local area or via the blood stream or lymphatics, i.e., gonococcal arthritis. This form of inflammation appears to be lower in incidence than the other types of arthritis.

*Osteoarthritis.* Osteoarthritis, or degenerative joint disease, which is said to develop to some degree in all persons past age 40, occurs primarily in the weight-bearing joints. The temporomandibular joint, however, may also be affected with the resultant bony "lipping." Popping and clicking as well as pain may be present during jaw movement.

*Rheumatoid Arthritis.* Rheumatoid arthritis, a process thought to be autoimmune in nature, involves the temporomandibular joint in about 20% of the cases. Areas of the joint membrane become inflamed, destroyed, and replaced by a vascular granulation tissue known as a pannus. The joint becomes swollen and painful and is usually treated with steroids and other antiinflammatory agents (64).

**MYOFASCIAL PAIN–DYSFUNCTION SYNDROME.** Perplexing to the patient and controversial to the practitioner, the myofascial pain–dysfunction syndrome has received much attention in recent years. The classic positive clinical findings are generally agreed upon as muscle tenderness, pain, clicking or popping of the temporomandibular joint with movement and limitation of jaw motion (33). Most reported series indicate a greater incidence in females (9). It is also significant that patients complaining of the syndrome show no evidence of organic disease in the joint proper and there is a lack of tenderness in the joint. These findings tend to substantiate a neuromuscular imbalance rather than joint disease. Occlusal disharmony, emotional factors, subconscious habits, etc. lead to chronic eccentric occlusion which in turn results in masticatory muscle spasm. The treatment is also controversial, but may consist of correction of obvious occlusal discrepancies, myotherapeutic exercises, drugs, and even psychotherapy (36).

## Injury and Repair

**HEALING OF EXTRACTION SITES.** Uncomplicated healing of an extraction site is basically a process of organization of the clot in the socket. Granulation tissue forms on the scaffolding of the clot until about the 3rd week, when young trabeculae of osteoid begin to form. Radiographic evidence of this new bone formation, however, may not become evident until the 6th–8th week following the extraction.

Alveolar osteitis, or the dry socket, is probably the most common complication in the wound healing process of an extraction site. The blood clot disintegrates, creating in the alveolar walls a focal type of osteomyelitis which is severely painful and has a foul taste and odor.

Another complication of the healing pattern in an extraction wound is failure of the granulation tissue to produce new bone, resulting in a fibrous healing, which, of course, persists on a radiograph as a radiolucent area.

The presence of a foreign body, such as a suture in a wound of the oral mucosa, may elicit a proliferation of multinucleated giant cells and granulation tissue, resulting in the formation of a foreign body granuloma.

**CHEMICAL INJURIES.** Caustic burns, such as those caused by silver nitrate or aspirin held against the mucosa, produce localized necrosis of the surface epithelium which usually appears white (35). This type of lesion should be included in a differential diagnosis when leukoplakia is suspected.

Chronic lead (plumbism) and bismuth ingestion produce pigmented lines in the marginal gingivae.

Argyrosis (amalgam tattoo) is the result of the incorporation of finely granular amalgam particles into the soft tissue, forming a clinically visible blue black pigmented area. Microscopically these usually evoke little or no inflammatory response.

**DRUG REACTIONS.** In 35 to 50% of patients receiving the drug diphenylhydantoin (Dilantin), a fibrous hyperplasia of the gingival tissues is produced (55). The degree of this hyperplasia is often in inverse proportion to the degree of meticulous oral hygiene.

Allergic drug reactions in the oral cavity are generally classified into two main divisions: 1) stomatitis venenata, a localized mucosal surface delayed hypersensitivity reaction to a drug or chemical compound and 2) stomatitis medicamentosa, a more diffuse mucosal reaction to a drug received systemically.

**DENTURE INJURIES.** The epulis fissurata (more correctly, inflammatory fibrous hyperplasia) is basically a connective tissue hyperplasia in response to irritation from the flange or border of an ill-fitting denture, most often encountered in the mandibular mucobuccal fold area. Papillary hyperplasia (papillomatosis) is an epithelial proliferation associated primarily with a maxillary denture, usually occurring in the center of the hard palate as red, bumpy or cobblestone papillary projections. In one rather large series of cases, a high correlation was found between the incidence of papillary hyperplasia and the amount of time that dentures were left in the mouth (60).

## Cysts

**RETENTION CYSTS.** The mucocele is thought to be formed by a pooling of mucus in connective tissue as the result of rupture of a minor salivary gland duct. It commonly occurs on the lower lip, where it presents as a dome-shaped, bluish, soft lesion. The mucocele may sometimes be confused clinically with a hemangioma, although it cannot be emptied by digital pressure (68).

A lesion with a similar pathogenesis is the ranula, but a larger gland and duct are involved. The lesion manifests as a fluctuant swelling in the floor of the mouth.

**TRAUMATIC BONE CYST.** The lesion referred to as a traumatic bone cyst is not a true cyst, although it resembles a cyst radiographically and is indeed a pathologic cavity. Usually discovered on routine radiographs, this asymptomatic lesion appears as a sharply outlined, but irregularly shaped radiolucency. It is most often found in the mandibular molar region (3). The radiolucent area is seen above the inferior alveolar canal and may scallop up between the roots of the overlying teeth. Bone expansion may or may not be present and the teeth are normally vital (29).

Several theories have been proposed concerning the etiology of this lesion, but the most generally accepted is that of intramedullary hemorrhage followed by resorption of bone and the formation of an empty cavity.

**ODONTOGENIC CYSTS.** The dentigerous or follicular cyst arises about the crown of an impacted tooth and usually contains the crown of the tooth. This cyst is potentially destructive to large areas of surrounding bone and may be the source of even more sinister neoplasms. (See also section on Periapical Cyst earlier in chapter.)

A primordial cyst is believed to represent the cystic degeneration of a tooth bud prior to any calcification and is usually found in the site of a missing or supernumerary tooth.

The odontogenic keratocyst is distinguished by having a high recurrence rate (8) and a rather unique, active epithelial lining. Multiple cysts of this type occur in conjunction with the jaw cyst–basal cell nevus–bifid rib syndrome (45).

**FISSURAL AND DEVELOPMENTAL CYSTS.** The globulomaxillary cyst appears on a radiograph as an "inverted pear" radiolucency between the roots of the maxillary lateral and cuspid incisors. Expansion of bone is uncommon, and associated teeth are usually vital (18) and asymptomatic. In many instances a globulomaxil-

lary cyst is coincidentally discovered on routine radiographic examination.

The incisive canal cyst (also called nasopalatine duct cyst or median anterior maxillary cyst) is seen radiographically between the roots of the maxillary central incisors as an ovoid or heart-shaped radiolucency. The associated teeth are vital as a rule. A visible clinical swelling may be noted in the palatine papilla area, particularly if the cyst is located primarily in the incisive foramen rather than in the canal. It is currently felt that surgical intervention is not warranted for this cyst in dentulous patients if it is small and asymptomatic (49).

The nasolabial cyst (nasoalveolar cyst) is a soft tissue cyst which occurs at the junction of the ala of the nose and upper lip, resulting in a visible clinical swelling. Radiographs may show evidence of secondary bone involvement if present.

### QUESTIONS

62. Which of the following oral cysts would be expected to have the highest rate of recurrence?
    1. Radicular cyst
    2. Nasolabial cyst
    3. Keratocyst
    4. Incisive canal cyst
    5. Eruption cyst

63. Which of the following bone diseases show hereditary patterns?
    a. Osteogenesis imperfecta
    b. Osteitis fibrosa cystica
    c. Cleidocranial dysostosis
    d. Cherubism
    e. Hand–Schüller–Christian disease
    1. a, c, and d
    2. a, d, and e
    3. b, c, and d
    4. b, d, and e
    5. c, d, and e

64. Myelophthisic anemia may be expected to occur in
    a. multiple myeloma
    b. eosinophilic granuloma
    c. osteopetrosis
    d. osteogenesis imperfecta
    1. b and c
    2. b, c, and d
    3. a and c
    4. All of the above
    5. None of the above

65. Because of similarities in microscopic and radiographic appearances of the conditions, the dentist who receives a biopsy report diagnosing a central giant cell granuloma should take further steps to rule out
    1. fibrous dysplasia
    2. osteitis deformans
    3. Albright's syndrome
    4. hyperthyroidism
    5. hyperparathyroidism

66. A single 4-mm pigmented lesion on the alveolar mucosa may represent
    1. an amalgam tattoo
    2. a melanoma
    3. argyrosis
    4. a nevus
    5. All of the above

67. The radiograph shown is from the maxilla of a 22-year-old female who has complained of pain in the bicuspid area for several months. Vitality tests were normal for all teeth. Oral hygiene is excellent, and there is no evidence of periodontal disease elsewhere. The clinical features and osteolytic area are most suggestive of

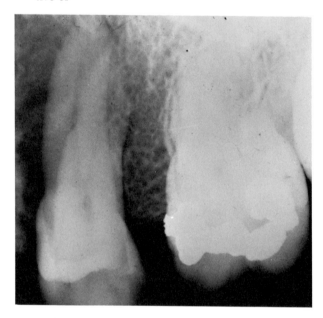

    1. fibrous dysplasia
    2. a lateral periodontal cyst
    3. osteosarcoma
    4. multiple myeloma
    5. hyperparathyroidism

68. A primary difference between rheumatoid arthritis and osteoarthritis of the temporomandibular joint is that rheumatoid arthritis
    1. is believed to be caused by wear and tear, whereas osteoarthritis is thought to be of autoimmune etiology
    2. responds to antiinflammatory therapy only, whereas osteoarthritis responds to steroids only
    3. can be treated medically with immobilization, heat, and cortisone, whereas osteoarthritis always requires surgical intervention in the joint
    4. is believed to be of autoimmune etiology, whereas osteoarthritis is thought to be caused by abnormal function or wear and tear

69. Which of the following neuralgias is characterized by a trigger zone which initiates a spasmodic lancinating pain in a sensory division of the fifth cranial nerve?

1. Trigeminal neuralgia
2. Causalgia
3. Glossopharyngeal neuralgia
4. Orolingual paresthesia

70. Spontaneous unilateral facial paralysis with drooping of the corner of the mouth and inability to close the eyelid strongly suggests
    1. Bell's palsy
    2. tic douloureux
    3. trigeminal neuralgia
    4. Stevens–Johnson syndrome

71. The second molar shown in the radiograph was loose and slightly tender. The patient, a 23-year-old female, had complained of a low-grade fever for several days. Her overall oral hygiene was good, and there was no other evidence of periodontal disease. The differential diagnosis should include

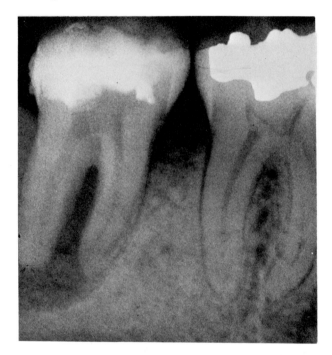

    a. periapical granuloma
    b. eosinophilic granuloma
    c. Garré's osteitis
    d. Albers–Schönberg disease
    1. a and b
    2. c and d
    3. a and c
    4. b and c
    5. b and d

72. Rheumatoid arthritis may cause a bilateral condylar ankylosis. If this has occurred in a 4-year-old boy, by 10 years of age, facial deformity will be characterized by a
    1. maxillary prognathism
    2. mandibular prognathism
    3. maxillary retrognathia
    4. mandibular retrognathia

73. Probably the most important etiologic factor in the development of the temporomandibular joint pain–dysfunction syndrome is
    1. rheumatoid arthritis
    2. loss of vertical dimension
    3. muscular strain and imbalance
    4. infection of the temporomandibular joint
    5. osteoarthritis

74. Of the following, which would be the most commonly occurring complication sequela to a tooth extraction?
    1. Condensing osteitis
    2. Alveolar osteitis
    3. Osteomyelitis
    4. Pulmonary abscess
    5. Alveolar abscess

75. The soft, fluctuant swelling on the mucosal surface of the lower lip shown below has been present for 1 week in this 20-year-old male. The most likely diagnosis is

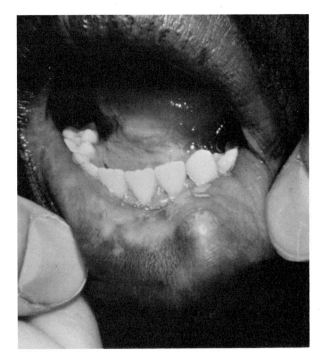

    1. hematoma
    2. mucocele
    3. traumatic cyst
    4. traumatic fibroma
    5. traumatic neuroma

76. Failure of osseous regeneration in an asymptomatic extraction wound is referred to as
    1. an internal callous
    2. an apical scar
    3. fibrous healing
    4. a dry socket
    5. alveolar osteitis

77. The healing mechanism after tooth extraction is basically described as

1. organization
2. resolution
3. suppuration
4. calcification
5. induration

78. Of the following cysts, which is the most potentially aggressive and destructive?
    1. Dentigerous cyst
    2. Globulomaxillary cyst
    3. Incisive canal cyst
    4. Periapical cyst

79. Multiple odontogenic keratocysts are associated with the
    1. Melkersson–Rosenthal syndrome
    2. basal cell nevus–bifid rib syndrome
    3. Plummer–Vinson syndrome
    4. Albright's syndrome

80. A 20-year-old female complains of a swelling in the palate. Examination reveals a soft, fluctuant area in the midline of the anterior hard palate. The incisors test vital and there is no evidence of periodontal disease. A radiograph, however, reveals a well-defined, heart-shaped radiolucency between the roots of the maxillary central incisors. These findings are most suggestive of a
    1. lateral periodontal cyst
    2. incisive canal cyst
    3. dentigerous cyst
    4. nasolabial cyst
    5. radicular cyst

81. Which of the following lesions is characterized by inflammatory fibrous hyperplasia in the flange area of an ill-fitting denture and is assumed to require surgical removal, as spontaneous regression is rare?
    1. Papillary hyperplasia
    2. Epulis fissurata
    3. Denture sore mouth
    4. Decubitus ulcer

82. A 3-cm ovoid radiolucent area is found on routine radiographic examination in the mandibular molar region of a 17-year-old male. The outline of the radiolucent area is consistent with a cyst, as the roots of the associated molars seem to extend into the area. The teeth, however, tested vital. Upon opening into the area, the oral surgeon found the area to be completely empty. Which of the following statements best applies to this situation?
    1. The lesion represents an embryonic bone defect and requires no treatment.
    2. The lesion represents a large radicular cyst, and all teeth in the area should be extracted or receive endodontic therapy.
    3. The lesion represents a traumatic bone cyst, and the surgical procedure of opening into the area will initiate healing.
    4. The lesion represents a dentigerous cyst, and treatment should consist of marsupialization.

83. Routine periapical radiographs of a young adult patient reveal a relatively large inverted pear-shaped radiolu-

*(Continued)*

cency situated between the roots of the right lateral incisor and canine. The roots of both teeth seem to be displaced away from the radiolucent area. Both teeth test vital. The condition most likely to be responsible for the area in question is a(n)

1. radicular cyst
2. periodontal cyst
3. incisive canal cyst
4. globulomaxillary cyst
5. nasolabial cyst

# REFERENCES

1. AEGERTER E, KIEKPATRICK JA: Orthopedic Diseases. Philadelphia, WB Saunders, 1975
2. BARTLETT RC, EVERSOLE LR, ADKINS RS: Autosomal recessive hypohydrotic ectodermal dysplasia: Dental manifestations. Oral Surg 33:736–742
3. BEASLEY JD: Traumatic cyst of the jaws: Report of 30 cases. J Am Dent Assoc 92:145–152, 1976
4. BEUMER J, TROWBRIDGE HO, SILVERMAN S, EISENBERG E: Childhood hypophosphatasia and the premature loss of teeth. Oral Surg 35:631–640, 1973
5. BHASKAR SN: Synopsis of Oral Pathology. St. Louis, CV Mosby, 1977
6. BOUDREAU GE, JERGE CR: The efficacy of sealant treatment in the prevention of pit and fissure dental caries: A review and interpretation of the literature. J Am Dent Assoc 92:383–387, 1976
7. BOWEN WH: Prospects for the prevention of dental caries. Hospital Practice. May:163–168, 1974
8. BRANNON RB: The odontogenic keratocyst. Oral Surg 42:54–72, 1976
9. BROOKE RI, STERN PG, KERRY JM: The diagnosis and conservative treatment of myofascial pain dysfunction syndrome. Oral Surg 44:844–852, 1977
10. BRUSTEIN HC, MAUTNER RL: Osteogenesis imperfecta. Oral Surg 42:42–52, 1976
11. BUDNICK SD: Compound and complex odontomas. Oral Surg 42:501–506, 1976
12. CHARBENEAU GT, DENNISON JB: Clinical success and potential failure after single application of a pit and fissure sealant: a four-year report. J Am Dent Assoc 98:559–564, 1979
13. CHERRICK HM: Trigeminal neuralgia. Oral Surg 34:714–726, 1972
14. CIPOLLARO AC: Cancer of the skin. Am J Nurs 66:2231–2237, 1966
15. DICK HM, SIMPSON WJ: Dental changes in osteopetrosis. Oral Surg 34:408–416, 1972
16. DICKSON VL, EICHNER ER: Clinical aspects of multiple myeloma. Resident and Staff Physician. Aug:46–51, 1975
17. EVERSOLE LR: Oral lesions as the initial sign in pemphigus vulgaris. Oral Surg 33:354–361, 1972
18. EVERSOLE LR: Clinical Outline of Oral Pathology. Philadelphia, Lea and Febiger, 1978
19. GARDNER AF: Pathology of Oral Manifestations of Systemic Diseases. New York, Hafner, 1972
20. GARDNER DG, MILLS DM: The widened periodontal ligament of osteosarcoma of the jaws. Oral Surg 41:652–656, 1976
21. GENCO RJ, EVANS RT, ELLISON SA: Dental research in microbiology with emphasis on periodontal disease. J Am Dent Assoc 78:1016–1036, 1969
22. GIBBONS RJ, VAN HOUTE J: Dental caries. Annu Rev Med 26:121, 1975
23. GOING RE, HAUGH LO, GRAINGER DA, CONTI AJ: Four-year clinical evaluation of a pit and fissure sealant. J Am Dent Assoc 95:972–981, 1977
24. GOLDSTEIN E, GOTTLIEB MA: Taurodontism: Familial tendencies demonstrated in eleven of fourteen case reports. Oral Surg 36:131–144, 1973
25. GORLIN RJ, CHAUDHRY AP, PINDBORG JJ: Odontogenic tumors. Cancer 14:73–101, 1961
26. GORLIN RJ, SEDANO H: Ehlers-Danlos syndrome. Mod Med Dec:104, 1971
27. GORLIN RJ, SEDANO H: Infantile cortical hyperostosis (Caffey-Silverman syndrome). Mod Med May:108, 1972
28. GREER RO, GOLDMAN HM: Oral papillomas. Oral Surg 38:435–440, 1974
29. HANSEN LS, SAPONE J, SPROAT RC: Traumatic cysts of jaws. Oral Surg 37:899–910, 1974
30. HIGH CL, FREW AL, GLASS RT: Osteosarcoma of the mandible. Oral Surg 45:678–679, 1978
31. HOFF M: Dental manifestations in Ehlers-Danlos syndrome. Oral Surg 44:864–871, 1977
32. KROLLS SO, HOFFMAN S: Squamous cell carcinoma of the oral soft tissues: A statistical analysis of 14,253 cases by age, sex, and race of patients. J Am Dent Assoc 92:571–574, 1976
33. LASKIN DM: Etiology of the pain-dysfunction syndrome. J Am Dent Assoc 79:147–153, 1969
34. LEHNER T: Oral candidosis. The Dental Practitioner 17:209–216, 1967
35. LUMMERMAN H: Essentials of Oral Pathology. Philadelphia, JB Lippincott, 1975
36. LUPTON DE: Psychological aspects of temporomandibular joint dysfunction. J Am Dent Assoc 79:131–136, 1969
37. MASSLER M, PAWLAK J: The affected and infected pulp. Oral Surg 43:929–947, 1977
38. MATTESON SR, CUTLER LS, HERMAN PA: Warthin's tumor. Oral Surg 41:129–134, 1976
39. MICHAUD M, BAEHNER RL, BIXLER D, KAFRAWY AH: Oral manifestations of acute leukemia in children. J Am Dent Assoc 95:1145–1150, 1977
40. MILLER R, SAKAMOTO E, ZELL A, et al: Cleidocranial dysostosis: A multidisciplinary approach to treatment. J Am Dent Assoc 96:296–300, 1978
41. MILLER WD: Microorganisms of the Human Mouth. Philadelphia, SS White, 1890
42. MILOBSKY L, MILOBSKY SA, MILLER GM: Adenomatoid odontogenic tumor (adenoameloblastoma). Oral Surg 40:681–685, 1975
43. NAIDORF IJ: Inflammation and infection of pulp and periapical tissues. Oral Surg 34:486–497, 1972
44. NOLTE WA: Oral Microbiology. St. Louis, CV Mosby, 1973
45. PAYNE TF: An analysis of the clinical and histopathological parameters of the odontogenic keratocyst. Oral Surg 33:538–546, 1972
46. RANKOW RM, POLAYES IM: Diseases of the Salivary Glands. Philadelphia, WB Saunders, 1976, pp 282–283
47. SCHERP HW: Dental Caries: Prospects for prevention. Science 173:1199–1205, 1971
48. SELTZER S: Classification of pulpal pathosis. Oral Surg 34:269–287, 1972
49. SHAFER WG, HINE MK, LEVY BM: A Textbook of Oral Pathology. Philadelphia, WB Saunders, 1974
50. SHAFER WG, WALDRON CA: Erythroplakia of the oral cavity. Cancer 36:1021, 1975
51. SHEPPARD IM, SHEPPARD SM: Subluxation of the temporomandibular joint. Oral Surg 44:821–829, 1977
52. SILVERMAN S, BEUMER J: Primary herpetic gingivostomatitis of adult onset. Oral Surg 36:496–503, 1973
53. SILVERMAN S, GRIFFITH M: Studies on oral lichen planus II. Oral Surg 37:705–710, 1974

54. SILVERSTONE LM: Preventive Dentistry. London, Update Books, 1978
55. SPOUGE JD: Oral Pathology. St. Louis, CV Mosby, 1973
56. TEN CATE AR: The epithelial cell rests of Malassez and the genesis of the dental cyst. Oral Surg 34:956–964, 1972
57. THOMAS JG: A study of dens in dente. Oral Surg 38:653–655, 1974
58. TOPAZIAN RG, COSTICH ER: Familial fibrous dysplasia of the jaws (cherubism). Oral Surg 23:559, 1965
59. TOTTEN RS: Tumors of the oral cavity, pharynx, and larynx. J Am Med Assoc 215:454–455, 1971
60. TUCKER KM, HEGET HS: The incidence of inflammatory hyperplasia. J Am Dent Assoc 93:610–613, 1976
61. WALDRON CA, GIANSANTI JS: Fibrous dysplasia of the jaws. Oral Surg 35:190–201, 1973
62. WALDRON CA, SHAFER WG: Leukoplakia revisited. Cancer 36:1386–1392, 1975
63. WEGE WR: Idiopathic internal resorption. Oral Surg 36:443–445, 1973
64. WEISSMAN G: Rheumatoid arthritis: How the new non-steroidal anti-inflammatory drugs work. Resident and Staff Physician. Dec:48–55, 1976
65. WEITZNER S, LOCKEY MW, LOCKARD VG: Adult rhabdomyoma of the soft palate. Oral Surg 47:70–73, 1979
66. WILNER D, SHERMAN RS: Roentgen diagnosis of Paget's disease (osteitis deformans). Dent Radiogr Photogr 43:47–59, 1970
67. WITKOP CJ, GORLIN RJ: Four hereditary mucosal syndromes. Arch Dermatol 84:104–113, 1961
68. WOOD NK, GOAZ PW: Differential Diagnosis of Oral Lesions. St. Louis, CV Mosby, 1975

## ANSWER KEY

| | | | |
|---|---|---|---|
| 1. 4 | 22. 3 | 43. 2 | 64. 3 |
| 2. 4 | 23. 5 | 44. 4 | 65. 5 |
| 3. 1 | 24. 2 | 45. 2 | 66. 5 |
| 4. 5 | 25. 4 | 46. 3 | 67. 3 |
| 5. 1 | 26. 2 | 47. 1 | 68. 4 |
| 6. 5 | 27. 3 | 48. 1 | 69. 1 |
| 7. 3 | 28. 3 | 49. 3 | 70. 1 |
| 8. 4 | 29. 4 | 50. 4 | 71. 1 |
| 9. 3 | 30. 1 | 51. 5 | 72. 4 |
| 10. 2 | 31. 2 | 52. 4 | 73. 3 |
| 11. 4 | 32. 5 | 53. 2 | 74. 2 |
| 12. 5 | 33. 2 | 54. 4 | 75. 2 |
| 13. 4 | 34. 3 | 55. 2 | 76. 3 |
| 14. 4 | 35. 5 | 56. 1 | 77. 1 |
| 15. 1 | 36. 5 | 57. 4 | 78. 1 |
| 16. 4 | 37. 4 | 58. 4 | 79. 2 |
| 17. 5 | 38. 2 | 59. 4 | 80. 2 |
| 18. 3 | 39. 2 | 60. 4 | 81. 2 |
| 19. 5 | 40. 5 | 61. 2 | 82. 3 |
| 20. 3 | 41. 4 | 62. 3 | 83. 4 |
| 21. 3 | 42. 2 | 63. 1 | |

# 12
# ORAL MEDICINE

## Willard G. Fischer

### DIAGNOSIS

Correct diagnosis is essential to proper treatment. Although some conditions are known to respond to empirical treatment, the primary objective of diagnosis is to establish the etiology of an abnormal condition so that rational therapy may be instituted.

### Signs of Abnormality

In order to recognize an abnormality it is necessary to have a knowledge of the wide range of conditions which affect patients and a knowledge of the diagnostic features of these conditions. Signs of abnormality provide diagnostic clues which involve consideration of:

1. color
2. consistency
3. function
4. hemorrhage
5. location
6. mobility
7. number
8. odor
9. shape
10. size
11. sounds
12. ulceration
13. abnormal deviation in any of the four vital signs

### QUESTIONS

1. Cyanosis of the lips is a common finding in all except
   1. cardiac congestion
   2. congenital heart defects
   3. iron deficiency anemia
   4. polycythemia

2. The most prominent oral sign of Gardner's or Peutz–Jeghers syndrome is
   1. the presence of numerous small polyps on the buccal mucosa
   2. small melanotic lesions on the lip and hard palate
   3. numerous small petechiae on the buccal mucosa
   4. ulcerations on the tongue

3. Minute yellow granules are readily detected on the buccal mucosa of approximately 80% of the population. These Fordyce's spots are one of the very few pathognomonic signs which enable a definitive diagnosis to be made because they are known to be
   1. aberrant tonsilar tissue
   2. hyperkeratoses due to trauma
   3. minor mucous glands
   4. ectopic sebaceous glands

4. A 38-year-old female brought her three teen-aged children for initial examination. On the buccal mucosa of each were detected white, corrugated, firm, non-tender lesions. Although histologic examination is necessary for definitive diagnosis, the strongest clinical suspicion to be entertained is that these lesions are
   1. hyperkeratotic
   2. an atypical form of lichen planus
   3. leukoedema
   4. white sponge nevi

5. Leukoedema, occasionally observed on the buccal mucosa, is characterized by a clinical appearance of
   1. raised, white lesions with an annular configuration
   2. erosions
   3. a milky white, translucent coloration of the mucosa with minute "hanging" folds of tissue
   4. white lesions with a lacelike configuration

6. Redness and enlargement of minor salivary gland orifices in the palate are clinical signs of early
   1. papillary inflammatory hyperplasia
   2. nicotinic stomatitis
   3. primary syphilis
   4. secondary syphilis

7. Prolonged antibiotic administration is known to result in the presence of a
   1. crenated tongue
   2. geographic tongue
   3. black hairy tongue
   4. median rhomboid glossitis

8. A 10-year-old female was brought in by her mother for restorative treatment. The history provided by the mother included a recent evaluation for emotional difficulties and problems with school work. She also reported that the girl had appeared rather listless for the past several years and that she was disposed to chew on

her painted toys rather than play with them. Clinical examination disclosed pallor of the oral mucosa and a grayish blue discoloration of the gingiva. These findings are most consistent with a clinical impression of

1. cherubism
2. cretinism
3. the Pierre Robin syndrome
4. plumbism

9. An 18-year-old female requested aesthetic improvement of her "brown teeth." She reported that two of her four brothers' teeth had a similar appearance. Some chipping of occlusal and incisal enamel, not attributable to caries or trauma, was apparent. Radiographs demonstrated an absence of pulp chambers and canals of most teeth and unusually short tapering roots. These findings are characteristic of

1. amelogenesis imperfecta
2. dentinogenesis imperfecta
3. erythroblastosis fetalis
4. fluorosis

10. Examination of a 4-year-old male patient's dentition revealed a pronounced yellow green discoloration of crowns of the entire dentition. The father reported multiple transfusions at the time of birth. These findings suggest that the most likely, although rare, cause of the patient's tooth discoloration is

1. amelogenesis imperfecta
2. dentinogenesis imperfecta
3. erythroblastosis fetalis
4. fluorosis

11. In the United States the most common cause of mottled enamel and tooth discoloration is

1. amelogenesis imperfecta
2. dentinogenesis imperfecta
3. erythroblastosis fetalis
4. endemic fluorosis

12. The earliest clinical sign of the initiation of dental caries, e.g., Class V caries, is most often

1. pain elicited by exploration
2. a change in color of the suspected area
3. an enamel defect detectable with an explorer
4. radiographic appearance

13. Amber-colored tooth translucency, blue sclerae, and bone fragility suggested by a history of skeletal bone fractures early in life are characteristic findings in

1. osteitis fibrosa cystica
2. osteitis deformans
3. osteogenesis imperfecta
4. osteoporosis

14. Match the pathologic condition listed in the right-hand column with its usual degree of consistency determined on palpation.

(a) firm     (1) pyogenic granuloma
(b) stony hard     (2) ranula
(c) rubbery     (3) irritation fibroma
(d) soft     (4) a lymph node involved with metastatic carcinoma

15. A 42-year-old female requested an evaluation of a "swelling" in the midline of the hard palate. She reported that she had noticed this about a month ago on self-examination and that she was fearful that it was malignant because her father "died from mouth cancer." Examination revealed a $3 \times 4$ cm, very hard elevation with an intact mucosa. Observation, rather than immediate removal or biopsy, is indicated because these findings are characteristic of

1. a cancer phobia on the part of the patient
2. an enostosis
3. a most common exostosis
4. a pleomorphic adenoma, the most common tumor of the palate

16. The chief complaint of a 19-year-old male was soreness in the area of the right temporomandibular joint and some pain on mastication. He reported having received a "bump on the jaw" in a minor automobile accident a week ago. A clinical sign of altered function which would substantiate the suspicion of a fracture on the right condyle is

1. an inability to protrude the mandible
2. a deviation of the mandible to the right, on opening
3. a deviation of the mandible to the left, on opening
4. inability to wink the right eye

17. In the absence of systemic disease, most infections originating within the oral cavity (e.g., pericoronitis, periapical abscesses and acute necrotizing ulcerative gingivitis) usually remain localized and respond well to mechanical forms of therapy alone. Signs and/or symptoms of systemic involvement which indicate treatment of these conditions with antibiotics include all except

1. lymphadenopathy
2. redness and tenderness of an operculum
3. elevation of temperature
4. trismus and/or pain on swallowing

18. A program of prevention is of utmost importance for the patient undergoing radiation therapy to the head and neck area because of the known development of rampant caries shortly after such therapy. Rampant caries is of high incidence in these patients because

1. of compromise of the blood supply to all the oral tissues
2. of the direct effect of radiation upon the teeth
3. gingival recession produced by the radiation exposes the cementum
4. xerostomia invariably occurs and persists for about a year following treatment

19. A 40-year-old male patient reported that a tumor had been removed from his parotid gland 2 months ago. He now experiences profuse sweating of a small area of the skin overlying his left temple. This occurs invariably when he eats the spicy foods he enjoys. These findings are most characteristic of

1. Albright's syndrome
2. Behçet's syndrome
3. the auriculotemporal, or Frey's, syndrome
4. Gardner's syndrome

20. A 28-year-old female in her third trimester of pregnancy complained of a "growth on her gum." She reported that it had been present for about 2 weeks. Clinical examination revealed a red, sessile, exophytic lesion involving the buccal gingiva in the area of the mandibular left first molar which bled readily upon moderate finger pressure. These findings are most characteristic of
   1. a gingival cyst
   2. a pyogenic granuloma
   3. an irritation fibroma
   4. pregnancy gingivitis

21. Some dilatation of capillaries in the facial skin is a common finding in middle-aged patients. However, development of multiple angiomas which may rupture spontaneously and are accompanied by a history of espistaxis are highly suggestive of
   1. Albright's syndrome
   2. Lobstein's syndrome
   3. the Rendu–Osler–Weber disease
   4. Trotter's syndrome

22. Petechiae involving the conjunctiva, yellow skin color, multiple unexplained bruises and a flushed, ruddy complexion are all clinical findings which suggest
   1. diabetes mellitus
   2. a predisposition for excessive bleeding following extractions
   3. hepatitis
   4. the onset of erythema multiforme

23. Angular cheilosis may be the result of infection, loss of vertical dimension, hypovitaminosis B₂, or iron deficiency anemia. When it is the result of infection, the biologic agent most often responsible is
   1. *Actinomyces bovis*
   2. a group A coxsackievirus
   3. *Candida albicans*
   4. viridans streptococcus

24. Fovea palatinae, located in the midline at the junction of the soft and hard palate, are the result of
   1. coalescence of mucous gland ducts
   2. fistula formation
   3. nicotinic stomatitis
   4. the development of small fissural cleft cysts

25. Multiple small vesicles and/or ulcerations which are characteristic of herpangina and infectious mononucleosis are most often limited to the
   1. buccal mucosa
   2. gingiva
   3. oropharynx and soft palate
   4. tongue

26. A 20-year-old female requested that her maxillary central incisor be replaced by a fixed bridge. She had been wearing a removable appliance for about 2 years. Clinical examination revealed a red area in the palate covered by the present appliance with long hairlike projections extending from it. These findings are characteristic of

1. multiple irritation fibromas
2. nicotinic stomatitis
3. papillary inflammatory hyperplasia
4. stomatitis venenata

27. Ulceration of the oropharynx and oral mucosal surfaces is often an early sign of
   1. anemia
   2. sensitivity to penicillin
   3. squamous cell carcinoma
   4. Vincent's infection

28. Persistence of the tuberculum impar in the course of development results in the presence of a smooth, red, diamond-shaped area on the posterior dorsal aspect of the tongue. The location, shape, and color of this area are characteristic of
   1. the circumvallate papillae
   2. foliate papillae
   3. erythema migrans or the geographic tongue
   4. median rhomboid glossitis

29. Foliate papillae and lingual tonsils are common developmental anomalies often found on the lateral border of the posterior third of the tongue. Their detection often arouses suspicion of a malignancy because
   1. of their color
   2. of their consistency
   3. they are often unilateral and in a site where a malignancy often develops
   4. of their size

30. An unusually high mandibular labial frenum attachment is often a primary etiologic factor in
   1. development of caries involving the mandibular central incisors
   2. development of an irritation fibroma
   3. gingival recession on the labial surface of the mandibular central incisors
   4. certain types of speech impairment

31. Examination of a 20-year-old male patient's dentition revealed that the maxillary right lateral incisor occupied the position normally occupied by the maxillary right cuspid and vice versa. The relative position of these two teeth represents a common form of
   1. malposition
   2. transposition
   3. apposition
   4. gemination

32. During surgical removal of a malposed maxillary third molar for a 28-year-old male patient, its root was found to be fused to that of one of the adjacent second molar roots. This condition is termed
   1. fusion
   2. apposition
   3. concrescence
   4. germination

33. Cervical radiolucencies, termed adumbration, are easily misconstrued as evidence of dental caries. One of the major reasons for the appearance of these radiolucencies is

1. the employment of faulty vertical angulation
2. the anatomy of the tooth in the area in which they appear
3. excessive exposure time
4. the "mach-band" effect

34. Least frequently involved in Stevens–Johnson syndrome is the
    1. eye
    2. genitalia
    3. oral mucous membrane
    4. skin

35. Secondary syphilis may be manifested clinically by
    1. lip ulceration
    2. perforation of the palate
    3. oral mucous patches and a maculopapular skin rash
    4. vesicles involving the oropharynx and soft plate

36. Clinical and radiographic examination of a 19-year-old male patient revealed a retained mandibular left second deciduous molar which was noncarious, vital, and nonmobile. A round, 1 cm, well-circumscribed, totally radiolucent area immediately 5 mm apical to the bifurcation was demonstrated on the radiographs. These findings are most suggestive of a(n)
    1. dentigerous cyst
    2. eruption cyst
    3. primordial cyst
    4. radicular cyst

37. Initial radiographic survey of a 32-year-old male revealed a well-circumscribed radiolucency between the maxillary left lateral incisor and cuspid roots. Slight deviation of the roots of these teeth suggested the presence of an expansile type of lesion. Pulpal pathology was ruled out by thorough examination. These findings suggest the presence of a
    1. lateral periodontal cyst
    2. globulomaxillary cyst relatively early in its development
    3. nasopalatine cyst
    4. primordial cyst associated with a supernumerary tooth

38. Radiographically the midpalatine, globulomaxillary, and median mandibular cysts are most similar in respect to their
    1. degree of radiolucency
    2. having a characteristic location
    3. size
    4. having a characteristic configuration

39. A routine radiographic survey may provide the initial evidence of Albers–Schönberg disease primarily because
    1. delayed eruption may be suggested
    2. the bone pattern is exceedingly dense with loss of trabecular spaces
    3. pulp canals are most often absent
    4. hypercementosis is a common feature

40. Fibrous ankylosis of the temporomandibular joint is most often associated with
    1. nocturnal bruxism
    2. congenital hypoplasia of the condyle
    3. a fracture of the condyle
    4. rheumatoid arthritis

41. An exceptionally far forward attachment of the lingual frenum is responsible for
    1. hypomobility due to ankyloglossia
    2. buccal caries
    3. glossopyrosis
    4. lingual varicosities

42. A 35-year-old male patient complained of increasing "soreness" of a tooth. Radiographs of this maxillary second bicuspid demonstrated a slight thickening of the periodontal ligament space in the apical area. The tooth was noncarious, 2° mobile, and reacted within normal limits to pulpal stimuli. No other signs of periodontal disease were present. The most likely cause of the patient's complaint on the basis of these findings is
    1. ankylosis of the tooth
    2. pulpal death due to anachoresis
    3. an occlusal discrepancy
    4. undiagnosed scleroderma

43. Ankylosis of a tooth is most definitely suggested by
    1. absence of the periodontal ligament space on radiographs
    2. a thickened periodontal ligament space on radiographs
    3. a clear, ringing sound upon percussion
    4. inability to move the tooth buccolingually

44. The sign which indicates that a tooth is most severely periodontally involved is:
    1. radiographic evidence of 50% bone loss
    2. depressibility and/or rotatability
    3. 3° mobility
    4. a pocket depth of 5 mm

45. Dryness of the skin, lips, and fingernails; thin sparse head and eyebrow hair; and congenital absence of numerous teeth are all associated with
    1. Albers–Schönberg disease
    2. Gardner's syndrome
    3. hereditary ectodermal dysplasia
    4. osteogenesis imperfecta

46. Precocious eruption of teeth is known to be associated with
    1. hyperparathyroidism
    2. hyperthyroidism and hyperpituitarism
    3. hypoparathyroidism
    4. excessive vitamin A intake

47. Acrodynia, hypophosphatasia, and progeria are rare conditions in which
    1. delayed eruption of teeth is common
    2. precocious eruption of teeth invariably occurs
    3. premature exfoliation of deciduous teeth is known to occur
    4. multiple supernumerary teeth are often present

48. Because it may involve bone only late in its development, the cyst which is least apt to be demonstrated by radiographic means is the
    1. follicular cyst
    2. globulomaxillary cyst
    3. nasoalveolar cyst
    4. nasopalatine cyst

49. The most common extraoral cause of halitosis is
    1. diabetes mellitus
    2. chronic sinusitis with postnasal drip
    3. indigestion
    4. kidney dysfunction

50. Match the systemic condition list in the right column with the type of halitosis it may produce.

    (a) acetone odor          1. rhinitis
    (b) "mousy" odor          2. kidney dysfunction
    (c) ozena                 3. severe diabetes
    (d) uremic odor           4. liver disease

51. The least objective clinical sign of periodontal disease is
    1. a pocket depth of 5 mm
    2. the presence of halitosis
    3. moderate mobility (2°) of teeth
    4. presence of a purulent discharge

52. Initial examination of a 35-year-old male patient disclosed a pedunculated, freely movable, 1 × 1.5 cm lesion on the buccal mucosa at the level of the occlusal plane. Its surface was intact and of the same color as the surrounding tissue. It did not blanch on finger pressure. The patient reported that it caused him no pain and that he had been aware of its presence for about 2 years. These findings are most characteristic of a(n)
    1. hemangioma
    2. irritation fibroma
    3. melanoma
    4. exophytic type of squamous cell carcinoma

53. A 35-year-old male complained of a "growth" in the floor of the oral cavity. He reported that he first noticed it about 3 weeks ago, but that it had not undergone any appreciable enlargement since. Clinically the lesion was observed to be to the right of the midline, slightly elevated, nonulcerated, and had a blue surface coloration. It was nontender, movable, and had a palpable border. A viscid fluid was obtained on aspiration. The most likely, but presumptive, diagnosis of this lesion is a(n)
    1. hemangioma
    2. mucocele
    3. ranula
    4. primordial cyst

54. A 73-year-old male was referred by his physician for evaluation of a lesion in the floor of the mouth. The history included smoking of three packages of cigarettes and consumption of a minimum of 10 oz. alcoholic beverage per day. There was also a history of syphilis, treated 20 years ago. Clinical examination revealed an indurated, white, nontender, 1.5 × 1.5 cm lesion to the right of the midline in the floor of the mouth. No nodes were palpable. Until proven otherwise by biopsy examination, this lesion must be considered a
    1. basal cell carcinoma
    2. fibrosarcoma
    3. dermoid cyst
    4. squamous carcinoma

55. A 23-year-old male complained of a swelling of the left cheek which had appeared "overnight." He reported no other symptoms. Palpation disclosed a fluctuant, nontender swelling without detectable borders. Clinical examination revealed a severely carious maxillary left molar, with radiographic evidence of pronounced periapical radiolucencies. These findings are most compatible with a diagnosis of
    1. cellulitis
    2. chronic alveolar abscess
    3. Ludwig's angina
    4. Vincent's angina

56. Defects in tooth structure in amelogenesis imperfecta are limited to the
    1. crown and root form
    2. crown and pulp chamber
    3. dentin and pulp
    4. color, shape, and size of the crown

57. Examination of a 9-year-old male patient's dentition revealed a bifid crown of the mandibular left lateral incisor. The two developmental disturbances which should be considered as the possible etiologies of this condition are
    1. dilaceration and fusion
    2. dilaceration and enamel hyperplasia
    3. fusion and gemination
    4. dilaceration and gemination

58. Examination of an 18-year-old male patient's dentition revealed a severe enamel hypoplasia of only the mandibular left second bicuspid. This Turner tooth is most likely to have developed as a result of
    1. congenital syphilis
    2. periapical infection of its deciduous predecessor
    3. an exanthematous fever during its calcification
    4. a vitamin B deficiency

59. Taurodontism is characterized by a radiographic appearance of teeth which possess
    1. bell-shaped crowns and short tapering roots
    2. large elongated pulp chambers and unusually short roots, particularly in the molar regions
    3. bifid root formation of teeth which are usually single rooted
    4. unusually large bulbous roots

60. Multiple unerupted teeth and deviations in size and shape of erupted permanent teeth are most commonly found in association with
    1. congenital syphilis and cleidocranial dysostosis
    2. cleidocranial and craniofacial dysostosis
    3. ectodermal dysplasia and cleidocranial dysostosis
    4. congenital syphilis and craniofacial dysostosis

61. Unerupted teeth which present a ghostlike radiographic appearance represent a form of
    1. amelogenesis imperfecta
    2. dentinogenesis imperfecta
    3. regional odontodysplasia
    4. shell teeth

62. Recent clinical study has suggested that the least reliable diagnostic feature of sickle cell anemia is
    1. a "hair-on-end" appearance of the calvarium
    2. a history of weakness, ready fatigability, headaches, and joint pain
    3. jaundice of the eyes
    4. a characteristic radiographic appearance of the trabecular pattern

63. Match the type of cyst listed in the right-hand column with the feature assisting in its diagnosis.

    (a) involves only the crown of a tooth
    (b) occasionally heart-shaped
    (c) a history of trauma to the area
    (d) may be pear-shaped

    1. hemorrhagic bone cyst
    2. globulomaxillary cyst
    3. nasopalatine and incisive canal cysts
    4. dentigerous cyst

64. Match the radiographic appearance listed in the right-hand column with the condition with which they may be associated.

    (a) ameloblastoma, cherubism
    (b) ossifying fibroma
    (c) osteogenic sarcoma
    (d) sickle cell anemia

    1. "ground-glass" radiopacity
    2. "hair-on-end" effect (of the calvarium)
    3. "soap bubble-like" radiolucencies
    4. "sun-ray" radiopacity

65. Lower facial asymmetry, café-au-lait discolorations of the skin, and irregular brown pigmentation of the lips are early signs of
    1. Addison's disease
    2. Albers–Schönberg disease
    3. Albright's disease
    4. Paget's disease

66. Marocheilia is one of the most common developmental anomalies of the lips. It may be associated with all of the following conditions except
    1. acromegaly
    2. cretinism
    3. hyperthyroidism
    4. myxedema

67. A maxillary labial frenum which extends exceptionally far lingually is often a primary etiologic factor in
    1. caries involving the maxillary central incisors
    2. a diastema between the central incisors
    3. labial gingival recession in the maxillary incisor region
    4. speech impairment

68. Characteristic clinical findings in hereditary gingival fibromatosis include all the following except
    1. firm gingival consistency
    2. generalized gingival enlargement
    3. spontaneous gingival hemorrhage
    4. a pink gingival color

69. Developmental disturbances which result in unusual size and/or shape of teeth most frequently occur in
    1. maxillary and mandibular incisors
    2. maxillary third molars and mandibular incisors
    3. third molars and maxillary lateral incisors
    4. third molars and mandibular second bicuspids

70. Congenital syphilis may be responsible for a variety of anomalies in the permanent dentition. The most constant of these is
    1. congenitally missing teeth
    2. Hutchinson's incisors
    3. relatively short mandibular first molar roots
    4. mulberry-shaped molars

71. Hypercementosis may be associated with
    1. acromegaly and Paget's disease
    2. osteogenic sarcoma
    3. histiocytosis X diseases
    4. von Recklinghausen's disease of bone

72. A 29-year-old female was hospitalized with complaints of coldness of the hands and ulceration of two of her fingers which had failed to heal. She was referred to the Dental Department for consultation. Her facial skin was observed to be taut and dry. A complete mouth radiographic survey demonstrated unusually wide periodontal ligament spaces throughout the dentition. These findings are most consistent with a diagnosis of
    1. fibrous dysplasia
    2. the Plummer–Vinson syndrome
    3. scleroderma
    4. Sjögren's syndrome

73. Crepitus (a crackling sound) elicited on palpation would be of greatest assistance in diagnosis of
    1. ankylosis of the temporomandibular joint
    2. a fracture of the mandible
    3. Paget's disease of bone
    4. von Recklinghausen's disease

74. A swishing or hissing sound detected at the initial opening and end of closing movements of the mandible is a finding most often associated with
    1. ankylosis of the temporomandibular joint
    2. hypoplasia of the condyles
    3. occlusal discrepancies
    4. osteoarthritis involving the temporomandibular joint

75. Solitary ulcerations of the oral mucosa are most often the result of
    1. chemical burns
    2. intake of excessively hot liquids or foods
    3. trauma
    4. radiation therapy

76. Oral ulcers which are characteristically painless are those associated with
    1. trauma
    2. tuberculosis
    3. primary herpes
    4. primary syphilis

77. Oral ulcerations which heal with clinical evidence of scarring are known to be associated with
    1. chemical burns, e.g., an aspirin burn
    2. herpangina
    3. periadenitis mucosa necrotica recurrens
    4. trauma

78. Match the condition listed in the right-hand column with the abnormal deviation in vital sign with which it may be associated.

    (a) tachycardia            1. diabetes mellitus
    (b) hypertension           2. primary herpetic
                                  gingivostomatitis
    (c) erratic respira-       3. hyperventilation
        tory rate
    (d) elevation of tem-      4. hyperthyroidism
        perature

79. Match the condition listed in the right-hand column with the abnormal deviation in vital sign with which it may be associated.

    (a) bradycardia            1. anxiety and/or
                                  syncope
    (b) hypotension            2. emphysema
    (c) dyspnea                3. myxedema
    (d) subnormal tem-         4. well-trained
        perature                  athlete

80. A 20-year-old male who was an outstanding athlete had an essentially negative physical evaluation except for a systolic blood pressure reading of 92. It is most likely that this latter finding is due to
    1. early cardiovascular disease
    2. apprehension
    3. an undiagnosed diabetic condition
    4. lack of a reliable history

81. A pronounced elevation of temperature is a major diagnostic feature of all except
    1. herpangina
    2. Ludwig's angina
    3. primary herpes
    4. recurrent aphthous ulcers

82. A subnormal temperature is common to all except
    1. angioneurotic edema
    2. aniline intoxication
    3. myxedema
    4. syncope

83. The most common condition encountered in dental practice in which a subnormal temperature is invariably found is
    1. aniline intoxication
    2. cretinism

3. myxedema
4. syncope

## Symptoms of Abnormality

Symptoms of abnormality are patients' reports of conditions. The diagnosticians should consider the following general symptoms:

1. bleeding
2. unusual color
3. unusual, or a change in, consistency
4. limited, or a change in, function
5. excessive, or a change in, mobility
6. pain or discomfort
7. unusual sounds
8. loss of, or unusual, sensation, e.g., paresthesia
9. a change in shape, e.g., swelling
10. loss of, or an unusual, taste sensation
11. xerostomia (dry mouth)

QUESTIONS

84. The most common complaint of gingival bleeding upon tooth brushing is the result of
    1. diabetes mellitus
    2. monocytic leukemia
    3. local irritating factors
    4. a vitamin C deficiency

85. A 20-year-old female complained of recent spontaneous gingival bleeding and "sore, tender gums." She reported that she had ceased any effort regarding oral hygiene because of this. Clinical examination revealed a white slough of the marginal gingiva throughout the mouth, and a fetid breath odor was obvious. There were no other remarkable findings. The most likely diagnosis of the patient's gingival bleeding is
    1. diabetic gingivitis
    2. leukemic gingivitis
    3. acute necrotizing ulcerative gingivitis
    4. marginal gingivitis

86. An 18-year-old male reported recent spontaneous gingival bleeding. Multiple petechiae were apparent on clinical examination of the oral mucosa. Local irritating factors seemed to be absent. Possible etiologies of the patient's gingival bleeding include all the following except
    1. drugs
    2. exposure to chemicals
    3. hemophilia
    4. leukemia

87. A 42-year-old female complained of "streaks of" blue and grayish black discoloration of the floor of the mouth, buccal mucosa, and palate. She reported a sudden appearance of these discolorations 2 days previously. Further questioning revealed that her physician had "taken her off cortisone for arthritis." These findings suggest that the reason for the patient's oral pigmentation is probably

1. hypoadrenalism
2. hypoparathyroidism
3. hypopituitarism
4. hypothyroidism

88. A 19-year-old male complained of a "soft piece of skin growing out of my tooth." Clinical examination revealed severe carious destruction of the maxillary left first molar with what appeared to be granulation tissue extending from the exposed pulp chamber. The correct diagnosis with these findings is
    1. acute pulpitis
    2. chronic suppurative pulpitis
    3. chronic open hyperplastic pulpitis
    4. an irritation fibroma involving the pulp

89. Patients that have been taking prescribed antihistamines (e.g., amphetamine sulfate [Benzedrine]), ataractics, (e.g., chlordiazepoxide hydrochloride [Librium]) or muscle relaxants (e.g., methocarbamol [Robaxin]) are most apt to report
    1. spontaneous gingival bleeding
    2. gingival swelling
    3. delayed healing following a recent extraction
    4. xerostomia

90. A 23-year-old female complained of bilateral stiffness and soreness in the area of the temporomandibular joint. Symptoms had occurred daily for the past week and were most pronounced on awakening in the morning but always diminished and disappeared during the day. History and physical findings were unremarkable. The most likely cause of the patient's problem is
    1. fibrous ankylosis of the temporomandibular joint
    2. nocturnal bruxism
    3. sudden development of a malocclusion
    4. early osteoarthritis

91. The primary complaints of a 19-year-old male were pain, mild trismus, and inefficiency in mastication which he believed to be due to an erupting mandibular third molar. Further questioning disclosed frequent headaches and some loss of hearing on the affected side. Clinical examination revealed congenital absence of third molars and no tooth or soft tissue pathology. Restricted movement of the soft palate was noted. These findings suggest prompt medical consultation because they are characteristic of
    1. Meniere's disease
    2. the Plummer–Vinson syndrome
    3. a tumor of the nasopharynx as a cause of Trotter's syndrome
    4. a psychogenic disturbance

92. A 28-year-old male complained of a right-side unilateral facial paralysis. Examination also revealed inability to wink the right eye and excessive lacrimation. He reported that the symptoms appeared quite suddenly 2 days ago on awakening. These are characteristic signs of
    1. angioedema
    2. the auriculotemporal syndrome

3. Bell's palsy
4. trigeminal neuralgia

93. The form of lichen planus which is most often responsible for symptoms of pain is the
    1. atrophic
    2. erosive
    3. keratotic
    4. vesiculobullous

94. A 50-year-old male complained of a "sore mouth" of 3 days duration. He had been on a prolonged course of penicillin prescribed by his physician. Clinical examination revealed ill-defined white areas on the buccal mucosa and soft palate. When these areas were wiped firmly with a gauze sponge, a raw, red, bleeding, tender surface was exposed. These findings are most consistent with a diagnosis of
    1. an idiosyncrasy
    2. candidiasis
    3. secondary syphilis
    4. a toxic reaction to penicillin

95. A 19-year-old male complained of pain and tenderness upon mastication in the area of an erupting mandibular third molar. He had been applying aspirin tablets to the area. The result of this was manifested clinically by a white excoriation of tissue overlying the erupting tooth. This type of chemical insult to the tissue is most accurately described as
    1. an allergic reaction
    2. a factitial injury
    3. an idiosyncrasy
    4. a toxic reaction

96. Periodontal abscesses, alveolar osteites following tooth extraction, and acute alveolar abscesses are most apt to develop without apparent cause in a patient with
    1. Albers–Schönberg disease
    2. diabetes mellitus
    3. Hand–Schüller–Christian disease
    4. Letterer–Siwe's disease

97. Bacterial invasion of the pulp as a result of caries is the most common general cause of pulpitis. The least common general cause is
    1. chemical irritation
    2. anachoresis or blood transmission of bacteria to the pulp
    3. thermal irritation
    4. trauma

98. A 20-year-old female complained of a severe "toothache" which she reported had kept her awake for the past two nights. Clinical examination revealed caries involving a mandibular bicuspid which was markedly sensitive to slight percussion. A radiograph disclosed no periapical radiolucency. These findings are sufficient to make a diagnosis of
    1. acute suppurative pulpitis
    2. acute pulpal hyperemia
    3. irreversible pulpal change with progression towards development of an alveolar abscess
    4. partial pulpitis

99. A 19-year-old male patient complained of a severe "toothache" involving a maxillary lateral incisor. The tooth was noncarious, but a deep cingulum pit was detected upon exploration. Radiographs demonstrated a pronounced periapical radiolucency and what appeared to be an extension of enamel into the middle third of the pulp canal. These findings are most characteristic of

1. concrescence
2. pulpal death as a result of a dens in dente
3. pulpal death as a result of denticle formation
4. pulpal death as a result of anachoresis

100. A 20-year-old male required postoperative care subsequent to extraction of a mandibular third molar 5 days ago. He reported onset of a dull, persistent pain in the area "yesterday" which was becoming increasingly severe. Clinical examination revealed exposed bone in the alveolus and a fetid breath odor. Treatment of this alveolar osteitis is

1. based on the assumption that the patient dislodged the clot
2. based on the assumption that the vasoconstrictor in the anesthetic solution prevented clot formation
3. of necessity empirical since no single cause of "dry socket" has yet been determined
4. based on the assumption that preexisting infection has prevented healing

101. A 43-year-old female complained of a dull persistent radiating pain in the site of her last extraction 3 years ago. She was now edentulous. Clinical examination of the mandibular right molar area revealed an incompletely healed extraction site from which a suppurative discharge could be expressed. A radiograph disclosed a 2 × 2 cm, ill-defined, "worm-eaten" area of bone. These findings are most compatible with a diagnosis of

1. an infected residual cyst
2. a chronic alveolar osteitis
3. chronic osteomyelitis
4. an osteogenic sarcoma

102. The most common cause of unilateral paresthesia of the lower lip is

1. impingement of an overextended denture flange upon the mental nerve
2. osteomyelitis
3. trauma to the inferior alveolar nerve in the course of extraction of a mandibular third molar
4. a tumor of the fifth nerve

103. A 28-year-old male patient complained of hyperesthetic sensations resulting from inadvertent biting of a small nodular swelling on the lower lip. Examination revealed a very firm, white, 0.5 × 0.5 mm, elevated growth on the lower lip in the area of the mandibular left lateral incisor. The patient reported first noticing the lesions about 2 months ago, shortly after he had a slight contusion in the area. These findings most suggest the presence of

1. an irritation fibroma
2. an hemangioma
3. a mucocele
4. a neuroma

104. A 32-year-old male complained of a swelling which involved the moist mucous membrane of the lower lip in the area of the left cuspid. He reported involuntary biting of this lesion twice during the past year which had caused it to "disappear for a while." Inspection and palpation revealed a spherical, well-defined, 0.5-cm, slightly elevated lesion which had a bluish green surface discoloration. These findings are most suggestive of a

1. residual cyst
2. mucocele
3. ranula
4. traumatic neuroma

105. A 42-year-old male requested reconstruction of a maxillary full denture which was now "loose." Clinical examination revealed a red, exophytic, fissured, 3 × 1 cm, nontender lesion in the maxillary anterior vestibule. A biopsy report would be expected to confirm a strong clinical impression of

1. an epulis fissuratum
2. papillomatosis
3. a pyogenic granuloma
4. squamous cell carcinoma

106. A 25-year-old male was in acute distress with pain, elevation of temperature, and a firm, bilateral mandibular swelling. This swelling apparently elevated the tongue and caused some difficulty in swallowing and breathing. He reported that his symptoms had appeared 3 days after he had an "abscessed" lower molar tooth extracted 1 week ago. These findings indicate prompt institution of antibiotic therapy because they are characteristic of

1. an alveolar osteitis
2. Ludwig's angina
3. herpangina
4. Vincent's angina

107. A 26-year-old female complained of a loud snapping or cracking sound when she opened her mouth. She produced this unusual sound only on extended or full opening. She reported that although pain was not associated with this condition, it was often socially embarrassing. Thorough clinical examination ruled out occlusal discrepancies as a possible cause. These findings suggest

1. ankylosis of the temporomandibular joint
2. hypoplasia of the condyles
3. that the head of the condyle is rapidly passing over a prominence of the meniscus
4. rheumatoid arthritis

108. A 32-year-old male complained primarily of pain in the area of the incisive papilla and an occasional "salty taste" in the mouth. He reported trauma and pain sensations primarily when he ate toast. Examina-

tion revealed an unusually large, slightly reddened incisive papilla and a spherical radiolucency close to the alveolar crest between the maxillary incisors. These findings are most characteristic of a

1. globulomaxillary cyst
2. median cyst
3. nasoalveolar cyst
4. nasopalatine cyst

109. The complaint of a metallic taste reported by dental patients is most frequently associated with
1. acute necrotizing ulcerative gingivitis
2. bismuthosis
3. galvanism
4. mercurialism

# METHODOLOGY

The diagnostic procedure essentially involves an information gathering process followed by an analysis of the findings. History taking and a physical examination constitute the primary methods of information gathering. Clinical findings may indicate the need for additional tests, such as microscopic examination of biopsied tissue, and the results of these often provide the most significant finding in establishing a diagnosis.

### QUESTIONS

110. The most important procedure in diagnosis is
1. elicitation of the chief complaint
2. conduct of a thorough examination
3. development of the case history
4. proper interpretation of radiographic findings

111. The primary purpose in obtaining an accurate history is to
1. determine how healthy the patient may be
2. uncover an undiagnosed systemic condition
3. provide a basis for determining how the patient's physical status may be affected by dental therapy
4. assist the physician in management of a medical problem

112. Correct diagnosis in which the examination findings play the major role are most often the result of
1. brilliance on the part of the examiner
2. a complete and thorough examination
3. skill in examination technique
4. perception of a particular finding as being abnormal

113. The significance of a positive examination finding is that it may
1. corroborate the history
2. be present in the absence of symptoms
3. be the first manifestation of an abnormal condition
4. All of the above

## Clinical Methods

General categories of information necessary to the development of a complete history include the

1. vital statistics
2. chief complaint
3. history of present illness
4. past medical history
5. family history
6. occupational history
7. personal and social histories
8. review of systems

### QUESTIONS

114. A patient with Letterer–Siwe's disease is not apt to consult a dentist because
1. the primary symptoms relate to skeletal bone destruction
2. the head and neck are never involved
3. this condition rarely occurs after the age of 2 years
4. this condition invariably runs a rapid and fatal course

115. Most commonly associated with trigeminal neuralgia is
1. a tumor of the fifth cranial nerve
2. involvement of the left side of the face
3. its occurrence after the age of 30
4. that attacks are separated by longer time intervals as the condition progresses

116. It is most rare for a male patient to have
1. acute necrotizing ulcerative gingivitis
2. chronic desquamative gingivitis
3. chronic gingivitis
4. periodontitis

117. Female patients are known to be far more predisposed to develop
1. dental caries
2. periapical cementifying fibromas (cementomas)
3. periapical abscesses
4. periodontitis

118. Ethnic background is a known predisposing factor in
1. hemophilia
2. iron deficiency anemia
3. pernicious anemia
4. thalassemia

119. In the elicitation of the chief complaint and throughout the history-taking procedure, it is most important for the examiner to
1. appear to be concerned
2. direct the questioning
3. be unhurried
4. be seated

120. The chief complaint should be recorded initially by a notation

*(Continued)*

1. concerning its mode of development
2. as to when the symptoms were first noticed
3. of it in the patient's own words
4. of any previous treatment of the symptoms

121. By far the most common (and often difficult to evaluate) chief complaint of the dental patient is
    1. glossodynia
    2. inability to wear their dentures
    3. inefficiency in mastication
    4. odontalgia

122. A 20-year-old female complained of a severe "toothache." She had been unable to sleep for the past two nights and had applied ice cubes to allay the pain. The mandibular left first molar was severely involved with caries and markedly sensitive to percussion. These are cardinal findings characteristic of
    1. acute pulpal hyperemia
    2. a developing periapical granuloma
    3. irreversible pulpal change
    4. mild periodontitis

123. Complaints of occasional sporadic sensitivity of a tooth to cold alone are most characteristic of
    1. irreversible pulpal change
    2. pulpal hyperemia
    3. an occlusal discrepancy
    4. a suppurative pulpitis

124. The chief complaint is best analyzed by obtaining a detailed history of the present illness. These details include all except
    1. the approximate date or time of onset of symptoms
    2. inciting factors and mode of development of symptoms
    3. a familial history of the condition
    4. any professional or attempted self-treatment

## Past Medical History

Significant elements of a past medical history which may be of assistance in oral diagnosis may include

1. allergies, particularly to medications
2. serious illnesses and/or hospitalizations
3. medications prescribed
4. blood transfusions

### QUESTIONS

125. A 20-year-old male developed urticaria approximately 8 days subsequent to parenteral administration of penicillin for a nose infection a year ago. This history is exceedingly important and should be made special note of because
    1. it indicates that the patient has a drug idiosyncrasy
    2. the patient may have received a toxic dose
    3. it suggests that a sensitizing dose was received and that an anaphylactic reaction could follow administration of penicillin in any form or by any other route

4. penicillin is the antibiotic of choice in treatment of the vast majority of oral infections

126. An asymptomatic red tongue lesion was detected in the course of initial examination of a 43-year-old female patient. The level of suspicion that this lesion might be a squamous cell carcinoma would be most increased with a past medical history of the
    1. auriculotemporal syndrome
    2. Papillon–Lefèvre syndrome
    3. Pierre Robin syndrome
    4. Plummer–Vinson syndrome

127. It is most important to limit treatment of the pregnant woman to emergency procedures only
    1. during the first trimester
    2. if there is a history of spontaneous abortion
    3. during the third trimester
    4. during the morning

128. A 28-year-old female brought her 5-year-old son for initial examination. The history provided by the mother included a report of rubella (German measles) during pregnancy. The condition most certain to be manifested in the child's dentition is
    1. dentinogenesis imperfecta
    2. moderate to severe enamel hypoplasia
    3. shell teeth
    4. taurodontism

129. A 45-year-old female reported a family history of a bleeding tendency and that her father was a hemophiliac. A week later, upon examination of a relative, indications were found for the extraction of two teeth. One would be most concerned and seek medical consultation prior to performing these extractions if this patient was the woman's
    1. brother
    2. mother
    3. sister
    4. son

130. Bakers, cooks, and food handlers most likely to develop
    1. gingival pigmentation
    2. rampant caries
    3. severe abrasion of teeth
    4. vague dental pain

131. Plumbism is a condition most commonly found in a patient whose occupation is that of
    1. mill worker
    2. painter
    3. plumber
    4. poultry farmer

132. The level of suspicion that a lesion might be a squamous cell carcinoma of the floor of the oral cavity would be most increased with a history of
    1. high alcoholic beverage consumption and syphilis
    2. syphilis and excessive smoking
    3. high alcoholic beverage consumption and excessive tobacco use
    4. diabetes and high alcoholic beverage consumption

133. Symptoms which suggest the presence of cardiovascular disease include all except
    1. ankle edema
    2. dyspnea on exertion
    3. jaundice of the eyes
    4. substernal chest pain

134. A history of frequent counseling for emotional problems is most often associated with all except
    1. acute necrotizing ulcerative gingivitis
    2. aphthous ulcers
    3. gingival pigmentation
    4. glossodynia and glossopyrosis

135. By far the greatest amount of diagnostic information is obtained by means of two of the four general classical methods of physical diagnosis. These two methods are
    1. inspection and palpation
    2. inspection and percussion
    3. palpation and percussion
    4. palpation and auscultation

136. Inspection of the patient's hands may provide clues to the diagnosis. Match the finding listed in the right-hand column with the condition with which it may be associated.
    (a) neurofibromatosis     1. bullae
    (b) Parkinson's disease    2. nodules
    (c) pemphigus              3. pigmentaion
    (d) Addison's disease      4. tremor

137. Match the sign listed in the right-hand column with the condition of the eyes with which it may be associated.
    (a) Bell's palsy           1. exophthalmos
    (b) Grave's disease        2. blue sclerae
    (c) congenital syphilis    3. inability to wink
    (d) osteogenesis           4. interstitial keratitis
        imperfecta

138. A 43-year-old male had a fistulating swelling of the left side of the neck. He reported intermittent fever and night sweats for the past month. He also reported that a mandibular left molar had been extracted 6 months ago. Firm palpation of the swelling revealed small yellow flecks in an exudate arising from the fistula. These findings are most suggestive of a
    1. cellulitis
    2. syphilitic lesion
    3. lesion of actinomycosis
    4. tuberculous lesion

139. At the present time the key to reducing the mortality rate as a result of oral malignancy is considered
    1. public education in the dangers of smoking and high alcoholic beverage consumption
    2. early detection
    3. the discovery of more effective chemotherapeutic agents
    4. improvement in surgical technique(s)

140. A 44-year-old male presented with a fractured lingual cusp of the maxillary left first bicuspid. Inspection revealed that the fracture was of the shearing type and that the tooth had apparently never been restored. The patient reported no history of severe trauma and that he had "broken it biting on a piece of bread." This common finding in mature patients is due to
    1. ankylosis and dentinal sclerosis of teeth
    2. development of a bruxing habit
    3. changes in the occlusion as a result of interproximal wear and increased brittleness of teeth
    4. dentinal sclerosis and pulpal calcification

141. A diagnosis of acute suppurative pulpitis can only be made by
    1. analysis of symptoms
    2. finding pus on opening into the pulp chamber(s)
    3. radiographic examination
    4. subjecting the tooth to thermal, electric, and percussive stimuli

142. Radiographic examination, which is an integral part of the examination of the dental patient, is essentially examination by means of
    1. auscultation
    2. inspection
    3. palpation
    4. percussion

143. In the right-hand column are listed the primary factors governing the diagnostic quality of the radiograph. Match them with the item which has the greatest influence on their production.
    (a) kilovoltage            1. density
    (b) incorrect              2. contrast
        angulation
    (c) exposure time          3. definition
    (d) object-film            4. distortion
        distance

144. Radiographs of patients with heavy, dense bone are apt to be insufficiently dense for diagnostic purposes. In order to produce radiographs of sufficient density for these patients, and at the same time minimize patient exposure, it is most desirable to
    1. increase the exposure time
    2. employ a high kilovoltage
    3. employ a long cone paralleling technique
    4. process the film for a longer period of time

145. If a radiograph possesses either excessive or insufficient density, it will also primarily
    1. present "blurred" images
    2. lack sufficient contrast quality for diagnosis
    3. require further fixing
    4. present marked distortion of images

146. In order to produce a radiograph of long gray scale contrast quality, it is necessary to
    1. decrease the exposure time
    2. employ a kilovoltage of 70 or greater
    3. employ a kilovoltage of less than 70
    4. employ a paralleling technique

147. Readability of radiographs produced by means of

(Continued)

high kilovoltage (70 or above) techniques is most enhanced by
1. maximum collimation
2. proper filtration
3. use of a long rather than a short cone
4. elimination of all incident light

148. A low (below 70) kilovoltage technique is most advantageous in demonstrating
1. alveolar crestal bone resorption
2. early or small carious lesions
3. periapical lesions
4. a retained root

149. Greater object–film distances are required in a paralleling technique than in a bisecting technique. As a result, the use of a long cone is indicated in order to
1. reduce exposure time
2. produce a radiograph of long gray scale contrast quality
3. minimize distortion
4. prevent loss of definition and/or detail

150. Definition and detail are terms which are often used synonymously. Technically, detail refers to
1. image density
2. lack of image distortion
3. reproduction of very small objects
4. image sharpness

151. Production and use of faster film has been a major factor in reducing patient exposure. However, the fastest film manufactured has not been used routinely by clinicians because
1. a long gray scale contrast cannot be obtained
2. the image(s) are often distorted
3. images appear granular and lack definition
4. it requires more careful processing

152. A major advantage of the periapical radiograph as compared with a pantomograph is that
1. distortion is totally absent
2. greater image sharpness can be obtained
3. it is quicker and easier to produce
4. landmarks are never superimposed

153. Marked elongation because the vertical angulation was insufficient is most apt to result in
1. burn-out of structures of minimum density
2. misinterpretation of alveolar crestal bone height as being less than it actually is
3. misinterpretation of alveolar crestal bone height as being greater than it actually is
4. production of tooth images which suggest very short root length

154. Marked foreshortening because the vertical angulation was excessive is most apt to result in
1. misinterpretation of alveolar crestal bone height as being greater than it actually is
2. burn-out of structures of maximum density
3. an appearance of osteoporosis of the trabecular pattern
4. misinterpretation of an abscess or granuloma

155. A paralleling technique produces a radiograph of greater diagnostic value than a bisecting technique does for all of the following reasons except one. Which one?
1. A more accurate anatomic relationship of structures is demonstrated.
2. Distortion of images is minimized.
3. Problems in film placement are reduced.
4. Superimposition of landmarks is less likely.

156. Excessive film fog which impairs the diagnostic quality of the radiograph is most often the result of
1. an inherent quality of the film
2. improper, too rapid processing at an excessively high temperature
3. employment of insufficient exposure time
4. improper storage of film prior and subsequent to exposure

157. Burn-out is a most significant factor in diagnosis of
1. the presence of an abscess, granuloma, or cyst
2. early small interproximal caries and integrity of the alveolar crest
3. carious exposure of the pulp
4. the presence or absence of a retained root

158. Aids in the differentiation of radiographic landmarks which are atypical in size, location, and/or shape from abnormal conditions include all except
1. the production of another radiograph at a markedly altered angulation
2. comparing the radiograph with one of the contralateral side
3. increasing the exposure time
4. employment of a paralleling technique in order to avoid superimposition

159. Panorex, Orthopantomograph, Panelipse, and Panex all
1. describe radiographic techniques involving employment of a moving source of radiation and film
2. are better techniques than the paralleling technique
3. are names of pantomographic machines
4. are names of radiographs

160. The most outstanding advantage of pantomography as compared with a periapical survey is that
1. there is greater definition of images
2. there is less image distortion
3. the anatomic scope of examination is greater
4. it is more useful in patient education

161. A pantomograph is of particular value in initial evaluation because it
1. is so easily and rapidly produced
2. demonstrates all structures with maximum definition
3. demonstrates all hard tissues of primary concern with minimum distortion
4. demonstrates all hard tissue of primary concern with a "reasonable" degree of definition and lack of distortion

162. On initial examination of a 20-year-old female, a pantomograph revealed a foreign body in the mandibular right molar region. Its configuration and the history suggested that it was a retained orthodontic wire. When attempts were made to localize it by means of the shift sketch technique, the object appeared to move distally (or posteriorly) as the area was radiographed from a 45° greater (anterior) horizontal angulation. This indicates that the object is
    1. more apical to the tooth than the pantomograph indicates
    2. buccal to the tooth
    3. in the cheek rather than in the bone
    4. lingual to the tooth

163. The most difficult and challenging technique for localization of fractures, cysts, tumors, foreign bodies, etc. to perform is production of a
    1. right angle view
    2. shift sketch
    3. sialogram
    4. stereoscopic view

164. The principal disadvantage of using a pointed cone rather than an open cone is that
    1. the primary beam cannot be adequately filtered
    2. patients are subjected to greater amounts of scatter radiation
    3. a paralleling technique cannot be used in conjunction with it
    4. the primary beam is decreased in intensity

165. Screens are commonly incorporated in extraoral film casettes primarily for the purpose of
    1. increasing the contrast quality
    2. enhancing image definition
    3. reducing distortion
    4. reducing patient radiation dosage

166. Protection of the patient from possible deleterious genetic effects of radiation is accomplished primarily by
    1. adequate collimation of the beam to a maximum of a 3-in. diameter at the skin entrance area
    2. proper filtration by addition of at least 0.5 mm aluminum
    3. draping the patient with a lead apron
    4. use of Class D film speed

167. The most frequent and definite indication for a sialogram is
    1. the presence of an acute submandibular swelling with no clue to its etiology
    2. suspected sialolithiasis
    3. the patient's complaint of a salty taste
    4. the patient's complaint of xerostomia

168. A sialogram may provide information of significance in diagnosis of Sjögren's syndrome because it may demonstrate
    1. cysts in the parotid gland
    2. characteristic reduction in end arborization of salivary acini
    3. malignant tumors of the parotid
    4. which salivary glands are involved

169. On initial examination of a 20-year-old male, palpable cervical lymph nodes were detected. The history and other physical findings were unremarkable. No oral lesions were detected. All of the following should be considered except
    1. acute leukemia
    2. angioedema
    3. infectious mononucleosis
    4. Hodgkin's disease

170. Patients who have received low level (e.g., 200–400 rad) radiation therapy to the head and/or neck should be given a most meticulous examination of the neck by means of palpation because
    1. they are known to develop Hodgkin's disease
    2. the incidence of thyroid malignancy is far greater in these patients than in the general population
    3. they are most prone to develop von Recklinghausen's disease
    4. they are predisposed to develop an osteogenic sarcoma

171. The least significant finding in palpation of the neck for nodes is
    1. their degree of firmness
    2. whether they are fixed or movable
    3. their size
    4. whether or not they are tender

172. A white, firm, slightly ulcerated lesion of the lower lip of a 55-year-old male was detected in the course of initial examination. The patient was fair-skinned and reported that he had worked out-of-doors most of his life. A sign which would raise the level of suspicion that this lesion is a squamous cell carcinoma is the presence of firm, palpable
    1. axillary nodes
    2. deep cervical nodes
    3. preauricular nodes
    4. submental nodes

173. A 1 × 1 cm, nontender, white lesion on the lateral border of the tongue was detected during initial examination of a 43-year-old female. Upon palpation, the lesion felt indurated and "bound down." This latter sensation suggests
    1. dyskeratosis
    2. hyperkeratosis
    3. infiltration of cells into the deeper tissues
    4. parakeratosis

174. A 44-year-old male complained of pain in the maxillary left quadrant. Several previous dental consultations had provided no solution, and his physician had ruled out sinusitis. Radiographs and clinical examination revealed no caries or periodontal disease, and all teeth responded within normal limits to electric and thermal tests. Careful questioning revealed that pain occurred primarily on mastication, with occasional

(Continued)

sporadic thermal sensitivity which had become increasingly severe over the course of the past 8 months. A most meticulous examination by means of exploration is indicated because these findings are commonly associated with

1. the auriculotemporal syndrome
2. the "cracked tooth" syndrome
3. the myofacial pain dysfunction syndrome
4. Trotter's syndrome

175. A tooth which is severely carious, markedly sensitive to percussion, and unresponsive to electric stimuli

1. may be reactive to cold stimuli
2. is indicated for extraction
3. may or may not possess a periapical radiolucency
4. invariably possesses a periapical radiolucency

176. Marked sensitivity of a tooth to percussion suggests that

1. a chronic alveolar abscess is present
2. a cyst has formed
3. the periodontal ligament and/or bone is already involved
4. the pulp is beginning to degenerate

177. A wheezy type of respiration is most often associated with

1. bronchial asthma
2. cardiovascular disease
3. emphysema
4. tuberculosis

178. Mediate auscultation is of greatest value in oral diagnosis in detection of

1. ankylosis of teeth
2. hypertension
3. inflammation of the periodontal ligament
4. most types of periapical pathology

179. If the percussion test with the handle of an explorer produces a clear ringing sound rather than a dull thud, the tooth is most likely to

1. be ankylosed
2. be periodontally involved
3. possess a periapical lesion
4. be a sound tooth with a viable periodontal ligament

180. The most favorable prognosis can be provided for a tooth which

1. responds within normal limits to electric stimulation
2. is sensitive to heat stimuli, but relieved by cold
3. is sensitive to percussion
4. is markedly responsive to cold only during time of application

181. A tooth which responds markedly to heat and cold only during time of application is considered to be affected by

1. an acute pulpitis
2. a chronic pulpitis
3. pulpal hyperemia
4. partial pulpitis

182. Odontalgia which is incited by heat stimulation but relieved by cold application provides evidence that the pulp

1. is acutely inflamed
2. is hyperemic
3. has undergone irreversible change
4. is beginning to necrose

183. Pain which persists following removal of thermal stimuli to a tooth is considered to be a cardinal sign of an irreversible pulpitis. However, these teeth have been successfully treated without resorting to endodontic therapy by

1. application of strontium chloride densensitizing paste
2. elimination of a high spot on a restoration, providing the tooth has been recently restored
3. treating a 5-mm pocket on the distal
4. treating a carious lesion with zinc oxide–eugenol

184. Electric pulp testing is of primary value in determining

1. the degree of pulp vitality
2. whether or not any pulp vitality remains
3. the type of pulpitis which may be present
4. whether or not pulp change may be reversible

185. A 43-year-old male was hospitalized with complaints of increasing frequency of headaches, sweating, and loss of libido. He had been taking tolbutamide (Orinase) for diabetes for the past 2 years. The patient reported increasing difficulty in mastication and incising. Photographs provided by the patient taken over the past 5 years suggested development of pronounced supraorbital ridges, enlargement of the nose and lips, and mandibular prognathism. These findings are consistent with an impression of

1. craniofacial dysostosis
2. acromegaly
3. hyperthyroidism
4. Paget's disease

186. Study models are of greatest value in

1. determining the presence of a malocclusion
2. evaluation of the extent of periodontitis
3. analyzing the forces of occlusion
4. determining whether a fixed or removable appliance is indicated

187. If a patient is suspected of being sensitive to acrylic, the test most helpful in diagnosis is the

1. heterophil antibody
2. patch
3. scratch
4. tourniquet

188. Formation of a bulla following stroking of intact skin or mucosa constitutes a positive reaction in the attempt to elicit

1. Babinski's sign
2. Chvostek's sign
3. Nikolsky's sign
4. Romberg's sign

189. Associate the condition listed in the right-hand column with the special method of examination which may assist in its diagnosis.

(a) dermatographia    1. thrombocytopenia
(b) Nikolsky's sign    2. sensitivity to denture base material
(c) patch test    3. angioedema
(d) tourniquet test    4. chronic desquamative gingivitis

190. Blood chemistry values determined by sequential multiple analyzer most often provide
1. cardinal signs of abnormality
2. information which contributes to a diagnosis
3. pathognomonic signs of disease
4. questionable information

191. Match the condition listed in the right-hand column with the abnormal deviation in blood chemistry with which it may be associated.

(a) elevated BUN (Blood Urea Nitrogen)    1. cardiovascular disease
(b) elevated cholesterol    2. diabetes
(c) elevated glucose    3. acute hepatitis
(d) elevated SGOT (Serum Glutamic Oxalacetic Transaminase)    4. renal disease

192. Match the condition listed in the right-hand column with the abnormal deviation in blood chemistry with which it may be associated.

(a) low BUN    1. Addison's disease
(b) low cholesterol    2. uncontrolled diabetes
(c) low glucose    3. epilepsy
(d) low SGOT    4. liver disease

193. Paget's disease, fibrous dysplasia, and hyperparathyroidism are most likely to provide blood chemistry findings of an elevated
1. serum calcium
2. serum calcium phosphatase
3. serum glutamic oxalacetic transaminase
4. uric acid

194. A 49-year-old male reported both a family history and symptoms suggestive of diabetes. The most reliable means of establishing a diagnosis is a
1. urinalysis
2. fasting blood sugar determination
3. glucose tolerance test
4. confirmation of the patient's history of polyuria by collection of a 24-hour urine sample

195. The glucose tolerance test is considered to indicate the presence of a mild diabetic condition when the blood sugar
1. returns to a normal value within 1 hour
2. returns to the base fasting level in 2 hours
3. reaches a peak level in 1 hour
4. is lower at the 2nd hour reading than the first

196. A 50-year-old female reported chronic thirst and frequent, vague chest and joint pain. A pantomograph demonstrated generalized osteoporosis and an elliptical 1 × 2 cm radiolucency in the body of the mandible. An elevated (greater than 13 mg/100 ml) calcium blood level would substantiate a clinical impression of
1. Albers–Schönberg disease
2. diabetes mellitus
3. hyperparathyroidism
4. rheumatoid arthritis

197. A 42-year-old female patient reported "gnawing" head pains, loss of weight, and ready fatigability over the course of the past 6 months. A pantomograph demonstrated multiple multilocular radiolucencies. Blood chemistry tests revealed high serum calcium, low serum phosphates, and a serum alkaline phosphatase within the range of normalcy. These findings are most compatible with a clinical impression of
1. Addison's disease
2. hyperparathyroidism
3. hypoparathyroidism
4. multiple myeloma

198. A 65-year-old male complained that his maxillary denture had become "tight" and no longer "fit." A pantomograph demonstrated an aberrant trabecular pattern suggestive of a cotton wool appearance. Laboratory studies revealing an elevated serum alkaline phosphatase and calcium and phosphate levels within the range of normalcy would substantiate the clinical impression of
1. Albers–Schönberg disease
2. hyperparathyroidism
3. Paget's disease
4. von Recklinghausen's disease of bone

199. Blood studies were requested for a 20-year-old female because the clinical findings suggested a possible bleeding tendency. The laboratory report included:

Hematocrit: 45%
WBC: 6240/ml
Platelets: 275,000
Differential: Segs: 64%   Monos: 3
             Bands: 2   Eos: 2
             Lymph: 28   Bas: 1

These findings suggest
1. acute infection
2. anemia
3. lymphocytic leukemia
4. no disease process since all of the findings are within the range of normalcy

200. The primary laboratory finding associated with agranulocytosis is a
1. decrease in white cell count
2. decrease in platelets
3. decrease in red cell count
4. increase in white cell count

201. Ninety-five percent of all disorders of hemostasis are detectable by means of

(Continued)

1. bleeding time determination
2. platelet count
3. both bleeding time determination and platelet count
4. prothrombin time determination

202. A clotting time within the range of normalcy, abnormal clot retraction, and prolonged bleeding time are associated with
   1. hemophilia A
   2. scurvy
   3. thrombocytopenia
   4. von Willebrand's disease

203. Prolonged clotting time is a manifestation of all the following except
   1. a fibrinogen deficiency
   2. hemophilia A
   3. Hageman (Factor XII) deficiency
   4. scurvy

204. A platelet deficiency is associated with all the following except
   1. acute myelogenous leukemia
   2. aplastic anemia
   3. hereditary hemorrhagic telangiectasia
   4. idiopathic thrombocytopenic purpura

205. Partial thromboplastin time (PTT) and prothrombin time (PT) tests will detect 95% of all coagulation disorders. A factor deficiency identification test (FDIT) is indicated when
   1. the PT is abnormal
   2. both the PT and PTT yield abnormal results
   3. the PTT is abnormal
   4. the PT and PTT yield normal results

206. A 37-year-old female reported spontaneous gingival bleeding of 3 months' duration. A platelet count disclosed 20,000/ml. The test result which would be expected to be within the range of normalcy is the
   1. bleeding time
   2. capillary fragility
   3. clot retraction
   4. prothrombin time

207. A vitamin K deficiency is indicated by
   1. an FDIT
   2. a low platelet count
   3. an increased PT
   4. a decreased PT

208. A 23-year-old student whose classmate was hospitalized 2 weeks ago with infectious mononucleosis complained of fatigue, headaches, and chills. Petechiae were clinically observable on the soft palate. If this patient had contracted the disease, a peripheral blood smear would likely demonstrate
   1. an increase in abnormal mononuclear cells
   2. an absence of lymphocytes
   3. hypochromic red cells
   4. macrocytic red cells

209. A diagnosis of infectious mononucleosis is most firmly established by a blood examination finding of
   1. abnormal mononuclear cells
   2. a high agglutination titer
   3. a white cell count of 10,000
   4. lymphocytosis

210. A definitive diagnosis of any periapical pathology is possible only by
   1. thorough and proper analysis of all clinical findings
   2. electric pulp testing
   3. microscopic examinationof a biopsy specimen
   4. a proper interpretation of radiographic findings

211. A firm, white, 2 × 2 cm white lesion involving the buccal mucosa of a 55-year-old male was biopsied. In this incisional biopsy a small piece of normal-appearing tissue was included in the specimen. Although the report was negative, a strong clinical suspicion of malignancy remained in the mind of the examiner because of the history and clinical appearance of the lesion. The examiner's next step should be to
   1. accept the report
   2. obtain an exfoliative cytology specimen
   3. perform another biopsy, preferably total excision
   4. request reexamination of the tissue

212. A white, keratotic, 2 × 3 cm lesion involving the buccal mucosa of a 55-year-old male was biopsied. A report of cellular change confirming the strong clinical suspicion of leukoplakia would include
   1. acanthosis
   2. dyskeratosis
   3. hyperkeratosis
   4. parakeratosis

213. A white lesion involving the buccal mucosa of a 62-year-old male was biopsied. A diagnosis of carcinoma-in-situ was reported. This condition is synonomous with
   1. Bowen's disease
   2. Fordyce's disease
   3. Grave's disease
   4. Pott's disease

214 A diagnosis of multiple myeloma is most accurately established by means of
   1. the history, because the symptomatology is always the same
   2. histopathologic examination of a lesion
   3. radiographic findings of typical, discrete radiolucencies in the mandible
   4. a urinalysis, since Bence Jones protein is invariably found

215. Exfoliative cytology has proved to be a most valuable aid in diagnosis of
   1. infections such as actinomycosis
   2. osteogenic sarcoma
   3. cancer of the uterine cervix
   4. verrucous lesions of the oral cavity

216. In obtaining an exfoliative cytology sample, it is most important to

1. use a tongue blade
2. properly stain the smear
3. remove the surface of suspicious hyperkeratotic lesions in order to sample the deeper layers
4. request examination by fluorescent microscopy

217. Incorporation of blood, debris, and necrotic tissue in an exfoliative cytology sample is most apt to
1. lead to a false-positive result and/or report
2. render staining impossible
3. obscure the cytologic picture for the examiner and lead to a false-negative result and/or report
4. require a longer time for examination

218. Although it is valuable as a screening test, a positive reaction to a Venereal Disease Research Laboratory (VDRL) test should be confirmed by a
1. Kahn test
2. Mazzini test
3. Fluorescent *Treponema* antibody (FTA) test
4. Wasserman

219. A 35-year-old male reported that he had been treated for syphilis 5 years ago. A positive result was returned following a request for a routine VDRL serology test. This finding could be
1. a false-positive result
2. present although the patient was adequately treated
3. evidence of reinfection
4. All of the above

220. Specific immunologic tests for syphilis include all the following except
1. an FTA
2. a *Treponema pallidum* immobilization (TPI)
3. Reiter protein complement fixation (RPCF)
4. a VDRL

221. A false-positive result of a serologic test would most likely occur in a patient that had
1. infectious mononucleosis
2. a maculopapular skin rash
3. oral mucous patches
4. a perforation of the palate

222. An elevated IgA would suggest the possibility of an increased response to oral antigen stimulation in
1. aphthous stomatitis
2. desquamative gingivitis
3. benign mucous membrane pemphigoid
4. periodontal disease

223. Hepatitis B can be diagnosed during the acute phase by demonstrating
1. a reduction of surface antigen by administration of γ-globulin
2. an increase of surface antigen ($HB_sAg$)
3. the presence of hepatitis B surface antigen
4. a rising antibody titer against the antigen

224. The immunologic test of greatest value in diagnosis of benign mucous membrane pemphigoid is the

1 complement fixation
2. hemagglutination
3. immunofluorescence
4. immune precipitation

225. Prescribing penicillin for control of dental caries is not recommended for all of the following reasons except that
1. it is known to be ineffective
2. mycotic infections of the oral cavity may ensue
3. resistant stains of organisms may develop
4. superinfections may result because of a change in oral flora

226. Caries activity and/or susceptibility tests in general
1. determine which teeth are involved
2. most often determine what is clinically evident
3. determine the number and extent of caries
4. are useful in determining the type of restoration indicated

227. The lactobacillus test for caries activity is a test which
1. determines the buffering capacity of the saliva
2. involves calorimetry
3. estimates the number or percentage of a bacterial population
4. determines the rate of enzymatic activity

228. The rationale for employing a culture technique in endodontic therapy is based upon the
1. need to determine the antibiotic of choice
2. need for determining which organism may be present
3. demonstrated higher percentage of clinical success when a culture technique is used
4. need for sterilizing the canal(s) prior to filling

229. In a case of suspected actinomycosis, a laboratory culture technique is indicated in order to determine the presence of
1. granulomatous tissue
2. actinomyces which constitute sulfur granules
3. sulfur granules themselves
4. pus

230. Antibiotic sensitivity testing is of greatest assistance in
1. diagnosis of actinomycosis
2. treatment of acute necrotizing ulcerative gingivitis
3. endodontic therapy
4. rational management of oral suppurative lesions

231. Phase contrast microscopic examination of a smear taken from the oral cavity is of assistance in determining the
1. morphology and/or motility of organisms present
2. number of organisms present
3. specific organisms present
4. viability of organisms present

232. A routine urinalysis may determine all of the following except
1. the specific amount of glucose present
2. that the patient is diabetic

(*Continued*)

3. the presence of bacteria
4. the presence of glucose

233. Paper strip reagents are useful in determining all of the following except
    1. the presence of albumin and protein
    2. the presence of blood
    3. dysfunctional disorders of the bladder and kidney
    4. the pH

## ANALYSIS

Diagnosis involves complex thought processes. Common difficulties may be overcome, at least in great measure, by recognizing that

1. pathognomonic signs and/or symptoms are a rarity
2. most often two or more characteristics of an abnormality contribute to a diagnosis
3. the range of normalcy is great
4. a particular finding often assumes greater or lesser significance when collated with other findings
5. not only may similar findings appear in different conditions, but markedly different findings may be present in the same condition, largely depending on its stage of development

Correct diagnoses can only be made on the basis of an analysis of *all* findings. An attempt to make a diagnosis by telephone without an adequate history and opportunity to perform an examination is particularly hazardous. For the same reason, many diagnoses made on the basis of clinical findings alone must be recognized as clinical "impressions."

### QUESTIONS

234. In the right hand-column are listed cardinal signs of some abnormalities. Match them with the description of the lesion which is characteristic of the condition with which it is associated.

    (a) bluish-white specks surrounded by a red halo, located on the buccal mucosa

    1. Bitot's spot (a characteristic finding in vitamin A deficiency)

    (b) a large, brilliant red spot on the skin of the trunk

    2. Fordyce's spots (pathognomonic of the presence of ectopic sebaceous glands)

    (c) a shiny, gray, triangular spot on the cornea

    3. Herald's spot (a cardinal finding in pityriasis rosea)

    (d) minute yellow granules located on the lip

    4. Koplik's spots (pathognomonic of rubeola)

235. Conditions in which a reduced or subnormal stature is a characteristic finding include all the following except
    1. achondroplasia
    2. acromegaly
    3. hereditary ectodermal dysplasia
    4. juvenile diabetes

236. In the right-hand column are listed signs of abnormality relative to the shape of the head and facial features. Match them with the condition with which it is associated.

    (a) congenital syphilis

    1. a pronounced beak-shaped nose

    (b) the Hallermann-Streuff syndrome

    2. depressed cheek bones, downward sloping palpebral fissures, and deformed pinnae (ears)

    (c) sickle cell anemia

    3. a saddle-shaped nose

    (d) Treacher Collins syndrome

    4. a tower-shaped skull

237. A smooth, slightly elevated area on the skin, which may be either pale or red compared with the surrounding tissue, is characteristic of all the following except
    1. the typical appearance of a wheal
    2. a lesion which invariably produces the symptom of itching
    3. the typical lesion of urticaria
    4. the most common clinical evidence of sensitivity

238. Dryness of the skin is common to all the following except
    1. ectodermal dysplasia
    2. hyperthyroidism
    3. hypothyroidism
    4. senile keratosis

239. The most common clinical dermatologic manifestation of an allergy is
    1. bullae formation
    2. formation of petechiae
    3. urticaria
    4. vesicle formation

240. Silver poisoning is exceedingly rare today, largely because the production and prescription of medications containing the metal has been discontinued. The most prominent clinical sign of argyria is
    1. facial dermatitis
    2. a marked bluish skin coloration, particularly of those portions exposed to sunlight
    3. keratosis of the facial skin
    4. a distinctive pigmentation of the attached gingiva

241. The most pronounced sign of von Recklinghausen's disease of the skin is
    1. the presence of numerous facial angiomas
    2. bulla formation
    3. a positive Nikolsky's sign

4. the presence of numerous nodular swellings on the skin of the face and neck

242. Raynaud's disease or syndrome frequently precedes, or is found in association with, scleroderma. Common findings in this condition include all the following except
   1. brittle fingernails
   2. trophic changes in the skin
   3. excessively moist skin
   4. ulceration of the digits and extremities

243. Presence of Heberden's nodes (as indicated by swelling of the terminal finger joints) is most characteristic of
   1. Albright's syndrome
   2. fibrous dysplasia
   3. osteoarthritis
   4. rheumatoid arthritis

244. The Argyll Robertson pupil, characteristic of neurosyphilis, refers to
   1. inflammation of the cornea
   2. lack of reactivity of the iris to light
   3. photophobia
   4. discoloration of the sclerae

245. Clinical signs of neuropathy are listed in the right-hand column. Match them with the nerve involved.

   (a) V-trigeminal    1. inability to wrinkle the nose
   (b) VII-facial    2. loss of taste sensation in the posterior ⅓ of the tongue
   (c) IX-glossopharyngeal    3. deviation of the mandible on opening
   (d) XII-hypoglossal    4. deviation of the tongue on protrusion

246. Pronounced microcheilia and micrognathia, which make dental therapy technically challenging, is most common to
   1. Crouzon's disease (craniofacial dysostosis)
   2. the Pierre Robin syndrome
   3. Sainton's disease (cleidocranial dysostosis)
   4. the Sturge–Weber syndrome

247. An oral examination of a 16-year-old male patient revealed hemangiomatous colorations involving the buccal mucosa, gingiva, and palate. Similar port wine marks were apparent on the left side of the face in areas supplied by the trigeminal nerve. These findings are most often associated with
   1. Albright's syndrome
   2. Gardner's syndrome
   3. Kaposi's syndrome
   4. the Sturge–Weber syndrome

248. Clinically the most definitive indication of the presence of Vincent's infection (also termed trench mouth, fusospirochetosis, and ANUG) is
   1. a history of spontaneous gingival bleeding
   2. a fetid breath odor

3. marginal gingivitis
4. necrosis of interdental papillae

249. Following self-application of aspirin to the oral soft tissues, the most common clinical sign observed is evidence of
   1. acanthosis
   2. blanching of tissue
   3. coagulation necrosis
   4. edema with accompanying swelling

250. Pronounced ptyalism is so common that it is nearly synonymous with
   1. argyria
   2. arsenism
   3. bismuthism
   4. mercurialism

251. Substernal chest pain is the most common initial symptom of
   1. angina pectoris
   2. congestive heart disease
   3. coronary disease
   4. hypertension

252. A 43-year-old female complained of a sharp, stabbing pain on the right side of the face. Although this had been occurring previously during eating, recently it had begun to occur spontaneously. Signs and symptoms of this pain were elicited by tapping the cheek immediately distal to the commissure of the lip, indicating a trigger zone. Pathology of the oral soft tissues and teeth was ruled out by thorough examination. The condition to be most suspected is
   1. Bell's palsy
   2. a neuritis involving the fifth nerve
   3. Parkinson's disease
   4. tic douloureux

253. A 23-year-old male complained of swelling of his upper lip "about twice a week." He reported that this occurred shortly after working hours on days that "unpleasant situations had arisen in the office." The swelling was never present the following morning. He also reported endodontic treatment of a maxillary anterior tooth just prior to the first occurrence of the swelling. Thorough examination revealed no evidence of pathology associated with the endodontically treated tooth. The evidence is sparse, but the strongest suspicion to be entertained is
   1. that the patient is allergic to something in the office
   2. angioedema
   3. that the patient is cancerphobic
   4. that the endodontically treated tooth is not responding to therapy

254. A 57-year-old male arrived for his scheduled 10 A.M. appointment slightly dazed and unable to concentrate. His skin was moist and clammy. The history had previously revealed that he was diabetic, insulin controlled. Questioning disclosed that he had missed eat-

(Continued)

ing his usual breakfast this morning because he was fearful of being late for his appointment. These are indications that

1. his diabetic condition is now uncontrolled
2. he is hypoglycemic and may go into insulin shock
3. he should be referred to his physician
4. he is more apprehensive than usual

255. Hyperthyroidism and anxiety are the most common causes of
    1. bronze skin discoloration
    2. dryness of the skin
    3. erythematous patches on the skin
    4. excessively moist skin

256. A history of trauma and/or recent tonsillectomy, pain elicited on palpation of the tonsillar fossa area, and radiographic evidence of an exceptionally long styloid process are most characteristic findings associated with the
    1. carotid artery syndrome
    2. Eagle syndrome
    3. myofacial pain dysfunction syndrome
    4. Plummer–Vinson syndrome

257. A patient with a history of multiple allergies is given xylocaine. The reaction most suggestive of sensitivity is manifested by
    1. a sudden rise in blood pressure
    2. mild tachycardia
    3. a sudden rise in temperature
    4. mild syncope

258. When the blood pressure of a 43-year-old male patient was taken, multiple petechiae appeared on the forearm. This is a likely occurrence in all the following except
    1. acute myelogenous leukemia
    2. hemophilia
    3. idiopathic thrombocytopenic purpura
    4. a vitamin C deficiency

259. Characteristic locations of the lymphoepithelial (branchial cleft) and thyroglossal cysts are, respectively, the
    1. submandibular and lateral areas of the neck
    2. lateral and midline areas of the neck
    3. midline and lateral areas of the neck
    4. midline and parotid areas of the neck

260. Yellow discoloration of the oral mucous membranes, as well as skin and eye sclerae, is a common finding in disorders of the liver. The eye is not affected in
    1. carotenemia
    2. pernicious anemia
    3. sickle cell anemia
    4. quinacrine hydrochloride therapy

261. A deviation of the mandible to the left on opening is most suggestive of
    1. a fracture of the right condyle
    2. unilateral hyperplasia of the right condyle
    3. osteoarthritis
    4. a form of subluxation

262. A 15-year-old male patient had gingival inflammation and pocket formation. Palmer hyperkeratosis was also apparent. Radiographs confirmed the suspicion of severe bone loss and a vertical type of bone resorption. These findings are most characteristic of
    1. chronic and recurrent acute ulcerative gingivitis
    2. dyskeratosis congenita
    3. the Papillon–Lefèvre syndrome
    4. the Pierre Robin syndrome

263. Least contributory to a tentative diagnosis of a lesion of the tongue being a squamous cell carcinoma is
    1. the presence of induration determined on palpation
    2. altered function or apparent hypomobility
    3. that it is $1.5 \times 1.5$ cm in size
    4. the presence of painless ulceration

264. A tooth with a carious lesion that had just begun to involve the dentin would most likely manifest
    1. a periapical rarefaction
    2. sensitivity to percussion
    3. a positive response to electrical stimuli
    4. extreme sensitivity to application of thermal stimuli

265. Extracapsular temporomandibular joint disorders, as compared with those involving intracapsular structure, far more frequently provide signs or symptoms of
    1. anxiety, stress, or nervousness of the patient
    2. clicking and/or crepitus
    3. deviation of the mandible on opening
    4. limited movement, e.g., trismus

266. A 57-year-old male patient requested an evaluation of white lesions on his tongue and buccal mucosa. He first noticed these about 2 weeks ago after reading about the desirability of oral self-examination. The past medical history revealed treatment of severely itching skin lesions on his forearm and lateral surfaces of both shins. He pointed out several of these lesions on his arm which appeared as firm, glistening, red papules. He also indicated several "healed spots" which possessed a brown pigmentation. The most common intraoral white lesions associated with these findings are those of
    1. leukoedema
    2. lichen planus
    3. candidiasis
    4. benign mucous pemphigoid

267. Examination of a 47-year-old male patient revealed marked redness and prominent minor mucous gland duct openings confined to a $2 \times 2$ cm area on the right side of the soft palate. It should be anticipated that the history would contain a report of
    1. cigarette smoking
    2. pipe smoking
    3. past treatment for syphilis
    4. tobacco chewing

268. Glossodynia, glossopyrosis, and numbness of the tongue are symptoms most often associated with

1. aplastic anemia
2. iron deficiency anemia
3. pernicious anemia
4. sickle cell anemia

269. Clinical research has indicated that emotional and/or stress factors are most closely associated with
    1. the black hairy and the fissured tongue
    2. erythema migrans and the black hairy tongue
    3. lichen planus and the geographic tongue
    4. median rhomboid glossitis and lichen planus

270. An oval, glistening, grayish white, slightly elevated area with an inflamed border best describes
    1. an aspirin burn
    2. a Koplik's spot
    3. a mucous patch
    4. an oral tuberculous lesion

271. Presence of a trigger area is a common finding in trigeminal neuralgia. Detection and/or location of such an area may also assist in and support a diagnosis of
    1. condylar hyperplasia
    2. ankylosis of the condyle on the side that the painful spasm of muscle is elicited
    3. the myofacial pain dysfunction syndrome
    4. unilateral subluxation

272. Firm, fixed neck nodes are most apt to be detected in association with
    1. an ameloblastoma
    2. a basal cell carcinoma
    3. an odontogenic fibroma
    4. a squamous cell carcinoma

273. A firm, freely movable, nontender mass in the submental region of the neck was detected on initial examination of a 64-year-old male patient. These clinical characteristics are most closely associated with
    1. acute lymphadenitis
    2. benign lymphoid hyperplasia
    3. a branchial cyst
    4. a squamous cell carcinoma of the lower lip

274. Periostitis and osteomyelitis, particularly of the mandible, are most commonly associated with
    1. argyria
    2. arsenism
    3. mercurialism
    4. phosphorous poisoning

275. A diabetic condition is most often associated with
    1. hyperpituitarism (acromegaly)
    2. hypothyroidism (cretinism)
    3. hyperthyroidism (Grave's disease)
    4. hyperparathyroidism (renal rickets)

276. The most common condition associated with mouth breathing is
    1. an anterior open bite
    2. chronic gingivitis, particularly in the anterior regions
    3. a high palatal vault
    4. macroglossia

277. External root resorption is most often associated with
    1. an eosinophilic granuloma
    2. a periapical granuloma
    3. a periapical cementifying fibroma
    4. an odontogenic fibroma

278. Radiographic evidence of occlusal caries is
    1. never of any diagnostic significance and should be disregarded
    2. occasionally of great assistance when clinical inspection and exploration yield questionable findings
    3. most often due to an artifact
    4. the primary means of diagnosis

279. Findings common to cherubism include all the following except
    1. bilateral enlargement of the posterior areas of the mandible
    2. multiple soap bubblelike radiolucencies
    3. paresthesia of the lower lip
    4. an apparent upward tilt of the eyes.

280. Hereditary gingival fibromatosis is differentiated from diphenylhydantoin (Dilantin) hyperplasia primarily on the basis of
    1. the examination
    2. the history
    3. microscopic examination of a biopsy specimen
    4. a serology

281. A 31-year-old female requested an evaluation of a maxillary lateral incisor. Her dentist (now deceased) had treated this tooth endodontically 3 years ago. The patient reported no untoward symptoms since treatment. Radiographs disclosed a 2 × 2 mm periapical radiolucency and an apparently well condensed, properly extended gutta percha root canal filling. Comparison with a radiograph in the patient's possession taken immediately following treatment demonstrated no increase in size or degree of radiolucency. These findings suggest the presence of a(n)
    1. chronic asymptomatic abscess
    2. unresolved granuloma
    3. periapical scar
    4. residual cyst

282. One of the criteria enabling differentiation of hypercementosis from periapical osteosclerosis and a periapical cementifying fibroma (cementoma) is that hypercementosis is characterized by
    1. a periodontal ligament space which appears to be present external to the bulbous root surface
    2. a positive response to electrical stimuli
    3. a history of trauma
    4. additional radiographic evidence suggestive of acromegaly or Paget's disease

283. Conditions which may present markedly different radiographic appearances depending upon their stage of development include all the following except
    1. a cementoma
    2. dilaceration

(Continued)

3. fibrous dysplasia
4. Paget's disease

284. Findings associated with cervicofacial actinomycosis include all the following except

1. dysphagia
2. submaxillary swelling
3. involvement of the tongue
4. previous tooth extraction

285. Signs which occur as late complications of neurosyphilis include all the following except

1. the Argyll Robertson pupil
2. eighth nerve deafness
3. a "slapping" type of gait
4. Romberg's sign

286. Garré's osteomyelitis is the most unusual form of osteomyelitis. A major distinction between it and all other forms is that

1. it usually occurs in children
2. the mandible is often involved
3. peripheral bone swelling occurs
4. sequestration and suppuration are common

287. A 20-year-old male presented with an ulcerated, nontender, round 1 × 1 cm lesion at the left commissure of the lip. He stated that it had been present for about 8 days. Submandibular and cervical nodes were palpable and nontender. A Kline test yielded a negative result. The most likely diagnosis on the basis of these findings is

1. actinomycosis
2. a lesion of primary syphilis
3. a traumatic ulcer
4. a tuberculous ulcer

288. A clinical diagnostic feature most helpful in differentiating an oral tuberculous ulcer from a lesion of syphilis is that the tuberculous ulcer

1. has a rolled border
2. invariably involves the lower lip
3. is red
4. is usually considerably more painful

289. Development of a hematoma following a posterior superior alveolar injection is a known complication in the use of local anesthesia. Differentiation between a hematoma and an early space infection, which must be considered, is assisted by the fact that the infection is

1. likely to be firm upon palpation
2. unlikely to be inflamed
3. rarely accompanied by a local increase in temperature
4. more apt to be tender upon palpation

290. Soft tissue lesions may be white for a variety of reasons. Match the lesion listed in the right-hand column with the cause of its coloration.

(a) color of a fungus      1. aspirin burn
(b) hyperkeratiniza-       2. leukoedema
    tion
(c) tissue necrosis        3. lichen planus
(d) water content of       4. candidiasis
    tissue

291. The most pertinent clues in differentiating between recurrent aphthous ulcerations and a traumatic ulcer of the oral mucosa are most often obtained by means of

1. meticulous clinical examination
2. exfoliative cytology examination
3. a probing history
4. blood chemistry examination

292. An amalgam tattoo

1. most often appears on the buccal mucosa
2. is readily differentiated from a junctional nevus on visual examination
3. is due to precipitation of protein in immature collagen fibers
4. invariably presents radiographic evidence of amalgam particles in tissue

293. A 42-year-old female requested a fixed bridge. The patient appeared nervous and "fidgety" but not apprehensive. Vital signs disclosed no hypertension or temperature elevation, but the pulse rate was 104. Some degree of exophthalmos was apparent. Medical consultation is clearly indicated prior to treatment because these findings indicate that the patient's condition is most likely

1. hyperparathyroidism
2. hyperpituitarism
3. hyperthyroidism
4. hypothyroidism

294. Cafe au lait spots on the skin are common findings in all the following except

1. Albright's syndrome
2. hyperthyroidism
3. hypothyroidism
4. neurofibromatosis

295. An 11-year-old male patient had a soft, fluctuant, nontender swelling on the crest of the alveolar ridge in the area of the mandibular right cuspid. Radiographs disclosed a pronounced radiolucency involving the crown of the permanent cuspid. (The deciduous cuspid had exfoliated approximately 6 months ago.) Analysis of the occlusion and status of eruption indicated that space was present for eruption of the tooth and that the dentition was neither precocious or retarded in its development. On the basis of these findings the diagnosis of the swelling is a(n)

1. ameloblastoma
2. dentigerous cyst
3. eruption cyst
4. lymphoepithelial cyst

296. Dentigerous and eruptive cysts are similar radiographically in that they both involve the crown of an unerupted tooth. Differentiation between them rests primarily on the

1. age of the patient
2. amount of soft tissue and/or bone overlying the unerupted tooth
3. potential of the tooth for eruption
4. particular tooth involved

297. On initial evaluation of a 67-year-old male patient, six well-defined radiolucent areas appeared on a pantomograph in the body and ramus of the right mandible. The medical history and physical findings were unremarkable. He did report removal of two "spots" in his jaw on the right side last year by an oral surgeon. These were reported to be nonmalignant and "some kind of cyst." Assuming the patient is accurate in his report of the type of lesion(s) removed, the most likely diagnosis of the radiolucencies now observed is
    1. aneurysmal bone cysts
    2. cysts associated with undiagnosed multiple myeloma
    3. odontogenic keratocysts
    4. primordial cysts

298. A 43-year-old female requested evaluation of a swelling in the right mandible. She reported that she had been referred to an oral surgeon 3 years ago when this lesion was "about half" its present size, but had neglected the consultation because she was fearful of a severe diagnosis. Intraoral examination revealed a pronounced buccal and lingual swelling from cuspid to first molar. No nodes were palpable. Radiographs demonstrated expansion and thinning of cortical bone and a multilocular soap bubblelike lesion confined to the bicuspid area. No root resorption was evident, and pulpal pathology was ruled out by thorough examination. Fluid was aspirated prior to biopsy. These findings are most consistent with a diagnosis of
    1. an ameloblastoma
    2. an eosinophilic granuloma
    3. multiple odontogenic keratocysts
    4. an osteogenic sarcoma

299. An ameloblastoma is most likely to develop from a
    1. dentigerous cyst
    2. radicular cyst
    3. residual cyst
    4. primordial cyst

300. A 20-year-old male presented with a firm, "rubbery," 2 × 2 cm, freely movable, nontender mass in the left side of the neck. Thorough clinical examination and laboratory studies failed to reveal any other abnormalities. The patient reported that he had first noticed the "little lump" about 4 months ago, that it had increased in size very slowly, but that it had not bothered him except that it was more difficult to shave over the area recently. These findings indicate that the swelling is most likely
    1. a metastatic carcinoma
    2. a lymphoepithelial cyst
    3. a tuberculous lesion
    4. a thyroglossal duct cyst

301. A patient with undiagnosed, asymptomatic leukemia would most likely develop
    1. spontaneous gingival bleeding
    2. cervical lymphadenopathy
    3. gingival enlargement
    4. ulcerations of the oral mucosa

302. A 74-year-old male complained of a "broken tooth." His gait was spastic, and movement of his left arm was limited. It was necessary for his wife to assist him into the dental operatory. Clinical findings included hypertension and an erratic pulse. It should be anticipated that the medical history would be most apt to include a report of
    1. a cerebrovascular accident
    2. severe diabetes
    3. liver disease
    4. grand mal seizures

303. Clinical diagnostic features of scleroderma include all the following except
    1. thinning of the skin of the hands
    2. Raynaud's phenomenon
    3. pain and stiffness of the finger joints
    4. hypertension

304. Mikulicz's disease is dissimilar to Sjögren's syndrome in that
    1. bilateral swelling of the parotid glands is common
    2. the lacrimal glands may be affected
    3. submaxillary pain is common in Mikulicz's disease
    4. xerostomia is a prominent clinical feature

305. Ocular manifestations, e.g., conjunctivitis, ulceration of the cornea, and photophobia, are most common and apt to result in impairment of vision in
    1. Darier's disease
    2. lupus erythematosus
    3. the Stevens–Johnson syndrome
    4. Sutton's disease

306. A bulbous lingual variocosity can usually be differentiated from a cyst by
    1. noting its dark blue color
    2. detecting fluctuation
    3. a reduction in size upon exerting firm finger pressure
    4. noting that the patient has similar varicosities elsewhere in the oral cavity

307. Size is rarely a criterion of value in diagnosis. However, it may be employed to assist in differentiation between
    1. an enostosis and exostosis
    2. malignant and benign white lesions because benign lesions are most often less than 2 cm in diameter
    3. a petechial hemorrhage, which is pinpoint in size, and an ecchymosis, which is 2 cm or larger in diameter
    4. radiolucent lesions of the maxilla because a lesion larger than 2 cm is usually a cyst

308. A ground glass, rather than cotton wool, radiographic appearance may be present in Paget's disease. In such a case, Paget's disease must be considered, but differentiated from
   1. an ameloblastoma
   2. hyperparathyroidism
   3. osteomyelitis
   4. sickle cell anemia

309. A periapical cementifying fibroma (cementoma) may present a very similar radiographic appearance to that of a granuloma. However, it differs from a granuloma in that it
   1. is radiopaque in its early stages and the involved tooth is vital
   2. is radiolucent in its earliest stage and the involved tooth is vital
   3. occurs most frequently in the mandibular molar region
   4. occurs most frequently in males

310. Routine dental therapy ought to be postponed for the child with impetigo for all of the following reasons except that
   1. the lesions could be spread into the intraoral environment
   2. the therapist may contract it
   3. the patient's already high temperature may be elevated by dental therapy
   4. dental treatment is likely to be most uncomfortable for the patient because the lesions are often perioral

311. Clinically the condition which most closely mimics gonorrhea, in that an itching, burning urethritis is a prominent symptom, is
   1. Behçet's disease
   2. Reiter's disease
   3. Stevens–Johnson syndrome
   4. Sutton's disease

312. A 55-year-old patient returned 48 hours subsequent to insertion of full dentures complaining of a "sore spot" on the crest of the mandibular ridge. Examination revealed a $2 \times 2$ mm ulceration. Eventual development of osteonecrosis is most likely if the patient's past medical history contained a report of
   1. a coronary
   2. diabetes
   3. radiation therapy for a nasopharyngeal tumor
   4. thrombocytopenic purpura

313. A 25-year-old black male patient had a severe pericoronitis involving a mandibular left third molar. Signs and symptoms indicated removal of the tooth and antibiotic coverage for the procedure. The patient's medical history contained a report of discovery of the sickle cell trait 3 years ago on routine examination. This patient would be most apt to experience a hemolytic crisis upon
   1. administration of an antibiotic
   2. IV barbiturate sedation
   3. administration of a local anesthetic
   4. administration of nitrous oxide anesthesia

314. In examination of a 55-year-old black male, the eye sclerae were observed to be slightly yellow. The medical history and physical findings were entirely unremarkable. Assuming a reliable history, this finding suggests
   1. liver dysfunction
   2. undiagnosed and untreated hepatitis
   3. a normal variation
   4. a malignancy of the gall bladder.

315. Radiation therapy and prompt surgical treatment are contraindicated because regression during puberty and spontaneous disappearance in adulthood are common to
   1. achondroplasia
   2. cherubism
   3. fibrous dysplasia
   4. osteogenesis imperfecta

316. Discoid lupus erythematosus, leukoplakia, and lichen planus are similar in that
   1. actinic sensitivity is a common finding
   2. white keratotic lesions may appear on the buccal mucosa
   3. ulceration of the oral mucosa is usually present
   4. they all produce pain.

317. Leukoedema is similar to lichen planus in that it
   1. is identical in configuration
   2. is frequently indurated
   3. appears as a white coloration of the buccal mucosa
   4. often produces pain

318. Because they are exophytic and possess a roughened surface, verrucae of the oral mucosa are most similar in clinical appearance to
   1. basal cell carcinomas
   2. fibromas
   3. Fordyce's granules
   4. papillomas

319. A ranula and a mucocele are often remarkably similar in clinical appearance. They occur in the following locations in the order named
   1. buccal mucosa and the moist mucous membrane of the lip
   2. moist mucous membrane of the lip and the sublingual space
   3. sublingual space and the moist mucous membrane of the lip
   4. sublingual space and the soft palate

320. Two conditions which appear most similar clinically are
   1. benign migratory glossitis and traumatic ulcers
   2. Bowen's and Fordyce's diseases
   3. diphenylhydantoin (Dilantin) hyperplasia and hereditary gingival fibromatosis
   4. herpangina and acute necrotizing ulcerative gingivitis

321. Acute necrotizing gingivitis and leukemic gingivitis are similar in symptomatology and clinical appearance in that there may be
1. necrosis and fibromatosis
2. swelling and apparent hyperkeratosis
3. spontaneous hemorrhage and necrosis
4. spontaneous hemorrhage and atrophy

322. The most common and outstanding similar finding in Mikulicz's and Sjögren's syndromes is
1. association with a connective tissue disease
2. conjunctivitis
3. enlargement of any of the salivary glands
4. xerostomia

323. All of the following are true of maxillary sinusitis as it relates to oral findings except that
1. a fetid breath odor is often present
2. a cloudy radiographic appearance of the sinus is both a common and reliable diagnostic criterion for diagnosis
3. symptoms of pulpitis involving the maxillary posterior teeth is a common finding
4. maxillary sinusitis may be the result of dental infection

324. A large multilocular unilateral radiolucency may suggest the possibility of all except
1. an ameloblastoma
2. central giant cell granuloma
3. cherubism
4. an odontogenic myxoma

325. A lingual mandibular bone concavity (also termed embryonic bone cyst, latent bone cyst, static bone cyst, static bone cavity) is similar in radiographic appearance to the submandibular fossa (fossa for the submaxillary gland) only in that it is
1. usually well defined
2. located below the level of the mandibular canal
3. generally radiolucent
4. usually bilateral

326. Periapical cementifying fibromas, fibrous dysplasia, osteomyelitis, and Paget's disease may be similar in radiographic appearance in that they
1. are primarily radiolucent
2. may present quite different radiographic appearances depending on their stage of development
3. are primarily radiopaque
4. invariably appear in a combined radiolucent–radiopaque form

327. Least helpful in diagnosis of a periapical cementifying fibroma (cementoma) is the
1. presence of a radiolucency in the mandibular anterior region
2. presence of a radiopacity in a female patient
3. degree of radiolucency and/or radiopacity
4. lack of response to electrical stimulation

328. The incisive fossa may suggest the presence of an area of decreased bone density (and therefore periapical pathology) in the region of the
1. mandibular incisors
2. maxillary central incisors, specifically
3. mandibular central incisors, specifically
4. maxillary lateral incisors

329. On the basis of radiographic appearance alone, periapical pathoses are most apt to be suggested by all the following except
1. the inferior alveolar canal
2. a lingual mandibular bone concavity
3. a pronounced mental fossa
4. a pronounced submandibular fossa

330. Because of their (radiographic) location, the anterior palatine and mental foramina may be suspected of being
1. condensing osteites
2. developmental defects
3. malignant growth
4. periapical pathoses

331. Because of its location and relative radiographic density, a talon cusp may appear most similar to
1. dilaceration
2. a supernumerary tooth
3. fusion
4. gemination

## REFERENCES

1. ALLING CC III, MAHAN PE: Facial Pain, 2nd ed. Philadelphia, Lea & Febiger, 1977
2. ARCHER WH: Oral and Maxillofacial Surgery, Vol II. 5th ed. Philadelphia, WB Saunders, 1975
3. BELL WE: Orofacial Pains—Differential Diagnosis. Deneco of Dallas, 1973
4. BHASKAR SN: Radiographic Interpretation For The Dentist, 2nd ed. St. Louis, CV Mosby, 1975
5. BHASKAR SN: Synopsis of Oral Pathology, 5th ed. St. Louis, CV Mosby, 1977
6. CALDWELL RC, STALLARD RE: A Textbook of Preventive Dentistry. Philadelphia, WB Saunders, 1977
7. CLEATON-JONES P: Essential Medicine For Dental Practice. Springfield, Il, C Thomas, 1971
8. COHEN L: A Synopsis of Medicine in Dentistry. Philadelphia, Lea & Febiger, 1972
9. EVERSOLE LR: Clinical Outline of Oral Pathology: Diagnosis and Treatment. Philadelphia, Lea & Febiger, 1978
10. GORLIN RJ, GOLDMAN HM (eds): Thoma's Oral Pathology, Vol 2, 6th ed. St. Louis, CV Mosby, 1970
11. GORLIN RJ, PINDBORG JJ, COHEN MM JR: Syndromes of The Head and Neck, 2nd ed. New York, McGraw-Hill, 1976
12. KAMARIN BB, KAMARIN MA: Handbook of Oral Diagnostic Concepts and Cues. New York, University Press of America, 1978
13. KERR DA, ASH MM, MILLARD HD: Oral Diagnosis, 4th ed. St. Louis, CV Mosby, 1974
14. LYNCH MA (ed): Burket's Oral Medicine, 7th ed. Philadelphia, JB Lippincott, 1977
15. MALMED SF: Handbook of Medical Emergencies In The Dental Office. St. Louis, CV Mosby, 1978
16. MANSON-HING LR: Panoramic Dental Radiography. Springfield, Il, CC Thomas, 1976
17. MCCALL JO: Principles of Periodontics. Philadelphia, JB Lippincott, 1964

18. MCCARTHY FM: Emergencies in Dental Practice, 2nd ed. Philadelphia, WB Saunders, 1972
19. MITCHELL DF, STANDISH SM, FAST TB: Oral Diagnosis/Oral Medicine, 2nd ed. Philadelphia, Lea & Febiger, 1971
20. PINDBORG JJ: Pathology of the Dental Hard Tissue. Philadelphia, WB Saunders, 1970
21. PINDBORG JJ: Atlas of Diseases of The Oral Mucosa, 2nd ed. Philadelphia, WB Saunders, 1973
22. ROBBINS SL: Pathologic Basis of Disease. Philadelphia, WB Saunders, 1974
23. SCOPP IW: Oral Medicine, 2nd ed. St. Louis, CV Mosby, 1973
24. SHAFER WG, HINE MK, LEVY BM: A Textbook of Oral Pathology, 3rd ed. Philadelphia, WB Saunders, 1974
25. SHKLAR G, MCCARTHY PL: The Oral Manifestations of Systemic Disease. Reading, Butterworths, 1976
26. SISKIN M: The Biology of the Human Dental Pulp. St. Louis, CV Mosby, 1973
27. STAFNE EC, GIBILISCO JA: Oral Roentgenographic Diagnosis, 4th ed. Philadelphia, WB Saunders, 1975
28. WOOD NK, GOAZ PW: Differential Diagnosis of Oral Lesions. St. Louis, CV Mosby, 1975
29. WORTH HM: Principles and Practice of Oral Radiologic Interpretation. Chicago, Yearbook Medical, 1963
30. WUEHRMANN AH, MANSON-HING R: Dental Radiology, 4th ed. St. Louis, CV Mosby, 1977

## ANSWER KEY

| | | | | | | | |
|---|---|---|---|---|---|---|---|
| 1. 3 | 30. 3 | 59. 2 | 88. 3 | 117. 2 | 171. 3 | 225. 1 | 279. 3 |
| 2. 2 | 31. 2 | 60. 2 | 89. 4 | 118. 4 | 172. 4 | 226. 2 | 280. 2 |
| 3. 4 | 32. 3 | 61. 3 | 90. 2 | 119. 3 | 173. 3 | 227. 3 | 281. 3 |
| 4. 4 | 33. 2 | 62. 4 | 91. 3 | 120. 3 | 174. 2 | 228. 3 | 282. 1 |
| 5. 3 | 34. 4 | 63. c,d,b,a | 92. 3 | 121. 4 | 175. 3 | 229. 2 | 283. 2 |
| 6. 2 | 35. 3 | 64. b,d,a,c | 93. 2 | 122. 3 | 176. 3 | 230. 4 | 284. 3 |
| 7. 3 | 36. 3 | 65. 3 | 94. 2 | 123. 2 | 177. 1 | 231. 1 | 285. 2 |
| 8. 4 | 37. 2 | 66. 3 | 95. 2 | 124. 3 | 178. 2 | 232. 2 | 286. 3 |
| 9. 2 | 38. 2 | 67. 2 | 96. 2 | 125. 3 | 179. 4 | 233. 3 | 287. 2 |
| 10. 3 | 39. 2 | 68. 3 | 97. 2 | 126. 4 | 180. 4 | 234. c,d,b,a | 288. 4 |
| 11. 4 | 40. 4 | 69. 3 | 98. 3 | 127. 2 | 181. 3 | 235. 2 | 289. 4 |
| 12. 2 | 41. 1 | 70. 3 | 99. 1 | 128. 2 | 182. 3 | 236. b,d,a,c | 290. c,d,b,a |
| 13. 3 | 42. 3 | 71. 1 | 100. 3 | 129. 4 | 183. 4 | 237. 2 | 291. 3 |
| 14. d,c,a,b | 43. 1 | 72. 3 | 101. 3 | 130. 2 | 184. 2 | 238. 2 | 292. 3 |
| 15. 3 | 44. 2 | 73. 2 | 102. 3 | 131. 2 | 185. 2 | 239. 3 | 293. 3 |
| 16. 2 | 45. 3 | 74. 3 | 103. 4 | 132. 3 | 186. 3 | 240. 2 | 294. 2 |
| 17. 2 | 46. 2 | 75. 3 | 104. 2 | 133. 3 | 187. 2 | 241. 4 | 295. 3 |
| 18. 4 | 47. 3 | 76. 4 | 105. 1 | 134. 3 | 188. 3 | 242. 3 | 296. 3 |
| 19. 3 | 48. 3 | 77. 3 | 106. 2 | 135. 1 | 189. d,c,a,b | 243. 3 | 297. 3 |
| 20. 2 | 49. 2 | 78. b,d,c,a | 107. 3 | 136. c,a,d,b | 190. 2 | 244. 2 | 298. 1 |
| 21. 3 | 50. c,d,a,b | 79. b,c,d,a | 108. 4 | 137. b,d,a,c | 191. b,c,d,a | 245. b,c,a,d | 299. 1 |
| 22. 2 | 51. 2 | 80. 2 | 109. 1 | 138. 3 | 192. c,d,b,a | 246. 2 | 300. 2 |
| 23. 3 | 52. 2 | 81. 4 | 110. 3 | 139. 2 | 193. 2 | 247. 4 | 301. 2 |
| 24. 1 | 53. 3 | 82. 1 | 111. 3 | 140. 3 | 194. 3 | 248. 4 | 302. 1 |
| 25. 3 | 54. 4 | 83. 4 | 112. 2 | 141. 2 | 195. 2 | 249. 3 | 303. 1 |
| 26. 3 | 55. 1 | 84. 3 | 113. 4 | 142. 2 | 196. 3 | 250. 4 | 304. 3 |
| 27. 2 | 56. 4 | 85. 3 | 114. 3 | 143. c,a,d,b | 197. 4 | 251. 3 | 305. 3 |
| 28. 4 | 57. 3 | 86. 3 | 115. 3 | 144. 2 | 198. 3 | 252. 4 | 306. 3 |
| 29. 3 | 58. 2 | 87. 1 | 116. 2 | 145. 2 | 199. 4 | 253. 2 | 307. 3 |
| | | | | 146. 2 | 200. 1 | 254. 2 | 308. 2 |
| | | | | 147. 4 | 201. 3 | 255. 4 | 309. 2 |
| | | | | 148. 2 | 202. 3 | 256. 2 | 310. 3 |
| | | | | 149. 4 | 203. 4 | 257. 3 | 311. 2 |
| | | | | 150. 3 | 204. 3 | 258. 2 | 312. 3 |
| | | | | 151. 3 | 205. 2 | 259. 2 | 313. 4 |
| | | | | 152. 2 | 206. 4 | 260. 1 | 314. 3 |
| | | | | 153. 2 | 207. 3 | 261. 2 | 315. 2 |
| | | | | 154. 1 | 208. 1 | 262. 3 | 316. 2 |
| | | | | 155. 3 | 209. 2 | 263. 3 | 317. 3 |
| | | | | 156. 2 | 210. 3 | 264. 3 | 318. 4 |
| | | | | 157. 2 | 211. 3 | 265. 1 | 319. 3 |
| | | | | 158. 3 | 212. 2 | 266. 2 | 320. 3 |
| | | | | 159. 3 | 213. 1 | 267. 2 | 321. 3 |
| | | | | 160. 3 | 214. 2 | 268. 3 | 322. 4 |
| | | | | 161. 4 | 215. 3 | 269. 3 | 323. 2 |
| | | | | 162. 2 | 216. 3 | 270. 3 | 324. 3 |
| | | | | 163. 4 | 217. 3 | 271. 3 | 325. 3 |
| | | | | 164. 2 | 218. 3 | 272. 4 | 326. 2 |
| | | | | 165. 4 | 219. 4 | 273. 2 | 327. 3 |
| | | | | 166. 3 | 220. 4 | 274. 4 | 328. 4 |
| | | | | 167. 1 | 221. 1 | 275. 1 | 329. 2 |
| | | | | 168. 2 | 222. 4 | 276. 2 | 330. 4 |
| | | | | 169. 2 | 223. 3 | 277. 4 | 331. 2 |
| | | | | 170. 2 | 224. 3 | 278. 2 | |

# 13

# DENTAL RADIOLOGY

### Lincoln R. Manson-Hing / David F. Greer

Questions on dental radiology can pertain to the physics of radiography, radiographic technique, radiation hazards, x-ray protection, and radiographic interpretation. Questions related to interpretation often contain clinical and microscopic aspects of pathologic conditions. This review of dental radiology is presented in three sections: 1) technical principles, 2) anatomy and interpretive recognition, and 3) radiation hygiene.

## TECHNICAL PRINCIPLES OF RADIOLOGY

The technical principles of radiology include numerous factors about which entire textbooks have been written. The following material is a brief summary of these principles as they relate to dental radiology.

### X-Radiation and Its Properties

X-radiation is a form of electromagnetic radiation and possesses the properties of that family of radiations. All of these radiations, including x-radiation, have neither mass nor charge and travel in wave forms at a speed of 186,000 miles/sec. Some special properties of x-radiation in addition to those of the electromagnetic spectrum include the abilities to 1) penetrate opaque objects, 2) cause ionization and/or excitation in the matter with which it interacts, 3) create chemical changes, and 4) create phosphorescence and fluorescence in a variety of materials.

### Production of X-Radiation in a Dental X-Ray Machine

X-radiation is produced in a dental x-ray machine by converting electrical energy to kinetic energy as a result of moving electrons. This kinetic energy in turn is converted to x-radiation and heat. The efficiency of this process is very low: less than 1% of the original electrical energy is converted to x-radiation, while the remainder is dissipated as heat.

The three steps involved in x-radiation production occur in the x-ray tube of the machine and include 1) the boiling off of electrons from the filament at the cathode; 2) the creation of a high difference in potential between the cathode and the anode (target), resulting in the passage of electrons from the cathode to the anode; and 3) the bombardment of the tungsten target by the accelerated electrons, resulting in the production of x-radiation and heat. The process of x-ray production can be altered in the x-ray machine to control the quality and quantity of the resultant x-ray beam.

KILOVOLTAGE. Beam quality (hardness, penetrability, effective wavelength or effective energy) may be altered by changing the kilovolt peak (kVp). Since an increase in the kVp produces a greater difference in potential between the cathode and the anode, the electron speed is accelerated across the tube and causes a greater impact with the target. The end result is the production of x-radiation of higher quality (shorter effective wavelength, greater effective energy, greater hardness, or greater ability to penetrate. The kVp also affects the efficiency of x-ray production; efficiency is increased as the kVp increases. This means that the number of x-ray photons produced is greater and results in an increase in beam quantity (the number of x-ray photons per unit area or unit time).

MILLIAMPERAGE. Beam quantity may also be altered by changing the milliamperage setting on the x-ray machine panel. An increase in milliamperage increases the amount of heat supplied to the filament and results in a greater number of electrons available to traverse the tube and bombard the target. As more electrons interact at the target, more x-ray photons are produced and beam quantity is thus increased. Conversely, a decrease in milliamperage results in a decrease of beam quantity.

### Beam Alterations

The x-radiation produced in the x-ray tube of an x-ray machine travels in all directions from the target. All the radiation emitted from the tube is referred to as primary radiation. That portion that passes through the window of the glass envelope around the tube, traverses the oil surrounding the envelope, and exits the aperture seal of the tube head is referred to as the useful beam. The useful beam is conical in shape and contains x-ray photons having many different energies (wavelengths).

The shape and size of the beam that exits the tube head is determined by a process called collimation. Collimation reduces the volume of tissue irradiated and may be accomplished in several ways. These include the placement of a lead washer just outside the aluminum filter, the use of a metal cylinder inside the position-indicating device (open-end cylinder or cone), or the use of a lead-lined position-indicating device. These collimating methods, which are the most commonly used, result in a circular beam; however, collimating devices forming a rectangular beam are also available. When circular collimation is employed, the beam should be no wider in diameter than 2.75 in. at the surface of the patient's face.

Since the unaltered useful beam contains x-ray photons having many different wavelengths or energies, it is called a heterogeneous beam. The process of filtration is used to remove a portion of the long wavelength, low energy photons which could not pass through anatomic structures to reach the film. Although there is a certain amount of inherent filtration built into x-ray machines by the window of the glass envelope, the oil around the envelope, and the aperture seal, additional filtration is usually required to achieve the correct amount of total filtration. Aluminum is used to provide the additional filtration. The recommended amount of total filtration, according to some guidelines, is 1.5 mm aluminum for kVp settings below 70 and 2 mm for kVp settings 70 and above. Others recommend 2 mm for kVp settings below 70 and 2.5 mm for kVp settings 70 and above.

### Exposure Factors

The exposure factors that may be varied in intraoral radiography include the kVp, milliamperes, exposure time, and target-film distance. An alteration of one of the above factors requires a change in one or more of the other factors to assure the production of diagnostically useful radiographs. Although any of the factors may be altered, the two factors most commonly altered are the exposure time and the distance. If the kVp and milliamperage settings are constant, an increase in distance requires an increase in exposure time. Since x-rays diverge from the source in straight lines, the inverse square law may be used to determine the intensity of the beam and to calculate the correct exposure time at various distances from the target. This means

that the intensity of a beam at a point 16 in. from the target would have one-fourth the intensity of the same beam at a point 8 in. from the target; therefore, an exposure time four times greater would be required at 16 in. than at 8 in. Conversely if the correct exposure time using a 16-in. target-film distance were 60 impulses, the correct exposure time at 8 in. would be 15 impulses.

### Radiographic Quality

Radiographic quality may be measured in terms of density (the overall blackness of a radiograph), contrast (the differences in densities between adjacent areas on a radiograph), and sharpness or detail (the ability of a radiograph to produce exact outlines or borders of an object). Each of these qualities is influenced by inherent film characteristics, as well as inherent object characteristics. The following comments are confined to alterations in the qualities that can be influenced by changes in the exposure factors.

The density of a radiograph is the result of the amount of radiation reaching the film if a constant film speed[*] is used. Density may be increased by increasing the exposure time, milliamperage, or kVp or by decreasing the target-film distance.

The exposure factor which most greatly influences contrast is the kVp. An increase in this factor results in a longer scale of contrast or more shades of grey between the black and white areas on the film. With a decrease in the kVp setting, the contrast is of shorter scale (very few shades of grey between black and white), and the resulting radiograph is sometimes referred to as being of high contrast or very "contrasty."

In addition to being affected by film and object characteristics, sharpness or detail is inherently influenced by the size of the focal spot in the x-ray tube. A smaller focal spot provides greater sharpness than a larger one. Other exposure factors related to sharpness include the target-to-object and object-to-film distances. Decreasing the object-to-film distance provides an increase in image sharpness.

### QUESTIONS

1. In x-ray equipment, milliamperage controls the
   a. energy of the radiation
   b. temperature of the cathode filament
   c. speed of the electrons
   d. amount of radiation produced
   e. penetrability of the radiation produced
   1. a, c and e
   2. b, c, and d

[*] There are currently three film speed classifications available for intraoral films. These include speed B or slow, speed C or intermediate, and speed D or fast film. The difference between the slowest and the fastest films available is approximately a factor of eight.

3. a and c
4. b and d
5. c and e

The milliamperage control in the x-ray machine regulates the amperage or amount of electrical energy that reaches the filament of the x-ray tube. The amount of current sent to the filament affects its temperature and therefore the number of electrons emitted by the filament. Since these electrons are used to carry the electrical potential between the cathode and anode to produce x-rays, the number of electrons available controls the amount of x-rays produced.

The speed of the electrons is controlled by the electrical potential (kilovoltage) between the cathode and anode. Because the speed of the electrons determines the amount of energy given to individual x-ray photons, it affects the wavelength and penetrating quality of the radiation produced. The total energy of an x-ray beam is a function of both the number of photons in the beam and the energy carried by individual photons and therefore is affected by both milliamperage and kilovoltage controls.

2. The wavelength of x-ray photons is determined by the
   1. kilovoltage
   2. milliamperage
   3. amount of heat supplied to the filament
   4. quantity of electrons in the cathode stream.

The wavelength of x-ray photons is determined by the kilovoltage between the cathode and anode in the x-ray tube. Milliamperage controls the amount of electricity supplied to the filament, the resultant temperature or heat of the filament, the subsequent number of electrons supplied to the electron or cathode stream in the x-ray tube, and the number or amount of x-ray photons produced by the x-ray tube.

3. Sharpness of the radiographic image is increased by
   1. decreasing filtration
   2. increasing the focal spot-object distance
   3. decreasing the milliamperage
   4. increasing the object-film distance

An indistinct image is basically a result of the penumbra which forms when the source of radiation in the x-ray tube is too close to the area being x-rayed. Increasing the focal spot-to-object distance reduces the penumbra and increases image sharpness.

4. The intensity of x-radiation at any given distance from the source of radiation varies
   1. inversely with the square of the distance
   2. directly with the square of the distance
   3. inversely with the kVp
   4. directly with the kVp

Intensity of an x-ray beam is generally thought of as the number of x-ray photons in a given area arriving at a particular distance from the source of radiation. How-

ever, intensity can also be considered in terms of the amount of x-ray energy arriving at the given area.

In terms of number of photons, x-ray intensity varies inversely with the square of distance when all other factors (e.g., milliamperage, exposure time, kVp) are kept constant. This is due to the fact that x-rays travel in straight lines and diverge from the x-ray source in all directions; they are thus spread to four times the area they expose when the distance from the x-ray source is doubled. Since the intensity ratio is according to the square of the distance and is inversely proportional, the x-ray intensity decreases as distance increases.

In terms of x-ray energy, an increase in kVp increases the amount of x-ray energy at a given distance from the source of radiation; however, each kVp increase does not produce the same amount of increase in x-ray energy.

5. The purpose of a step-up transformer in an x-ray machine is to increase the
   1. heat to the filament
   2. wavelength of the x-rays
   3. voltage to the tube's filament circuit
   4. voltage to the tube's anode–cathode circuit
   5. milliamperage of the x-ray machine.

The step-up transformer is connected to the anode–cathode electric circuit of the x-ray tube, not to the filament circuit. It produces higher electric potentials and x-rays with shorter wavelengths. A transformer changes voltage, not amperage.

6. The quality of an x-ray beam can be described by stating the
   1. kilovoltage and milliamperage
   2. milliamperage and half-value layer
   3. exposure time and kilovoltage
   4. half-value layer and milliamperage
   5. kilovoltage and half-value layer.

Milliamperage and exposure time control the total number of x-ray photons produced. Kilovoltage controls the electrical energy potential between the anode and cathode of the x-ray tube (the energy with which x-rays are created) and therefore affects the quality of the x-ray beam. The half-value layer indicates the ability of an x-ray beam to penetrate an x-ray absorbing material and is used to measure the quality of an x-ray beam.

7. The paralleling intraoral radiographic technique fulfills which of the following basic principles of shadow casting?
   a. The source of radiation should be as small as possible.
   b. The distance from the radiation source to the object should be as great as possible.
   c. The distance from the object to the film should be as short as possible.
   d. The object and the film should be parallel.

e. The radiation should strike both the object and the film at right angles.

1. a, c, and e
2. b, d, and e
3. d and e
4. a, b, d, and e
5. All of the above

8. Of the following, which are characteristic of an aluminum filtered primary x-ray diagnostic beam?

    a. The filtered beam contains a greater number of shorter wavelength x-ray photons than a nonfiltered beam.
    b. The filtered beam contains a lesser number of longer wavelength x-ray photons than a nonfiltered beam.
    c. The filtered beam is comprised of fewer x-ray photons that are less penetrating than is the nonfiltered primary beam.
    d. The filtered beam has a higher half-value layer than the nonfiltered beam.

1. b, c, and d
2. a, b, and c
3. d, b, and a
4. d, c, and a
5. All of the above

The purpose of filtration is to remove long wavelength x-ray photons from a beam of x-radiation. These photons have less energy and are less penetrating than shorter wavelength photons. Following filtration, the beam is more penetrating and has a higher half-value layer (the amount of aluminum required to reduce the intensity of the beam by one-half) than the incident beam.

Since long wavelength photons with a low ability to penetrate are removed from the beam by filtration, the filtered beam contains fewer long wavelength photons than does a nonfiltered beam, which means it is comprised of fewer photons of low penetrability than the nonfiltered primary beam. In other words, a filtered beam has a higher half-value layer than a nonfiltered beam.

9. Intensifying screens are used in radiographic examinations in order to

1. improve detail
2. decrease the exposure time
3. protect the film from scatter radiation
4. increase the quantity of x-radiation necessary to produce a certain photographic effect on silver
5. improve definition.

Intensifying screens are sometimes used in radiographic examinations to reduce the exposure time required to produce diagnostically useful radiographs. When exposure time is reduced, the amount of scattered radiation which reaches the film is reduced, although not entirely deleted. The effect of intensifying screens on detail and definition varies with the speed of the screens used, and although sharpness is not improved, it may be easier for the interpreter to perceive detail because of the decrease in film fog.

10. The paralleling intraoral radiographic technique using the extension cone, compared with the bisection of the angle technique, involves

    a. greater vertical angulations
    b. greater object-to-film distances
    c. greater developing time
    d. greater anode-to-film distances

1. a and b
2. a and c
3. b and c
4. b and d
5. c and d

The paralleling intraoral technique involves placing the film parallel to the long axis of the object being x-rayed (the teeth and/or other oral structures), then directing the central ray of the x-ray beam at right angles to both the film and the object. The vertical angulation therefore is less than it would be when the bisecting technique is employed. The bisecting technique requires that the film be positioned immediately adjacent to the teeth being radiographed and the central ray is directed at right angles to the bisector of the angle formed by the plane of the film and the long axis of the teeth.

The object-to-film distance is obviously less when using the bisecting technique. The anode-to-film distances most commonly used for intraoral radiography are 8 and 16 in. The former is used primarily for the bisecting technique, while the latter may be employed for either. The 16-in. distance is much preferred for the paralleling technique since it requires a relatively greater object-to-film distance.

The developing time and all other processing procedures are the same for radiographs using either technique.

11. Exposure time for the maxillary molar region at an 8-in. target-film distance is 30 impulses, using 10 ma and 60 kv. The exposure time for the same area using the same factors but increasing the target-film distance to 16 in. would be

1. 45 impulses
2. 60 impulses
3. 90 impulses
4. 120 impulses
5. 150 impulses

According to the inverse square law, the intensity of a beam of radiation is inversely proportional to the square of the distances from the source (target) to points of radiation intensity measurements. In this case the distance is doubled and the intensity at 16 in. would be one-fourth that at 8 in. Therefore, four times as much exposure time would be needed at 16 in. to achieve the same radiographic density.

12. The quality of radiographs can be expressed in terms of overall density, contrast, and definition. Assuming equivalent density, how is the detail and contrast of the radiographic image affected by the factors of focal distance, kilovoltage peak, and/or millampere seconds?

    a. Focal distance directly affects definition.
    b. Focal distance directly affects contrast.
    c. The kVp directly affects contrast.
    d. The milliamperage directly affects definition.

  1. a and b
  2. a and c
  3. b and c
  4. b and d
  5. a, b, and c

The terms definition, detail, and sharpness are frequently used synonymously to describe the ability of a radiograph to record images accurately. For intraoral radiographs, definition is affected mainly by the object-to-film distance and target-to-object distance. For optimal definition the object-to-film distance should be as small as possible, while the target-to-object distance should be as great as possible.

Contrast is defined as the differences in density between adjacent areas appearing on a radiograph. Where there are few shades of grey between totally black and totally white areas, the contrast is described as high or short scale. When there are many shades of grey, the contrast is described as low or long scale. Increases in kVp produce long-scale contrast, while decreases in kVp produce short-scale contrast.

13. To increase only the penetrative quality of x-radiation, an operator should increase the

  1. exposure time
  2. kilovoltage
  3. milliamperage
  4. collimation
  5. anode-to-film distance.

The penetrative quality of x-radiation is determined by the effective wavelength of the beam; the shorter the effective wavelength, the more penetrating the beam. The effective wavelength is determined by the difference in electrical potential between the anode and cathode in the x-ray tube and may be altered by changing the kVp selector switch on the x-ray machine. An increase in kVp results in an increase in electrical potential and produces a beam with a shorter effective wavelength and greater penetrability.

Exposure time, milliamperage and anode-to-film distance affect the quantity of radiation produced rather than its penetrative quality. Collimation determines only the shape and size of the beam for a given distance and has no effect on beam penetrability.

## ANATOMICAL AND INTERPRETIVE RECOGNITION

In addition to the patient's history, examination, clinical and microscopic findings, radiographs are extremely important in arriving at a definitive diagnosis and treatment plan. A thorough understanding of the radiographic appearance of normal anatomic landmarks is necessary to be able to discern between normal and abnormal radiographic findings (Table 13–1).

Variations are commonly seen in the size, shape, location, and the degree of radiolucency or radiopacity of anatomic structures. When radiographic variations

**Table 13-1.  Normal Appearance of Anatomic Landmarks on Intraoral Radiographs**

| SITE | RADIOLUCENT | RADIOPAQUE |
|------|-------------|------------|
| Maxilla | Sinus | Hamular process |
| | Incisive foramen | Tuberosity |
| | | Coronoid process of mandible |
| | Nasal cavity | Floor of maxillary sinus |
| | Nutrient canals in sinus wall | Sinus septa |
| | | Zygoma |
| | Median maxillary suture | Floor of nasal cavity |
| | Lateral fossa | Inferior concha |
| | | Walls of median maxillary structure |
| | | Anterior nasal spine |
| | | Nasal septum |
| | | Soft tissue of the nose |
| Mandible | Submandibular fossa | External oblique ridge |
| | Mental foramen | Mental protuberance |
| | Incisive foramen | Genial tubercles |
| | Mental fossa | Mylohyoid ridge |
| | Nutrient canals | Cortex of the inferior border of the mandible |

exist, a confirmation that the structure is normal can usually be obtained by examining the appearance of the same landmark on the opposite side of the oral cavity since such variations ordinarily occur bilaterally.

When radiographic findings are abnormal, a definitive diagnosis should not be attempted without considering the patient's history and the clinical examination. However, from an abnormal radiographic finding it is usually possible to arrive at a radiographic differential diagnosis. When establishing a tentative diagnosis, the practitioner should remember that, although it is possible to divide most entities into radiolucencies, radiopacities, or combinations of them, the sizes and shape of lesions as well as their relationship to other structures are of utmost importance.

## QUESTIONS

14. In certain bone diseases localized or generalized radiopacities which reflect an increase of bone mineralization or a decrease in bone resorption may be noted. Which of the following diseases produce localized or generalized radiopacities?
    - a. Condensing osteitis
    - b. Cherubism
    - c. Albers–Schönberg disease
    - d. Sickle cell anemia
    - e. Chronic sclerosing osteomyelitis

    1. a, b, and c
    2. a, c, and e
    3. a, d, and e
    4. b, c, and d
    5. b, d, and e
    6. All of the above

Condensing osteitis is a bone infection characterized by sclerosis, which produces radiopacities. Chronic sclerosing osteomyelitis is a chronic process that is similar to condensing osteitis in that it produces radiopaque lesions. Albers–Schönberg disease is characterized by calcification of the marrow spaces of bones and produces radiopaque lesions. Cherubism produces bilateral lesions characterized by the replacement of bone with fibrous tissue, which produces radiolucencies. Sickle cell anemia produces radiolucent lesions because the bone marrow expands to manufacture more blood cells, resulting in resorption of the calcified parts of bone.

15. Of the restorative materials used in dentistry today, which are the most difficult to distinguish radiographically from caries?
    - a. Zinc oxide
    - b. Composite resin
    - c. Methyl methacrylate
    - d. Zinc phosphate cement
    - e. Calcium hydroxide

    1. a and b
    2. a and c
    3. b and d

    4. c and e
    5. d and e

Dental caries results in a loss of calcified material in the crowns of teeth; such losses are seen radiographically as radiolucent lesions within the radiopaque images of tooth crowns. Both zinc oxide and zinc phosphate cement are radiopaque materials and therefore should not be confused with caries. The other three materials listed are radiolucent.

16. Which of the following anatomic structures appear as radiopacities in periapical radiographs?
    - a. Hamular process
    - b. Anterior nasal spine
    - c. Zygoma
    - d. Submandibular fossa
    - e. Mylohyoid ridge
    - f. Mental foramen
    - g. Lateral fossa

    1. a, b, c, and d
    2. d, e, f, and g
    3. a, b, c, and e
    4. a, c, f, and g
    5. c, d, e, and f

Depressions, fossas, canals, and foramina are parts of bones that present less x-ray absorbing material in the path of the x-ray beam and are therefore radiolucent. Whole calcified structures such as the zygoma and calcified projections such as processes, spines, and ridges produce radiopaque images.

17. Which of the following conditions is most likely if a radiograph shows a dense, diffuse radiopacity at the apex of the distal root of the mandibular left first molar having a filled root canal and widening of the periodontal space at the apex of the mesial root?
    1. Osteoma
    2. Cementoma
    3. Dental granuloma
    4. Sclerosing osteitis
    5. Odontoma

Dental granulomas are radiolucent. Odontomas, osteomas, and cementomas show varying amounts of calcification at different stages of development. Odontomas and osteomas produce relatively well-organized calcified structures and are not usually attached to the apices of teeth; even more rarely do they affect both roots of a tooth. The cementoma is most commonly found at the apices of mandibular anterior teeth. The presence of a root canal filling in the tooth indicates a past infective or traumatic condition. The radiographic evidence that both root apices have undergone diffuse, radiopaque changes strongly suggests sclerosing osteitis.

18. A 19-year-old patient shows a relatively large spherical radiolucency in the left third molar region of the mandible. The patient has a full complement of posterior

teeth with the exception of the mandibular left third molar. The patient says he never had a "wisdom tooth" on that side. Although a definitive diagnosis cannot be made on the basis of radiographic evidence alone, which of the following is suggested?

1. Periodontal cyst
2. Extravasation cyst
3. Primordial cyst
4. Embryonal bone cyst
5. Dentigerous cyst

Both periodontal and dentigerous cysts are associated with existing teeth. Only the primordial cyst is associated with a tooth organ that failed to develop into a tooth. The extravasation cyst is related to trauma, does not usually occur in the third molar region, and usually is not spherical. The embryonal bone cyst is not listed as a dental condition in most textbooks (the designer of a question using this term is probably referring to the idiopathic bone cavity described by Stafne). This lesion is most commonly seen near the angle of the mandible and is located below the mandibular canal.

19. All of the following may have similar radiographic findings except
    1. an ameloblastoma
    2. giant cell lesion
    3. a complex odontoma
    4. an eosinophilic granuloma
    5. a lateral periodontal cyst

Of the five pathologic conditions listed, four produce radiolucent lesions. Only the complex odontoma produces calcified dental tissues which are radiopaque.

20. All the following anatomic structures are usually recognized on intraoral periapical radiographs except the
    1. mental foramen
    2. mylohyoid ridge
    3. coronoid process
    4. pterygoid hamulus
    5. mandibular foramen
    6. infraorbital foramen

The mental foramen and the mylohyoid ridge occur in the body of the mandible and are easily seen on intraoral radiographs. The coronoid process of the mandible and hamulus of the pterygoid plate are commonly seen in maxillary molar radiographs. The mandibular foramen is located in the ramus of the mandible and very rarely appears in mandibular molar radiographs; however, when it does appear the foramen is easily recognized. The infraorbital foramen does not appear on intraoral radiographs since it lies superior to the maxillary sinus.

21. Numerous areas of radiolucency in bones are common to each of the following except
    1. multiple myeloma
    2. hyperparathyroidism
    3. Albers–Schönberg disease
    4. metastatic tumors of bone
    5. malignant melanoma

All of the disease entities listed can produce multiple radiolucent bone lesions except Albers–Schönberg disease. This disease, also known as osteopetrosis, results in sclerosis of the marrow spaces and produces radiopaque lesions. All three neoplastic conditions listed produce multiple areas of bone destruction. Hyperparathyroidism is a generalized condition that is associated with destructive cystlike bone lesions called brown tumors.

22. A periapical radiograph of a mandibular second premolar reveals a sharp right angle deviation of the apical one-third of the root. This is diagnostic of
    1. dilaceration
    2. concrescence
    3. gemination
    4. dens in dente
    5. taurodontism

Dilaceration is a change in the direction of root formation and is usually due to trauma during tooth development. Concrescence is a condition where teeth are joined together by cementum. Gemination results in the formation of a large tooth. Dens in dente shows an invagination of enamel and dentin into the pulp chamber. Taurodontism shows a tooth with a large body and short roots.

23. Multiple discrete apical radiolucencies associated with vital asymptomatic mandibular anterior teeth are most suggestive of
    1. periapical cysts
    2. dental granulomas
    3. immature cementomas
    4. odontogenic cysts
    5. nutrient canals

Multiple periapical cysts in one area would be relatively rare occurrences, while immature cementomas are rather commonly found at the apices of mandibular incisor teeth. Dental granulomas and nutrient canals tend to be associated with trauma and/or infection and may or may not be associated with symptomatic teeth.

24. During a routine dental radiographic examination, a radiolucency is observed at the apex of the mandibular right central incisor. The patient has no subjective symptoms, but the tooth pulp gives no response when tested with ice and with the vitalometer. When the tooth is removed, a firm mass is found attached to its apex. A histologic examination of the mass reveals fibrovascular connective tissue infiltrated with lymphocytes and plasma cells. The microscopic findings in this case are most compatible with a diagnosis of
    1. granuloma
    2. abscess
    3. radicular cyst
    4. apical scar
    5. cementoma

The histologic findings do not include epithelium or a great infiltration of polymorphonuclear leukocytes, which rules out a diagnosis of cyst or abscess. Cementoma is not a probable diagnosis because the tooth was nonvital. The firmness of the mass and its attachment to the tooth upon extraction supports a clinical impression of granuloma.

25. Radiographs of a young adult show that all permanent teeth have small roots and obliterated pulp chambers. These findings are indicative of
   1. achondroplasia
   2. amelogenesis imperfecta
   3. cleidocranial dysostosis
   4. dentiogenesis imperfecta

Permanent teeth with small roots and obliterated pulp chambers are common findings in dentinogenesis imperfecta. Radiographic findings in cleidocranial dysostosis include many supernumerary and unerupted teeth. Amelogenesis imperfecta shows normal dentin and root formation but poorly calcified or thin enamel. Achondroplasia is a condition affecting bone, not teeth.

26. An 18-year-old man complains of a painful swelling in the palate. Examination reveals a soft, fluctuant, tender mass in the midline of the hard palate. The teeth test vital, and there is no evidence of periodontal disease. Radiographs, however, reveal a well-defined radiolucency between the roots of the maxillary central incisors. The clinical and radiographic findings are compatible with the diagnosis of a
   1. lateral periodontal cyst
   2. residual cyst
   3. incisive canal cyst
   4. nasoalveolar cyst

The location in the midline eliminates a nasoalveolar cyst, which would be located in soft tissue lateral to the ala or wing of the nose. Since the maxillary central incisor teeth are present, the midline lesion could not correctly be called a residual cyst. A lateral periodontal cyst located on the mesial of one of the central incisors could conceivably produce the described radiographic and clinical picture, but it probably would not extend upward into the hard palate. The best possibility listed is the incisive canal cyst, which would indeed be located in the midline in the hard palate region.

27. The radiographic examination of a patient 20 years old disclosed a circumscribed radiolucent lesion 2 cm in diameter in the mandibular right molar region. The lesion was sharply outlined but lacked a radiopaque periphery, was somewhat irregularly shaped and extended 5–6 mm above the apices of the molars and 10 mm inferiorly toward the lower border of the mandible. There was no evidence of involvement of the cortex or expansion of the bone, and the lesion was asymptomatic. All teeth tested within a normal vitality range. These findings would suggest

   1. dentigerous cyst
   2. primordial cyst
   3. residual focus of hematopoiesis
   4. hemorrhagic bone cyst

The lack of a radiopaque border and the irregular shape of the lesion indicate that the lesion is unlikely to be a cyst. The noninvolvement of the cortex and the lack of bone expansion do not necessarily rule out a cyst since these changes depend on the size of the lesion. Since the lesion is located apically, it cannot be a dentigerous cyst, which by definition is attached to the crown of an unerupted tooth. The data indicate that the lesion is associated with a tooth; this rules out primordial cyst, which by definition is not attached to a calcified tooth. Both a residual focus of hematopoiesis and a hemorrhagic bone cyst can produce the described radiographic picture; however, residual hematopoiesis is rare in a 20-year-old person and extremely rare at the apex of a tooth, while hemorrhagic lesions are relatively common. Thus hemorrhagic bone cyst is the best selection of the four lesions listed.

28. Tooth vitality is determined radiographically by
   1. abnormal appearance of tooth tissues
   2. the presence of secondary dentin
   3. closeness of caries to pulp
   4. periapical involvement
   5. None of the above

Tooth vitality cannot be determined radiographically. However, radiographs are useful in determining periapical involvement. As in other situations, the practitioner should use them as an adjunct to clinical findings and symptoms to reach a definitive diagnosis.

29. The first radiographic evidence of apical pathology following acute pulpitis is
   1. rarefaction of the alveolar bone
   2. inflammation of the periodontal tissues
   3. condensation of the alveolar bone
   4. thickening of the periodontal space

There is usually no radiographic evidence of changes at the apex during an acute pulpitis because bone destruction has not progressed sufficiently to appear on radiographs. After a period of several days, the first radiographic finding is usually a widening of the periodontal ligament space. This change may or may not be followed by a loss of the apical lamina dura. If there is such a loss, it may be followed in time by condensation of alveolar bone in the region. Neither rarefaction of bone nor inflammation of the periodontal tissues are seen radiographically in the initial stages of acute pulpitis.

30. A radiograph reveals a radiolucent shadow at the apex of the right central incisor. There is no break in the continuity of the lamina dura, and the tooth responds normally to the pulp tester. There are no clinical signs or

symptoms. What is the most probable explanation of the radiolucent shadow?

1. Periapical pathology of unknown etiology
2. Infection
3. Nutrient canal
4. Normal anatomic landmark

If a radiolucent shadow at the apex of an asymptomatic incisor is noted on a radiograph, the first possibility that should be considered is that the shadow is the incisive foramen. The foramen appears as a radiolucency in that area and may be superimposed upon the apex of either central incisor. Observing radiographs taken from different horizontal angles will usually show that the radiolucency changes its relationship to the apex and is not associated with the tooth in question.

Nutrient canals are rarely seen in the maxillary incisor area but occasionally may be seen near the apex of the maxillary cuspid. An infection normally produces signs or symptoms, and it is not evident radiographically unless it is of long duration. Periapical pathology of unknown etiology must be considered if radiographic confirmation of the presence of the incisive foramen cannot be obtained.

31. When a globulomaxillary cyst is present, certain abnormalities appear on a radiograph. The most likely of these is that the cyst
    1. is located lateral to tooth roots
    2. is located at the apex of the tooth
    3. contains the crown of a tooth
    4. contains a mass of calcified material
    5. All of the above

The globulomaxillary cyst appears as a radiolucency between the maxillary lateral incisor and cuspid and in some instances may push these teeth apart. The shape of the radiolucency is sometimes referred to as pear-shaped. There are typically no radiopacities such as tooth crowns or masses of calcified material associated with the radiolucency.

32. A patient, age 45, has pain in the mandible. On radiographic examination, several small, regular, distinct, radiolucent lesions are seen. The laboratory tests show Bence–Jones protein in the urine. The patient probably has
    1. eosinophilic granuloma
    2. malignant melanoma
    3. multiple myeloma
    4. metastatic carcinoma

The radiolucencies described, plus the Bence–Jones protein in the urine, would most strongly suggest multiple myeloma. Similar radiolucent lesions could also be anticipated in the ribs, spinal column, sternum, and skull.

Eosinophilic granuloma may also produce radiolucencies in the mandible, but they are usually not the regular, distinct lesions described here. Intraoral lesions of malignant melanoma are usually confined to the soft tissues; when they are found in the mandible or maxilla, their radiographic appearance is similar to that of lesions resulting from metastatic carcinoma, that is, they are ill-defined polymorphic radiolucencies.

33. Bilateral, asymptomatic, cystlike radiolucent lesions occurring in the bone at the angles of the mandible in a 7-year-old child are most likely related to a condition called
    1. cherubism
    2. static bone cavities
    3. embryonic bone cysts
    4. latent bone cysts
    5. idiopathic bone cavities

All of the above entities may produce radiolucencies at or near the angle of the mandible. However, the only one that usually produces bilateral radiolucencies is cherubism. Static bone cavities or latent bone cysts are radiolucencies which occur in the area of the angle of the mandible but are not open inferiorly. Embryonic cysts or idiopathic bone cavities produce similar unilateral radiolucencies, but they are open inferiorly.

34. A person who has sickle cell anemia may show certain radiographic changes in the bone of the skull. These changes may be
    1. "honeycomb" appearance of bone
    2. pear-shaped radiolucencies
    3. generalized widening of the periodontal spaces
    4. "hair on end" effect
    5. "sunburst" appearance of bone

Radiographic manifestations of certain abnormal conditions are frequently given descriptive names. Examples of such names are the "honeycomb" or "soap bubble" appearance found in some cases of ameloblastoma, the pear-shaped radiolucency of the globulomaxillary cyst, the "sunburst" or "sunray" appearance seen in some cases of osteogenic sarcoma, and finally, the "hair on end" effect sometimes demonstrated in cases of sickle cell anemia. A generalized widening of the periodontal spaces is most often associated with scleroderma.

On lateral or posteroanterior skull radiographs of patients with sickle cell anemia, the "hair on end" effect is due to the loss of the outer cortical plate of the calvaria with the diploë appearing to radiate outward from the inner cortical plate. Some radiologists have also suggested that a further radiographic finding in some cases of this condition is the so-called "stepladder" effect in which the trabeculae appear horizontally parallel to each other. This effect may be seen on intraoral radiographs in the mandibular posterior areas.

35. An occlusal radiograph of a patient's maxillary arch shows a relatively large radiolucent area between the roots of the left lateral incisor and the left canine. The roots of both teeth are displaced laterally. Both teeth

(Continued)

respond positively to pulp vitality tests. On the basis of the information provided, which of the following conditions is most likely?

1. Nasoalveolar cyst
2. Nasopalatine cyst
3. Incisive canal cyst
4. Globulomaxillary cyst

The nasoalveolar cyst is a soft tissue cyst which is located where the maxillary, lateral nasal, and medial nasal processes joined during the development of the face. It is not usually seen radiographically unless there is bone resorption adjacent to the cyst. The nasopalatine or incisive canal cyst is seen as a round to pear-shaped radiolucency in the midline of the maxilla where the palatal shelves of the maxillary processes and the premaxilla united during development. The globulomaxillary cyst is typically seen radiographically as a somewhat pear-shaped radiolucency between the maxillary lateral and cuspid teeth where the globular and maxillary processes united during development.

36. The anatomic structure most commonly superimposed over the apices of the mandibular premolars and interpreted as a pathologic condition is the

1. lingual foramen
2. mental foramen
3. submandibular fossa
4. mandibular canal

All of the above structures appear as radiolucencies or relative radiolucencies on radiographs. When the lingual foramen is seen on radiographs, it appears in the midline of the mandible as a small round radiolucency. The mental foramen appears as a rounded radiolucency in the area of the mandibular premolars and in some instances appears to be superimposed upon the apices of those teeth (particularly the second premolar). The submandibular fossa appears as a relatively radiolucent area, bounded superiorly by the more opaque mylohyoid image (internal oblique ridge) and inferiorly by the inferior cortex of the mandible. The mandibular canal appears as a radiolucent band which horizontally traverses the submandibular fossa.

## RADIATION HYGIENE

In the early years following the discovery of the x-ray in 1895, many dentists suffered the loss of one or more fingers due to the then common practice of holding the films in the patient's mouth and exposing their fingers to repeated doses of x-radiation. Today there is much evidence that x-rays can bring about changes in body chemicals, cells, tissues, and organs and that the effects of the radiation may not become evident for several years after the x-rays have been absorbed. This time lag is called "the latent period."

## Basic Effect of X-Radiation on Living Tissue

X-rays ionize atoms and break chemical bonds. They affect water, for example, by producing free oxygen, hydrogen, and hydoxyl radicals. Recombination of the radicals may produce hydrogen peroxide ($H_2O_2$), or the water parts may combine with other chemicals in the area to form new chemicals that may be foreign to the body and may be poisonous.

## Effect of X-Rays on Structure of Living Things

Cells exposed to radiation can show visible damage. Some cells may have broken chromosomes or vacuoles in the nucleus or cytoplasm. Tissues that grow rapidly and have many cells undergoing mitotic division are more susceptible or sensitive to x-rays and show greater radiation effects. For this reason, oral cancers are often treated with x-rays. However, tissue which has healed after x-ray treatment shows fewer, smaller blood vessels, impaired cell function, and a poor ability to repair itself. X-ray damaged bone and soft tissues are very susceptible to infection and may die, resulting in osteoradionecrosis. The amount of reaction to irradiation depends greatly upon the amount and rate of the dose delivered as well as the volume of tissue irradiated. Damaged tissues can be repaired as long as they have not completely degenerated, although they do not return to their original state. Any irreparable damage is cumulative for repeated doses of x-rays.

Clinical effects may be seen on patients who have undergone radiation therapy or received large doses of x-rays. The tanning and scarring of exposed skin is often referred to as a "radiation burn." A dry mouth and a rampant form of caries often result when the salivary glands are involved. Possible population effects of increased x-ray exposure include an increased incidence of cancer (especially leukemia), birth defects, cataracts, and a shorter life expectancy.

X-rays can cause mutations in all cells, including the germ cells of the reproductive organs. Damage to the genes in the somatic cells is removed from the population when the affected organism dies, but the damage in the germ cells of males or females may be passed on to succeeding generations.

A dose–response curve may be used to plot the effect of the x-ray dose and may show either a threshold or linear type of response. Most somatic effects due to x-rays are thought to produce a threshold dose–response curve which implies that the earliest evidence does not occur until a minimum or threshold dose is reached. The prevailing concept is that genetic effects, however, follow a linear dose–response curve and that any amount of radiation given to the germ cells produces a mutagenic response. Most geneticists agree that almost all mutations are harmful.

## Radiation Dose to the Patient

X-ray dose to the patient can be reduced by a factor of 20 in some cases where good radiation hygiene has not been practiced previously. Fast films require much less radiation to produce a latent image.

X-rays that cannot penetrate teeth and bone are unable to reach the film and are not clinically useful; they are an unnecessary part of the x-ray. However, they do contribute to the dose received by the patient. To remove these useless x-rays the x-ray beam is filtered. Filtration levels are shown in the section on Beam Alterations.

Reducing the size of the x-ray beam also reduces the amount of tissue being irradiated by the primary x-ray beam. Most dental radiologists recommend that the beam size at the patient's skin be collimated to no more than 2.75 in. in diameter.

## Guides for Radiation Protection

A gonadal shield should be used to cover the patient's reproductive tissues. Most dental x-ray shields have x-ray absorbing abilities that are the equivalent of 0.25 mm lead. The shield absorbs the scattered x-rays originating in both the x-ray machine and the irradiated dental area of the patient and prevents these rays from reaching the gonadal area.

Another type of protection involves the open-end cone.

When an open-end cone is used, it is not necessary for the x-ray beam to pass through any plastic material and there is no scattered radiation from primary x-rays.

Dental x-ray machine operators should stay out of the primary x-ray beam, should never hold films for the patient, and should move away from the patient's head a minimum distance of 6 feet. If unable to move 6 feet away from the patient, the operator should stand behind an adequate barrier. The operator may further reduce exposure by standing in areas of less scatter, for example, at right angles to the x-ray beam and towards the back of the patient. The operator should not hold the x-ray tube head during film exposure because a small amount of leakage radiation passes through every dental x-ray machine tube head. The National Council on Radiation Protection (USA) recommends that radiation workers not be exposed to more than 5 roentgens of X-rays per year or approximately 100 milliroentgens per week.

### QUESTIONS

37. The basic effect of x-radiation upon living tissues is
   1. cauterization
   2. precipitation
   3. ionization
   4. agglutination

X-rays are absorbed by the electrons of atoms. The result is usually a free electron (charged negative) and an atom minus an electron (charged positive). The process of forming positive and negative ions is called ionization.

38. The rays which are most likely to be absorbed by the skin and produce an x-ray injury are the
   1. central rays
   2. penetrating x-rays
   3. aluminum filtered x-rays
   4. x-rays of long wavelength
   5. x-rays of short wavelength.

Except for their direction, the x-ray photons in the central ray differ little from photons in other parts of the x-ray beam. Deep penetrating, higher energy (short wavelength) x-rays are absorbed less by the surface skin. Aluminum filtered x-rays have had most of the long wavelength, less penetrating x-rays removed from the x-ray beam.

39. Which of the following statements about radiation are correct?
   a. Roentgen rays can affect the structure of all biologic forms
   b. Developing, young, biologically active cells are particularly susceptible to ionizing radiation.
   c. In dental roentgenography, only the primary, direct beam of radiation is of practical importance as a potential hazard.
   d. In normal adult cells changes which may be brought about by radiation are of short duration, and the effects are soon dissipated.
   1. a and b
   2. b and c
   3. b, c, and d
   4. a and c
   5. All of the above

40. The radiation protection guide advocates that the x-ray dose to operators of dental x-ray machines should not exceed
   1. 100 milliroentgens per week
   2. 10 roentgens per week
   3. 100 roentgens per week
   4. 300 roentgens per week

41. Effective means of reducing patient radiation dose include
   a. proper collimation
   b. increased filtration
   c. fast films
   d. higher kilovoltage
   1. a, b, and c
   2. a and b
   3. b, c, and d
   4. b and c
   5. All of the above

Proper collimation, which restricts the size of the x-ray beam, reduces the amount of the patient's tissue irradiated by the x-ray beam. Increased filtration removes the less energetic and less penetrating x-rays from the beam and thus reduces patient x-ray exposure during radiography. Since fast films require less x-ray energy to expose them, the patient is exposed to significantly less x-radiation when these films are used. Higher kilovoltage produces a beam with more penetrating x-rays and reduces the x-ray dose to tissues between the film and x-ray tube. Higher kilovoltage reduces patient x-ray dose in extraoral radiography; however, there is some debate as to its effectiveness in reducing patient dose in intraoral radiography because, while the entrance dose is reduced, the depth dose is increased.

42. In most states, radiation protection laws or codes require that the diameter of dental x-ray beams measured at the patient's face be of no more than
   1. 2.75 in
   2. 2.5 in.
   3. 2.25 in.
   4. 2 in.

The beam produced by a dental x-ray machine should be no greater than 2.75 in. in diameter at the patient's face. This is stated in radiation protection guides as follows: "For intraoral radiography the beam *should* be no greater than 2.75 inches in diameter and *shall* be no greater than 3.00 inches." The reason for restricting beam size is to limit the volume of tissue exposed to primary radiation. A diameter of 2.75 in. restricts the beam to an area of 7.6 in., while a beam of 3 inches results in the exposure of 9 inches, which is an 18.5% increase in the area exposed.

43. The cells of the body which are least susceptible to x-radiation are
   1. lymphocytes
   2. mature bone
   3. erythroblasts
   4. epithelial cells
   5. connective tissue cells

The various types of cells of the human body have different sensitivities to x-radiation. In general the more rapidly dividing (immature) and the less differentiated a cell is, the greater its sensitivity to x-radiation. Lymphocytes, erythroblasts, and certain reproductive cells are the most sensitive of mammalian cells. Epithelial cells are less sensitive to x-radiation than the three mentioned but more sensitive than connective tissue cells. The least susceptible (most radioresistant) cells in the body of the adult mammal are bone and nerve cells.

44. The reason for adding an aluminum disk in the primary x-ray beam is to
   1. reduce exposure time
   2. reduce long wavelength radiation
   3. reduce the developing time
   4. increase density of exposed film
   5. reduce the diameter of the primary beam

## SUGGESTED READING

ALCOX RW: Dental Radiology—a special area of dental practice. Oral Surg 32:990, 1971

American Dental Association: Radiation hygiene and practice in dentistry, I to V. J Am Dent Assoc 74:1032, 1967; 75:1197, 1967; 76:115, 363, 602, 1968

American Dental Association Council on Dental Materials and Devices: New American Dental Association Specification No. 26 for dental x-ray equipment. J Am Dent Assoc 89:386, 1974

American Dental Association Council on Dental Materials and Devices: Recommendations in radiographic practices. J Am Dent Assoc 90:171, 1975

American Dental Association Council on Dental Materials and Devices: Acceptance program for rapid processing devices for dental radiographic film. J Am Dent Assoc, 91:611, 1975

American Dental Association, Alcox RW: Diagnostic radiation exposures and doses in dentistry. J Am Dent Assoc 76: 1066, 1968

BACHMAN L: Pedodontic radiography. Dent Radiogr Photogr 44:51, 1971

BERKMAN MD: Pedodontic radiographic interpretation. Dent Radiogr Photogr 44:27, 1971

BHASKAR SN: Synopsis of Oral Pathology, 4th ed. St. Louis, CV Mosby, 1975

BHASKAR SN: Roentgenographic Interpretation for the Dentist. 2nd ed. St. Louis, CV Mosby, 1975

Diagnostic x-ray systems—rules and regulations. Federal Register 37:16461, 1972

FREY NW, WUEHRMANN AH: Radiation dosimetry and intraoral radiographic techniques. I. X-ray beam patterns within the head. Oral Surg 38:151, 1974

FREY NW, WUEHRMANN AH: Radiation dosimetry and intraoral radiographic techniques. II. Internal and external dose measurements. Oral Surg 38:639, 1974

GOLDSTEIN IL, MOBLEY WH, CHELLEMI SJ: The observer process in the visual interpretation of radiographs. J Dent Educ 35:485, 1971

GORLIN RJ, GOLDMAN HM: Thoma's Oral Pathology, 6th ed. St. Louis, CV Mosby, 1970

KASLE MJ: An Atlas of Dental Radiographic Anatomy. Philadelphia, WB Saunders, 1973

LEE W: Comparative radiation doses in dental radiography. Oral Surg 37:962, 1974

LUND TM, MANSON-HING LR: Relations between booth positions and focal troughs of panoramic machines. Oral Surg 40:285, 1975

MANSON-HING LR: On the evaluation of radiographic techniques. Oral Surg 27:631, 1969

MANSON-HING LR: Panoramic Dental Radiography. Springfield, IL, CC Thomas, 1976

MENA CA: Taurodontism. Oral Surg 32:812–823, 1971

MESCHAN I: Analysis of Roentgen Signs in General Radiology. Philadelphia, WB Saunders, 1973

National Academy of Sciences: The effects on populations of exposure to low levels of ionizing radiation. Washington DC, National Research Council, 1972

National Council on Radiation Protection and Measurements: Dental x-ray protection, NCRP report No. 35. Washington DC, NCRP Publications, 1970

National Council on Radiation Protection and Measurements: Basic radiation protection criteria, NCRP report No. 39. Washington DC, NCRP Publications, 1971

National Council on Radiation Protection and Measurements: Review of the current state of radiation protection philosophy, NCRP report No. 43. Washington DC, NCRP Publications, 1975

Principles of Dental Radiography. Milwaukee, General Electric, 1977

RICHARDS AG: Radiation barriers. Oral Surg 25:701, 1968

SHAFER WG, HINE MK, LEVY BM: A Textbook of Oral Pathology, 2nd ed. Philadelphia, WB Saunders, 1963

STAFNE EC: Oral roentgenographic diagnosis. Philadelphia, WB Saunders, 1958

USPHS Department of HEW: Fast film exposure and processing in dental radiography. Washington DC, US Government Printing Office, 1970

WUEHRMANN AH, MANSON-HING LR: Dental Radiology, 4th ed. St. Louis, CV Mosby, 1977

X-rays in Dentistry. New York, Eastman Kodak, 1972

**ANSWER KEY**

| | | | |
|---|---|---|---|
| 1. 4 | 12. 2 | 23. 3 | 34. 4 |
| 2. 1 | 13. 2 | 24. 1 | 35. 4 |
| 3. 2 | 14. 2 | 25. 4 | 36. 2 |
| 4. 1 | 15. 4 | 26. 3 | 37. 3 |
| 5. 4 | 16. 3 | 27. 4 | 38. 4 |
| 6. 5 | 17. 4 | 28. 5 | 39. 1 |
| 7. 2 | 18. 3 | 29. 4 | 40. 1 |
| 8. 1 | 19. 3 | 30. 4 | 41. 5 |
| 9. 2 | 20. 6 | 31. 1 | 42. 1 |
| 10. 4 | 21. 3 | 32. 3 | 43. 2 |
| 11. 4 | 22. 1 | 33. 1 | 44. 2 |

# 14
# ORAL SURGERY AND PAIN CONTROL

## Marvin E. Revzin

## ORAL SURGERY

### Preoperative Evaluation

The several ways of determining the health status of a patient prior to surgery range from a complete classical health history obtained by verbal or written questions to a series of computerized laboratory tests performed as a battery by sophisticated machines. Whichever method is used, the doctor must be able to apply the gathered information in an intelligent and purposeful way. The major reason for any preoperative evaluation is to determine what is wrong with the patient and whether the patient is able to withstand the contemplated testing and curing procedures. The parts of any preoperative evaluation then must include some form of a health history supplemented by either diagnostic laboratory tests, radiographs, study models, if necessary, and, of course, a physical examination. Although a diagnosis and/or evaluation are similar, the two are not identical. A diagnosis implies no judgment, whereas an evaluation is all judgment.

Preoperative evaluation therefore includes a working diagnosis obtained by all the aids described, plus a judgment about the physiologic and psychologic condition of the patient's ability to handle the recommended plan of treatment of the diagnosed disease process. The major physiologic categories to be considered in the patient who requires oral surgery are cardiovascular, respiratory, endocrine, neurologic, renal, and hematopoietic. Preoperative evaluation must also include a current assessment of the psychologic or emotional status of the patient. The vital signs of blood pressure, pulse, respiration, weight, and temperature as well as the patient's physical appearance, color, stance, gait, and general signs of being alert and mentally aware, are the base line for evaluation. All doctors must be observant; they must be able to detect color, shape, and symmetry accurately and to note variations in size, texture of skin, mucosa, and hair because sometimes even slight changes may be clues that deserve additional attention in assessing a patient's condition. Such signs as shortness of breath, when it occurs, a cough,

swellings due to fluid retention are important in the evaluation process. So, too, are pains and irregularities in the vital signs.

A thorough understanding of the normal physiologic processes is a requirement in understanding how diseases may affect a patient's ability to undergo surgical procedures. It is not enough to know that a patient has "heart disease." It is essential to know what kind and how it interferes with routine activities. For example, a patient with heart disease who has either no limitation of activity or only mild restriction may usually be managed successfully even as an ambulant patient, whereas one who is short of breath with modest exertion or one who has severe limitations placed on normal activities requires consultation and extra caution before being treated, if at all, for any elective procedure. Respiratory disease signs and symptoms may be associated with cardiovascular problems, and the originating causes of such symptoms as chest pain, shortness of breath, and cough must be identified. Lung diseases such as emphysema or obstructive illnesses such as asthma and bronchiectasis require thorough assessment before any anesthetic is given or any surgery is performed.

Neurologic and psychologic evaluation are often conducted at the same time even though they are frequently independent of each other. Evaluation of the neurologic system, particularly the diseases of the cranial nerves or the central system that affect the patient's ability to withstand the surgery, must include assessments of the effect of medications and the patient's ability to understand and cooperate with the doctor. Seizure disorders and those which interfere with conscious motor control are important examples of this kind.

Patients with urinary system disease may have a condition that would be seriously compromised if kidney function is interfered with or, on the other hand, may have a simple urinary tract infection that responds readily to antibiotic treatment by the physician before the oral surgery is scheduled. Renal disease may be primary, or it may be a consequence of other systemic problems such as hypertension or diabetes. In either case, the type and severity is important to the patient's ability to accept oral surgery safely.

Although many systems might affect surgery, a bleeding disorder usually causes special concern to the surgeon. If a patient tells of previous bleeding episodes due to trauma or surgery, a thorough evaluation is mandatory. Patients with bleeding disorders are classified according to the deficiency they have, and these deficiencies may range from a vitamin K deficiency to classic hemophilia, a Factor VIII (antihemophilic globulin) deficiency, or hemophilia B, a Factor IX deficiency in Christmas disease. Patients with von Willebrand's disease, sometimes called vascular hemophilia, may bleed severely after one surgical procedure and only normally after another, which makes this disease difficult to detect by history alone. Bleeding disorders that result from medication such as heparin or other anticoagulants, e.g., coumarin, present solvable problems if the patient is evaluated properly. Patients with advanced liver disease are at risk because this organ is involved in the manufacture of several of the coagulation factors. The various anemias may have an impact on contemplated procedures because deficiencies may impede healing, increase anesthetic risks, or make these patients more susceptible to infections. Serious malignant changes in the hematopoietic systems, such as the various forms of leukemia, complicate the intended, necessary oral surgery because of the patient's higher risk of infections, spread of the disease, or inability to heal.

The most common endocrine disorder is diabetes, an endocrine–metabolic disorder which ranges from minor to serious involvement of the body's ability to regulate the metabolism of carbohydrates, lipids, and proteins. It also affects the body's acid–base balance. The cause is unknown, but treatment is directed at regulating carbohydrate metabolism either by diet, oral hypoglycemic agents, or insulin, each chosen by the physician depending upon the degree of metabolic disharmony. Patients with diabetes are at increased risk in regard to infection and stress. The dentist should be aware that the stress of oral surgery may precipitate hypoglycemia that requires treatment with orange juice given orally or with intravenous glucose. Other endocrine disorders of importance to patients undergoing dental surgery are thyroid and adrenal problems. In each, the patient's physician should be consulted, for these endocrine system aberrations may have a considerable effect on the patient before, during, and after any surgical procedure.

## QUESTIONS

1. A patient is taking a coumarin drug and requires the extraction of two teeth. This may be safely performed when
   1. the prothrombin time is three times the normal control
   2. the prothrombin time a week prior to surgery was two times the normal control
   3. the prothrombin time the day before surgery was two times the normal control
   4. the coumarin was discontinued an hour before surgery
   5. the coumarin dose was increased before surgery to prevent a thrombus from forming

2. A young white male gives a history of prolonged bleeding following previous cuts and complains of swollen knee joints. Complete blood studies most probably will indicate that he suffers from which of the following hematopoietic disorders?
   1. Christmas disease
   2. Von Willebrand's disease
   3. Sickle cell anemia
   4. Factor VIII deficiency
   5. Stuart–Power factor deficiency

3. A patient who gives a history of heavy alcohol use is at increased risk of prolonged bleeding following surgery because
   1. alcoholism affects the liver, which is the site of coagulation factors
   2. alcoholism affects the snythesis of vitamin C
   3. the alcoholic patient will not follow postoperative instructions
   4. sickling traits are frequently found in alcoholics
   5. Factor IX deficiencies are increased in heavy alcohol users

4. Vitamin K is useful in the treatment of postextraction hemorrhage when the cause of the bleeding is determined to be due to
   1. Christmas disease
   2. prolonged prophylactic antibiotic therapy
   3. a prothrombin deficiency
   4. thrombocytopenic purpura
   5. lowered platelet count

5. A 25-year-old white man presents with a slightly mobile lower molar and a swelling in the submaxillary triangle. He complains of weakness and anorexia. His hemogram is

   Hb: 11g
   WBC: 100,000
   Neutrophils: 90%
   Lymphocyte: 9%
   Monocyte: 1%
   Eosinophils: 0%

   The most probable diagnosis is
   1. infectious mononucleosis
   2. myelogenous leukemia
   3. sickle cell crisis
   4. infection of dental origin
   5. thrombocytopathia

6. Patients with heart disease who have some limitations placed upon their normal activity are best managed for surgical procedures by
   1. compulsory hospitalization and a general anesthetic
   2. indefinite delay of all surgery

(Continued)

**Table 14-1.   Suggested Laboratory Tests for Selected Diseases and Conditions**

ABSCESS
  White blood cell and differential counts
  Culture and sensitivity

ADDISON'S DISEASE
  Blood Glucose

ANEMIAS
  Hematocrit

BACTERIAL INFECTIONS
  Culture and sensitivity

BENIGN TUMORS
  Biopsy

BONE MARROW DEPRESSION
  White blood cells and differential counts

CANDIDIASIS
  Biopsy
  Culture and sensitivity
  Exfoliative cytology (PAS Stain)

CHRISTMAS DISEASE
  Clotting time
  PTT (partial thromboplastin time)

CHRONIC GRANULOCYTIC LEUKEMIA
  White blood cell and differential counts
  Philadelphia chromosome

DIABETES INSIPIDUS
  Urinalysis

DIABETES MELLITUS
  Blood glucose
  Cholesterol
  Triglycerides

DICUMAROL THERAPY
  PT (prothrombin time)

EXCESS VITAMIN D
  Calcium
  Phosphorus

FUNGAL INFECTIONS
  Biopsy
  Culture
  Intradermal tests

HEMOPHILIA
  Clotting time
  PTT (partial thromboplastin time)

HEPARIN THERAPY
  Clotting time

HEPATITIS
  BSP (bromsulphalein dye)
  HAA (hepatitis associated antigen)
  Alkaline phosphatase
  Cholesterol
  Triglycerides

HERPES SIMPLEX
  Biopsy
  Exfoliative cytology

HYPERINSULINISM
  Blood glucose

HYPERPARATHYROIDISM
  Calcium
  Phosphorus

HYPERTHYROIDISM
  PBI (protein bound iodine)
  $T_3$ (triiodothyronine)
  $T_4$ (total thyroxine)
  Blood glucose
  Cholesterol
  Triglycerides

HYPOFRIBINOGENEMIA
  Clotting time
  Protein electrophoresis

HYPOPARATHYROIDISM
  Calcium
  Phosphorus

HYPOPROTHROMBINEMIA
  PT (prothrombin time)

HYPOTHYROIDISM
  (same as for hyperthyroidism)

INFECTIONS
  White blood cell and differential counts
  Blood glucose
  Culture and sensitivity

IRON DEFICIENCY ANEMIA
  Hematocrit

JAUNDICE
  Alkaline phosphatase
  HAA (hepatitis associated antigen)

LEUKEMIA
  White blood cell and differential counts

LUPUS ERYTHEMATOSUS
  LE prep
  ANA (antinuclear antibody)

MALIGNANT TUMORS
  Biopsy

PERNICIOUS ANEMIA
  Hematocrit

POLYCYTHEMIA
  Hematocrit

RECURRENT SQUAMOUS CELL CARCINOMA
  Exfoliative cytology

RHEUMATIC FEVER
  ASO (antistreptolysin O titer)

SICKLE CELL ANEMIA
  Hematocrit
  Sickledex
  Hemoglobin electrophoresis

SYPHILIS
  RPR (rapid plasma reagin)
  VDRL (veneral disease research laboratory)
  FTA-ABS (fluorescent Treponema antibody absorption)

TUBERCULOSIS
  Mantoux test
  Fluorescent antibody techniques

VITAMIN K DEFICIENCY
  PT (prothrombin time)

3. selective surgery performed after consultation with patient's physician
4. the use of local anesthetic without vasoconstrictors

7. A patient has an extremely painful tooth which requires extraction. Her blood pressure is 170/100. The proper way to proceed would be to
   1. refer the patient to a physician but give her an analgesic prescription
   2. determine whether the patient is under treatment for hypertension, use anesthetic agents compatible with any drugs being taken, and remove the tooth
   3. refer the patient to an oral surgeon because the patient should have a general anesthetic
   4. use a local anesthetic without a vasoconstrictor and remove the tooth
   5. use mild sedation, with local anesthetics compatible with patient's medication, and remove the tooth

8. A patient reports that he has had anginal chest pains and that he has his own nitroglycerin tablets. He needs to have a single tooth extracted. Which of the following should the dentist do?
   1. Simply remove the tooth under local anesthesia and send him on his way.
   2. Use supplemental oxygen and a tablet of nitroglycerin prior to the local anesthetic and then proceed.
   3. Postpone all surgery until the physician gives permission
   4. Admit the patient to the hospital and remove the tooth under general anesthesia in the operating room.
   5. Consult with physician, have oxygen available, use preoperative nitroglycerin tablets as indicated, use local anesthesia, and extract the tooth.

9. A medical history reveals that the patient has the following signs and symptoms: polyuria, polydipsia, and weight loss. What is the possible diagnosis?
   1. Polynephritis
   2. Diabetes mellitus
   3. Hyperthyroidism
   4. Infection of dental origin
   5. Addison's disease

10. Prior to performing an extraction for a new patient, the dentist should
    a. obtain a complete medical history
    b. record temperature, blood pressure, pulse, and respiration
    c. obtain a complete blood count, plus bleeding and coagulation times
    d. order an electrocardiogram and chest x-ray
    e. Consult with the patient's physician if a significant medical problem exists
    1. a, b, and c
    2. a, c, and d
    3. b, c, and d
    4. a, b, and e
    5. a, b, c, and e

11. A 45-year-old man requests the extraction of his ten remaining maxillary teeth in order to have a denture constructed. The medical history reveals that he suffered a myocardial infarction 4 months previously. He is on anticoagulant medication which keeps his prothrombin time at 30 sec and a control of 12 sec. The proper course of treatment is to
    1. hospitalize the patient for proposed extractions
    2. consult the physician to reduce anticoagulants
    3. perform extractions under heavy sedation
    4. delay the elective extractions for a minimum of 6 months after the infarction
    5. extract the teeth, but take proper precautions to prevent postoperative bleeding

12. Exophthalmos is a sign of which of the following endocrine disorders?
    1. Hypoparathyroidism
    2. Hypothyroidism
    3. Hypoadrenalism
    4. Hyperthyroidism
    5. Hyperinsulinism

13. Patients who have rheumatic or congenital valvular heart disease are given prophylactic antibiotics before oral surgery to
    1. prevent recurrent rheumatic fever
    2. prevent subacute bacterial endocarditis
    3. reduce circulating bacteria
    4. prevent myocardial infarcts
    5. prevent arrhythmias

14. A hypoglycemic episode might occur in a patient taking 20 units of insulin and undergoing an extraction because the patient
    1. omitted breakfast
    2. ate cake before the extraction
    3. had an infection
    4. walked to the office
    5. had no exercise at all that morning

15. Patients with adrenal insufficiency and those who are treated with steriods for prolonged periods of time are an increased surgical risk because
    1. shock caused by increased stress stimulates epinephrine flow
    2. shock is not reversed by vasoconstrictors such as epinephrine
    3. steriods are useless in reversing the shock
    4. tissues heal more slowly due to higher glucose content in the blood stream

## Diagnosis

Although preoperative evaluation and diagnosis may become one and the same, there are sufficient differences to warrant a few words to distinguish the two. While preoperative evaluation is concerned with the total patient, diagnosis focuses on a specific item or group of items. Diagnosis describes lumps and bumps, as well as deviations from expected norms of function and form. It includes the mental as well as the physical state of health and disease. In effect, the diagnosis is made by establishing the chief complaint of the patient and then using all the clinical and laboratory tests required to reach a presumptive or working diagnosis; sometimes a list of possible diagnoses, called a differential diagnosis, is made. The final diagnosis may range from a simple infected tooth whose owner's chief complaint was that "it hurts" to an occult, difficult to label, and unusual process which defies a final diagnosis.

In order to make the diagnosis, the standard methods of physical examination—inspection, palpation, percussion, and auscultation—are modified for use in and about the oral cavity. Bimanual palpation of structures in the mouth conveys useful information regarding any masses encountered. A stethoscope is used on the temporomandibular joints to pick up sounds diagnostic of arthritic changes. Visual inspection of the tissues in the oral cavity and percussion of the teeth in their arches are standard procedures. These clinical methods are augmented by radiographic examinations, and differential diagnoses are frequently made possible by the kinds and locations of images. Study models, pulp tests, and the whole gamut of chemical laboratory examinations are also available. Biopsies of hard and soft tissues and the examination of body fluids and secretions may often be the only way to arrive at a definite diagnosis.

To make a diagnosis, which means to distinguish, the dentist must be able to distinguish the normal from the abnormal in that which is being studied.

## QUESTIONS

16. A patient's chief complaint is that a painless, soft lesion has been present on the mucous membrane side of the lower lip. It has varied in size and has a slight blue color to it. This describes a(n)
    1. fibroma
    2. hemangioma
    3. mucocele
    4. cystic carcinoma
    5. lymphangioma

17. A patient complains of significant discomfort in all the left maxillary posterior teeth. All these teeth are sensitive to percussion, but react normally to vitality testing. Palpation in the mucobuccal fold produces discomfort. The most probable diagnosis is
    1. an acute periapical abscess with referred pain to the remaining teeth
    2. generalized periodontal disease
    3. acute maxillary sinusitis
    4. tic douloureux

18. A patient has an abscessed second mandibular molar with a firm swelling beneath the mandibular border, trismus, and a temperature of 102° F. The infection has spread to the
    1. sublingual space
    2. infratemporal space
    3. submental space
    4. submandibular space below the mylohyoid muscle
    5. temporal space below the masseter M. attachment

19. A 48-year-old man complains of a pain in the left mandible. Clinical examination shows no dental caries, periodontal disease, or expansile lesions of the mandible; the teeth are vital. Radiographs reveal a radiolucent area enveloping the left mandibular second premolar. History is negative for recent trauma, but it reveals that a similar lesion of the calvaria was treated 2 years previously as an eosinophilic granuloma. The most probable diagnosis of the mandibular lesion is
    1. hyperparathyroidism
    2. histiocytosis
    3. squamous cell carcinoma
    4. osteoma
    5. osteomalacia

20. A cytologic smear of a suspicious-looking lesion is reported back as negative. Which of the following should be done?
    1. Place the patient on antibiotics.
    2. Repeat the smear in 30 days.
    3. Perform a biopsy of the lesion.
    4. Place the patient on a semiannual recall.
    5. Refer the patient for a complete blood count.

21. A small (0.4 cm) pedunculated, nonpainful firm growth has been present on the patient's buccal mucosa, along the tooth line, for about 2 months. The patient occasionally bites it accidentally. This is best treated by
    1. incisional biopsy
    2. total excision and histologic examination of the specimen
    3. correcting the occlusion to prevent biting
    4. irradiation of less than 3000 rads
    5. semiannual observation and reassurance

22. Squamous cell carcinoma of the lower lip can best be diagnosed by
    a. incisional biopsy
    b. cytologic smear
    c. excisional biopsy
    d. toluidine blue staining
    1. All of the above
    2. Both a and b
    3. Both b and c

23. A sudden swelling of the lip which comes and goes without apparent cause is most likely
    1. a mucocele
    2. angioneurotic edema
    3. a lymphangioma
    4. a hemangioma
    5. an aneurysm

24. A 50-year-old man has a slow enlargement of his maxilla and a gradual loss of hearing and vision. A differential diagnosis should include
    1. ossifying fibroma
    2. Paget's disease
    3. ameloblastoma
    4. eosinophilic granuloma
    5. osteomalacia

25. A 12-year-old boy complains of a severe sore throat; then his extremity joints became swollen and painful at times. These signs and symptoms suggest
    1. rheumatic fever
    2. osteoarthritis
    3. rheumatoid arthritis
    4. rubella
    5. rubeola

26. A patient has numerous radiolucent areas in the mandible and the facial bones. Laboratory tests reveal an elevated Bence–Jones protein. Differential diagnosis should include
    1. general lymphomatosis
    2. Hodgkin's lymphoma
    3. multiple myeloma
    4. hyperparathyroidism
    5. histiocytosis X

27. A patient has a sharp excruciating pain localized in the left canine fossa. The pain can be elicited by simply touching the area lightly; the teeth are free of pathosis. The patient most likely has
    1. sphenopalatine neuralgia
    2. a typical neuralgia
    3. Eagle's syndrome
    4. trigeminal neuralgia
    5. Bell's palsy

28. A patient whose eosinophil count is markedly elevated may have any of the following except
    1. allergic reaction
    2. parasitic infections
    3. asthma
    4. pemphigus
    5. acute dental abscess

29. Radiographic examination is useful in diagnosing all but one of the following cysts.
    1. Globulomaxillary
    2. Nasoalveolar
    3. Traumatic bone
    4. Follicular
    5. Radicular

30. A patient with a serious infection of dental origin has eyelid and periorbital edema, ptosis, and paresis of the third, fourth, and sixth cranial nerves. A differential diagnosis must include
    1. superior temporal space infection
    2. cavernous sinus thrombosis
    3. masticator space infection
    4. Ludwig's angina
    5. maxillary sinus infection

## Surgical Principles and Treatment

There are several major areas of concern to those who practice the full scope of oral and maxillofacial surgery: 1) the extraction of erupted and impacted teeth; 2) the preparation of the mouth for prostheses; 3) the management of benign and malignant tumors of the oral cavity; 4) the treatment of affectations of the salivary glands; 5) the surgical and supportive therapy of infections; 6) trauma to the teeth, arches, and jaws, as well as the contiguous soft tissues; 7) the surgical correction of acquired and congenital craniofacial deformities; and 8) the diagnosis and treatment of pathosis of the temporomandibular joints and their articulations. Principles of treatment depend upon an accurate diagnosis of the problem, a thorough understanding of the physiology of the pathosis involved, an understanding of the anatomy of the area involved, and an appreciation for the patient's psychic and physical reaction both to the condition and to the proposed therapy.

In line with the often repeated adage of surgery, "First, do no harm," successful surgery requires good anesthesia, excellent visibility, good access to the area, gentle handling of the tissues, excellent hemostasis, and concern for the total patient. In addition, the surgeon must have excellent vision and manual dexterity. Reduced to the basics all surgery involves a working diagnosis to remove, correct, eradicate, or restore. An incision is made, parts are removed or reassembled, and the wound is closed or treated so that the natural processes of repair may proceed as rapidly as possible. Normal tissue must not be compromised without good reason, but pathologic tissue must be entirely removed whenever possible.

Planning for the reconstructive phase of the process must occur at the time of the ablative surgery. Even in such a common dental surgical procedure as the extraction of a single tooth, thought must be given to the prosthetic replacement that will occupy its space. The extraction must be carried out in such a way as to leave an appropriate ridge for reconstruction.

### QUESTIONS

31. Principles of correct surgical flap design should include
    a. broad flap bases
    b. flaps which contain mucosa, submucosa, and periosteum
    c. incisions placed over bone
    d. vertical or diagonal releasing incisions
    e. incisions through mucosa followed by elevation of submucosa and periosteum
    1. All except b and c
    2. All except d
    3. All except e
    4. a and e
    5. a, b, and c

32. The Caldwell–Luc procedure is an approach to the
    1. masticator space
    2. maxillary sinus
    3. ethmoid sinus
    4. mediastinum
    5. submandibular space

33. The principal deterrent to normal wound healing is
    1. poor nutrition
    2. torn wound edges
    3. infection
    4. excessive bleeding
    5. inadequate suturing

34. A patient dislocated her left mandibular condyle 12 hours ago. Attempts at reducing the dislocation are unsuccessful. Probably the major reason is a(n)
    1. acute spasm of the masseter muscle
    2. mechanical obstruction caused by an articular eminence that is too large
    3. acute spasm of the external pterygoid muscle
    4. acute spasm of the internal pterygoid muscle
    5. acute spasm of the temporalis muscle

35. A closed fracture is one which is characterized by
    1. a lack of bone displacement
    2. an intact periosteum
    3. a lack of communication between the fracture site and an external surface
    4. communication between the fracture site and the oral cavity only
    5. an overlapping of the fractural bone edges

36. A horizontal fracture of the maxilla below the level of the orbits is classified as a
    1. Le Fort I fracture
    2. Le Fort II fracture
    3. Le Fort III fracture
    4. Zygomatico-maxillary complex fracture
    5. Caldwell–Luc fracture

37. A painful arthritic temporomandibular joint is treated with an injection of hydrocortisone. Its effect is to
    1. increase blood supply to the area
    2. decrease external pterygoid muscle spasm
    3. provide an antiinflammatory response
    4. remove bone spurs from the condyle
    5. lubricate the synovial lining

38. Bony ankylosis of the temporomandibular joint is treated by
    1. steroid injections into the joint
    2. surgical procedures
    3. immobilizing the jaws with wires
    4. rest, soft diet, heat, and aspirin
    5. occlusal equilibration

39. A 50-year-old man has a maxillary second molar that is the only remaining posterior tooth on that side. It has served as an abutment, but now it must be extracted. Care must be taken during the extraction to prevent
    1. postoperative osteitis
    2. displacement into the infratemporal fossa
    3. removing the floor of the maxillary sinus with the tooth
    4. pushing the palatal root into the nasal cavity
    5. the patient's swallowing the tooth

40. In the problem described in question 39, the best way to proceed would be to

    1. use a number 88 beaked forceps
    2. prepare a flap and remove the tooth surgically
    3. use a suitable forceps with the major forces directed toward the palate
    4. use a suitable forceps and direct a strong, sudden force down and out
    5. use a suitable forceps and direct a strong rotary force to twist the tooth from its socket

41. Swelling beneath the eye due to an abscessed maxillary canine tooth occurs because
    1. maxillary bone is very porous
    2. venous drainage takes place in that direction
    3. the root apex of the tooth lies above the attachment of the levator labii superioris and the caninus muscles
    4. an allergic reaction to the infection is present
    5. the maxillary antrum is involved

42. Differential blood studies to indicate an acute pyogenic bacterial infection would show
    1. increased lymphocytes
    2. increased eosinophils
    3. neutrophilic leukocytosis
    4. neutrophilic leukopenia
    5. decreased lymphocytes

43. Trismus due to dental infection occurs because one of the following anatomic spaces is involved. Which?
    1. Masticator
    2. Retropharyngeal
    3. Lateral pharyngeal
    4. Sublingual
    5. Submental

44. A fracture of the mandibular condyle may be drawn forward and medially because of the pull of which of the following muscles?
    1. Deep masseter
    2. External pterygoid
    3. Internal pterygoid
    4. Temporalis
    5. Digastric

45. Hemorrhage, a major consideration in emergency maxillofacial injuries can usually be controlled by
    1. clamping and tying the torn vessels
    2. suturing the largest available flaps
    3. applying pressure on the wound
    4. tying the major arteries of the area, e.g., the external carotid
    5. administering fresh whole blood

46. Mandibular impacted third molars are classified according to the
    a. relation of the impaction to the ramus
    b. relation of the impaction to the long axis of the second mandibular molar
    c. depth of the impaction in the mandible
    d. direction of the crown of the impaction in relation to the occlusal table
    e. relation of the impacted molar to the inferior alveolar canal

1. a and b
2. a and c
3. All but c
4. All but e
5. c, d, and e

47. The pterygomandibular space may be approached intraorally in order to drain a purulent abscess. Which of the following muscles is most likely to be incised in order to gain access to this space?
    1. Masseter
    2. Temporalis
    3. Buccinator
    4. Medial pterygoid
    5. Inferior pharyngeal constrictor

48. Alveoloplasties following extractions should adhere to which of the following principles?
    1. Conserve bone.
    2. Suture tightly to approximate cut gingiva.
    3. Use only absorbable sutures.
    4. Use bone wax to build contours.
    5. Reduce tuberosities to sinus floor levels for denture access.

49. The proximal segment of an edentulous mandibular angle fracture is usually displaced
    1. posteriorly
    2. inferiorly
    3. anteriorly and inferiorly
    4. anteriorly and superiorly
    5. medially only

50. The root most likely to be pushed into the maxillary sinus during a dental extraction is
    1. buccal root of the maxillary second premolar
    2. palatal root of the maxillary first molar
    3. palatal root of the maxillary second molar
    4. mesiobuccal root of the maxillary first molar
    5. mesiobuccal root of the maxillary second molar

## Intraoperative and Postoperative Treatment and Complications

The scope of oral surgery includes, but is not limited to, extraction of normally erupted, malposed, and impacted teeth; the preparation of the mouth by surgical procedures to receive prosthetic appliances; the surgical and supportive treatment of infections of local and systemic origins which appear in and about the oral cavity; the treatment of trauma to the soft and hard tissues of the teeth, jaws, and surrounding areas; the surgical management of tumors, benign and malignant; the treatment of sinus problems caused by dental disease; the surgical management of growth and development malfunctions by the appropriate orthognathic procedures; treatment of temporomandibular joint problems by surgical and adjunctive means; the restoration of form and function following the loss of bone and soft tissues of the jaws; the surgical treatment of congenital defects such as cleft lip and palate; and the

treatment of neurologic disorders such as those found in trigeminal neurologies

QUESTIONS

51. A patient with classic signs of postextraction infection requires antibiotics. The microorganisms are resistant to all antimicrobials except chloramphenicol. With what undesirable side-effects has this medication been associated?
    1. Eighth nerve destruction
    2. Bone marrow depression
    3. Pemphigoid eruptions of skin
    4. Hypersplenism
    5. Loss of speech

52. Proper treatment for postextraction alveolitis, "dry socket," should consist of
    1. thorough curettage of the socket
    2. irrigation with Monsel's solution
    3. gentle removal of debris, irrigation, and dressing of the socket with an obtundent
    4. gentle anesthetization of the area and use of a bur to place holes in the socket and start fresh bleeding
    5. cleaning of debris from socket and placing of sulfa crystals in wound

53. A patient returns 6 hours after a lower molar extraction bleeding from the extraction site. Bright red blood continues to emerge from the alveolus. The dentist should
    a. ligate the facial artery
    b. call an ambulance and admit the patient to a hospital
    c. use an aspirator to evacuate blood, place pressure gauze packs over wound, and reanesthetize with a local anesthetic containing a vasoconstrictor
    d. determine where bleeding is coming from and place pressure packs and sutures appropriately
    e. try to lower blood pressure to reduce bleeding
    1. a and e
    2. b and c
    3. c and d
    4. d and e
    5. All of the above

54. Following the removal of a lower molar tooth, the patient complains of numbness of the lip on the same side even after 10 days have passed. The dentist should explain that
    1. all lower molar extractions result in temporary numbness and that it will get better
    2. there must have been an infection at the root ends and that the numbness will disappear when the wound is completely healed
    3. numbness is a sign of a tumor and the patient should see a specialist
    4. the nerve was traumatized during the extraction and will heal in a month or so
    5. the patient didn't follow postoperative instructions and an infection developed following the extraction

55. A patient who received a tumoricidal dose of external radiation for a laryngeal malignant tumor 4 months

*(Continued)*

earlier needs to have a lower molar tooth extracted. The most likely consequence of an extraction for this patient is

1. nothing eventful
2. delayed return of sensation to the jaws
3. a localized osteitis
4. an osteoradionecrosis
5. unusual and prolonged bleeding

56. During the extraction of a maxillary molar a snap is heard and the tooth in the forceps shows that the palatal root has not been removed with the rest of the tooth. Attempts are made to retrieve the root but it disappears. The dentist is certain that it is in the maxillary sinus. In order to retrieve it the dentist must

1. enlarge the alveolus opening with a large bur and rongeurs
2. place ¼-in. gauze strips into the sinus and try to trap the root
3. close the socket opening with sutures and tell the patient what happened
4. have the patient close the nostrils and attempt to blow the root tip out of the socket
5. close the wound and open the maxillary sinus through the canine fossa

57. Primary consideration in the emergency treatment phase of patients with facial trauma should be to

1. administer antibiotics and a titetanus medication
2. observe patient closely for 24 hours prior to beginning definitive treatment
3. take care of airway, stop any hemorrhage, and watch neurologic status
4. reduce bone fractures and suture soft tissue
5. reduce fractures in order to stop bleeding

58. An apicoectomy is performed on a maxillary lateral incisor. The surgeon must be careful not to damage the

1. maxillary sinus
2. nasal floor
3. incisive canal contents
4. labial frenum
5. anterior alveolar nerve

59. Fractures of the mandible body that have a fairly complete dentition are best treated by

1. intraosseous wiring via external approach
2. intraosseous wiring via intraoral approach
3. Kirschner wire skewering
4. closed reduction via intermaxillary wiring
5. cast-cap splints

60. The most accepted way of treating a patient with trismus and an elevated temperature from acute pericoronitis of an impacted mandibular third molar is to

1. administer a general anesthetic and remove the tooth
2. irrigate the tooth socket, administer antibiotics and palliative treatment until the acute stage has subsided, and remove the tooth
3. remove the opposing maxillary third molar
4. perform an extraoral I and D and place the patient on antibiotics

5. perform an intraoral I and D and place the patient on antibiotics

61. A 5-year-old boy fell and struck his chin on the sidewalk. He can open his mouth only with difficulty, and his chin deviates to the right side when he does so. Clinical and radiographic examination confirms a fracture of the right subcondylar ramus. No other injuries are present. Treatment should consist of

1. circummandibular wiring of the mandibule for 6 weeks
2. intermaxillary fixation for 6–8 weeks
3. intermaxillary arch bars placed to guide occlusion, but no immobilization, and observation for 3 weeks
4. extra-skeletal pin fixation for 6 weeks
5. no treatment other than observation

62. The distal root of a mandibular second molar is pushed into a soft tissue space during an attempt to remove it. The most likely place for it to be is the

1. pterygomandibular space
2. sublingual space
3. submaxillary space below the mylohoid muscle
4. parapharyngeal space
5. temporal space

63. Mandibular bone is best restored by

1. autogenous bone
2. homogenous bone
3. Freeze-dried bone
4. β-lypholized bovine bone

64. A 20-year-old man has a true prognathous relationship between his maxilla and his mandible. Which of the following procedures could be helpful in restoring the arch relationship to normal?

1. Le Fort I advancement
2. Sagittal split osteotomy of the mandible
3. Bone graft to the molar eminences
4. C advancement of the mandible
5. Menton reduction genioplasty

65. Some patients may have prolonged bleeding episodes following surgery because of certain drugs they have been taking. Which of the following could cause such hypoprothrombinemia?

   a. Meprobamate
   b. Sodium bicarbonate
   c. Sodium or acetyl salicylates
   d. Tetracyclines
   e. Vitamin K

1. a and b
2. b and d
3. c and d
4. a and e
5. All of the above

## Hospital Protocol

Some dentists may find it necessary, prudent, or convenient to conduct a part of their practice in a hospital setting. Unlike their medical colleagues, who receive their major clinical education in hospitals, dentists have very little exposure to hospitals as undergraduate students. In fact, hospital dentistry has not occupied a major part of the predoctoral curriculum, and only recently have a significant number of postdoctoral residencies become available. Hospitals have rules and regulations which are enforced in order to protect the patients and to ensure a smooth working relationship among all those who practice in the hospital. These rules and regulations conform to the *Guidelines for Approval of the Joint Commission on Accreditation of Hospitals (JCAH)*, an overseeing and accrediting agency composed of the following member organizations: the American Medical Association, the American College of Surgeons, the American College of Physicians, the American Dental Association, and the American Hospital Association.

Dentists are now officially part of the JCAH, and they have a significant role in developing guidelines for the practice of dentistry in hospitals. In general, patients who have serious preexisting systemic health problems which preclude surgical treatment on an outpatient basis are admitted to hospitals for oral surgery. These patients must have the same preoperative medical care as all other patients and must also have physician care for any postsurgical medical problems which arise during the hospitalization. Such patients include those who have mental and emotional problems as well as physical ones.

When there is a large department of dentistry in the organization chart of the hospital, oral surgery is usually placed in this department administratively, but oral surgeons are responsible to the chief of surgery for surgical directions and governance. Dentists obtain privileges to practice in hospitals in the same manner as do physicians, that is, by application to the staff and by presenting documents attesting to licensing and specialty training certification. Privileges must be earned, and there is an increased sense of responsibility on the part of hospital boards to ensure qualifications by all who would practice in their hospitals. A knowledge of admission procedures; preparation for the use of the operating room; an understanding of the dentist's responsibility in regard to the anesthesiologist, nurses, and other staff; the ability to provide postoperative orders; and above all, the willingness to seek adequate and reliable consultation for admitted patients are all requisite attributes to be learned by the dentist using hospitals to treat patients. In addition, the dentist must be available to respond to consultation requests from other services.

It must be remembered that the physical environment of the hospital does not expand the scope of the dentist's capabilities. Additional education and training are the only ways of becoming more capable. A dentist who is incapable of managing fractured mandibles because he or she lacks the advanced training to do so will not be able to treat these fractures simply because they present themselves in the hospital. The hospital is no substitute for further training.

### QUESTIONS

66. The Joint Commission on Accreditation of Hospitals says that its approved hospitals must require which of the following for all dental patients admitted?
    1. A CBC and EKG on all patients prior to surgery
    2. The same medical evaluation given to all patients
    3. Chest x-rays prior to surgery
    4. Isolation for women pregnant more than 3 months
    5. Full mouth radiographs before dental extractions

67. Hospitals use standard abbreviations on order charts. The abbreviation t.i.d. means
    1. twice a day
    2. three times a day
    3. immediately before meals
    4. only at bedtime
    5. at 6, 12, and 6

68. Which of the following patients should be admitted to the hospital for necessary extraction of teeth?
    a. A patient who is 4 months pregnant and is doing well in her pregnancy
    b. A hemophiliac (Factor VIII) 18-year-old male
    c. A hyperthyroid patient not well controlled
    d. A patient with a radiolucent area around the teeth to be extracted where a bruit is heard
    e. The patient who is 66-years old and has no medical problem

    1. a and c
    2. b and c
    3. c and d
    4. b, c, and d
    5. a, b, and e

69. To prevent inadvertent contamination hospital operating room protocol prescribes that when a sterile-gowned surgeon and nurse need to pass each other, they should do so in which of the following manners?
    1. Back to back
    2. Back to front
    3. Side to side
    4. Front to front
    5. Never at all

70. The JCAH suggests that dentists be granted which of the following types of hospital staff memberships?
    1. Courtesy staff only
    2. Status comparable to other medical staff members
    3. Consultation staff only
    4. Limited
    5. Inactive, but on call

## PAIN CONTROL

### Local Anesthesia

ANATOMY AND ADMINISTRATION. One of the most common methods to control pain is the injection of suitable drugs into the tissues close to the nerves that conduct painful stimuli to the final receptor site in the central nervous system. These drugs prevent depolarization of nerve fibers, thus preventing the conduction of impulses along the nerves to the brain.

The main sensory nerve that supplies sensation to the teeth, jaws, and soft tissues of the oral cavity is the fifth cranial nerve or trigeminal nerve. It is the largest cranial nerve, and its sensory root arises from the semilunar (gasserian) ganglion in Meckel's cavity. It gives off three major branches, the ophthalmic, the maxillary, and the mandibular, which emerge through the superior orbital fissure, the foramen rotundum, and the foramen ovale, respectively. Each of these major divisions branch further and supply areas of major concern to the dentist desiring to block painful stimuli with a local anesthetic.

The administration of local anesthetics must follow well-established principles in order to obtain adequate anesthesia and to avoid undesirable side-effects. Both intraoral and extraoral techniques to block the maxillary and mandibular divisions are available. Most of the branches that need to be anesthetized for dentistry are usually blocked intraorally. Good accessibility, good light, and proper equipment are all important to the safe and efficient deposition of an anesthetic solution.

Sharp, properly sized disposable needles used on aspirating syringes, carrying suitable cartridges of anesthesia with or without vasoconstrictors, should be used. They should be firm enough to pass through tissues without deflecting, they should be long enough to reach their targets without being buried to their hubs, and they should be of large enough gauge to aspirate with ease so that the anesthetic is not injected into blood vessels.

All injections must be made slowly, whether the patient is awake or under sedation or general anesthesia, to prevent a large bolus of anesthetic with its vasoconstrictor from being directed rapidly to the heart in the event of an inadvertent intravascular injection. In an awake patient, a slow injection is less painful because there is no sudden extension of tissue by the fluid.

Sterile care of the instruments is mandatory to prevent infections from being deposited deep into the final nerve site and to prevent cross contamination between patients. Those parts of the armamentarium used for local anesthesia which are not disposable and presumed sterile must be sterilized by autoclaving or by the use of gas sterilization. The threat of hepatitis being transmitted in the dental office can be lowered by strict observance of sterilizing procedures.

### QUESTIONS

71. Which of the following branches of the maxillary nerve should be anesthetized to remove a maxillary first molar?
    a. Anterior palatine
    b. Posterior palatine
    c. Middle superior alveolar
    d. Anterior superior alveolar
    e. Posterior superior alveolar
    1. a, d, and e
    2. b, c, and d
    3. c, d, and e
    4. a, c, and e
    5. b, d, and e

72. Which of the following anatomic landmarks are used when an intraoral infraorbital nerve block is given?
    a. Pupil of the eye looking forward
    b. Infraorbital notch
    c. Midzygomatic notch
    d. Maxillary lateral incisor
    e. Maxillary second bicuspid
    1. a, b, and e
    2. b, c, and d
    3. c, d, and e
    4. a, c, and d
    5. a, c, and e

73. The intraoral infraorbital block anesthetizes which of the following nerves
    1. Posterior and middle superior
    2. Anterior superior and nasopalatine
    3. Anterior and middle superior
    4. Nasopalatine and lateral nasal
    5. Anterior palatine and posterior palatine

74. The best kind of needles for dental anesthetic injections are
    1. palladium autoclavable 23-gauge 1 in.
    2. iridium autoclavable 23-gauge 1⅝ in.
    3. sterile disposable 23-gauge 1 to 1⅝ in.
    4. sterile disposable 23-gauge ¾ to 1 in.
    5. stainless steel, sharp, 23-gauge 1¾ in.

75. Following a mandibular intraoral block injection the patient has difficulty closing the eyelid on the side of the injection. The probable cause is
    1. anesthesia of the motor branch of the mandibular nerve
    2. anesthesia of the facial nerve within the parotid gland
    3. an allergic response to the anesthetic
    4. anesthesia of an aberrant branch of the cervical colli nerve
    5. blocking of the vidian nerve because the injection was too high

**PHARMACOLOGY.** Local anesthetic drugs are for the most part synthetics which are divided into two groups, the esters and the amides. Both contain an aromatic lipophilic group plus a hydrophilic amino group which forms water-soluble salts when combined with acids. They differ from each other in that one forms an intermediate chain containing an amide linkage while the other forms an intermediate chain containing an ester linkage.

Monheim lists the following properties of an ideal anesthetic:

1. Its action must be reversible.
2. It must be nonirritating to the tissues and produce no secondary local reaction.
3. It should have a low degree of systemic toxicity.
4. It should have a rapid onset and be of sufficient duration to be advantageous.
5. It should have a potency sufficient to give complete anesthesia without the use of harmful concentrated solutions.
6. It should have sufficient penetrating properties to be effective as a topical anesthetic.
7. It should be stable in solution and undergo biotransformation readily within the body.
8. It should be relatively free from producing allergic reactions.
9. It should be either sterile or capable of being sterilized by heat without deterioration [1].

The esters have three divisions—the benzoic acid esters, the para-aminobenzoic acid esters, and the meta-aminobenzoic esters. The amide group has two divisions—the amines and the anilides. The drugs most commonly used in each are, procaine, tetracaine, and propoxycaine hydrochloride in the ester group and lidocaine, mepivacaine, and prilocaine hydrochloride in the amide group. People who are allergic or who have undesirable reactions to drugs in one group are likely to have the same reactions to other drugs in the same group, but they are unlikely to have bad reactions to anesthetics belonging to the opposite drug family.

Because the action of local anesthetics depends on the ability of the salt to liberate a free alkaloid base, a low pH such as that found in infected tissues, when the pH may be 5.5 or 5.6, prevents good anesthesia.

The use of a vasoconstrictor in the solution helps retard absorption of the anesthetic, thus increasing its duration of action and permitting a smaller amount of anesthetic to be used. By slowing absorption, the vasoconstrictor also helps reduce the toxic effects of the solution.

In the relatively small amounts of anesthetic used in dentistry, the only organ systems likely to be affected are the vessels in the immediate injection area, provided the concentrations and volumes used are controlled. Accidental intravascular injections of even small amounts, however, may result in several undesirable effects such as hypertensions, tremors, pallor, tachycardia, headache, and fibrillation. Once again, this indicates the necessity for aspirating and injecting very slowly. As with all drugs, an absolute mastery of the pharmacology of the agents used in dentistry, the advantages, disadvantages, side-effects, and above all, the knowledge of safe dosages is essential to their safe use.

## QUESTIONS

76. A patient presents with a periapical abscess of the maxillary second molar. A posterior superior alveolar block, a middle superior alveolar block, and a palatine injection are given. The patient still experienced pain when an attempt was made to remove the tooth. The most probable cause for this pain was that
1. an additional infraorbital block should have been given
2. an increased concentration of vasoconstrictor should be used
3. an ester type anesthetic should have been used
4. the pH of the abscess prevented adequate anesthesia
5. the above blocks were inappropriate and should have been supplemented by sedation.

77. How much anesthetic does 100 cc 2% lidocaine solution contain?
1. 2 mg
2. 20 mg
3. 200 mg
4. 2 g
5. 20 g

78. Local anesthetics have both lipophilic and hydrophilic properties. These are used to
1. limit free base and decrease diffusion into lipid-rich nerves
2. precipitate free base and increase diffusion into lipid-rich nerves
3. retard the solution's diffusion through interstitial tissues
4. increase the shelf life of the solution

79. Which of the following commonly used vasoconstrictors is most efficient when used with dental anesthetic solutions?
1. Norepinephrine
2. Nordefrin hydrochloride
3. Levonordefrin
4. Phenylephrine hydrochloride
5. Epinephrine

80. For patients who are particularly susceptible to untoward reactions to epinephrine, even a small amount may result in
a. marked elevation of blood pressure
b. tachycardia
c. cardiac arrhythmias
d. severe headaches
e. All of the above
1. a and c
2. a only
3. b and d
4. e
5. a, b, and d

**COMPLICATIONS.** Complications range from those which are slightly annoying and very transient to those which have serious, prolonged, and even irreversible consequences. They may be the result of human error (a lack of knowledge or faulty technique on the dentist's part, improper sterilization, inattention to necessary precautions), faulty equipment, or the patient's physiologic reactions to the medications being used. Undesirable physiologic reactions result from absorption of

**Table 14–2. Maximum Allowable Anesthetic Dose***

| WEIGHT IN POUNDS | 2% CARBOCAINE | 3% CARBOCAINE |
|---|---|---|
| 20 | 54 mg (1.5 Carpules) | 54 mg (1.0 Carpules) |
| 40 | 108 mg (3.0 Carpules) | 108 mg (2.0 Carpules) |
| 60 | 180 mg (5.0 Carpules) | 175 mg (3.25 Carpules) |
| 80 | 180 mg (5.0 Carpules) | 243 mg (4.5 Carpules) |
| 100 | 180 mg (5.0 Carpules) | 270 mg (5.0 Carpules) |
| 150 | 180 mg (5.0 Carpules) | 270 mg (5.0 Carpules) |

| WEIGHT IN POUNDS | LIDOCAINE 2% WITH 1:100,000 EPINEPHRINE |
|---|---|
| 20 | 63 mg (1.75 cartridges) |
| 40 | 135 mg (3.75 cartridges) |
| 60 | 207 mg (5.75 cartridges) |
| 80 | 279 mg (7.75 cartridges) |
| 100 (or over) | 300 mg (8.33 cartridges) |

* From Symposium on Anesthesia, sponsored by the Southern California Society of Oral and Maxillofacial Surgeons, Los Angeles, Calif., 1978, and modified in accordance with Bennett CR (ed): Monheim's Local Anesthesia and Pain Control in Dental Practice, 6th ed. St. Louis, Mosby, 1978, p 149.

the anesthetic and may be due to drug toxicity, the patient's idiosyncrasy to the drug, an allergic response, or an overwhelming anaphylactic reaction. These are systemic complications. Local reactions or complications are those such as prolonged pain, swelling, trismus, prolonged anesthesia, hematoma formation, irritation of the local tissues, sloughing of tissues, and broken needles. A psychologic reaction such as syncope as a result of local anesthesia is a frequent complication that can be avoided by consideration of the apprehensive patient.

Most complications may be minimized or avoided completely by a careful preanesthetic evaluation of the patient and by attention to the details of selecting the best anesthetic and its vasconstrictor, assembling the required equipment properly, and using appropriate techniques. Treatment of complications involves removing the cause and reversing the undesirable effects. Every dental office should be equipped with an oxygen delivery system and an emergency kit properly stocked with devices and drugs necessary to treat both local and systemic complications, and every dentist should be educated to use the appropriate measures to correct complications.

### QUESTIONS

81. Following an inadvertent intravascular injection of 2% lidocaine with 1:100,000 epinephrine, which of the following would indicate that a toxic overdose had been given?

    a. Hypertension
    b. Tachycardia
    c. Bradycardia
    d. Hypotension
    e. Headache

  1. a, c, and e
  2. a, b, and c
  3. a, b, and e
  4. c, d, and e
  5. b, d, and e

82. Two minutes after an injection of a local anesthetic with vasoconstrictor there is a total absence of pulse beat and respirations have stopped. The patient has had

  1. a syncopal attack
  2. an idiosyncratic reaction
  3. an anaphylactic reaction
  4. a toxic reaction
  5. an anginal attack

83. The proper measure for the dentist to take in case of an anaphylactic reaction is to

  1. begin cardiopulmonary resuscitation at once
  2. start an IV with 5% dextrose in water
  3. begin steroid injections at once
  4. give 10 mg 1:1000 epinephrine sublingually
  5. perform an emergency tracheotomy

84. If trismus follows an intraoral inferior alveolar nerve block injection, the cause is most likely to be that

  1. the needle was inserted too far superiorly
  2. the solution irritated the nerve sheath of the motor branch of the Vth nerve
  3. the needle passed through the medial pterygoid and irritated the muscle
  4. the needle traumatized the bone because it was inserted too quickly
  5. a vessel was accidentally pierced

85. Treatment of a hematoma which developed following a posterior superior alveolar nerve injection should be to

  1. incise and drain the area at once
  2. apply heat in the form of a hot pad to the area
  3. apply pressure and cold to the side of the face over the hematoma
  4. aspirate the area intraorally
  5. administer steroids to hasten diffusion of the trapped blood

### Conscious Sedation

Sometimes local anesthesia alone may be insufficient to relieve the patient of pain, discomfort, or most frequently the anxiety brought to the dental office. Agents are available to alter the consciousness level in such a manner that good regional (local) anesthesia can be used to extract a tooth or to perform other painful procedures. While the local anesthetic is the agent which interrupts the pain pathways and obtunds pain effectively and completely, some patients simply cannot submit to this as the sole method of pain control. Conscious sedation or medication by drugs and agents is used to help such patients undergo surgical procedures with both physical and mental comfort.

Sedation is not a general anesthetic stage, for the patient retains all protective reflexes and is easily aware of the surroundings. The patient may become amnesic to all unpleasant stimuli and may even regard everything with euphoria. The goals of conscious sedation techniques are to reduce anxiety in the patient, to raise the pain thresholds, to permit the use of good local anesthetic techniques, to help protect normal physiologic responses of the cardiovascular and respiratory systems, and to do these things with safety and comfort.

It is essential to evaluate the width of the patient's safety spectrum when using sedation. For ambulatory or outpatient use, the classification of physical status as defined by the American Society of Anesthesiology is useful:

I: A patient without systemic disease; a normal healthy patient.
II: A patient with mild systemic disease.
III: A patient with severe systemic disease that limits activity but is not incapacitating. There are three more categories, each more serious in regard to survival, so patients in these categories would not be acceptable risks.

The agents used for sedation are antianxiety drugs such as diazepam and other ataractics like promethazine hydrochloride (Phenergan), hydroxyzine hydrochloride (Atarax), and chlorpromazine. Barbiturates such as sodium pentobarbital (Nembutal) secobarbital (Seconal) are both hypnotics and sedatives, while the narcotics such as meperidine hydrochloride (Demerol) and morphine have strong analgesic properties. The ultrashort-acting barbiturates like sodium methohexital (Brevital) and sodium pentothal are useful in the hands of those well trained in general anesthesia, but these have limited use as conscious sedation agents when the operator is not so trained. The anticholinergic drugs such as atropine and scopolamine each have some usefulness as premedication agents, but their unique actions must, of course, be considered. For example, atropine must not be used for patients with glaucoma because it closes the aqueous drainage canals of the eyes. Scopolamine helps produce amnesia, but it sometimes makes old people agitated. The best inhalation agent for conscious sedation currently available is

nitrous oxide. It is often used in combination with one of the drugs already mentioned.

The major routes of administration of sedative agents are the oral, parenteral, either intramuscular or intravenous, and the inhalation route. Oral medication is the least reliable and least predictable in its results, for many factors weigh against assuring a given level of antianxiety and relaxation. The variability of gastric contents, delayed emptying of the stomach due to the very anxiety the medication is being offered for, inability to swallow, retching, and vomiting all make for a haphazard level of sedation. The intravenous route offers the best control because the medications may be titrated into the body and the results immediately observed. The doses may be tailored specifically and precisely for the purpose at hand. Techniques for IV administration of medications can be mastered as can any technique which requires dexterity, understanding, and attention to detail.

Modern technology has revived an interest in the use of nitrous oxide ($N_2O$) as an analgesic; machines have been developed to maintain a physiologic level of oxygen in the gas mixture at all times. This, plus the safety and ease of administering it as a supplement to local anesthesia, has made $N_2O$ a very useful adjunct in the fight against pain. By itself $N_2O$ produces unconsciousness and anesthesia in anoxic concentrations, and techniques using this gas formerly required an oxygen concentration level as low as 7%–10%. Today's analgesia machines are safety rigged to prevent an anoxic or even a hypoxic concentration of oxygen from being delivered to a patient. Fail-safe devices are incorporated to shut off the flow of $N_2O$ completely should the system run out of oxygen. Flow meters should be accurate to within 5% of indicated concentrations, and the machine should be capable of delivering 100% oxygen as a flush in emergency situations. Although $N_2O$ reduces anxiety, painful stimuli are still perceived by patients unless good local anesthesia is used to block the pain.

There are few contraindications to the use of this inhalation sedation technique. Because it depends upon gaseous uptake, crying, colds, and upper respiratory illness which dilute the gases render this method useless or at least much too complicated. Teratogenic effects in the first trimester of pregnancy for a single administration of the gases have not been proved, but it would be wise not to use $N_2O$ at this time. For various reasons, epileptics, asthmatics, and psychotics do not do well under nitrous oxide–oxygen ($N_2O$–$O_2$) sedation.

It should be clear that analgesia and early signs of anesthesia under $N_2O$–$O_2$ sedation are not the same, but sedation can lead to anesthesia whenever it is possible to increase the $N_2O$ concentration above analgesia levels. Current technology should prevent this from occurring, but the dentist should know the signs and symptoms of these two distinct stages. Analgesia is characterized by tingling sensations (paresthesias) in the tongue, lips, fingers, a ringing in the ears, sleepiness, and dissociation followed by dreams which indicate early anesthesia. The latter are sometimes sexual. The concentration of $N_2O$ in the blood creates the stages of analgesia, and while fairly common, not all patients experience all the symptoms described. Patients are apprehensive when they begin to lose control, and this indicates too deep a level—one which is almost anesthesia. Warmth, euphoria, and amnesia are the analgesic symptoms sought in this technique. An unpleasant, occasional consequence is nausea, usually an indication that the concentration of $N_2O$ is too great. This can be prevented by careful monitoring of the concentrations and by observing whether the patient is beginning to sweat, a sign that frequently precedes nausea.

Anesthesia, which can occur if too great a percentage of $N_2O$ is delivered in spite of precautions, should be recognized when the patient begins to hold the breath, grunts, rolls the eyeballs, and has increased pulse rate and blood pressure. Test the eyes then to see whether the eyelids resist opening and whether large pupils which respond to light are present. If these signs are present, the patient is no longer in an analgesic state, but has passed to true anesthesia; the dentist should be prepared to lighten the $N_2O$ concentration. Recovery from $N_2O$–$O_2$ sedation used without intravenous or oral adjuncts is very rapid.

Prolonged use of $N_2O$ in dental offices must be undertaken with precautions to scavenge the gas so that ambient concentrations are within safe limits for the operator and personnel subjected to repeated and prolonged episodes of $N_2O$, for it has been shown that undesirable effects, although still to be completely proved, may occur under these circumstances.

Complications which may arise because sedation is used occur because of coincidence, human error, or untoward circumstances. They may be related to the use of the particular modality, as the phlebitis which occurs occasionally when diazepam is used, or they may be due to preexisting patient susceptibility. It is important therefore to evaluate each patient prior to each episode of sedation and to know thoroughly what the patient's physical and emotional status is each time. Knowledge of a previous visit is insufficient to provide the ultimate measure of safety. Complications due to drug dosage, sensitivity, and allergy pertain in an increased measure when drugs are used for sedation parenterally, because reactions occur much more rapidly in these situations.

Inhalation agent complications are not usually serious, especially when $N_2O$–$O_2$ is used. When signs and symptoms of inhalation sedation do not appear according to expectations, the machine used to deliver the gases must be checked. In spite of all fail-safe devices built in, such as the pin system to prevent attaching delivery hoses to the wrong gas, i.e., the $N_2O$ hose to the $O_2$ outlet, malfunction may occur. If the signs are wrong, everything must be disconnected and the patient permitted to breath room air! The dentist must not proceed until everything checks out correctly.

Complications involving the intravenous routes may be much more serious, for in addition to the rapidity of drug reactions, human error such as a mistake in calculating dose concentrations can multiply the original mistakes many times over. It is possible to push IV sedation to IV anesthesia rapidly, and the dentist must be trained and equipped to manage such a situation. When combinations of routes are used, such as when both IV and inhalation sedation are employed, the complications inherent in each route become distinct possibilities. These combinations are not recommended for practitioners who have not had extensive education and training in general anesthesia.

## QUESTIONS

86. When a patient is told to take a 5-mg tablet of Valium 1 hour before the scheduled dental appointment, the major instruction should be to
   1. be accompanied by an adult who can drive
   2. have nothing by mouth from midnight on
   3. eat a substantial breakfast to prevent irritating the stomach
   4. All of the above
   5. None of the above

87. The onset of sedative action of secobarbital given by mouth depends upon the
   a. acidity of the gastric contents
   b. amount of anxiety present
   c. time since food was ingested
   d. blood circulation to the stomach's sphincter
   e. contents of the small intestines
   1. a, d, and e
   2. a, b, and c
   3. b, c, and d
   4. c, d, and e
   5. a, c, and d

88. Nitrous oxide, oxygen sedation is *not* recommended for
   a. psychotics
   b. epileptics
   c. Class I physical status
   d. Class III physical status
   e. first trimester pregnant women
   1. c, d, and e
   2. a, b, and e
   3. b, c, and d
   4. b, c, and e
   5. None of the above

89. One of the early symptoms of $N_2O$ analgesia is
   1. irregular breathing
   2. enlarged pupils which react to light
   3. gross muscular activity

4. erotic dreams
5. tingling of the finger tips

90. Which of the following are characteristics of diazepam (Valium) when it is used as intravenous sedation?
    a. Thrombophlebitis is an occasional undesirable side-effect.
    b. Diazepam may cause respiratory depression even in very small doses.
    c. Large doses (in excess of 10 mg) are excellent analgesics.
    d. Large doses (in excess of 10 mg) cause muscle relaxation that paralyzes swallowing movements.
    e. It is a good amnesic drug.

    1. a, c, and e
    2. a, b, and e
    3. b, d, and e
    4. b, c, and d
    5. c, d, and e

91. Which of the following is the proper administration of intravenous diazepam (Valium) sedation?
    1. A predetermined dose is administered based upon the patient's age, weight, and physical condition.
    2. A slow drop of Valium and 5% dextrose is administered throughout the procedure.
    3. A bolus of Valium of 5 mg is injected every 5 min until the desired level of sedation is reached.
    4. Valium is injected slowly, not more than 5 mg/min, until the desired level of sedation is reached.
    5. Ten milligrams of Valium as a single bolus will adequately sedate most patients with an additional 5 mg injected as necessary.

92. An intravenous overdose of a barbiturate used for sedation may cause death because the
    1. respiratory system is depressed
    2. circulatory system is depressed
    3. heart goes into ventricular fibrillation
    4. brain becomes ischemic
    5. platelets form a thrombus

93. While administering a mixture of $N_2O$–$O_2$ for sedation, the dentist notices that the patient is becoming agitated, the pupils are enlarged, and the eyelids are heavy. The flow meters read 60% $N_2O$ and 40% $O_2$. What is happening?
    1. The patient is just extra apprehensive and requires increased $N_2O$ concentration.
    2. This is a normal sequence of events.
    3. There is a flow meter error, and the patient is going into light anesthesia.
    4. The gas hoses are reversed, and the patient is too lightly sedated.
    5. The gas tanks are empty, and the patient is emerging from analgesia.

94. Scopolamine, 0.4 mg, is used as part of an intravenous drug mixture which includes 50 mg sodium pentobarbital (Nembutal) and 25 mg meperidine hydrochloride (Demerol) given to a 70-year-old man in Class II physical status. Soon after the operation the patient becomes disoriented, agitated, and hysterical. The reason for his behavior is that
    1. meperidine hydrochloride and pentobarbital cause this upon emergence
    2. scopolamine causes disassociative behavior in some elderly people
    3. the concentrations of the drug combination were inapprorpiate for a 70-year-old man
    4. the patient had an allergic response to the combination of medications
    5. Class II physical status patients behave this way with IV sedation

95. The minimal concentration of oxygen that should be used with $N_2O$ analgesia is
    1. 10%
    2. 20%
    3. 30%
    4. 40%
    5. 50%

## General Anesthesia

General anesthesia carries the alteration of consciousness beyond the stages of analgesia and depresses the central nervous system in what is believed to be an orderly fashion. It affects first the most highly developed brain centers in the cerebrum and then the most recently developed centers in the medulla. Neurophysiologic investigations reveal that the system is highly complex, and new information is being sought constantly.

It is generally agreed that the inhalation or intravenous routes of anesthetic administration are preferable to other modes of delivery because the results may be obtained more precisely than when the agent is administered orally, rectally, or intramuscularly. Agents should be nontoxic and reversible by means of an antagonist, should have minimal untoward side-effects, such as nausea or vomiting, should have a high safety factor, and should be excreted without major harmful metabolic changes. If the agent is an inhalation agent, it should be nonirritating, should have good patient acceptance, should be compatible with oxygen, and should be nonflammable or explosive.

The inhalation methods of delivery include the open drop, semiopen drop, insufflation, semiclosed and closed methods. Each utilizes a special armamentarium suitable for the task. One of these methods may be used in conjunction with the intravenous route to maintain suitable anesthetic levels.

In order to assess the depth or profoundness of anesthesia Guedel described the signs created when ether was used as the sole anesthetic agent. These were divided into four stages: 1) analgesia; 2) delirium; 3) surgical opportunity, which was further divided into three planes, depending upon the degree of relaxation required; and finally 4) respiratory paralysis followed by

**Table 14–3. General Anesthetic Agents and Routes of Administration**

INHALATION ANESTHETICS
*Gases*
    Cyclopropane
    Ethylene
    Nitrous oxide
*Volatile liquids*
    Chloroform
    Diethyl ether (ether)
    Enflurane (Ethrane)
    Ethyl chloride
    Halothane (Fluothane)
    Methoxyfluorane (Penthrane)
    Trichloroethylene (Trilene, Trimar)
    Vinyl ether (Vinethene)
INTRAVENOUS ANESTHETICS
    Fentanyl with droperidol (neurolept) (Innovar)
    Ketamine (dissociative) (Ketalar, Ketaject)
    Methohexital sodium (Brevital)
    Thiamylal sodium (Surital)
    Thiopental sodium (Pentothal)

death. The intravenous agents telescope these stages so that they no longer are the guides to the depth of anesthesia. In fact, each agent has its own set of signs to indicate the level of unconsciousness, and these must be understood by the dentist. In each set, however, respiratory, eye, and muscular signs are important. Respiratory signs include rate, volume, and regularity, while eye signs include the reflex of the lids, eyeball movements, and pupillary responses. Muscle responses depend upon the degree of relaxation in the skeletal muscles and in the presence or absence of the reflexes of the pharynx and larynx. Thus, the most important way to monitor the condition of the patient under general anesthesia is close observation of all physical signs. Of course, preanesthetic base line readings of pulse, blood pressure, respiratory rate, and color must be obtained prior to administration of the anesthetic.

It is essential that the dentist have adequate training before administering any anesthetic agent. This must be obtained in a recognized training program such as is offered in residency programs. The employment of general anesthesia to perform surgery is a discipline in itself.

### QUESTIONS

96. An inhalation agent used for general anesthesia should
    a. support combustion
    b. be compatible with oxygen
    c. be able to initiate the laryngeal reflex to protect the body
    d. produce few undesirable effects such as nausea
    e. have rapid induction times.

    1. a, c, and d
    2. b, d, and e
    3. b, c, and e
    4. a, d, and e
    5. c, d, and e

97. General inhalation agents may be administered by the
    a. open drop method
    b. closed method
    c. semiclosed method
    d. insufflation
    e. semipermeable method

    1. None of the above
    2. All of the above
    3. All but d
    4. All but e
    5. c, d, and e

98. Nasoendotracheal intubation is used frequently for moderate to long dental cases. The major advantage of this procedure is that it
    1. permits the dentist to operate without anesthestic equipment in the way
    2. permits the anesthesiologist to monitor the patient without getting in the dentist's way
    3. insures a patient's airway function at all times
    4. prevents saliva from accumulating in the buccal vestibules
    5. insures a clear, dry working area around the maxillary teeth

99. During general anesthesia induced by sodium pentothal and oxygen, the patient begins to make wheezing, crowing sounds and appears to be having difficulty inspiring. Which of the following may be taking place?
    a. Bronchospasm
    b. Laryngospasm
    c. Cardiospasm
    d. Simple cough reflex action
    e. Anaphylactic reaction

    1. a and b
    2. b and c
    3. a and c
    4. c and e
    5. d and e

100. The appropriate therapy for bronchospasm is to
    1. give 1 mg IV epinephrine 1:1000
    2. give $O_2$ by full-face mask
    3. give IV succinylcholine plus $O_2$ by face mask
    4. deepen the anesthetic stage
    5. suction the oral cavity of excessive saliva

### REFERENCES

1. MONHEIM L: General Anesthesia in Dental Practice, 4th ed. St. Louis, CV Mosby, 1974, p 122

### SUGGESTED READINGS

#### PREOPERATIVE EVALUATION AND DIAGNOSIS

KILLEY HC, SEWARD GR, KAY LW: An Outline of Oral Surgery, Part II. BRISTOL, WRIGHT and SONS, 1971, pp 1-54
PRIOR J, SILBUSTEIR J: Physical Diagnosis. St. Louis, CV Mosby, 1973

REVZIN M: Patient Evaluation. In Goldman HM, Forrest SP, Byrd DL, Mcdonald RE (eds): Current Therapy in Dentistry, Vol. II. St. Louis, CV Mosby, 1966, pp 323–330

STEINER RB, THOMPSON RD: Oral Surgery and Anesthesia. Philadelphia, WB Saunders, 1977, pp 1–17, 89–116, 117–131, 211–233, 234–268

WAITE DE: Textbook of Practical Oral Surgery. Philadelphia, Lea & Febiger, 1972, pp 18–33

## SURGICAL PRINCIPLES, TREATMENT AND COMPLICATIONS

ARCHER HW: Oral and Maxillofacial Surgery Vol I, Philadelphia, WB Saunders, 1975, pp 15–250, 405–409

ARCHER HW: Oral and Maxillofacial Surgery, Vol. II. Philadelphia, WB Saunders, 1975, pp 1540–1678

KILLEY HC, KAY LW: The Impacted Wisdom Tooth. London, E & S Livingstone, 1975

KILLEY HC, SEWARD GR, KAY LW: An Outline of Oral Surgery, Part I. Bristol, Wright & Sons, 1970, pp 17–52, 151–157

KRUGER G: Textbook of Oral Surgery, 4th ed. St. Louis, CV Mosby, 1974, pp 1–110, 314–385

STEINER RB, THOMPSON RD: Oral Surgery and Anesthesia. Philadelphia, WB Saunders, 1977, pp 211–268

WAITE DE: Hemorrhage and Shock. In Waite DE (ed): Textbook of Practical Oral Surgery. Philadelphia, Lea & Febiger, 1972, pp 431–440

## HOSPITAL PROTOCOL

ARCHER HW: Oral and Maxillofacial Surgery, Vol I. Philadelphia, WB Saunders, 1975, pp 419–437

DOUGLAS BL, CASEY GJ (eds): A Guide to Hospital Dental Procedure. Chicago, Council on Hospital Dental Service, American Dental Association, 1964

HOOLEY JR: Hospital Dentistry. Philadelphia, Lea & Febiger, 1970

## PAIN CONTROL

ALLEN GA: Dental Anesthesia and Analgesia. Baltimore, Williams & Wilkins, 1972

ALLING CC III, MAHAN PE (eds): Facial Pain, 2nd ed. Philadelphia, Lea & Febiger, 1977, pp 45–56

BENNETT CR (ed): Monheim's Local Anesthesia and Pain Control in Dental Practice. St. Louis, CV Mosby, 1978

MCCARTY FM: The Prevention of Selected Complications with Local Anesthesia Alone and With the Adjuvants: Anesthesia Progress 26:37–42, 1979

MONHEIM L: General Anesthesia in Dental Practice, 4th ed. St. Louis, CV Mosby, 1974

## ANSWER KEY

| | | | |
|---|---|---|---|
| 1. 3 | 26. 3 | 51. 2 | 76. 4 |
| 2. 4 | 27. 4 | 52. 3 | 77. 4 |
| 3. 1 | 28. 5 | 53. 3 | 78. 2 |
| 4. 3 | 29. 2 | 54. 4 | 79. 5 |
| 5. 2 | 30. 2 | 55. 4 | 80. 4 |
| 6. 3 | 31. 3 | 56. 5 | 81. 3 |
| 7. 5 | 32. 2 | 57. 3 | 82. 3 |
| 8. 5 | 33. 3 | 58. 2 | 83. 1 |
| 9. 2 | 34. 3 | 59. 4 | 84. 3 |
| 10. 4 | 35. 3 | 60. 2 | 85. 3 |
| 11. 4 | 36. 1 | 61. 3 | 86. 1 |
| 12. 4 | 37. 3 | 62. 3 | 87. 1 |
| 13. 2 | 38. 2 | 63. 1 | 88. 2 |
| 14. 1 | 39. 3 | 64. 2 | 89. 5 |
| 15. 2 | 40. 3 | 65. 3 | 90. 2 |
| 16. 3 | 41. 3 | 66. 2 | 91. 4 |
| 17. 3 | 42. 3 | 67. 2 | 92. 1 |
| 18. 4 | 43. 1 | 68. 4 | 93. 3 |
| 19. 2 | 44. 2 | 69. 1 | 94. 2 |
| 20. 3 | 45. 3 | 70. 2 | 95. 2 |
| 21. 2 | 46. 4 | 71. 4 | 96. 2 |
| 22. 3 | 47. 3 | 72. 1 | 97. 4 |
| 23. 2 | 48. 1 | 73. 3 | 98. 3 |
| 24. 2 | 49. 4 | 74. 3 | 99. 1 |
| 25. 1 | 50. 2 | 75. 2 | 100. 3 |

# 15

# PHARMACOLOGY

## Thomas J. Pallasch

In its broadest sense a drug is any chemical which interacts with a biologic system to alter the level of physiologic activity within that system. The particular biologic system may range from a single cell and its subcellular components such as enzymes, to an intact organ system, onto the most incredibly complicated of all systems, the human being.

In order to be therapeutically useful in the prevention or treatment of disease, a drug must possess certain properties: selectivity, potency, reversibility of action, and the chemical ability to interact with biologic systems. If a drug were to interact with most or all of the available chemical components within the human organism, its multiplicity of actions would render it essentially useless. Therefore, a useful drug is one which alters the activity of only a few of these systems (no drug ever exerts a single pharmacologic effect) for the betterment of the target organism.

Potency is the milligram amount of the drug necessary to produce the pharmacologic action. It must be possible to administer the drug in a sufficient amount to produce its effect. If a drug were so impotent that pounds of the chemical were required to induce an effect, it would be essentially useless. Potency is relatively unimportant when compared to drug efficacy, which is the inherent ability of the drug to effect physiologic change. The formulation of a more efficacious drug is an important therapeutic advance, whereas the introduction of a more potent drug simply means that a lesser milligram dosage is required.

Most therapeutically useful drugs are reversible in action because they are metabolized in the liver and excreted by the kidneys. Although an irreversible general anesthetic would hardly be desirable, there are a few useful drugs which have an irreversible effect (an alcohol block of the fifth cranial nerve in trigeminal neuralgia).

Finally, a drug must be chemically capable of interacting with biologic systems. It must be water- and fat-soluble to some extent so that it can dissolve in tissue fluids and pass body membranes that are essentially lipid in nature. It must also possess a chemical structure complementary to its receptor site, which is that por-

tion of the biologic system with which the drug interacts to produce its effect.

Drugs may produce their physiologic alterations by a number of mechanisms: enzyme stimulation or inhibition, alteration in the amount of substrates available for enzyme action, release of endogenous chemicals such as antimetabolites, and the control of metabolic processes. Drugs acting on endogenous enzyme systems (acetylcholinesterase, adenyl cyclase, phosphodiesterase, monoamine oxidase) control the metabolic processes dependent upon these enzymes. An increase or decrease in the substrates available for these enzymes also alters physiologic activity. Antimetabolites such as the sulfonamides and some anticancer drugs produce a deficiency of a metabolite essential to a physiologic process. The amphetamines release norepinephrine from adrenergic nerve terminals. It is probable that the majority of drugs act at the cell membrane or within the cell, particularly with enzyme systems.

It is imperative to remember that drugs only alter those inherent functions within the system and cannot confer new functions upon that endogenous system. Drugs may inhibit enzymes, alter heart rate and contractility, block nerve conduction, or increase renal sodium excretion, but they cannot create new enzymes or cause the heart to take over the functions of the brain.

Since all drugs possess more than one pharmacologic effect, their use is always associated with unwanted actions. These have been grouped under the broad term adverse effects, which range from merely annoying side-effects to frankly harmful (toxic) ones. The major goal of rational therapeutics is to maximize the therapeutic benefits and minimize the adverse effects of a given drug. Unfortunately the lay public is convinced that efficacious drugs can be formulated to produce only good. Such a drug has never existed and never will. Since all organisms are to some extent genetically different (the principle of biologic variation), even those of the same species, drug effects may vary from animal to animal. Therefore, it is not scientifically sound to extrapolate research findings routinely from one animal species to another. An awareness of the biologic variation inherent in all species is essential to knowledgeable drug use.

## GENERAL PRINCIPLES

### Prescription Writing

A prescription is a written or verbal instruction by a licensed practitioner (dentist or physician) to a pharmacist concerning the dispensation of medication to a patient. It also contains directions to the patient regarding the use of the medication. Virtually all (greater than 98%) prescriptions are written for precompounded or proprietary substances formulated by drug manufacturers.

PHYSICAL FORM OF THE PRESCRIPTION. The prescription should contain the following information: the practitioner's name, title, address, telephone number, and registration number with the Drug Enforcement Administration (DEA); the date; and the patient's name, address, and age. (The DEA number indicates that the practitioner is approved and licensed by the Drug Enforcement Administration to administer and prescribe Schedule drugs.) By tradition the prescription is written in a certain manner and contains four component parts: 1) the superscription ($R_x$), which is a symbol for the Latin word recipio meaning take thou; 2) the inscription, which is the name of the drug or drugs and the individual unit dose of that drug; 3) the subscription, which contains directions to the pharmacist regarding the form of the drug (capsule, tablet, liquid) and the number of units of the drug to be administered to the patient; and 4) the signature, which instructs the patient regarding drug dosage and the time intervals between each dose. The prescription should also contain a mechanism to denote the number of refills desired, if any. Some states allow only a written prescription; some, an oral prescription for certain types of drugs; and others, a written prescription to follow one delivered orally. The prescription is a medicolegal document.

CHOICE OF DRUG. Drugs are identified by a variety of names and can be prescribed in three ways: 1) the official, chemical name (United States Pharmacopeia, National Formulary), 2) the generic (nonproprietary) name (United States Adopted Name), or 3) the proprietary (brand) name coined by the manufacturer. If the generic name is prescribed, the pharmacist may dispense any of the preparations of the drug regardless of brand name. It is commonly assumed that generic prescribing assures that the patient will receive the cheapest effective drug. Most pharmacists work on a percentage mark-up on drugs, however; the more costly the

drug to them, the greater the retail percentage mark-up. Therefore, this assumption may be fallacious in some instances.

LANGUAGE, WEIGHTS, AND MEASURES. The use of the Latin language and abbreviations is no longer in vogue, and it is perfectly acceptable to write the prescription in longhand English. Drugs are prescribed on the basis of a milligram per kilogram (or pound) of body weight. The metric system should always be utilized. The most important weights and measures in comparing the apothecary and metric systems are 1) 1 grain equals 60 mg, 2) 1 teaspoon equals 5 ml, 3) 1 tablespoon equals 15 ml. and 4) a 1% solution equals 1g/100 ml (10 mg/ml).

THE CONTROLLED SUBSTANCES ACT OF 1970 The provisions of the Controlled Substances Act, which replaced the Harrison Narcotic Act of 1914 and the Drug Abuse Control Amendments of 1965, were put into effect in May of 1971. The Bureau of Narcotics and Dangerous Drugs was originally responsible for the enforcement of this law, but it was merged into the DEA in 1973. The Controlled Substances Act requires 1) annual registration with the DEA of any individual who manufactures, distributes, prescribes, administers, or dispenses controlled drugs; 2) gradations in legal penalties for the illegal sale of controlled drugs; 3) maintenance of office records (date, patient, drug, and amount) if controlled substances are dispensed, as by a pharmacist; 4) maintenance of the invoices for all purchased controlled drugs; and 5) placement of controlled substances into five Schedules.

Schedule I drugs are experimental hallucinogens and opioids for which there is no approved medical use. Schedule II drugs are those of high abuse potential: opioids, amphetamines and congeners, and short-acting barbiturates. Schedule III drugs are narcotics, primarily codeine, in combination with aspirin or acetaminophen and other sedative–hypnotics with supposedly less abuse potential. Schedule IV drugs include other sedative–hypnotics (chloral hydrate, ethchlorvynol), minor tranquilizers (meprobamate and the benzodiazepines) and propoxyphene (Darvon). Schedule V drugs include codeine cough preparations and some opium-containing agents.

All prescriptions for controlled substances must contain the full name and address of the patient, the full name and address of the dentist or physician, the DEA number, and the date. Schedule II drug prescriptions may not be refilled, and other schedule drugs (III–V) may only be refilled up to five times within 6 months after the initial date of issuance.

DRUG REFERENCE SOURCES. Two of the best general reference sources for drugs of any and all types are

*AMA Drug Evaluations, 3rd edition* (Publishing Sciences Group, Inc, 1977, Littleton, Massachusetts) and *Facts and Comparisons* (111 West Port Plaza Drive, St. Louis, Missouri 63141).

Dental Drug Service Newsletter (P.O. Box 1912, Glendale, California, 91209) is an excellent and economical monthly publication which is designed specifically for dentists and provides a constant update on clinical dental pharmacology.

### QUESTIONS

1. Which of the following statements are true regarding the Controlled Substances Act of 1970?
   a. It places drugs in various Schedules according to abuse potential.
   b. It is administered by the Bureau of Narcotics and Dangerous Drugs.
   c. It requires that office records be kept for controlled substances.
   d. It prohibits a dentist from prescribing Schedule II narcotics.
   e. It limits the number of refills on Schedule drugs.
   1. a, b, and c
   2. b, c, and d
   3. c, d, and e
   4. a, c, and e
   5. All of the above

2. Which of the following statements are true regarding a prescription?
   a. It must be written utilizing Latin abbreviations
   b. It must contain the proprietary (brand) name of the drug.
   c. It should use the Apothecary system of weights and measures
   d. It is a medicolegal document.
   e. It contains instructions to both the pharmacist and patient.
   1. a, b, and c
   2. b, c, and d
   3. c, d, and e
   4. a and b
   5. d and e

## Toxicity

Drug toxicity is the harmful effect of a chemical upon biologic systems. Toxicology is the study of such harmful effects. Many terms such as side-effect, drug-induced diseases, or secondary effects have been used to denote drug toxicity; however, the most common term in present use is the adverse effect or adverse experience.

CLASSIFICATION OF ADVERSE EFFECTS. Serious toxicity produced by a drug is due to an overdosage of the drug. Either too great a dosage was employed, or the individual should never have received the drug. As previously stated, however, no drug ever possesses only one pharmacologic effect. Even though a low incidence of adverse effects is associated with a drug's usage, it may be impossible even with the soundest pharmacologic judgment to divorce totally a drug's therapeutic benefit from its side-effects. Adverse effects to drugs can be classified into three general types: 1) toxicity due to a direct extension of the drug's pharmacologic effects, 2) toxicity due to an altered recipient of the drug, and 3) drug allergy.

TOXICITY DUE TO DIRECT EXTENSION OF PHARMACOLOGIC EFFECTS. Based upon the known pharmacology of a drug, predictable adverse effects may occur. These may be due to an absolute overdosage of the drug, such as local anesthetic-induced convulsions or serious respiratory depression with morphine. Some drugs, by their very chemical nature, are highly irritant to skin and mucosa, i.e., the aspirin burn. Nausea and vomiting from the narcotics, motor incoordination from sedative–hypnotic agents, and gastric irritation from aspirin occur under the best of circumstances. The wise practitioner advises patients of such side-effects; the foolish practitioner overdoses a patient with a drug to the point of serious toxicity. The incidence and extent of adverse drug reactions essentially resides in the hands of the drug user (see Drug Abuse) and the drug administrator.

TOXICITY DUE TO AN ALTERED RECIPIENT OF THE DRUG. Many types of adverse drug effects occur in patients who are "different" from the vast majority of other patients in that some alteration in normal physiologic processes is present. When the drug and defect combine, toxicity occurs. For example, patients with liver or renal disease may not be fully capable of metabolizing or excreting a drug at the normal rate, leading to toxic blood levels even with customary dosages (drug cumulation). Latent emotional disturbances may be exposed when a mind-altering drug is added to the system. A depressed individual may become suicidal when exposed to the central nervous system depressants; a psychotic episode may be precipitated upon exposure to hallucinogenic drugs (LSD, phencyclidine). Serious toxicity may also occur when one drug is administered to a patient receiving other drugs for other conditions (see Drug Interactions).

A patient may possess genetic aberrations which pose no problem except when a given drug is present. A patient deficient in serum cholinesterase will do very well until succinylcholine chloride (Anectine) is administered. Because succinylcholine is metabolized by serum cholinesterase, a deficiency in this enzyme allows the level of succinylcholine to become high enough to induce apnea. It is possible that many blood dyscrasias (agranulocytosis, hemolytic anemia, thrombocytopenia, and aplastic anemia) are caused not only by direct drug toxicity, but also by some combination of a drug with a genetic deficiency in the bone marrow.

A very special form of toxicity occurs in pregnant women; it affects not the mother, but the fetus. Teratology is the study of damage to the fetus during the first trimester of pregnancy, the critical period of organogenesis in the human. Many drugs have been suspected of being teratogens, but only a few have proven to be so: thalidomide, some anticancer drugs, methylmercury, and possibly ethyl alcohol and phenytoin. The inhalation anesthetic agents and diazepam are suspect. The wise practitioner knows that there is no such thing as a placental barrier to drugs; any drug given to the mother is given to the fetus. Local anesthetics, analgesics, and sedative–hypnotics have never been implicated as teratogens.

**DRUG ALLERGY.** For a drug to induce an allergic reaction, there must first be a sensitizing dose and then a subsequent challenge dose. Due to their low molecular weight, drugs are not allergenic per se but must combine with tissue proteins (the vast majority in the skin) to form a drug–protein complex which then promotes antibody formation, a process which requires deoxyribonucleic acid–ribonucleic acid (DNA–RNA) protein synthesis over at least 5–7 days. A drug is termed a hapten and the drug–protein complex the complete or functional hapten. When the challenge dose of the drug is given, antibodies are present to interact with the drug–protein complex, and the allergic reaction occurs. Both the sensitizing and challenge doses would be present if the drug were given continuously over a long enough period of time, and the allergic symptoms would appear during the course of treatment with the drug. Since the sensitizing dose ellicits no allergic symptoms, patients are often unaware of their drug allergy. Individuals may also be sensitized without their knowledge ("but I never had penicillin before") since some drugs such as penicillin occur naturally in the environment. The wise practitioner assumes all patients to be allergic until proven otherwise.

The symptoms of drug allergy are highly variable, but the principal shock organ of drug allergy in man is the skin (erythema, itching, angioedema, urticaria, photosensitivity, contact and exfoliative dermatitis). Other shock organs of drug allergy are the liver, bone marrow, and smooth muscle, both vascular and bronchial (systemic anaphylaxis). The majority of drug allergies are of the immediate type, occurring within seconds to a few hours after drug exposure.

It is theoretically possible for any chemical to produce allergy; however, the vast majority of drug allergies are produced by only a few drugs. Penicillin is by far the most allergenic of all drugs. Other drugs known to produce a high incidence of allergy include the sul-

fonamides, procaine-type local anesthetics, streptomycin, the tetracyclines, aspirin, the phenothiazines, heavy metals, and iodine.

QUESTIONS

3. Drugs produce their teratogenic effects during the second trimester of pregnancy because the fetus is protected from chemicals during the first trimester by the placental barrier.
    1. Both statement and reason are correct and related.
    2. Both statement and reason are correct but not related.
    3. The statement is correct, but the reason is not.
    4. The statement is not correct, but the reason is an accurate statement.
    5. Neither statement nor reason is correct.

4. Hepatic or renal impairment during drug administration may produce drug
    1. allergy
    2. cumulation
    3. idiosyncrasy
    4. tolerance
    5. None of the above

5. Which of the following are signs and symptoms of an acute allergic reaction?
       a. Urticaria
       b. Skin erythema
       c. Bronchoconstriction
       d. Hypotension
       e. Itching
    1. a, b, and c
    2. b, c, and d
    3. c, d, and e
    4. a and b
    5. All of the above

6. Some drugs do not produce any toxic effects because some drugs produce only one pharmacologic effect.
    1. Both statement and reason are correct and related.
    2. Both statement and reason are correct but not related.
    3. The statement is correct, but the reason is not.
    4. The statement is not correct, but the reason is an accurate statement.
    5. Neither statement nor reason is correct.

## Dose–Response

The dose–response (dose–effect) is the relationship of a given dose of a drug to a specific effect either therapeutic or toxic. The dosage of a drug is the amount (in mgs.) of that drug administered during a given period of time.

There are two types of dose–response (effect) curves which graphically demonstrate the effects of increasing drug dosage upon a single biologic unit or a group of such units: 1) the graded (quantitative) and 2) the quantal (all or none). The graded dose–response curve takes the form of a gradually rising curve which illustrates the degree of response seen in a single biologic unit (one cell, one human) to a given dose of a drug. As the dose is increased, the response of the unit becomes greater and greater until a maximum effect, either therapeutic or toxic, is reached. The response of the organism is gradual (graded), but doubling the dose does not necessarily double the effect.

The quantal dose–response curve takes the form of a sigmoid curve or the classic gaussian (frequency) distribution curve. It illustrates the relationship between increasing drug dosage and the proportion (percent) of biologic units in a population of such units which display the pharmacologic or toxicologic effect at a given dose. It is all or none since, at a given dose, a unit in the population either does or does not show the effect. Those individuals reacting to the drug at a very low dose are termed hypersensitive; those reacting only at very high doses, hyposensitive. The majority of units (individuals) respond at the median or average dose of the drug.

The quantal dose–response curve is used to determine the margin of safety of a drug by comparing the quantal curves for therapeutic efficacy and toxicity. This relationship is expressed as the therapeutic index (TI), a comparison of the dose at which 50% of the test animals respond therapeutically is known as the effective dose ($ED_{50}$) and the dose at which 50% of the animals die is known as the lethal dose ($LD_{50}$). The TI is derived from the equation: $TI = LD_{50}/ED_{50}$. The higher the number, the greater the safety of the drug.

### QUESTIONS

7. The therapeutic index of a drug indicates the maximum effective dose of the drug because the therapeutic index compares therapeutic and lethal doses of a given drug to express its margin of safety.
   1. Both statement and reason are correct and related.
   2. Both statement and reason are correct but not related.
   3. The statement is correct, but the reason is not.
   4. The statement is not correct, but the reason is an accurate statement.
   5. Neither statement nor reason is correct.

8. Dose–response curves are utilized to express the
   a. therapeutic index of a drug
   b. median effective dose of a drug
   c. minimal effective dose of a drug
   d. median lethal dose of a drug
   e. minimal lethal dose of a drug

   1. a, b, and c
   2. b, c, and d
   3. c, d, and e
   4. d and e
   5. All of the above

## Structure Action

The structure–activity relationship is the effect of the particular chemical structure of a drug on its specific tissue receptor. The drug receptor is that portion of the biologic system with which the drug interacts to produce its therapeutic or toxic effect. Drug–receptor interactions are highly specific and are determined by the complementary chemical structures of the drug and the receptor site (the key in the lock analogy).

Two general theories have been formulated to explain the drug–receptor process: 1) Clark's occupational theory (1, 2) and 2) Paton's rate theory (3, 4).

OCCUPATIONAL THEORY.　According to the occupational theory, the degree of drug effect is proportional to the number of receptors occupied; the drug effect occurs according to the law of mass action. As long as some receptors are occupied, an effect will be discernible and the maximum effect occurs when all receptors are occupied. Not all receptor sites must be occupied for the maximum effect to occur, however; it occurs when only a critical amount of the total number of receptors are occupied by the drug.

The occupational theory also proposes that an effective drug must possess affinity and/or intrinsic activity. Drug affinity, the inherent ability of the drug to attach to its receptor, is critically dependent upon complementary chemical structures. Intrinsic activity is the ability of the drug to produce a physiologic change during drug–receptor interaction. These two terms have allowed for a classification of drugs into three types: 1) an agonist, possessing both affinity and intrinsic activity, 2) an antagonist, possessing affinity but no intrinsic activity, and 3) a partial agonist (dualist), possessing affinity but less intrinsic activity than the agonist.

Depending upon its concentration at the receptor site, a partial agonist may function either as an agonist or an antagonist. Most therapeutically useful drugs are agonists, and variances in their affinity and intrinsic activity may render some members of a common group of drugs more beneficial than others. Most antagonists are inhibitors of the action of endogenous chemicals (acetylcholine, histamine, norepinephrine) and are useful as antidotal agents (epinephrine and antihistamines in anaphylactic shock induced by histamine) or as therapeutic agents (atropine, curare, adrenergic blocking drugs).

RATE THEORY.　The rate theory holds that the magnitude of a drug's effect is proprotional, not to the number of receptors occupied, but to the rate at which the drug and receptor combine. An agonist drug associates quickly with and then rapidly dissociates from the receptor so as to be able to reassociate again. An antagonist associates with the receptor but dissociates much more slowly and therefore has a very slow reassociation rate. The rate-limiting step is the rate of dissociation of the drug from the receptor, since reassociation (and receptor activation) can only occur again after drug dissociation from the receptor.

### QUESTIONS

9. The chemical structure of a drug is critically important to its interaction with its receptor site because a drug and its receptor site chemically interact to alter physiologic processes.
    1. Both statement and reason are correct and related.
    2. Both statement and reason are correct but not related.
    3. The statement is correct, but the reason is not.
    4. The statement is not correct, but the reason is an accurate statement.
    5. Neither statement nor reason is correct.

10. According to the occupational theory of drug–receptor interaction,
    a. drugs act according to the law of mass action
    b. an antagonist possesses intrinsic activity but no affinity
    c. a partial agonist possesses affinity but no intrinsic activity
    d. the drug effect is proportional to the number of receptors occupied
    e. an agonist possesses affinity and intrinsic activity

    1. a, b, and c
    2. b, c, and d
    3. c, d, and e
    4. a, d, and e
    5. c and e

## Biotransformation

Biotransformation is the metabolic alteration of a drug to a different chemical structure.

**MECHANISMS OF BIOTRANSFORMATION.**  A drug may either be metabolized from an inactive to an active pharmacologic or toxicologic form or, more commonly, from an active to an inactive pharmacologic form. The principal organ involved in biotransformation reactions is the liver, which utilizes both its microsomal and nonmicrosomal enzyme systems. A secondary and minor site of biotransformation is the blood plasma, where drugs such as ester types of local anesthetics (procaine) and succinylcholine (Anectine) are metabolized by serum (pseudo) cholinesterase.

The prime function of the liver biotransformation mechanisms is to convert a drug to a lipid-insoluble, ionized form which is more readily excreted by the kidney. The conversion of a drug to a more toxic metabolite is of considerable importance and plays a major role in chemical carcinogenesis. It also explains the tha-

lidomide tragedy of the 1960s, which occurred because essentially only one species (man) biotransformed thalidomide into a teratogen. The major chemical reactions involved in biotransformation are oxidation, reduction, hydrolysis (Phase I reactions), and conjugation with glucuronic acid (Phase II reactions). Most of these chemical modifications are very minor in nature, implying that drug–receptor interaction must be highly specific.

**FACTORS ALTERING BIOTRANSFORMATION.**  The rate at which a chemical is biotransformed or the type of metabolite formed may be altered by genetics, age, nutrition, and a number of drugs. The interspecies and intraspecies differences in rate and type of metabolite vary enormously; genetic and species differences in the rate of drug metabolism may result in 10 to 20-fold or greater variances (6). Surely the fact that the metabolic rates and patterns of lower animals may not always be extrapolable to man has been responsible for the loss of potentially useful drugs, the inaccurate labeling of a drug as toxic, and the failure to detect potentially toxic chemicals (thalidomide). The neonate and the aged may not possess all the liver enzymes necessary to metabolize chemicals adequately. The gray baby syndrome occurs in newborn infants due to their inability to metabolize the antibiotic chloramphenicol. Certain drugs, such as sedative–hypnotics, alcohol, tranquilizers, and antihistamines, in chronic usage stimulate the liver microsomal enzymes to increase their own rate of metabolism and that of other drugs (see Drug Interaction).

### QUESTIONS

11. The principal site of biotransformation of a drug is the
    1. plasma
    2. spleen
    3. gastrointestinal tract
    4. liver
    5. reticuloendothelial system

12. Drugs are usually metabolized to their lipid-insoluble, ionized form because drugs are not metabolized to a more toxic form.
    1. Both statement and reason are correct and related.
    2. Both statement and reason are correct but not related
    3. The statement is correct, but the reason is not.
    4. The statement is not correct, but the reason is an accurate statement.
    5. Neither statement nor reason is correct.

## Absorption, Distribution, and Metabolism

Every drug introduced into an intact animal necessarily goes through the same sequence of events. It is absorbed, is distributed to its receptor site, interacts with that receptor to produce a response, is detoxified, and finally is eliminated from the animal.

The method by which the drug is administered to the animal may greatly affect the onset of its action. Drugs may be administered intravenously, intraarterially, intrathecally (within the spinal cord), subcutaneously, intramuscularly, topically, orally, or by inhalation. Drug administration via a syringe is termed parenteral. The parenteral administration of a drug bypasses the membranes of the skin and gastrointestinal mucosa, resulting in a more rapid onset of action. Only a few drugs such as the general anesthetics, amyl nitrite, nicotine, and marihuana are well absorbed through the lung alveoli. Pollutants of the atmosphere are also absorbed in this manner. Some drugs such as aspirin and ethyl alcohol are well absorbed through the gastric mucosa; however, most drugs are absorbed more quickly and extensively in the first few feet of the small intestine.

The rate of absorption and distribution of a drug is critically dependent upon its ability to transverse membranes; this ability is in turn dependent upon the drug's pKa (pH at which 50% of the drug is ionized and 50% is unionized) and lipid solubility. Highly ionized drugs pass through membranes with great difficulty; therefore, it is not surprising that most useful drugs are weak acids and bases, since their physiologic pH is close to neutral (pH 6–8). A basic drug is more highly ionized at an acidic pH and vice versa. According to the fluid mosaic model (7) cell membranes are essentially lipid in nature (with interspaced proteins) and therefore the greater the lipid solubility of a drug, the greater its ability to transverse membranes. The lipid solubility of highly ionized drugs is poor.

The onset of action of a drug is dependent upon its route of administration and its ability to transverse membranes to reach its receptor site. Its onset of action, magnitude of effect, and to some extent its duration of action are all dependent upon a critical amount of drug molecules interacting with tissue receptors (see Structure Action). The pKa of the drug and its lipid solubility play a major role in drug distribution to the receptor site.

Drugs are primarily excreted by the kidney, either in their original state or as biotransformed metabolites. Since the pH of the urine is acidic, basic drugs are more highly ionized and undergo less renal reabsorption. That portion of the drug not absorbed through gastric or intestinal mucosa is excreted in the feces. General anesthetics are excreted through the lungs, and minute amounts of some drugs may be found in the saliva, sweat, and breast milk.

## QUESTIONS

13. The principal route of drug excretion is via the
    1. feces
    2. saliva
    3. urine
    4. bile
    5. sweat

14. Highly ionized drugs transverse membranes poorly because lipid-soluble drugs are usually highly ionized.
    1. Both statement and reason are correct and related.
    2. Both statement and reason are correct but not related.
    3. The statement is correct, but the reason is not.
    4. The statement is not correct, but the reason is an accurate statement.
    5. Neither statement nor reason is correct.

15. Which of the following routes of drug administration are termed parenteral?
    a. Oral
    b. Inhalation
    c. Intramuscular
    d. Intravenous
    e. Subcutaneous
    1. a, b, and c
    2. b, c, and d
    3. c, d, and e
    4. a and b
    5. All of the above

## Drug Interactions

A drug interaction occurs when one drug interferes with the action of another drug through any of the following mechanisms: 1) altered gastrointestinal absorption, 2) competition for plasma protein binding sites, 3) altered hepatic microsomal enzyme activity (metabolism or biotransformation), 4) interference with drug–receptor interaction (synergism or antagonism), and 5) altered renal excretion.

GENERAL ASPECTS. The list of drug interactions is myriad, but fortunately only a limited number are of serious clinical significance (9). The list is even smaller for medical–dental drug interactions (drugs administered by the dentist to a patient receiving medication for a systemic disease). Most drug interactions interfere with drug absorption, distribution, metabolism, and excretion (AOME or pharmacokinetic interactors). A few are of the pharmacodynamic type which involve synergistic or antagonistic actions on similar receptors or physiologic systems.

ALTERED GASTROINTESTINAL ABSORPTION. Various antacids containing calcium, magnesium, and aluminum interfere with the absorption of the tetracyclines, and kaolin–pectin (Kaopectate) interferes with lincomycin absorption.

**COMPETITION FOR PLASMA PROTEIN BINDING SITES.** Aspirin displaces the coumarin anticoagulants, oral hypoglycemics, and methotrexate from plasma proteins, thereby increasing their free blood concentrations and potential toxicity. Sedative–hypnotic agents also displace coumarins from plasma protein.

**ALTERED HEPATIC MICROSOMAL ENZYME ACTIVITY.** Extended (not sporadic) use of various sedative–hypnotics (barbiturates, alcohol) stimulates microsomal enzyme activity and increases the metabolism of the coumarin anticoagulants, tetracyclines, tricyclic antidepressants, corticosteroids, phenytoin, quinidine, and other sedative–hypnotics. The monoamine oxidase inhibitors (MAOI) block hepatic enzymes as well as norepinephrine metabolism in the adrenergic nerve terminal, thereby increasing the depressant effects of narcotics and general anesthetics and increasing sympathetic nerve activity after administration of indirect adrenergic amines such as tyramine and amphetamine.

**INTERFERENCE WITH DRUG–RECEPTOR INTERACTIONS.** All central nervous system depressants (alcohol, barbiturates, nonbarbiturate sedatives, narcotics, antihistamines, tranquilizers, and general anesthetics) are synergistic. The combination of bacteriostatic with bactericidal antibiotics is antagonistic since bacteriostatic agents prevent bacterial multiplication and bactericidal antibiotics affect only dividing organisms. Aspirin increases the ulcerogenic potential of the corticosteriods and enhances the anticoagulant effect of the coumarins by inhibiting platelet agglutination. The halogenated hydrocarbon general anesthetics and cyclopropane sensitize the heart to the arrhythmic effects of epinephrine. Adrenergic amines may also enhance the arrythmic effects of digitalis.

QUESTIONS

16. Aspirin is contraindicated in the presence of
    a. adrenocorticosteriods
    b. coumarin anticoagulants
    c. oral antidiabetic agents
    d. penicillin
    e. codeine
    1. a, b, and c
    2. b, c, and d
    3. c, d, and e
    4. a and d
    5. b and e

17. The combination of bactericidal and bacteriostatic antibiotics results in antagonism because bactericidal antibiotics affect only replicating microorganisms.

1. Both statement and reason are correct and related.
2. Both statement and reason are correct but not related.
3. The statement is correct, but the reason is not.
4. The statement is not correct, but the reason is an accurate statement.
5. Neither statement nor reason is correct.

# CENTRAL NERVOUS SYSTEM

## Sedative–Hypnotics

The sedative–hypnotics are drugs which produce sedation (drowsiness) or hypnosis (sleep), depending on the drug dosage. In higher doses the drugs produce anesthesia (defined as hypnosis, the inability to respond to command, and loss of protective laryngeal reflexes), coma, and death.

**CLASSIFICATION.** The sedative–hypnotics are divided into two types, based upon their chemical structure: 1) barbiturates and 2) nonbarbiturates. Their pharmacologic effects are essentially the same, although the nonbarbiturates are less potent (a greater milligram amount is required to produce the desired effect). The two chemical types are not cross-allergenic.

**MECHANISM OF ACTION.** The sedative–hypnotics probably act at synaptic membrane surfaces within the central nervous system (CNS), possibly in the same manner as inhalation general anesthetics (see Anesthetics) (10). The most sensitive area of the CNS to the action of the sedative–hypnotics is the reticular-activating system (RAS) which functions to keep us awake.

**PHARMACOLOGIC EFFECTS.** The sedative–hypnotics, which act primarily on the CNS, produce sedation, hypnosis, anesthesia, coma, and death as the dosage is increased. Death is due to medullary respiratory depression. There is little effect on the cardiovascular system in normal doses. Rapid eye movement (REM, dreaming) sleep is diminished. The sedative–hypnotics do not suppress the pain pathways of the spinal cord and therefore do not possess any analgesic properties; indeed they produce hyperalgesia (heightened response to pain). The sedative–hypnotics stimulate the liver microsomal enzyme system to increase the metabolism of many other drugs. Because they also stimulate the synthesis of the porphyrins, they are contraindicated in patients with porphyria.

**ABSORPTION, DISTRIBUTION, METABOLISM, AND EXCRETION.** All the various sedative–hypnotics are well absorbed from the gastrointestinal tract. Their onset of action is dependent upon their ability to enter the CNS and therefore their lipid solubility. The barbiturates are classified according to their fat solubility as well as their onset and duration of action: 1) ultrashort-acting, 2) short-acting, 3) intermediate-acting and 4) long-acting. Most of these agents depend upon liver metabolism for their detoxification. The very short duration of action of the ultrashort agents such as thiopental and methohexital is due to redistribution of the drug from the brain to fat and other tissues and not their liver metabolism.

**TOXIC EFFECTS.** The adverse effects of the sedative–hypnotics are a direct extension of their pharmacologic properties: drowsiness, ataxia, hypnosis (if undesired), coma, and death due to respiratory depression. They also exacerbate the symptoms of porphyrism, leading to cranial and peripheral nerve damage. The intravenous agents do not appreciably suppress laryngeal reflexes; they allow for reflex stimulation by saliva, blood, and pain resulting in laryngospasm. Allergy to the barbiturates is not uncommon. Continual use of the sedative–hypnotics may produce a form of drug dependence and subsequent withdrawal symptoms very similar to alcohol (see Drug Abuse). Paradoxical excitement (idiosyncrasy) to the sedative–hypnotics is less common than previously thought, but hyperactivity during emergence from the intravenous agents is common. Although death from normal hypnotic doses is unknown, combination with other CNS depressants is synergistic and very dangerous (see Alcohol).

**THERAPEUTIC USES.** The sedative–hypnotics are useful for preoperative sedation, nighttime hypnosis, and general anesthesia induction. Pentobarbital (Nembutal), is a component of the commonly employed Jorgensen technique of intravenous sedation, and thiopental (Pentothal) and methohexital (Brevital) are employed for anesthesia induction. Phenobarbital (Luminal) is useful in the therapy of epilepsy (cortical focal, grand mal). The use of the sedative–hypnotics as anticonvulsants (acute administration) and daytime antianxiety medication has been totally supplanted by the benzodiazepines (diazepam). Flurazepam (Dalmane) is currently the drug of choice for nighttime sleep induction.

**REPRESENTATIVE AGENTS.** The barbiturates include the ultrashort-acting thiopental (Pentothal) and methohexital (Brevital), the short-acting secobarbital (Seconal) and pentobarbital (Nembutal), the intermediate-acting amobarbital (Amytal) and butabarbital (Butisol), and the long-acting phenobarbital (Luminal). The nonbarbiturate sedative–hypnotics include chloral hydrate (Noctec), glutethimide (Doriden), ethchlorvynol (Placidyl) and the common drug of abuse, methaqualone (Quaalude). Flurazepam (hydrochloride) (Dalmane), a benzodiazepine with significant hypnotic effects, can also be placed in this category.

QUESTIONS

18. Which of the following disease states is an absolute contraindication to the use of the sedative–hypnotic agents?
   1. Liver disease
   2. Renal impairment
   3. Angina pectoris
   4. Porphyrism
   5. Epilepsy

19. Which of the following statements are *true* regarding the sedative–hypnotic agents?
   a. They produce sleep by an effect on the reticular activating system.
   b. They do not produce analgesia.
   c. They may induce drug dependence similar to ethyl alcohol.
   d. Intravenous agents predispose the patient to laryngospasm.
   e. They produce death by respiratory depression.
   1. a, b, and d
   2. b, c, and d
   3. c, d, and e
   4. a and d
   5. All of the above

20. Chloral hydrate should not be administered to a patient allergic to the barbiturates because the barbiturates and nonbarbiturate sedative–hypnotics are cross-allergenic.
   1. Both statement and reason are correct and related.
   2. Both statement and reason are correct but not related.
   3. The statement is correct, but the reason is not.
   4. The statement is not correct, but the reason is an accurate statement.
   5. Neither statement nor reason is correct.

## Anticonvulsants

Anticonvulsants are drugs which prevent or abolish seizure activity in the central nervous system.

**GENERAL ASPECTS OF ANTICONVULSANT DRUGS.** The vast majority of anticonvulsant drugs are employed primarily in the therapy of epilepsy (antiepileptics). For many years the barbiturates were the only drugs available to terminate acute seizure episodes (strychnine intoxication, status epilepticus, local anesthetic-induced convulsions). The barbiturates are no longer used for this purpose since their respiratory and cardiovascular depressant effects are a distinct hazard to individuals recovering from poststimulation CNS depression. The benzodiazepines, notably diazepam (Valium), are now the drugs of choice for termination of most convulsions of whatever origin (see Central Nervous System, Stimulants).

**MECHANISMS OF SEIZURE ACTIVITY.** Epileptic seizures are electrical "explosions" in the brain characterized by high frequency action potential bursts and loss of inhibitory postsynaptic potentials (IPSP). They are characterized by brief, spontaneous seizures; disturbances of consciousness; possible convulsions; and autonomic hyperactivity (12). The seizure is maintained by reentry of excitatory impulses in a closed feedback pathway.

**MECHANISM OF ACTION OF ANTIEPILEPTICS.** Phenytoin (diphenylhydantoin) reduces the duration of neuronal after-discharge, stabilizes neuronal membranes, and limits the spread of seizure activity. The molecular mechanism of phenytoin action is unknown but may involve decreased sodium or calcium permeability or inhibition of Na, K-activated adenosinetriphosphatase. Diazepam terminates local anesthetic-induced seizures by an action on the amygdala portion of the limbic system.

**PHARMACOLOGIC EFFECTS.** All the anticonvulsants produce varying degrees of CNS depression as manifested by ataxia and drowsiness. Phenytoin is useful in terminating certain cardiac arrhythmias.

**CLASSIFICATION OF EPILEPTIC SEIZURES.** The various forms of epilepsy are classified, according to the electroencephalogram patterns and clinical signs and symptoms, into two types: 1) partial seizures—cortical focal (Jacksonian), temporal lobe, and psychomotor; and 2) generalized seizures—absence (petit mal), tonic–clonic (grand mal), and status epilepticus (repeated tonic–clonic seizures for an indefinite period of time) (13).

**TOXIC EFFECTS.** The adverse effects of the antiepileptic drugs are 1) cerebellar and vestibular—ataxia, vertigo, diplopia, 2) behavioral—hyperactivity, confusion, drowsiness; 3) gastrointestinal—anorexia, nausea, vomiting, and 4) allergic—skin lesions, erythema multiforme, blood dyscrasias. Phenytoin is a possible teratogen. There are essentially no adverse effects of diazepam.

**THERAPEUTIC USES.** Diazepam (Valium) is the drug of choice for the termination of all acute seizure activity. Phenytoin (Dilantin) and phenobarbital (Luminal) are the mainstay of therapy in cortical focal and grand mal seizures, primidone (Mysoline) and phenytoin in temporal lobe and psychomotor seizures, and ethosuximide (Zarontin) and trimethadione (Tridione) in absence seizures.

QUESTION

21. Which one of the following anticonvulsant drugs is the agent of choice in terminating most tonic–clonic seizures?
    1. Primidone (Mysoline)
    2. Phenobarbital (Luminal)
    3. Phenytoin (Dilantin)
    4. Diazepam (Valium)
    5. Trimethadione (Tridione)

## Narcotics

A narcotic analgesic is any drug chemically related to morphine or possessing morphinelike properties and the potential for inducing morphinelike drug dependence. The various narcotic drugs include morphine as the prototype, meperidine (Demerol), codeine, oxycodone (Percodan), fentanyl (Sublimaze), methadone (Dolophine), alphaprodine (Nisentil), and diacetylmorphine (heroin). Synonymous terms for the narcotics are opiates or opioids.

**SOURCE.** Morphine and codeine are naturally occurring constituents of opium derived from the milky exudate of the unripe poppy plant (*Papaver somniferum*). Other narcotics are chemical derivatives of morphine or codeine, or synthesized in the laboratory. Opium contains two pharmacologically active alkaloid groups: 1) the phenanthrene (morphine and codeine) and 2) the benzylisoquinolene, principally papaverine, a smooth muscle relaxant without narcotic properties. Opium is formulated as tinctures (alcohol as the solvent) in laudanum and paregoric useful in the treatment of diarrhea.

**MECHANISM OF ACTION.** The opiate (opioid) receptor was first demonstrated in nerve tissue by Pert and Synder in 1973 (14). Opioid receptors in the central nervous system are primarily located in the limbic system, area postrema, solitary nuclei, and the substantia gelatinosa of the spinal cord (15). The location of opioid receptors in the limbic system (amygdala, corpus striatum, and hypothalamus) explains the effect of morphine on the emotional (reaction) component of pain; the location in the area postrema, its tendency to induce nausea and vomiting; and the solitary nuclei location, its suppression of the cough reflex and gastric secretions. The substantia gelatinosa is the "gate" in the gate control theory of pain as espoused by Melzack and Wall (16, 17); the localization of morphine in the substantia gelatinosa lends credence to this theory.

The sodium ion plays an important role in the binding of the opioids or their antagonists to the receptor sites. A high concentration of the sodium ion increases the binding of narcotic antagonists but decreases receptor binding of the narcotic agonists. The opioid receptor may exist in two different configurations (allosteric) regulated by the sodium ion (18).

Opiates probably interact with neruonal or synaptic membrane surfaces to alter ion flow, but the precise mechanisms by which the opioids produce narcosis (analgesia, drowsiness, mood alteration, mental clouding, and anesthesia) is unknown. Some possible mechanisms are 1) decreased tissue levels of adenosine monophosphate (cAMP), 2) increased tissue levels of guanosine monophosphate (cGMP), 3) inhibition of prostaglandins, 4) increased brain catecholamines, or 5) decreased brain acetylcholine levels (15).

The most interesting recent development in narcotic research has been the identification by Hughes, Kosterlitz and colleagues (19) of endogenous opioidlike substances which produce effects similar to morphine. These endogenous opioids have been termed the enkephalins and endorphins. The enkephalins are very short peptides (five amino acids): methionine enkephalin and leucine enkephalin. This recent discovery has led to speculation that individuals who tolerate pain very well may indeed be capable of "turning on" these natural opioids to relieve their pain.

**PHARMACOLOGIC EFFECTS.** Morphine produces analgesia, sedation, euphoria, dysphoria, emesis, constipation, miosis, and respiratory depression. It also releases histamine from the mast cell and reduces or eliminates cough (antitussive). Morphine affects both the objective component of the pain response (pain perception) and the subjective component (pain reaction), the latter probably through an action on the limbic system. The individual may indeed still feel the pain but may be emotionally indifferent to it. Morphine can produce surgical anesthesia in sufficient dosage. Morphine in therapeutic doses has little effect on the cardiovascular system and is not liver toxic. In therapeutic doses codeine produces little euphoria or dysphoria but is analgesic, antitussive, and emetic. Because meperidine possesses anticholinergic effects, it must be used with caution in patients with glaucoma and prostatic disease.

**ABSORPTION, DISTRIBUTION, METABOLISM, AND EXCRETION.** Only a few narcotic agents (codeine, oxycodone, and methadon) produce satisfactory analgesia when administered orally. Morphine and meperidine are best employed parenterally. Codeine is metabolized to morphine.

**TOXICITY.** The most serious adverse effect of the opioids is respiratory depression, leading to a rise in blood carbon dioxide, which poses problems for patients with head injuries. Respiratory depression is the usual cause of death in overdosage. The opioids may also release histamine and therefore may exacerbate asthma. Other side-effects are nausea and vomiting, dizziness, dysphoria, constipation, delirium, and insomnia. Chronic opioid use may result in serious drug dependence (see Drug Abuse). The opioids are relatively contraindicated in patients with hypothyroidism, Addison's disease, diminished respiratory reserve, and asthma, as well as in patients concomitantly receiving other CNS depressants, monoamine oxidase inhibitors and the tricyclic antidepressants.

**REPRESENTATIVE AGENTS.** The narcotic analgesics are the drugs of choice for both moderate and severe pain of whatever origin. Codeine, which is the drug of choice for orofacial pain, is increasingly effective as the dose is increased. Its drug dependence liability is extremely low. Oxycodone (Percodan) is a multiple drug preparation consisting of oxycodone, acetylsalicylic acid–phenacetin–caffeine (ACP), and atropine, but it is probably no more effective than any other codeine–aspirin formulation. Meperidine (Demerol) is less potent than morphine but is equiefficacious in proper dosage. Methadone (Dolophine) is the most efficacious oral narcotic analgesic, but its use has been restricted because it has been abused in methadone maintenance programs for opioid dependence. Fentanyl (Sublimaze) is 50 times more potent than morphine and is a component of Innovar used in neuroleptic analgesia.

**NARCOTIC ANTAGONISTS.** Until recently the only drugs available to treat narcotic intoxication were partial agonists such as nalorphine (Nalline) and levallorphan tartrate (Lorfan). Naloxone (Narcan) is a complete antagonist of the opioid receptor, possessing none of the pharmacologic effects of morphine. Although naloxone is the drug of choice in the treatment of narcotic overdosage, it is imperative to remember that, because its duration of action is much shorter than that of narcotic agents, it allows the patient to return to the narcotic state if the opioid has not been metabolized or excreted. Naltrexone is a complete narcotic antagonist possessing a long (up to 72 hours) duration of action.

## QUESTIONS

22. The pharmacologic effects of morphine include
   - a. sedation
   - b. emesis
   - c. constipation
   - d. histamine release
   - e. euphoria

   1. a, b, and c
   2. b, c, and d
   3. c, d, and e
   4. a, b, and e
   5. All of the above

23. Codeine is an effective analgesic for mild to moderate pain because codeine may induce serious narcotic drug dependence.
    1. Both statement and reason are correct and related.
    2. Both statement and reason are correct but not related.
    3. The statement is correct, but the reason is not.
    4. The statement is not correct, but the reason is an accurate statement.
    5. Neither statement nor reason is correct.

## Nonnarcotic Analgesics

Nonnarcotic analgesics are drugs which reduce somatic pain but do not possess any significant central nervous system depressant effects like the narcotics do. Many of the agents in this group (aspirin, phenylbutazone, and indomethacin) are termed the nonsteroidal antiinflammatory agents or drugs (NSAIAs, NSAIDs).

**CLASSIFICATION.** Nonnarcotic analgesics can be classified as 1) analgesics with antiinflammatory and/or antipyretic properties (aspirin, phenacetin, and acetaminophen); and 2) analgesics chemically related to the narcotics (propoxyphene, ethoheptazine, and pentazocine). These drugs can also be classified as 1) peripherally acting (at the source of pain) and 2) centrally acting (on the CNS). The locus of action of the analgesic drug is important, since drugs acting at different sites are synergistic in their analgesic effect.

**MECHANISM OF ACTION.** The prostaglandins, lipid substances which are found in most tissues, possess a multiplicity of effects. They are one of the chemical mediators of inflammation and pain. Part of the mechanism of action of aspirin is to inhibit their tissue synthesis by blocking the enzyme prostaglandin synthetase (Cyclooxygenase). Acetylsalicylic acid (aspirin) and acetaminophen (Tylenol) also affect the hypothalamus and prostaglandin synthesis in the brain to reduce fever (antipyresis). Acetaminophen is a very poor inhibitor of prostaglandin synthesis peripherally. The centrally acting nonnarcotic analgesics (propoxyphene and pentazocine) produce their effects by essentially unknown mechanisms but probably at synapses similar to the narcotics.

**PHARMACOLOGIC EFFECTS.** Aspirin is analgesic, antipyretic, antiinflammatory, antirheumatic (is effective in rheumatic fever), uricosuric (increases uric acid secretion), and keratolytic (destroys keratin). It is deacetylated in the liver to its major active form, salicylic acid. Aspirin prevents platelet agglutination and platelet adhesion to collagen during blood clotting by preventing the release of adenosine diphosphate (ADP) from platelets and by inhibiting collagen glycosyl-

transferase and thromboxane $A_2$ synthesis from arachidonic acid (see Prostaglandins). The possible prophylactic benefits of aspirin in the prevention of arterial clotting diseases (myocardial infarction) is presently unknown (20). Acetaminophen (Tylenol) is analgesic, and equally effective as an antipyretic as aspirin. The centrally acting nonnarcotic analgesics possess essentially the same range of effects as the narcotics, although in much reduced form: analgesia, sedation, drowsiness, dysphoria, and euphoria.

**TOXIC EFFECTS.** In high doses, aspirin is hypoprothrombinemic and may induce gastric bleeding and ulceration, hepatic damage, and salicylism (drowsiness, tinnitus, sweating, hyperventilation, restlessness, delirium, hallucinations, convulsions, and coma). Alkalinization of the urine with sodium bicarbonate is common antidotal therapy to increase the concentration of ionized, excretable drug. Aspirin is allergenic, although there is a higher incidence of allergy to aspirin in patients with nasal polyps.

Acetaminophen does not possess any of the adverse effects of aspirin on the gastric mucosa and blood clotting mechanism, but it may induce fatal hepatic necrosis with acutely high doses (7 g in adults and 3 g in children) (21). Phenacetin and/or aspirin have been implicated as toxic to the kidneys (analgesic nephropathy), but this is yet unproven. Large doses of propoxyphene and pentazocine produce a narcoticlike syndrome: sedation, ataxia, euphoria or dysphoria, cardiovascular and respiratory depression, coma, and death. Their severe toxic effects are treated in a manner similar to narcotic overdosage (see Narcotic Antagonists). Due to their mood-altering properties, both propoxyphene and pentazocine are potential drugs of abuse, and individuals are known to have become dependent on these drugs. Pentazocine (Talwin) was formulated in an attempt to produce a "nonnarcotic narcotic" and possesses slight narcotic antagonist effects. Its use is associated with a high incidence (approximately 6%) of perceptual changes and dysphoria. None of the nonnarcotic or narcotic analgesics are teratogenic.

**THERAPEUTIC USES.** The nonnarcotic analgesics are useful in the control of mild to moderate pain. The major question is the relative efficacy of one drug versus another. After the consideration of numerous clinical studies designed to determine the relative efficacy of the nonnarcotic analgesics, the following conclusions can be drawn: 1) a 600-mg dose of aspirin is effective as an analgesic, and greater doses produce greater analgesia; 2) 650 mg acetaminophen (Tylenol) is equiefficacious with 600 mg aspirin, and 325 mg acetaminophen is no better than a placebo; 3) APC is no more effective than aspirin alone; 4) propoxyphene (Darvon) in 32-mg doses is no better than a placebo, and in 65-mg doses is usually more effective than a placebo; 5) pentazocine (Talwin) in 50-mg oral doses is comparable in efficacy to 60 mg codeine. It is imperative to remember that peripherally and centrally acting analgesics are synergistic; therefore, the combination of aspirin or acetaminophen with codeine, propoxyphene, or pentazocine is quite rational.

### QUESTIONS

24. The antiinflammatory and antipyretic effects of aspirin are related to its inhibition of the synthesis of
   1. adrenocorticosteroids
   2. bradykinin
   3. histamine
   4. prostaglandins
   5. substance P

25. Which of the following statements are true regarding acetylsalicylic acid?
   a. It is synergistic with codeine.
   b. It prevents platelet agglutination during blood clotting.
   c. Tinnitus is a symptom of aspirin intoxication.
   d. It may induce gastric ulceration and bleeding.
   e. Alkalinization of the urine increases it excretion rate.
   1. a, b, and c
   2. b, c, and d
   3. c, d, and e
   4. a and d
   5. All of the above

26. High doses of acetaminophen may produce severe liver damage because acetaminophen is as effective as an antipyretic as aspirin.
   1. Both statement and reason are correct and related.
   2. Both statement and reason are correct but not related.
   3. The statement is correct, but the reason is not.
   4. The statement is not correct, but the reason is an accurate statement.
   5. Neither statement nor reason is correct.

## Psychotropics

Psychotropic drugs are agents which affect mood and mental processes (behavior) through an action on the central nervous system. These agents are properly employed in the treatment of various mental diseases or emotional disorders.

**CLASSIFICATION OF MENTAL DISEASE.** There are two broad classes of mental disease amenable to drug therapy: 1) functional psychoses (schizophrenia and manic–depressive psychosis) and 2) affective disorders (anxiety and depression). Schizophrenia is characterized by abnormal thought patterns, delusions, paranoid behavior, and a loss of contact with reality. Manic–de-

pressive psychosis, which is usually bipolar (both mania and depression), is characterized by the alteration of extreme elation and motor hyperactivity with depressive episodes. Some authorities classify manic–depression as an affective disorder.

Anxiety is a hyperreaction to external stimuli which should not ordinarily provoke such emotional responses. In contrast, fear is a normal response to threatening stimuli. The common symptoms of anxiety include apprehension, nervousness, panic, sweating, frequent urination, worry, fear, and muscle tension. Depression can be classified as either exogenous or endogenous. Exogenous (reactive) depression occurs in response to definite external stimuli: a major illness, death of a loved one, business or professional failure, or a severe loss of self-esteem. Although such reactions should not be considered abnormal, they may pose a medical problem if they continue for periods long enough to affect social behavior seriously. Endogenous depression begins at a specific period of time (usually later in life) and is unrelated to any specific external stimulus. It is characterized by feelings of guilt and worthlessness, persistent bodily complaints, and loss of energy and appetite. Symptoms of anxiety are very commonly seen in depressive states and vice versa, and a differential diagnosis may be very difficult.

**DRUG THERAPY OF MENTAL DISEASE.** Schizophrenia is treated by the antipsychotic agents (major tranquilizers): phenothiazines and butyrophenones); manic–depressive psychosis, by lithium carbonate and the phenothiazines; anxiety states, by the antianxiety agents (minor tranquilizers), notably the benzodiazepines); and depression, by the tricyclic antidepressants (dibenzazepines), the monoamine oxidase inhibitors, and electroshock therapy.

### Antipsychotic Agents

*Classification.* The antipsychotics (major tranquilizers) are of two chemical types: 1) the phenothiazines and 2) the butyrophenones. Reserpine can also be classed as a major tranquilizer but is now employed only in the treatment of essential hypertension since other antipsychotics are more effective. The phenothiazines include the prototype chlorpromazine (Thorazine) and others such as promazine (Sparine), thioridazine (Mellaril), and prochlorperazine (Compazine). Promethazine (Phenergan) is technically a phenothiazine by chemical structure but is not antipsychotic; it is essentially an antihistamine with sedative properties useful as antianxiety preoperative medication. The butyrophenones include haloperidol (Haldol) and droperidol (Inapsine).

*Mechanism of action.* The mechanism of action by which the antipsychotics reduce or eliminate psychotic behavior is still essentially unknown. The amine hypothesis of schizophrenia states that this disease is due to an abnormal level (either too much or too little) of certain brain amines within the central nervous system, and the amines norepinephrine, serotonin, and dopamine have been studied in this regard. The antipsychotics are known to block dopaminergic neurons within the central nervous system, and also inhibit dopamine-sensitive adenylate cyclase in the limbic system.

*Pharmacologic Effects.* The antipsychotics possess a multiplicity of effects on the central and autonomic nervous systems. Effects on the central nervous system include sedation, reduction in psychotic behavior, emotional quieting, decrease in convulsive thresholds (possibily precipitating convulsions), and alteration in hypothalamic temperature-regulating mechanisms. The phenothiazines are also α-adrenergic blocking drugs, anticholinergics, antihistamines, local anesthetics, and antiemetics (blocking the chemoreceptor trigger zone in the CNS). The antipsychotics also potentiate the analgesic effects of narcotics and droperidol if combined with Sublimaze (fentaryl) in the combination drug, Inouar, for neuroleptic analgesia.

*Toxic Effects.* It can be expected that any drug group possessing such a wide variety of pharmacologic effects also produces a number of adverse effects. The use of the antipsychotics is associated with sedation, endocrine alterations (gynecomastia, lactation, impotence, cessation of ovulation, loss of libido), skin pigmentation, hypotension, disturbances in equilibrium, and allergic reactions (skin lesions, obstructive jaundice, and blood dyscrasias). A most serious form of toxicity associated with the antipsychotics is the extrapyramidal syndrome (involuntary motor movements) probably due to blockade of dopaminergic neurons in the basal ganglia. The syndrome consists of tremors, seizures, akathisia, dyskinesia, and a state resembling Parkinson's disease. Tardive dyskinesia occurs after very long term use of the major tranquilizers and is irreversible.

*Therapeutic Uses.* The antipsychotics are used in the treatment of functional psychoses (schizophrenia and the manic phase of manic–depressive psychosis), chemically induced nausea, alcoholism, LSD intoxication, and for narcotic potentiation.

### Antimania Drugs

*Classification.* Two distinct drug groups are of benefit in the treatment of manic–depressive psychosis: the phenothiazines and lithium carbonate. Lithium was first used for this purpose in 1949.

*Mechanism of Action.* The precise biochemical mechanisms by which the lithium ion suppresses the manic phase of manic–depressive psychosis is unknown but may involve antagonism of adrenergic synapses within the CNS or polypeptide hormones and their effect on adenylate cyclase. The emotion-quieting effects of the phenothiazines are probably responsible for their efficacy in manic states.

*Pharmacologic Effects.* The lithium ion is without substantial pharmacologic actions other than its effectiveness in manic–depressive psychosis.

*Toxic Effects.* Normal side-effects to the lithium ion include nausea and vomiting, diuresis, diarrhea, fatigue, and tremor. Severe intoxication results in tremors, confusion, restlessness, seizures, coma, and possible death.

*Therapeutic Uses.* Lithium carbonate (Eskalith, Lithane, Lithonate) is extremely effective in the treatment of the manic phase of manic–depressive psychosis and in the prophylactic prevention of the manic phase in the bipolar form of the disease. Since its onset of action is slow (4–7 days), a combination of antipsychotics (for control of the manic phase) and lithium (for its long-term benefits) is commonly used.

### Antianxiety Agents

*Classification.* The only two antianxiety agents (minor tranquilizers) of any clinical importance today are the propanediols (meprobamate) and the benzodiazepines. By far the most important of these is the benzodiazepines: diazepam (Valium), chlordiazepoxide (Librium), oxazepam (Serax), chlorazepate (Azene) and flurazepam (Dalmane), lorazepam (Avitan), and prazepam (Vestran).

*Mechanism of Action.* The major locus of action of the benzodiazepines is probably the limbic system, an area of the brain which plays a prominent role in the emotions. The mechanism of action of the benzodiazepines may involve facilitating the inhibitory effects of the neurotransmitter γ–aminobutyric acid (GABA) possibly by facilitating the interaction between GABA and its receptor site (22). The benzodiazepines may then function to potentiate the physiologic actions of GABA.

*Pharmacologic Effects.* The pharmacologic effects of the benzodiazepines, other than the relief of anxiety, are remarkably few. Sedation may occur but it is at least theoretically possible to separate sedation from the tranquilizing effects of these drugs (23). This is not possible with the sedative–hypnotics. The benzodiazepines also relax skeletal muscle by affecting both the brain and the polyneurons of the spinal cord. Diazepam is the drug of choice for terminating most convulsions of whatever origin.

*Absorption, Distribution, Metabolism, and Excretion.* A most important clinical factor in the use of the benzodiazepines is their very slow liver metabolism and the production of active metabolites. Diazepam has a minimal half-life of 20–50 hours, and its metabolite, desmethyldiazepam, may possess an even longer half-life. Flurazepam hydrochloride has a half-life of 50–100 hours; oxazepam possesses the shortest half-life, 3–21 hours. Obviously, the potential for cumulation is very great with drugs which are so slowly metabolized. Peak blood levels are seen at 2 hours with diazepam and at 4 hours with chlordiazepoxide. Diazepam is very poorly and slowly absorbed after intramuscular administration.

*Toxic Effects.* Even in high doses the benzodiazepines produce little cardiovascular or respiratory depression. Sedation is the principal adverse effect. They are mild anticholinergics and may be teratogenic. Long-term, excessive use may induce a form of drug dependence resembling the alcohol–barbiturate type. Paradoxical excitement may be seen in some individuals due to the release of anxiety-bound hostility, aggression inhibited by fear or anxiety. The removal of this anxiety by the benzodiazepines allows for the anxiety–bound hostility to become manifest.

*Therapeutic Uses.* The minor tranquilizers are used in the treatment of anxiety states, convulsions, some forms of epilepsy, and as preoperative medication.

## Antidepressants

**CLASSIFICATION.** There are two types of drugs available for the treatment of either exogenous or endogenous depression: 1) the tricyclic antidepressants (dibenzazepines) and 2) the monoamine oxidase inhibitors (MAOI). The former are used almost exclusively since the MAOI are considerably more toxic.

**MECHANISMS OF ACTION.** The tricyclics block the reuptake of norepinephrine and 5-hydroxytryptamine (serotonin) in adrenergic nerve terminals in the CNS, and this in turn may be responsible for their antidepressant effects. The monoamine oxidase inhibitors interfere with the metabolism of norepinephrine, epinephrine, dopamine, and serotonin in the CNS and the adrenergic nerve terminal. The slow onset of action of these drugs (2–3 weeks) indicates that their effectiveness may be dependent upon depletion of endogenous chemicals.

**PHARMACOLOGIC EFFECTS.** The tricyclics possess strong anticholinergic effects and also block norepinephrine uptake in the heart. The monoamine oxidase inhibitors inhibit many enzymes in the liver, thereby slowing the metabolism of many drugs.

**TOXIC EFFECTS.** The adverse effects associated with the tricyclic antidepressants include hypotension, cardiac arrhythmias, tachycardia, delusions, hallucinations, tremors, mild parkinsonism, sweating, jaundice, and blood dyscrasias. Acute toxicity due to the tricyclics results in hyperpyrexia, hypertension, convulsions, and coma; these effects may be reversed to some extent by physostigmine.

The monoamine oxidase inhibitors are extremely toxic drugs and may induce liver damage, confusion, tremor, insomnia, hallucinations, hypotension, and convulsions. The ingestion of certain foods containing tyramine (beer, cheese, wine) may induce hypertensive crisis in patients taking the monoamine oxidase inhibitors. The inhibition of liver microsomal enzymes by monoamine oxidase inhibitors retards the metabolism of CNS depressants (sedative–hypnotics, narcotics, general anesthetics).

**THERAPEUTIC USES.** The tricyclic antidepressants are the mainstay of therapy for mental depression, particularly of the endogenous type. Unfortunately their slow onset of action (2–3 weeks) renders them useless in the treatment of acute depression so that electroshock therapy may be the treatment of choice. The monoamine oxidase inhibitors are used in the treatment of depressive states unresponsive to any other treatment modalities.

**REPRESENTATIVE AGENTS.** Commonly employed tricyclic antidepressants (imipraminelike drugs, dibenzazepines) are imipramine (Tofranil, Presamine), amitriptyline (Elavil), and doxepin (Sinquan). The monoamine oxidase inhibitors include isocarboxazid (Marplan), tranylcypromine (Parnate), phenelzine (Nardil), and pargyline (Eutonyl). The benzodiazepines are also commonly used in depressive states associated with anxiety.

### QUESTIONS

27. Drugs used in the treatment of mental depression include
    a. sedative–hypnotics
    b. monoamine oxidase inhibitors
    c. dibenzazepines
    d. phenothiazines
    e. reserpine
    1. a, b, and c
    2. b, c, and d
    3. c, d, and e
    4. a and e
    5. b and c

28. The phenothiazine tranquilizers are
    a. α-adrenergic blocking agents
    b. antiemetics
    c. antipsychotic agents
    d. important antianxiety agents
    e. potentiate narcotic agents
    1. a, b, and c
    2. b, c, and d
    3. c, d, and e
    4. a, b, c, and e
    5. a and e

29. Which of the following statements are true regarding the benzodiazepines (diazepam)?
    a. They are antipsychotic agents.
    b. They have a low therapeutic index.
    c. They are skeletal muscle relaxants.
    d. They have very long biologic half-life.
    e. Their locus of action is the limbic system.

1. a, b, and c
2. b, c, and d
3. c, d, and e
4. a and e
5. All of the above

30. Which of the following drugs is used in the treatment of manic–depressive psychosis?
    1. Diazepam
    2. Reserpine
    3. Phenytoin
    4. Lithium carbonate
    5. Phenobarbital

## Alcohol

Ethyl alcohol is a chemical substance produced by the fermentation of sugar by yeast. It possesses pharmacologic and toxic actions on the 1) central nervous system, 2) gastrointestinal tract, 3) cardiovascular system, 4) kidneys, 5) liver, and 6) endocrine system.

### LOCI OF ACTION

*Central Nervous System.* The principal locus of action of ethyl alcohol is the brain. Alcohol does not, at any dose level, stimulate the central nervous system; rather it produces a progressive dose-dependent depression of the CNS. The initial effect is on the reticular activating system and the cerebral cortex. The first mental processes affected are those dependent upon previous experience and training, those that produce sobriety and self-restraint. As the dose of alcohol is increased, the following effects occur: 1) loss of attention, judgment, memory, and concentration; 2) loss of self-restraint and inhibition; 3) impaired visual and motor coordination; 4) impaired heavy muscle function; 5) sleep, 6) coma, and 7) respiratory depression resulting in death. Ethyl alcohol possesses significant analgesic properties.

*Gastrointestinal Tract.* Ethyl alcohol increases the secretion of saliva and gastric juice by a direct stimulant effect and psychic (pleasurable) stimulation. Alcoholics commonly suffer from chronic gastritis. Alcohol has an emetic effect because it directly irritates the gastrointestinal tract and because it acts on the nausea center, the chemoreceptor trigger zone (CTZ) in the area postrema, in the brain.

*Cardiovascular System.* Ethyl alcohol is a vasodilator and prevents the vasoconstrictive response of skin blood vessels to cold. Moderate doses produce only minor changes in blood pressure, pulse rate, and cardiac output. Acute intoxication results in severe cardiovascular depression. Large chronic doses damage the heart.

*Kidneys.* Alcohol produces a diuresis by inhibiting antidiuretic hormone secretion. An individual's increased liquid intake when drinking alcoholic beverages is also a factor.

*Liver.* In excessive amounts alcohol increases the fat content of the liver and may induce cirrhosis.

*Endocrine System.* Alcohol releases catecholamines from the adrenal medulla resulting in hyperglycemia, increased blood pressure, and mydriasis.

ABSORPTION, DISTRIBUTION, METABOLISM, AND EXCRETION. Although ethyl alcohol is rapidly absorbed from the stomach, it is primarily absorbed from the small intestine. Food in the stomach effectively retards alcohol absorption by slowing its passage into the duodenum. Alcohol is distributed evenly throughout the body according to total body water, and 90%–98% is metabolized in the liver to acetaldehyde, acetyl coenzyme A (CoA), and $CO_2$. Disulfiram (Antabuse), used in the treatment of alcoholism, inhibits the conversion of acetaldehyde to acetyl coenzyme A, thus producing the most unpleasant effects of acetaldehyde intoxication. Since the liver metabolism of alcohol is constant at the average rate of 10 ml/hour (0.01%), 4 oz (120 ml) of a 100-proof beverage (proof value is double the percent of alcohol by volume) would require 6 hours to metabolize completely.

TOXIC EFFECTS. The beginning acute lethal dose of ethyl alcohol is approximately 0.50% (500 mg/100 ml blood) and is produced by ingestion of 12–15 oz pure alcohol drunk rapidly by a 150-lb person. Most states accept a 0.10% blood–alcohol concentration as proof of intoxication while driving an automobile. Chronic alcoholism results in 1) chronic alcoholic deterioration (dilated facial capillaries, bloated appearance, flabby muscles, emotional instability, memory impairment) 2) psychoses (delirium tremens), and 3) peripheral tissue damage (fatty liver, cirrhosis, myocarditis, neuropathy).

CONTRAINDICATIONS. Ethyl alcohol is contraindicated in the presence of 1) peptic ulcer, 2) severe hepatic or renal disease, 3) epilepsy, 4) porphyrism 5) Hodgkin's disease, 6) previous drug dependence on alcohol, and 7) other central nervous system depressants. The concomitant ingestion of alcohol and barbiturates may reduce the blood–alcohol level which would be fatal by 30%.

THERAPEUTIC USES. Ethyl alcohol is therapeutically employed as a sedative (preoperative), hypnotic (sleep), analgesic, and local anesthetic (to produce permanent nerve damage in neuralgia disorders).

### QUESTION

31. Which of the following statements regarding ethyl alcohol is false?
    1. It is primarily absorbed in the stomach.
    2. It is metabolized at a constant rate.
    3. It possesses analgesic effects.

(*Continued*)

4. It does not produce central nervous system stimulation.
5. It stimulates gastric secretions.

## Stimulants

Stimulants which increase nerve activity in the CNS are manifested by mood elevation, wakefulness, increased motor activity, and potential hallucinations and convulsions. An old term for these drugs is analeptics. The central nervous system stimulants constitute a chemically heterogeneous group of drugs including the amphetamines, the xanthines, strychnine, tetanus toxin, picrotoxin, nikethamide, pentylenetetrazol, and newer drugs such as doxapram and methylphrenidate.

MECHANISM OF ACTION. The amphetamines produce their central effects by releasing norepinephrine from nerve terminals and by a norepinephrinelike effect on the postjunctional membrane (both indirect and direct adrenergic effects). Strychnine and tetanus toxin block postsynaptic nerve inhibition. Strychnine is an antagonist of glycine, an inhibitory nerve transmitter in the CNS. Picrotoxin blocks presynaptic nerve inhibition. Most other CNS stimulants enhance synaptic excitation. In effect nerve impulses travel unrestricted throughout the central nervous system; homeostasis is maintained by a balance between excitatory and inhibitory nerve transmission. The central mechanism of action of the xanthines is unknown, but their peripheral effects are largely the result of increasing tissue concentrations of cyclic adenosine monophosphate (cAMP) by inhibition of the enzyme phosphodiesterase which metabolizes cAMP to the pharmacologically inactive 5 AMP.

PHARMACOLOGIC EFFECTS. Strychnine produces complete contraction of all voluntary muscles and opisthotonos (body arched so that only the head and feet are touching the ground). Tetanus toxin produces varying degrees of convulsions. The amphetamines induce euphoria, aggression, paranoid behavior, and severe mental depression after their use is discontinued. Methylphenidate is chemically and pharmacologically related to the amphetamines. The xanthines constrict cerebral blood vessels and peripherally (outside the CNS) produce increased myocardial contraction, diuresis, relaxation of bronchial and other smooth muscles, and increased gastric secretions.

TOXIC EFFECTS. The adverse effects of the CNS stimulants are directly related to their pharmacologic actions: inability to sleep, irritability, restlessness, tremors, aggravation of peptic ulcers (xanthines), hyperpyrexia, hypertension, tachycardia, mental disturbances, and convulsions. Intravenous diazepam (Valium) is effective antidotal therapy in terminating the convulsions.

THERAPEUTIC USES. Stimulants such as pentylenetetrazol (Metrazol) have been used to stimulate respiration in patients intoxicated with CNS depressants (barbiturates). However, this practice is no longer employed since the margin of safety between respiratory stimulation and the convulsions is very narrow. Doxapram (Dopram) possesses a higher therapeutic index and is used to treat respiratory depression induced by general anesthetics. The xanthines (caffeine, theophylline, and theobromine) as found in numerous beverages (coffee, tea, colas, and cocoa) are used as social stimulants and as drugs (theophylline) in the treatment of bronchial asthma and congestive heart failure. The amphetamines have little, if any, present therapeutic usefulness but have been employed in the treatment of obesity (as anorexants), mental depression, narcolepsy, and Parkinson's disease. Methylphenidate (Ritalin) is effective in the treatment of the minimal brain dysfunction syndrome.

QUESTION
32. Theophylline is useful in the treatment of bronchial asthma because the xanthines are direct $\beta$-adrenergic receptor stimulants.
   1. Both statement and reason are correct and related.
   2. Both statement and reason are correct but not related.
   3. The statement is correct, but the reason is not.
   4. The statement is not correct, but the reason is an accurate statement.
   5. Neither statement nor reason is correct.

## AUTONOMIC NERVOUS SYSTEM

Since the autonomic nervous system (ANS) regulates the physiologic activities of organ structures and systems not under voluntary control, such as the heart, blood vessels, glands, viscera, and smooth muscle, it controls respiration, circulation, digestion, metabolism, body temperature, sweating, salivation, and endocrine function. The hypothalamus is the principal locus of integration of the ANS. There are two distinct divisions of the ANS: 1) parasympathetic (cholinergic) and 2) sympathetic (adrenergic). Most structures innervated by these systems are affected in an opposite manner (stimulatory vs. inhibitory, contraction vs. relaxation). The parasympathetic nervous system is primarily involved in homeostasis; the sympathetic nervous system, in emergency and stress situations. Stimulation of the parasympathetic nervous system results in miosis, reduced heart rate and force of myocardial contraction, vasodilation, bronchial smooth muscle contraction, increased gastric secretions and intestinal muscle tone and release of catecholamines from the adrenal medulla via ganglionic stimulation. Excitation of the sympathetic nervous system results in mydriasis; increased heart rate and force of myocardial contraction; either vasodilation or vasoconstriction, depending on the location of the blood vessels; bronchial smooth muscle relaxation; relaxation of intestinal smooth muscle; and glycogenolysis.

## Neurohumoral Transmission

A clear understanding of the concept of neurohumoral transmission is vital to appreciate the manner in which drugs alter the activity of the ANS.

MECHANISM. In neurotransmission the activity of nerve cells and the structures they innervate are regulated by endogenous chemical mediators released by nerve stimulation at nerve synapses or neuroeffector junctions (where the nerve innervates the particular organ system). Nerves therefore transmit their information (impulses) across synapses and neuroeffector junctions by means of these specific chemicals known as neurotransmitters. The prime neurotransmitters in the ANS are acetylcholine, norepinephrine, and epinephrine. Additional neurotransmitters located in the CNS are dopamine, serotonin, histamine, γ-aminobutyric acid, and the amino acids glycine, glutamic acid, and aspartic acid.

SEQUENCE OF EVENTS. A number of individual steps are essential to the completion of the sequential events occurring in nerve transmission:

1. Synthesis of the chemical mediators. Acetylcholine is synthesized in the cholinergic nerve terminal from choline and acetyl CoA by the enzyme choline acetylase; norepinephrine is synthesized in the adrenergic nerve terminal from phenylalanine and tyrosine via the intermediate dopamine.
2. Binding and storage of mediators. Acetylcholine is stored within vesicles in the nerve terminal in a highly concentrated ionic form; norepinephrine is bound to adenosine triphosphate and a protein.
3. Release of chemical mediators. The nerve action potential causes acetylcholine- and norepinephrine-containing vesicles to fuse with the presynaptic membrane and discharge their contents.
4. Diffusion across the synaptic cleft. The released chemical mediator acetylcholine or norepinephrine diffuses across the synaptic cleft or neuroeffector junction to combine with receptors in the postjunctional (postsynaptic) membrane.
5. Interaction with the postjunctional (postsynaptic) membrane. Activation of the receptor by the neurotransmitter produces either an excitatory

postsynaptic potential or an inhibitory postsynaptic potential to continue nerve transmission.
6. Termination of action of the mediator. The postjunctional action of acetylcholine is terminated by metabolism by the enzyme acetylcholinesterase; the action of norepinephrine, by diffusion into the surrounding tissue and reuptake into the adrenergic nerve terminal.
7. Repolarization of the postjunctional (postsynaptic) membrane. Termination of chemical mediator action allows for the return of the receptor to its original state and reexcitation.

## Neuropharmacologic (autonomic) Receptors

There are two types of autonomic receptors: 1) cholinergic (interact with acetylcholine) and 2) adrenergic (interact with norepinephrine and epinephrine). The cholinergic receptor is divided into two types: muscarinic and nicotinic. The muscarinic cholinergic receptor is located at the neuroeffector junction of the parasympathetic nervous system (where the nerve fiber innervates the organ system). The nicotinic receptor is located at all autonomic ganglia (both parasympathetic and sympathetic) and at the voluntary neuromuscular junction (not part of the ANS). Stimulation of the muscarinic receptor results in stimulation of the enzyme guanyl cyclase which in turn increases the tissue concentration of $3'5'$ guanosine monophosphate (cGMP).

The adrenergic receptor is also divided into two types: α (alpha) and β (beta). Stimulation of the α receptor results in vasoconstriction, mydriasis, and gastrointestinal smooth muscle relaxation. Excitation of the β adrenergic receptor results in vasodilation, increased heart rate and force of myocardial contraction, bronchial smooth muscle relaxation, and glycogenolysis. Beta adrenergic stimulation results in increased tissue levels of cyclic AMP (cAMP) through stimulation of the enzyme adenylate cyclase. Therefore, the β receptor is closely associated with or identical to adenylate cyclase located at the neuroeffector junction.

## Sites of Drug Action in the ANS and CNS

Numerous drugs act at all the various steps involved in neurohumoral transmission to either increase or decrease the effects of the neurotransmitters. Hemicholinium decreases the synthesis of acetylcholine, and botulinus toxin prevents the release of acetylcholine, resulting in diminished cholinergic response. Anticholinesterase drugs such as the organophosphate insecticides inhibit the enzyme acetylcholinesterase, thereby preventing the termination of acetylcholine action. The belladonna alkaloids (atropine and scopolamine) are cholinergic blocking drugs which occupy the muscarinic receptor site and prevent its excitation by acetylcholine. Epinephrine is released from the adrenal medulla during stress and interacts with both $\alpha$ and $\beta$ receptors. Tyramine and the amphetamines release norepinephrine from the adrenergic nerve terminal, and the norepinephrine in turn interacts with adrenergic receptors. Phentolamine and propranolol are $\alpha$ and $\beta$ blocking drugs, respectively, and prevent the excitation of these receptors by norepinephrine and epinephrine. Reserpine and guanethidine deplete norepinephrine in the adrenergic nerve terminal and prevent its reuptake, thereby reducing adrenergic tone to blood vessels. Nicotine and mecamylamine hydrochloride are stimulants and depressants of autonomic ganglia, respectively. In the CNS the antidepressant drug imipramine blocks norepinephrine reuptake into the nerve terminal; chlorpromazine, a major tranquilizer, blocks the receptor for dopamine; and strychnine is an antagonist of the inhibitory neurotransmitter, glycine.

### Classification of ANS Drugs

The drugs affecting the ANS are classified according to the effects they produce: 1) adrenergic, 2) cholinergic, 3) adrenergic blocking, 4) cholinergic blocking, and 5) ganglion stimulating and blocking.

ADRENERGICS. The effects of adrenergic drugs are similar to those of the sympathetic (adrenergic) nervous system stimulants. In addition, many of these agents possess stimulatory effects on the CNS. Adrenergic is synonymous with sympathomimetic.

*Classification.* The adrenergic drugs can be classified according to either their chemical structure or their mechanism of action. The chemical classification depends upon whether the drug contains the catechol (o-dihydroxybenzene) structure or not. The catecholamines are only four: norepinephrine, epinephrine, isoproterenol, and dopamine. The noncatecholamines (lacking one of the hydroxyl groups on the benzene ring) include: the amphetamines, ephedrine, metaraminol (Aramine), mephentermine (Wyamine), methoxamine hydrochloride (Vasoxyl), and phenylephrine hydrochloride (Neo-Synephrine).

The drugs are classified according to their mechanism of action as to whether they are 1) direct acting (interact directly with the $\alpha$ and/or $\beta$ receptors in the postjunctional membrane), 2) indirect acting (release norepinephrine from the adrenergic nerve terminal), or 3) mixed-acting (both direct and indirect action). All of the catecholamines are direct acting adrenergic amines. Most of the noncatecholamines are also direct acting. Tyramine is an indirect acting adrenergic amine, and the amphetamines are mixed-acting. Most drugs in both categories possess highly varying degrees of both $\alpha$- and $\beta$-adrenergic stimulation. Phenyl-

ephrine is solely an $\alpha$ drug, norepinephrine is almost exclusively an $\alpha$ drug, and isoproterenol is solely a $\beta$-adrenergic stimulant. Epinephrine is both an $\alpha$ and $\beta$ drug but is the most potent of the $\alpha$-adrenergic stimulants.

*Mechanism of Action.* The direct acting adrenergic drugs interact with either the $\alpha$ or $\beta$ receptor or both at the neuroeffector junction of the sympathetic nervous system. Indirect adrenergic amines release norepinephrine from the adrenergic nerve terminal; the norepinephrine then interacts primarily with the $\alpha$ receptor. Drugs with a mixed action possess both direct and indirect actions.

*Pharmacologic Effects.* The concept of the $\alpha$- and $\beta$-adrenergic receptors (see Neuropharmacologic (Autonomic) Receptors) is best understood by comparing the effects of norepinephrine, epinephrine, and isoproterenol on the cardiovascular system under controlled conditions. Norepinephrine (almost solely an $\alpha$ drug) produces increased systolic pressure, increased diastolic pressure, increased mean pressure, decreased heart rate, decreased cardiac output, and increased peripheral resistance. Epinephrine (both an $\alpha$ and $\beta$ drug) produces an increased systolic pressure, decreased diastolic pressure, stable mean pressure, increased cardiac output, increased heart rate, and decreased peripheral resistance. Isoproterenol (solely a $\beta$ drug) produces increased systolic pressure, decreased diastolic pressure, decreased mean pressure, increased heart rate, increased cardiac output, and decreased peripheral resistance. The noncatecholamines possess variable $\alpha$ and $\beta$ effects, but most produce vasoconstriction. The $\alpha$ effects of epinephrine dominate at higher doses. Drugs possessing $\alpha$ effects induce mydriasis; those with $\beta$ actions, glycogenolysis and bronchial smooth muscle relaxation.

*Toxic Effects.* The adverse effects of the adrenergic drugs are generally those of sympathetic (adrenergic) nerve stimulation: fear, anxiety, restlessness, headache, tremor, tachycardia, pallor, and respiratory difficulty. Higher doses may induce cerebral hemorrhage and cardiac arrhythmias. A number of general anesthetics (see Anesthetics, General) sensitize the heart to the arrhythmic effects of the adrenergic drugs. The amphetamines (Benzedrine, Dexedrine, and Methedrine) given intravenously may induce convulsions and hallucinations.

*Therapeutic Uses.* Drugs possessing an $\alpha$-adrenergic effect are used to produce vasoconstriction. Epinephrine (Adrenalin) possesses a very potent $\alpha$ effect on the blood vessels of skin and mucosa and is a drug of choice to control hemorrhage and to reduce absorption of local anesthetics. Drugs possessing a $\beta$ effect (epinephrine, ephedrine, and isoproterenol) are most useful in bronchial asthma, and epinephrine is the drug of choice for the severe bronchoconstriction seen in systemic anaphylactic shock. Alpha drugs such as norepinephrine (Levophed), metaraminol (Aramine) and methoxamine (Vasoxyl) are sometimes used in hypotensive states to elevate blood pressure by vasoconstriction although this practice may be irrational since these drugs reduce blood flow to vital organs such as the brain. Other $\alpha$ drugs (phenylephrine and its congeners) are useful as nasal decongestants. The amphetamines have been employed in the treatment of obesity (anorexia), narcolepsy, mental depression, Parkinson's disease, and epilepsy, but better and safer drugs are available.

**CHOLINERGICS.** Cholinergic drugs produce effects similar to those of acetylcholine, both muscarinic and nicotinic, and effects similar to those of drugs which activate the parasympathetic nervous system. The cholinergic agents are divided into two types: acetylcholinelike types and anticholinesterases. Cholinergic drugs are sometimes called cholinomimetic.

*Mechanism of Action.* Drugs with an acetylcholinelike effect act directly on the cholinergic receptor (both muscarinic and nicotinic). Anticholinesterase agents possess a greater affinity for the enzyme acetylcholinesterase than for acetylcholine and block the enzymes active sites, thereby causing acetylcholine to continue functioning as a neurotransmitter. Anticholinesterase drugs are divided into two types, reversible and irreversible, depending on their duration of action (hours versus days) in blocking acetylcholinesterase. Both types of cholinergic drugs produce essentially the same pharmacologic effects but, obviously, by different mechanisms.

*Pharmacologic Effects.* Cholinergic drugs induce vasodilation, decreased rate and force of myocardial contraction, increased gastric secretions and intestinal muscle tone, bladder and bronchial constriction, miosis, increased glandular secretions, and stimulation and later depression of autonomic ganglia and the neuromuscular junction.

*Toxic Effects.* The signs and symptoms of intoxication with cholinergic drugs are termed cholinergic crisis: flushing and warmth of the skin (vasodilation), tachycardia (adrenal release of epinephrine), extreme salivation, lacrimation and sweating, cardiovascular collapse, coma, and convulsions. Death from such intoxication is due to a depolarizing paralysis of the muscles of respiration (diaphragm and intercostal muscles).

*Therapeutic Uses.* The principal use of acetylcholinelike drugs such as bethanechol chloride (Urecholine) is as a smooth muscle stimulant in the treatment of urinary retention, postoperative abdominal distention, and gastric atony after vagotomy. The shorter acting anticholinesterases such as neostigmine (Prostigmin) are used in the treatment of glaucoma and myasthenia gravis. Physostigmine may reverse the CNS effects of diazepam and the tricyclic antidepressants. The long acting acetylcholinesterase (organophosphates) such as parathion are employed as insecticides and nerve gases. Pilocarpine, one of the cholinomimetic alkaloids (along with muscarine), is used as a miotic and as a stimulant for salivary secretions. Muscarine has only toxicologic interest as the causative agent of rapid mushroom (*Amanita muscaria*) poisoning.

**ADRENERGIC BLOCKING DRUGS.** Adrenergic blocking drugs suppress (inhibit) activity within the sympathetic (adrenergic) nervous system.

*Classification.* Drugs which inhibit the sympathetic nervous system are divided into two types, adrenergic blocking and adrenergic neuron blocking, depending upon their mechanism of action. Adrenergic blocking drugs act at the postjunctional (neuroeffector) membrane to block either the $\alpha$ or $\beta$ receptor, but not both. Therefore, they are classified as $\alpha$–adrenergic blocking drugs or $\beta$–adrenergic blocking drugs. Adrenergic neuron blocking drugs act prejunctionally, at the adrenergic nerve terminal, to interfere with the storage and release of norepinephrine. Therefore, they affect both $\alpha$ and $\beta$ responses, but primarily $\alpha$, since norepinephrine is predominantly an $\alpha$ drug.

*Mechanism of Action.* Adrenergic blocking drugs are competitive inhibitors of either the $\alpha$ or $\beta$ adrenergic receptor at the neuroeffector junction of the sympathetic nervous system. Adrenergic neuron blocking drugs affect the adrenergic nerve terminal by one of the following mechanisms: 1) blocking adrenergic nerve transmission, 2) preventing the release of norepinephrine, 3) preventing vesicular (granular) uptake of norepinephrine, and 4) depleting norepinephrine in the nerve terminal. Guanethidine sulfate (Ismelin) possesses all four effects, whereas reserpine only depletes norepinephrine in the adrenergic terminal and prevents its granular reuptake. Some of the drugs (methyldopa) act on the CNS to reduce blood pressure.

*Pharmacologic Effects.* The effects of the drugs which suppress adrenergic nerve activity are highly variable, depending upon the relative degree of $\alpha$ or $\beta$ control of a given organ system and the level of stimulation at the time the drug is given. Alpha blocking drugs induce hypotension, reflex tachycardia, miosis, and nasal stuffiness. Beta blocking drugs increase airway resistance in the bronchi, produce hypotension (mechanism unknown), and may induce heart failure ($\beta$ blockade). The adrenergic neuron blocking drugs produce a transient increase in blood pressure, followed by a decline in blood pressure, along with the other adrenergic blocking effects.

*Toxic Effects.* The adverse effects of the adrenergic blocking drugs are essentially the same as their pharmacologic effects, since all may interfere with processes in the CNS and result in depression, lassitude, sedation, nightmares, and hallucinations. The mental depression induced by reserpine may be so great as to promote suicidal behavior.

***Therapeutic Uses.*** The beneficial effects of the adrenergic blocking drugs have been limited. The α–blocking drugs have been disappointing in the treatment of essential hypertension, but they are useful in the management of shock because they increase blood flow to vital organs. The β–blocking drug propranolol (Inderal) is used in the treatment of cardiac arrhythmias, hypertension, and angina pectoris. Guanethidine sulfate (Ismelin), methyldopa (Aldomet), and reserpine (Serpasil) are only employed in the treatment of essential hypertension. The ergot alkaloids which are both α–stimulating and α–blocking agents are used in the treatment of migraine headaches and as oxytocics to decrease postpartum bleeding.

**CHOLINERGIC BLOCKING DRUGS.** Cholinergic blocking drugs inhibit the action of acetylcholine at the neuroeffector junction of the parasympathetic nervous system. These drugs are classic antimuscarinic agents. Some of the synonyms for the cholinergic blocking drugs are anticholinergics, antiparasympathetics, and parasympatholytics.

***Classification.*** The cholinergic blocking drugs are classified as 1) the belladonna alkaloids (atropine and scopolamine) and 2) synthetic anticholinergics (methantheline and propantheline).

***Botanical Sources.*** The belladonna alkaloids have been used pharmacologically and toxicologically for centuries. They are naturally occurring compounds in the deadly nightshade plant (*Atropa belladonna*), jimson weed (*Datura stramonium*) and henbane (*Hyoscyamus niger*).

***Mechanism of Action.*** The cholinergic blocking drugs are classic competitive antagonists (inhibitors) of acetylcholine at the neuroeffector junction of the parasympathetic nervous system.

***Pharmacologic Effects.*** The cholinergic blocking drugs produce the following effects (in decreasing order of sensitivity) through inhibition (blockade) of the parasympathetic nervous system: 1) decreased secretions (salivary, bronchial, sweat), 2) mydriasis and cycloplegia, 3) increased heart rate due to vagal blockade (in higher doses) 4) decreased gastrointestinal tone and motility, and 5) decreased gastric secretions.

***Toxic Effects.*** The adverse effects of the cholinergic blocking drugs in toxic doses include: dry, burning mouth; marked thirst; blurred vision; widely dilated pupils; tachycardia; flushing of the skin; and central effects of restlessness, excitement, delirium, and psychotic behavior. Toxic doses of atropine also produce central nervous system effects of restlessness, irritability, delirium, disorientation, and hallucinations. Sco

polamine differs from atropine in normal usage because it produces central nervous system depression resulting in sedation and amnesia; in toxic doses, however, it produces stimulant effects similar to those of atropine. The anticholinergics are contraindicated in patients with glaucoma or prostatic disease.

***Therapeutic Uses.*** The cholinergic blocking drugs are used in the treatment of Parkinson's disease, gastrointestinal spasms, peptic ulcer. They are used as antidotes for anticholinesterase and mushroom intoxication and as mydriatics and cycloplegics in opthalmology. They can also be used to reduce salivary and bronchial secretions in dentistry and anesthesiology.

**GANGLIONIC BLOCKADE** Ganglion-blocking drugs are agents which inhibit (block) all autonomic ganglia, both sympathetic and parasympathetic. Hexamethonium was the first ganglion-blocking drug developed, but it is no longer used therapeutically. Atropine and curare also block autonomic glanglia, but only in toxic doses.

***Mechanism of Action.*** Ganglion blockers are competitive antagonists of acetylcholine at the postsynaptic (postjunctional) membrane of autonomic ganglia.

***Pharmacologic Effects.*** The ganglion-blocking drugs generally produce 1) hypotension, 2) increased heart rate, 3) atony of the bladder and gastrointestinal tract, 4) reduction in gastric secretions, 5) mydriasis and cycloplegia, and 6) reduced perspiration and salivation (xerostomia).

***Toxic Effects.*** The adverse effects of ganglion blocking drugs are identical to their pharmacologic effects.

***Therapeutic Uses.*** Ganglion-blocking drugs are therapeutically employed only to produce hypotension. They are used to 1) produce controlled hypotension and subsequent hemorrhage reduction during surgical procedures and 2) to reduce blood pressure in hypertensive crisis.

***Representative Agents.*** The drugs in this category currently available are mecamylamine (Inversine), pentolinium (Ansolysen), and trimethaphan (Arfonad).

### QUESTIONS

33. Stimulation of the β adrenergic receptor results in
    a. vasoconstriction
    b. mydriasis
    c. increased heart rate
    d. bronchial relaxation
    e. glycogenolysis

    1. a, b, and c
    2. b, c, and d
    3. c, d, and e
    4. a and d
    5. All of the above

34. The β adrenergic receptor is closely related to which of the following enzymes?

1. Phosphodiesterase
2. Adenosinetriphosphatase
3. Adenylate cyclase
4. Monoamine oxidase
5. Acetylcholinesterase

35. One of the following drugs partially produces its effects by releasing norepinephrine from the adrenergic nerve terminal. Which one?
    1. Isoproterenol (Isuprel)
    2. Amphetamine
    3. Phenylephrine (Neo-Synephrine)
    4. Dopamine
    5. None of the above

36. Epinephrine is used as a vasoconstrictor in local anesthetic solutions because epinephrine has an α effect on the blood vessels of skin and mucosa.
    1. Both statement and reason are correct and related.
    2. Both statement and reason are correct but not related.
    3. The statement is correct, but the reason is not.
    4. The statement is not correct, but the reason is an accurate statement.
    5. Neither statement nor reason is correct.

37. Epinephrine and norepinephrine are direct acting adrenergic drugs because epinephrine and norepinephrine interact with α and β receptors at the adrenergic neuroeffector junction.
    1. Both statement and reason are correct and related.
    2. Both statement and reason are correct but not related.
    3. The statement is correct, but the reason is not.
    4. The statement is not correct, but the reason is an accurate statement.
    5. Neither statement nor reason is correct.

38. Atropine and scopolamine produce identical therapeutic effects because atropine and scopolamine block the muscarinic cholinergic receptor.
    1. Both statement and reason are correct and related.
    2. Both statement and reason are correct but not related.
    3. The statement is correct, but the reason is not.
    4. The statement is not correct, but the reason is an accurate statement.
    5. Neither statement nor reason is correct.

39. The muscarinic cholinergic receptor is located at the
    1. neuroeffector junction of the sympathetic nervous system
    2. neuroeffector junction of the parasympathetic nervous system
    3. sympathetic autonomic ganglia
    4. parasympathetic autonomic ganglia
    5. neuromuscular junction

40. Propranolol (Inderal) is a β–adrenergic blocking drug useful in the treatment of
    a. hypertension
    b. angina pectoris
    c. cardiac arrhythmias
    d. cardiac arrest
    e. bronchial asthma
    1. a, b, and c
    2. b, c, and d
    3. c, d, and e
    4. a and d
    5. d and e

41. One of the earliest and most prominent signs of intoxication with cholinergic drugs is
    1. pallor
    2. vasoconstriction
    3. convulsions
    4. bradycardia
    5. extreme salivation

42. Reserpine is useful in the treatment of essential hypertension because reserpine depletes norepinephrine in the adrenergic nerve terminal.
    1. Both statement and reason are correct and related.
    2. Both statement and reason are correct but not related.
    3. The statement is correct, but the reason is not.
    4. The statement is not correct, but the reason is an accurate statement.
    5. Neither statement nor reason is correct.

43. Ganglion-blocking drugs are useful in the treatment of hypertensive crisis because ganglion-blocking drugs increase parasympathetic tone on blood vessels.
    1. Both statement and reason are correct and related.
    2. Both statement and reason are correct but not related.
    3. The statement is correct, but the reason is not.
    4. The statement is not correct, but the reason is an accurate statement.
    5. Neither statement nor reason is correct.

44. The adrenergic drugs are used therapeutically to
    a. reduce hemorrhage
    b. reduce nasal congestion
    c. terminate convulsions
    d. relax bronchial smooth muscle
    e. induce hypotension
    1. a, b, and c
    2. b, c, and d
    3. c, d, and e
    4. a, b, and d
    5. None of the above

45. The following statements regarding atropine are true.
    a. It is a competitive antagonist of norepinephrine.
    b. It produces xerostomia.
    c. It induces mydriasis.
    d. It produces tachycardia.
    e. It is an inhibitor of acetylcholinesterase.
    1. a, b, and c
    2. b, c, and d
    3. c, d, and e
    4. a and e
    5. All of the above

# CARDIOVASCULAR SYSTEM

## Cardiac Glycosides

The term cardiac glycosides is a generic term for a group of drugs chemically related to digitalis which are effective in the treatment of congestive heart failure and atrial cardiac arrhythmias.

**HISTORY.** The pharmacologic actions of the foxglove plant (*Digitalis purpurea*) were known to the ancient Egyptians. They were first published in medical literature in 1785 by Withering, who described the plant's effects on dropsy (congestive heart failure).

**PATHOPHYSIOLOGY OF CONGESTIVE HEART FAILURE.** Starling's law states that the force of contraction of the heart increases as the systolic fiber length increases; therefore, the heart enlarges to compensate for diminished efficiency. The essential pathology in congestive heart failure is a progressive loss in efficiency of cardiac muscle, resulting in cardiac enlargement, through activation of Starling's law, and peripheral edema. The peripheral edema results from 1) increased hydrostatic pressure in capillaries and veins, 2) reduced cardiac output allowing for greater renal sodium reabsorption, and 3) increased secretion of the adrenal mineralocorticoid, aldosterone.

**MECHANISM OF ACTION.** The prime therapeutic effect of digitalis in congestive heart failure is an increase in the force of myocardial contraction (positive inotropic effect), which is due either to an increase in energy supply to the myocardial contractile mechanism or improved efficiency in the conversion of chemical to mechanical energy. The cardiac receptor for digitalis is probably the membrane enzyme, $Na^+$, $K^+$-activated APT–ase. There is a positive correlation between the positive inotropic effect of digitalis and the degree of inhibition of ATP–ase. Through its ATP–ase inhibition, digitalis increases calcium entry into the sarcoplasm, resulting in a more rapid rate of increase in muscle tension. The beneficial effect of digitalis in terminating atrial arrhythmias is principally due to an increase in the refractory period of cardiac muscle (essentially true for all antiarrhythmic drugs).

**PHARMACOLOGIC EFFECTS.** All the beneficial affects of digitalis in congestive heart failure can be attributed to a single pharmacologic action: an increase in the efficiency of the cardiac muscle which results in an increase in the force of myocardial contraction. This increase in myocardial efficiency improves the cardiac output and negates the need for cardiac enlargement. It results in 1) increased stroke volume, 2) decreased residual diastolic volume, 3) decreased heart size, 4) decreased venous pressure, 5) decreased blood volume, and 6) increased sodium excretion and diuresis. Digitalis also decreases nerve impulse formation at the sinoatrial node (a negative chronotropic effect), decreases nerve impulse conduction at the atrioventricular node, and increases the refractory period of cardiac muscle (negative dromotropic effects). These actions on the rate of impulse formation and conduction velocity may terminate atrial cardiac arrhythmias but also allow for the production of ventricular arrhythmias by encouraging ectopic foci formation.

**TOXIC EFFECTS.** Digitalis is one of the most widely prescribed drugs, even though it carries a very low margin of safety. Toxicity usually occurs due to the cumulation of maintenance doses or from large doses used to terminate cardiac arrhythmias. The signs and symptoms of digitalis intoxication include 1) gastrointestinal (usually the initial symptoms)—anorexia, nausea and vomiting; 2) neurologic—headache, fatigue, malaise, delirium, hallucinations, and, importantly, pain to the lower third of the face; 3) visual—blurred vision and yellow green vision; and 4) cardiac—extrasystoles, atrioventricular nodal blockade and ventricular arrhythmias. The cause of death is usually ventricular fibrillation. The molecular mechanism of digitalis-induced cardiac arrhythmias is potassium loss due to inhibition of membrane-bound $Na^+$, $K^+$-activated ATP–ase. The treatment of digitalis toxicity entails drug withdrawal, potassium administration, and the use of antiarrhythmic drugs such as phenytoin, lidocaine, and propranolol.

**THERAPEUTIC USES.** Digitalis is the mainstay of therapy in congestive heart failure. It is also extensively employed in the treatment of atrial cardiac arrhythmias such as atrial flutter, atrial fibrillation, and paroxysmal atrial tachycardia.

**REPRESENTATIVE AGENTS.** The various cardiac glycosides include digitoxin (Crystodigin, Purodigin), digoxin (Lanoxin), lanatoside C (Cedilanid), and deslanoside (Cedilanid-D). The various preparations differ only in onset and duration of action.

### QUESTIONS

46. Digitalis is used in the treatment of congestive heart failure because digitalis increases the force of myocardial contraction.
    1. Both statement and reason are correct and related.
    2. Both statement and reason are correct but not related.
    3. The statement is correct, but the reason is not.
    4. The statement is not correct, but the reason is an accurate statement.
    5. Neither statement nor reason is correct.

47. Which of the following statements are true regarding the cardiac glycosides?
   a. They inhibit Na, K-activated ATP-ase.
   b. They are useful in the treatment of atrial cardiac arrhythmias.
   c. Toxic doses induce ventricular fibrillation.
   d. They produce diuresis by inhibition of aldosterone.
   e. They increase impulse formation at the sinoatrial node (positive chronotropic effect).

   1. a, b, c
   2. b, c, d
   3. c, d, e
   4. a and b
   5. a and e

## Antiarrhythmics

Antiarrhythmic drugs are agents which terminate and/or prevent disorders of cardiac rhythm (cardiac arrhythmias and dysrhythmias).

**PATHOPHYSIOLOGY OF CARDIAC ARRHYTHMIAS.** As yet, there is no general agreement as to the underlying pathogenesis of disorders of impulse generation or conduction in the heart. With cardiac arrhythmias, the normal conduction pattern (sinoatrial node, atrioventricular node, and Purkinje's fibers) in the heart becomes asynchronous, and the efficiency of the heart is greatly diminished.

There are three main theories as to the origin of cardiac arrhythmias: 1) ectopic pacemaker activity, 2) circus movement, and 3) reciprocal activation. Ectopic foci appear when the repetitive rhythm of cardiac muscle fibers exceed the rhythm of the normal cardiac pacemaker. Circus movement is initiated when an impulse traveling around an obstacle (atrial orifices, infarcted tissue, or refractory tissue) becomes self-propagating. This self-propagation occurs when the perimeter of the obstacle is long enough, the muscle refractory period short enough, or the conduction velocity slow enough so that the circular impulse constantly encounters tissue no longer in its refractory period and capable of stimulation. Reciprocal activation occurs when adjacent cardiac muscle fibers excite each other to the point of contraction. The list of conduction irregularities in the heart include extrasystoles (premature contractions), paroxysmal atrial tachycardia, atrial flutter, atrial fibrillation, ventricular tachycardia, and ventricular fibrillation.

**MECHANISM OF ACTION.** Cardiac muscle is unique in that it cannot be stimulated while in its refractory period, this property is exploited in the use of antiarrhythmic agents. The prime mechanism by which antiarrhythmics supress abnormal cardiac rhythm is by increasing the duration of the refractory period of cardiac muscle. The aberrant impulses then reach cardiac muscle which cannot contract, and the abnormal rhythm is terminated. Many of the agents also suppress ectopic pacemaker activity and are general depressants of all muscle tissue, cardiac included.

**TOXIC EFFECTS.** The adverse reactions associated with the antiarrhythmic agents include 1) neurological—tinnitus, vertigo, visual disturbances; 2) gastrointestinal—nausea and vomiting, cramps, diarrhea; 3) central nervous system—psychosis, convulsions; 4) hematologic—blood dyscrasias; 5) allergic—thrombocytopenia purpura, anaphylaxis; and 6) cardiovascular—hypotension, embolism, cardiac arrhythmias (myocardial depression promotes ectopic escape mechanisms).

**THERAPEUTIC USES.** Quinidine and procainamide are employed in artial and ventricular arrhythmias, digitalis in atrial arrhythmias, propranolol in atrial tachycardia and digitalis-induced arrhythmias, lidocaine in ventricular conduction disturbances (particularly after myocardial infarction), and phenytoin in atrial, ventricular, and digitalis-induced arrhythmias.

**REPRESENTATIVE AGENTS.** The currently employed antiarrhythmic agents are digitalis, quinidine (Quinora, Quinidex), procainamide (Pronestyl), propranolol (Inderal), lidocaine (Xylocaine), and phenytoin (Dilantin).

### QUESTIONS

48. The prime mechanism by which antiarrhythmic agents terminate cardiac arrhythmias is to
   1. slow impulse formation at the sinoatrial node
   2. block the $\beta$ adrenergic receptor
   3. block conduction in the Purkinje fibers
   4. increase the refractory period of cardiac muscle
   5. slow nerve conduction through the atrioventricular node

49. Drugs employed in the treatment of atrial cardiac arrhythmias are
   a. lidocaine (Xylocaine)
   b. phenytoin (Dilantin)
   c. digitalis
   d. quinidine (Quinora)
   e. warfarin (Coumadin)

   1. a, b, and c
   2. b, c, and d
   3. c, d, and e
   4. a and d
   5. All of the above

## Antihypertensives

Antihypertensive drugs reduce the pathologically elevated blood pressure in essential hypertension and hypertensive crisis.

**PATHOPHYSIOLOGY OF ESSENTIAL HYPERTENSION.** This disease of unknown etiology is initially manifested by elevated systolic and/or diastolic blood pressure. It progresses to pathologic changes in peripheral vasculature (optic fundi) and essential organ systems (brain, kidney). It is generally agreed that chronically elevated blood pressure is associated with increased morbidity and mortality and that various measures which reduce the blood pressure also reduce its attendant pathology.

One or more of the following factors have been implicated in the etiology of essential hypertension: 1) hyperactivity of the central nervous system (stress), 2) abnormalities in the sympathetic (adrenergic) nervous system, 3) pathology in vascular smooth muscle, 4) excess reabsorption or impaired excretion of sodium, and 5) activation of the renin–angiotension–aldosterone system. There are differences of opinion as to the parameters for mild, moderate, and severe hypertension, but it appears reasonable to define mild hypertension as a diastolic pressure greater than 100 mm mercury with slight optic changes and no cardiac or renal involvement and to define severe hypertension as a diastolic pressure greater than 130 mm mercury with cardiac and renal decompensation, renal damage and/or optic fundi hemorrhage. Moderate hypertension lies somewhere between the two. Hypertensive crisis is characterized by an extremely high blood pressure due to known disease states such as acute heart failure, hypertensive encephalopathy, pheochromocytoma, toxemia of pregnancy, and acute glomerular nephritis.

**MECHANISM OF ACTION.**    Blood pressure is regulated via the interaction of a number of physiologic systems. Rapid alterations in pressure are moderated by the CNS baroreceptors, the sympathetic nervous system, adrenal release of epinephrine and norepinephrine, and the hormones angiotensin and vasopressin. The long-term regulation of blood pressure is dependent on kidney alterations in sodium and water excretion as well as changes in diameter of the blood vessels themselves. The principal therapy of essential hypertension involves weight reduction, reduced intake and increased secretion of sodium, and reduction in adrenergic vascular tone. It is becoming increasingly common to employ multiple therapy regimes simultaneously to eliminate as many etiologic factors as possible.

**PHARMACOLOGIC EFFECTS.**    The drug therapy of essential hypertension is directed towards two therapeutic benefits: 1) sodium excretion and 2) reduction in adrenergic vascular tone. The following drugs are included in the antihypertensive armamentarium: diuretics, reserpine (Serpasil), methyldopa (Aldomet), hydralazine (Apresoline), propranolol (Inderal). Clonidine (Catapres), and guanethidine (Ismelin). The benzothiazide diuretics increase sodium excretion, produce direct relaxation of ateriolar smooth muscle, and are the mainstay of antihypertensive therapy. Reserpine reduces adrenergic tone by depleting norepinephrine in the adrenergic nerve terminal and decreasing its reuptake. Methylodopa, clonidine and possibly propranolol reduce vascular tone by affecting the CNS. Hydralazine is a direct smooth muscle relaxant, and guanethidine sulfate is an adrenergic neuron blocking drug which prevents norepinephrine release, depletes it in the adrenergic nerve terminal and prevents its granular reuptake.

**TOXIC EFFECTS.**    The following adverse effects are associated with the antihypertensive agents: 1) benzothiazides—loss of potassium; 2) reserpine—mental depression, nasal stuffiness, hypotension; 3) methyldopa—allergy, edema, sedation, hypotension; 4) hydralazine—nasal congestion, muscle tremors, systemic lupus erythematosus; 5) propranolol—exacerbation of asthma, hypotension, heart failure; 6) clonidine—acute hypotension, bradycardia, xerostomia, impotence; and 7) guanethidine—nasal congestion, hypotension, bradycardia.

**THERAPEUTIC USES.**    The thiazide diuretics are the mainstay of therapy in essential hypertension; however, combination drug therapy is increasingly encountered. The regimens for current therapy are 1) mild hypertension—a benzothiazide diuretic alone and/or reserpine; 2) moderate hypertension—a thiazide diuretic and/or reserpine, with the addition of either methyldopa, hydralazine, or propranolol; and 3) severe hypertension—combinations of the drugs mentioned plus guanethidine sulfate or clonidine hydrochloride. A mild hypertensive crisis may be terminated by resperine or methyldopa; severe hypertensive emergencies, by diazoxide (hyperstat), nitroprusside, trimethaphan or another ganglion-blocking drug.

## QUESTIONS

50. Which of the following drugs are commonly used in the treatment of mild to moderate essential hypertension?
    - a. Guanethidine (Ismelin)
    - b. Clonidine (Catapres)
    - c. Hexamethonium
    - d. Reserpine
    - e. Hydrochlorothiazide
    1. a, b, and c
    2. b, c, and d
    3. c, d, and e
    4. a and b
    5. d and e

51. The benzothiazide diuretics are effective in the treatment of essential hypertension because the benzothiazides possess a direct relaxant effect on vascular smooth muscle.

1. Both statement and reason are correct and related
2. Both statement and reason are correct but not related.
3. The statement is correct, but the reason is not.
4. The statement is not correct, but the reason is an accurate statement.
5. Neither statement nor reason is correct.

52. The drugs which are effective in the treatment of essential hypertension because they reduce sympathetic (adrenergic) tone to blood vessels are

    a. methyldopa (Aldomet)
    b. chlorothiazide
    c. hydralazine (Apresoline)
    d. guanethidine sulfate (Ismelin)
    e. propranolol (Inderal)

1. a, b, and c
2. b, c, and d
3. c, d, and e
4. a, d, and e
5. b and e

## Coronary Dilators

Coronary vasodilators are drugs useful in the treatment of angina pectoris and certain peripheral vasoconstrictive diseases due to their nonspecific vasodilating properties.

MECHANISM OF ACTION. Coronary vasodilators relax smooth muscle irrespective of type of innervation or a response to neurotransmitters whether acetylcholine or norepinephrine. They are collectively termed nitrites or nitrates; the nitrates are reduced to the nitrite ion which interacts with the muscle receptor.

PHARMACOLOGIC EFFECTS. The most prominent action of the coronary vasodilators is on the cardiovascular system: 1) flushing of the head and neck, 2) dilation of meningeal vessels (pulsating headache), 3) transient dilation of large coronary vessels, and 4) dilation of large systemic capacitance vessels. These drugs also relax bronchial and biliary smooth muscle.

ABSORPTION, DISTRIBUTION, METABOLISM, AND EXCRETION. Amyl nitrate is absorbed by inhalation from crushable ampules; nitroglycerin, through the buccal or sublingual mucosa; and the longer acting nitrates, by the oral route. Tolerance develops rapidly with repeated use.

TOXIC EFFECTS. All the side-effects of these drugs are related to their cardiovascular actions: headache, dizziness, weakness, syncope, and hypotension. The nitrate ion produces methemoglobinemia with chronic use.

THERAPEUTIC USES. Vasodilating (smooth muscle relaxant) drugs are useful in the treatment of paroxysmal nocturnal dyspnea, Raynaud's disease, biliary colic, and most importantly, angina pectoris. Nitroglycerin is primarily effective in the treatment of angina not because of its effect on coronary vessels but because of its vasodilating action on larger systemic blood vessels. This action decreases venous return and left ventricular diastolic volume, resulting in a reduced myocardial oxygen requirement and decreased cardiac work.

REPRESENTATIVE AGENTS. Nitroglycerin is used to terminate anginal attacks and longer acting drugs such as erythrityl tetranitrate (Cardilate) and isosorbide dinitrate (Isordil) to prevent anginal symptoms prophylactically. The most recent significant advance in the long-term management of the anginal patient is the increasingly common use of the $\beta$–adrenergic blocking drug, propranolol (Inderal).

QUESTION

53. Nitroglycerin is used in the treatment of angina pectoris because nitroglycerin reduces cardiac output.

1. Both statement and reason are correct and related.
2. Both statement and reason are correct but not related.
3. The statement is correct, but the reason is not.
4. The statement is not correct, but the reason is an accurate statement.
5. Neither statement nor reason is correct.

## Diuretics

Diuretics are drugs which increase the rate of urine formation by increasing urine volume and loss of solute and water.

PATHOPHYSIOLOGY OF EDEMA. A net increase in the extracellular fluid (edema) is directly related to faulty excretion of the sodium ion. Edema may result from such diverse diseases as congestive heart failure, hepatic and renal disease, and secretion of the sodium-retaining corticosteroid, aldosterone.

MECHANISM OF ACTION. The most effective diuretics are saluretic, that is, they increase sodium excretion. The various agents are classified according to their mechanism of action in producing the diuresis: 1) osmotic agents, 2) carbonic anhydrase inhibitors, 3) organomercurials, 4) sulfonamides, 5) high ceiling (loop) diuretics, and 5) potassium-sparing agents. Osmotic diuretics (mannitol) decrease solute content by reducing sodium and water reabsorpotion in the loop of Henle. Carbonic anhydrase inhibitors reduce carbonic anhydrase-mediated sodium bicarbonate reabsorption. The organomercurials reduce chloride absorption in the loop of Henle, which reduces sodium reabsorption. The sulfonamides (benzothiazides) inhibit sodium reabsorption in the loop of Henle. The loop diuretics (furosemide, ethacrynric acid) also reduce sodium reabsorption by decreasing chloride transport in the ascending limb of the loop of Henle. The potassium-sparing diuretics (spironolactone, triamterene) decrease sodium reabsorption in the convoluted tubules. Digitalis and theophylline also produce diuresis by increasing the glomerular filtration rate and thus reducing sodium reabsorption.

**TOXIC EFFECTS.** The adverse effects of the diuretics include malaise, dehydration, hyponatremia, hypokalemia (potassium loss), alkalosis, and potentiation of digitalis intoxication because of potassium depletion.

**THERAPEUTIC USES.** Diuretics are useful in the treatment of edematous states of whatever origin: cardiac, renal, or hepatic. In addition the benzothiazides are the prime initial therapy in the treatment of essential hypertension.

**REPRESENTATIVE AGENTS.** The benzothiazide diuretics are the most commonly used drugs and include chlorothiazide (Diuril) and hydrochlorothiazide (Esidrix). The high ceiling (loop) diuretics are the most potent agents and include furosemide (Lasix) and ethacrynic acid (Edecrin). The prototype of the carbonic anhydrase inhibitors is acetazolamide (Diamox). The mercurial diuretics are only administered intravenously. The combination of several diuretics in one preparation is very common.

### QUESTIONS

54. Which of the following diuretics is commonly used in the treatment of hypertension?
    1. Organomercurials
    2. Carbonic anhydrase inhibitors
    3. Benzothiazides
    4. Aldosterone antagonists
    5. None of the above

55. Diuretics are effective in the treatment of edema because they promote the excretion of
    1. potassium
    2. chloride
    3. mercury
    4. sodium
    5. hydrogen

## Anticoagulants

Anticoagulants are drugs which inhibit the action or synthesis of one or more clotting factors to prevent the formation of a normal blood clot or suppress the extension of an existing clot.

**THEORIES OF BLOOD COAGULATION.** There are two major theories of blood clot formation: 1) the cascade (sequential) theory and 2) the autoprothrombin theory. According to the cascade theory, the initial event in clot formation is activation of Factor XIII (Hageman factor) by contact with a "foreign" surface which then activates factor XI (plasma thromboplastin antecedent) to produce a progressive cascade, culminating in the conversion of prothrombin to thrombin. In the autoprothrombin theory, the autoprothrombins consisting of Factors VII (proconvertin), IX (plasma thromboplastin component), and X (Stuart factor) are derived from prothrombin by autocatalysis. Prothrombin is changed to an intermediate "prethrombin" which is converted to thrombin by activated Factor X. All factors must be converted to their activated form.

Both theories agree on the necessity for platelet activation of Factor X, the importance of calcium in a number of the stages, and intrinsic thromboplastin generation by the interaction of platelets and Factors V (proaculerin), VIII (antihemophilic factor), IX, X, XI, and XII, as well as extrinsic thromboplastin generated by the contact between tissue extract and Factors V, VII, and X. Numerous inhibiting factors are available for the various stages of the clotting sequence, including antithrombin, important to the mechanism of action of heparin.

**CLASSIFICATION OF ANTICOAGULANTS.** There are two types of anticoagulants: 1) parenteral heparin and 2) oral anticoagulants (the coumarins and indandiones).

**MECHANISM OF ACTION.** The anticoagulant effect of heparin requires a plasma α-globulin (heparin cofactor) which is probably identical to the normal plasma antithrombin (antithrombin III). The prime effect of heparin is to prevent thrombin formation from prothrombin by facilitating complexes of heparin cofactor with activated Factors IX, X, XI, and XII. Heparin also prevents platelet aggregation induced by thrombin. The oral anticoagulants block the liver formation of Factors II (prothrombin), VII, IX, and X by interference with the action of vitamin K, possibly by converting K to a less active form. It is commonly held that coumarins are competitive inhibitors of vitamin K but this is probably no longer a fact (24).

**PHARMACOLOGIC EFFECTS.** The oral anticoagulants are without pharmacologic actions other than their effects on blood coagulation. Heparin is bound to histamine in mast cells and is released during anaphylaxis, but its role in acute allergy is unknown. Heparin also reduces the fat content of the blood, but its role in lipid metabolism is also unknown.

**TOXIC EFFECTS.** The adverse effects of the anticoagulants are all related to their effects on the clotting process: bleeding from skin, mucosa, and gastrointestinal surfaces; and bleeding into joints (hemarthrosis). The coumarins interact with a number of other drugs (see Drug Interactions). From a dental viewpoint its interaction with aspirin is most important, because aspirin increases the anticoagulant effect of the coumarins.

**LABORATORY CONTROL OF ANTICOAGULANT DOSAGE.** The correct dosage of heparin is determined by the whole blood clotting time or the partial thromboplastin time; the dosage of the oral anticoagulants, by the one-stage prothrombin time (Quick Time).

**THERAPEUTIC USES.** The anticoagulants are used in the prevention or treatment of thromboembolic diseases: 1) venous thrombosis, 2) pulmonary embolism, 3) postmyocardial infarction embolism, 4) rheumatic heart disease, and 5) cerebrovascular disease. The coumarins are much less effective than heparin in arterial clotting disorders since arterial clots are critically dependent upon the initial aggregation of platelets (platelet plug) which is unaffected by the coumarins. Heparin is reserved for acute parenteral hospital use, whereas the oral agents are most useful for chronic outpatient medication. The most important and efficacious use of the anticoagulants is in the prevention and treatment of venous and pulmonary emboli. The drugs are also employed to prevent embolism in rheumatic heart disease. Heparin is used to prevent peripheral venous thrombosis and pulmonary emboli after acute myocardial infarction.

**REPRESENTATIVE AGENTS.** Heparin is formulated for intravenous injection (Lipo-Heparin, Panheparin) or as a repository form (Depo-Heparin). The most common coumarin derivatives in use are sodium warfarin (Coumadin, Panwarfin and bishydroxycoumarin (Dicumarol).

## QUESTIONS

56. Which of the following statements are true regarding the coumarin anticoagulants?
    a. They are primarily useful in venous clotting disorders.
    b. The site of action is the liver.
    c. They reduce the physiologic actions of Vitamin K.
    d. They affect platelet agglutination in arterial clotting.
    e. Dosage is determined by whole blood clotting time.
    1. a, b, and c
    2. b, c, and d
    3. c, d, and e
    4. a and d
    5. All of the above

57. Heparin is effective in the prevention of arterial clotting disorders because heparin prevents platelet agglutination.
    1. Both statement and reason are correct and related.
    2. Both statement and reason are correct but not related.
    3. The statement is correct, but the reason is not.
    4. The statement is not correct, but the reason is an accurate statement.
    5. Neither statement nor reason is correct.

# ANESTHETICS

## General Anesthetics

The ideal general anesthetic would produce simultaneous analgesia (loss of pain), amnesia (loss of memory), and hypnosis (loss of wakefulness), as well as skeletal muscle relaxation. It would also inhibit reflexes, in a reversible manner, allowing for surgical intervention. This ideal is rarely attained with the drugs presently available, however. In its broadest sense general anesthesia is simply defined as hypnosis (sleep) and loss of protective laryngeal reflexes (cough). The ensuing discussion concerns only inhalation (gaseous) anesthetics.

**PHYSICAL PROPERTIES.** Most inhalation anesthetics are organic compounds which are relatively inert chemically and are minimally metabolized. General anesthetics pass through tissues by passive diffusion (higher concentration to lower concentration) to achieve a critical gaseous partial pressure within the brain. Inhalation anesthetics exist in two forms at room temperature: volatile liquids and gases.

**PRODUCTION OF GENERAL ANESTHESIA.** There are three phases of general anesthetic administration: 1) induction (onset to desired surgical plane), 2) maintenance (performance of surgery), and 3) emergency (patient recovery). Satisfactory general anesthesia occurs when the concentration (partial pressure) of the gas in the brain allows for safe and effective surgical anesthesia.

The depth of anesthesia is directly related to the partial pressure of the gas in the CNS which is dependent upon the 1) partial pressure of the anesthetic in the inspired gas, 2) rate and depth of pulmonary ventilation, 3) transfer of gas from the alveoli to blood, 4) loss of gas from blood to other tissues, and 5) solubility of the gas in the blood (Ostwald's coefficient, blood–gas solubility coefficient). The greater the solubility of the gas in the blood, the more gas that must be dissolved to attain the critical partial pressure. Highly lipid-soluble drugs (high Ostwald's coefficient) such as diethyl ether have a very slow induction and emergence time, whereas drugs with a low blood–gas solubility coefficient such as cyclopropane and nitrous oxide possess a very rapid induction and emergence time. The Ostwald's coefficient of an anesthetic gas is not necessarily related to its potency or efficacy.

**MECHANISM OF ACTION.** There is as yet no satisfactory explanation as to how general anesthetics produce their effects. The various drugs (inhalation and intravenous) possess diverse chemical and physical properties, and yet all produce a CNS depression which allows for loss of consciousness and surgical intervention. Various theories have been developed to explain the mechanism of action of general anesthetics:

1. Meyer–Overton: the potency of the gas is proportional to its lipid solubility.
2. Surface tension: the potency of the gas is proportional to its ability to lower surface tension.
3. Cell permeability: anesthetics produce changes in the permeability of cells in the brain.
4. Miller and Pauling's hydrate microcrystal: anesthetics produce water microcrystals in the brain which interfere with neuronal excitability.
5. Biochemical: inhalation anesthetics inhibit oxygen consumption, calcium uptake or NADH oxidation in the brain.

It is probable that the locus of action of inhalation anesthetics is the synaptic membrane, particularly in the reticular activating system, where the drugs alter membrane pore size and subsequent ion flow.

**STAGES OF GENERAL ANESTHESIA.** It is common practice to employ multiple inhalation agents along with intravenous barbiturates, narcotics, anticholinergics, and neuromuscular blocking drugs to obtain an optimal stage of safe and effective anesthesia. It is therefore rare to observe the classic signs and symptoms of ether anesthesia as described by Guedel: stage I (analgesia)—onset of anesthesia to loss of consciousness; stage II (delirium)—involuntary excitement to loss of eyelid reflex; stage III (surgical anesthesia)—regular respiration and fixed eyeballs to onset of paralysis of respiratory muscles; stage IV (medullary paralysis)—cessation of weakened respiration to circulatory failure and death. In practice the depth of anesthesia is determined by the character of the respiration, eyeball movements, pupillary size,and the presence or absence of certain reflexes.

**ANESTHETIC AGENTS.** Inhalation general anesthetics are classified into 1) volatile (ethers and halogenated hydrocarbons) and 2) gaseous (nitrous oxide, ethylene, and cyclopropane). All agents possess desirable and undesirable properties.

*Volatile Agents.* The popularity of diethyl ether has declined, and divinyl ether, once used as an induction agent for diethyl ether by the open-drop method, is no longer employed. Diethyl ether possesses a very slow induction and emergence time; it is explosive, nauseating, and irritating to mucous membranes, but it produces little respiratory or cardiovascular depression in the surgical stage. The halogenated hydrocarbons of which the prototype is halothane (Fluothane) are extensively employed. All the halogenated hydrocarbons possess four common properties: 1) progressive reduction in blood pressure, 2) moderate to marked respiratory depression, 3) tendency to produce cardiac arrhythmias (sensitize the heart to epinephrine), and 4) tendency to produce liver damage.The most common halogenated hydrocarbons presently used are halothane (Fluothane), methoxyflurane (Penthrane), enflurane (Ethrane), and isoflurane (Forane). Chloroform and trichloroethylene (Trilene) are no long utilized.

*Gaseous Agents.* Cyclopropane and ethylene are rarely employed; nitrous oxide is the most common general anesthetic in use today. Nitrous oxide is not used as the single anesthetic agent since surgical anesthesia cannot be attained at concentrations which are not hypoxic (less oxygen than room air). Nitrous oxide, which possesses a rapid induction time, is an excellent analgesic. It is nonflammable, does not irritate mucosa, and produces little nausea and vomiting (pleasant odor), respiratory depression, or cardiovascular depression. Highly explosive, cyclopropane produces frequent nausea and cardiac arrhythmias but possesses a rapid induction and emergence time; it produces little respiratory or cardiovascular depression. Ethylene possesses a more rapid induction time that nitrous oxide and produces little respiratory or cardiovascular depression, but it is explosive.

QUESTIONS

58. Which of the following drugs are classified as halogenated hydrocarbon general anesthetics?

    a. Cyclopropane
    b. Halothane (Fluothane)
    c. Nitrous oxide
    d. Ethylene
    e. Enflurane (Ethrane)

1. a, b, and d
2. b, c, and d
3. c, d, and e
4. a and d
5. b and e

59. All inhalation general anesthetics are gases at room temperature because inhalation anesthetics pass into and out of the central nervous system by passive diffusion.

1. Both statement and reason are correct and related.
2. Both statement and reason are correct but not related.

3. The statement is correct, but the reason is not.
4. The statement is not correct, but the reason is an accurate statement.
5. Neither statement nor reason is correct.

60. The area of the central nervous system which is most sensitive to the action of the inhalation general anesthetics is the
   1. cerebral cortex
   2. medullary respiratory center
   3. reticular activating system
   4. hypothalamus
   5. limbic system

61. Which of the following statements are true regarding nitrous oxide?
   a. It is explosive.
   b. Induction time is rapid.
   c. It has analgesic properties.
   d. It has a pleasant odor.
   e. It is a potent respiratory depressant.
   1. a, b, and c
   2. b, c, and d
   3. c, d, and e
   4. a and d
   5. b and e

62. Epinephrine administration is contraindicated when halogenated hydrocarbon general anesthetics are used because halogenated hydrocarbons sensitize the heart to the arrhythmic effects of epinephrine.
   1. Both statement and reason are correct and related.
   2. Both statement and reason are correct but not related.
   3. The statement is correct, but the reason is not.
   4. The statement is not correct, but the reason is an accurate statement.
   5. Neither statement nor reason is correct.

63. One of the following statements is not true regarding general inhalation anesthetics. Which one?
   1. They act at nerve synaptic membranes.
   2. A critical partial pressure of gas must be attained in the brain.
   3. They undergo little liver metabolism.
   4. They produce death by medullary respiratory and cardiovascular depression.
   5. Highly lipid-soluble agents possess a rapid induction time.

## Local Anesthetics

Local anesthetics are chemical substances that block nerve conduction reversibly when applied locally to the nerve tissue. Substances such as alcohol are employed to produce permanent nerve damage in the treatment of intractable pain, but they are not clinically useful in dental anesthesia.

TYPES OF LOCAL ANESTHESIA. There are essentially three types of local anesthesia: 1) topical, 2) infiltration, and 3) nerve block. Topical anesthetics are applied to nerve terminals in skin and mucous membrane. Infiltration anesthesia is analogous to a subcutaneous injection and affects small nerve fibers or nerve terminals. In nerve block anesthesia, the drug is deposited along the nerve trunk at some distance from the area of operative manipulation.

CHEMICAL AND PHYSICAL PROPERTIES. Local anesthetics are weak bases (pH of 8–9) possessing secondary or tertiary amine groups and are either derivatives of paraaminobenzoic acid (esters) or aniline (amides). Ester derivatives are not cross-allergenic with amide derivatives. All of the common dental anesthetics used presently are of the amide type. The solutions are stored as hydrochloride salts in the dental cartridge (to increase chemical stability and prolong shelf-life). Once injected into tissue, they are hydrolyzed to the free base form necessary for passage through tissue to the receptor site. The charged (cationic) form of the molecule is necessary for receptor interaction and nerve blockade. Any reduction in tissue pH (infection) increases the amount of charged anesthetic and decreases the amount of free base, thereby limiting the total amount of anesthetic at the receptor site and preventing adequate local anesthesia.

MECHANISM OF ACTION OF LOCAL ANESTHETICS. The site of action of local anesthetics is the nerve membrane. The drugs prevent the generation of the nerve action potential and maintain the nerve in a state of polarization by preventing the influx of sodium ions necessary for depolarization. The nerve receptor for local anesthetics is closely related to the phospholipids of the nerve membrane. Local anesthetics probably attach to two negatively charged phosphate groups forming a stable bridge complex which prevents the opening of the sodium channels (pores) and generation of the nerve action potential (25).

INDUCTION AND DURATION OF ANESTHESIA. The induction time for nerve block anesthesia varies inversely with the drug concentration (the greater the local anesthetic concentration, the shorter the onset of action) and directly with the square root of the radius of the nerve (the larger the nerve fiber, the slower the onset of action). The degree and duration of the nerve block is dependent upon 1) the total drug dosage, 2) the affinity of the drug for the receptor, and 3) the inherent ability of the drug to produce local anesthesia. The latter two properties vary greatly among drugs.

ABSORPTION, DISTRIBUTION, METABOLISM, AND EXCRETION. Local anesthetics are very well absorbed parenterally. The ester type are metabolized partially in the blood by serum (pseudo) cholinesterase and partially in the liver; the amide type are metabolized solely in the liver and excreted partially unchanged by the kidney.

### MISCELLANEOUS PHARMACOLOGIC ACTIONS.

In therapeutic doses local anesthetics are essentially devoid of any pharmacologic effects other than anesthesia. Most, except cocaine, are vasodilators; however, mepiuacaine is a cardiac and skeletal vasoconstrictor and prilocaine is neither a vasodilator nor a vasoconstrictor (26). Local anesthetics depress all muscle tissue.

### TOXICITY OF LOCAL ANESTHETICS.

Toxic symptoms from local anesthetic overdosage are due to an action upon the cardiovascular system and the central nervous system. The symptoms of cardiovascular depression are vasodilation, hypotension, and cardiac arrest. Toxic effects on the CNS are usually first noted as stimulation (nervousness, muscle twitching, tonic–clonic convulsions) followed by drepression (loss of consciousness, cardiovascular and respiratory depression). Death is due to respiratory depression and/or cardiac arrest. All toxic effects are due to a massive overdosage of the drug and are prevented by attention to dosage, use of a vasoconstrictor, and avoidance of intravascular injection.

The toxic symptoms are treated by support of vital physiologic functions, particularly proper patient oxygenation. Diazepam (Valium) is a direct antidote for local anesthetic-induced convulsions when administered intravenously, but it is rarely necessary because the stimulation phase is usually of very short duration. The use of intravenous barbiturates to terminate convulsions is contraindicated since their respiratory depressant effects potentiate the postseizure depression.

### VASOCONSTRICTORS.

Drugs which increase blood vessel constriction are included in local anesthetic solutions to antagonize the vasodilatory actions of local anesthetics. They decrease the rate of local anesthetic absorption, which increases their efficacy (greater drug concentration of the nerve membrane) and decreases their toxicity (slower vascular absorption). Epinephrine (Adrenalin) is the most potent and efficacious vasoconstrictor. Other drugs occasionally used are norepinephrine (Levophed), phenylephrine (Neo-Synephrine), and levonordefrin (Neo-Cobefrin).

### REPRESENTATIVE AGENTS.

The ester type of local anesthestics include procaine (Novocain), tetracaine (Pontocaine), and propoxycaine (Ravocaine). The amide type include lidocaine (Xylocaine), mepivacaine (Carbocaine), prilocaine (Citanest), and bupivacaine (Marcaine).

### QUESTIONS

64. The inclusion of vasoconstrictors in local anesthetic solutions is therapeutically useful to

    a. reduce the irritant effect of local anesthetics on blood vessels
    b. produce a greater amount of the cationic form of the local anesthetic
    c. increase the local anesthetic concentration at the nerve membrane
    d. slow the vascular absorption of the local anesthetics
    e. antagonize the vasodilation produced by local anesthetics

1. a, b, and c
2. b, c, and d
3. c, d, and e
4. a and d
5. All of the above

65. Some of the local anesthetics classified as the amide type are

    a. lidocaine (Xylocaine)
    b. procaine (Novocain)
    c. prilocaine (Citanest)
    d. propoxycaine (Ravocaine)
    e. mepivacaine (Carbocaine)

1. a, b, and c
2. b, c, and d
3. c, d, and e
4. a, c, and e
5. b and d

66. Which of the following statements are true regarding local anesthetics?

    a. Amide and ester derivatives are cross-allergenic.
    b. They are stored in cartridges as citrate salts.
    c. Amide type anesthetics are metabolized solely in the liver.
    d. The charged (ionized) form is necessary for receptor interaction.
    e. They are depressants of all muscular function.

1. a, b, and c
2. b, c, and d
3. c, d, and e
4. a and b
5. d and e

67. Local anesthetics are less effective in areas of infection because reduced tissue pH produces a greater amount of the cationic (charged) form which limits receptor access.

1. Both statement and reason are correct and related.
2. Both statement and reason are correct but not related.
3. The statement is correct, but the reason is not.
4. The statement is not correct, but the reason is an accurate statement.
5. Neither statement nor reason is correct.

68. Tremors, muscle twitching, and convulsions are symptoms of local anesthetic toxicity on the

1. cardiovascular system
2. neuromuscular system
3. central nervous system
4. autonomic nervous system
5. None of the above

69. The most important antidotal therapy for local anesthetic toxicity is
    1. intramuscular diazepam
    2. intramuscular pentobarbital
    3. nitrous oxide–oxygen inhalation
    4. support of vital functions
    5. intravenous vasopressor

70. Which of the following statements are true regarding the mechanism of action of local anesthetics?
    a. They act at the nerve (axon) membrane.
    b. They maintain the nerve in depolarized state.
    c. Receptor–drug interaction involves phosphate groups.
    d. They are competitive inhibitors of acetylcholine.
    e. They prevent generation of the nerve action potential.

    1. a, b, and c
    2. b, c, and d
    3. c, d, and e
    4. a, c, and e
    5. b and e

## ANTIINFECTIVES AND ANTIBIOTICS

### Sulfonamides

The sulfonamides were the first reasonably nontoxic antiinfective agents to be employed systemically in man. Due to the development of antibiotics superior to the sulfonamides and the emergence of many resistant bacteria, their use is now restricted to only a few disease states. They are commonly combined today with a newer drug, trimethoprim, which is synergistic with the sulfonamides.

**MECHANISM OF ACTION.** The sulfonamides are competitive antagonists of paraminobenzoic acid and prevent bacterial incorporation of paraminobenzoic acid into folic acid necessary for one carbon transfer (methyl groups) in amino acid synthesis. Mammalian cells obtain their folic acid from the diet, but some bacteria must synthesize their own folic acid. Therefore, the sulfonamide-induced folic acid deficiency is lethal to these bacteria. Trimethoprim is an inhibitor of dihydrofolate reductase, which reduces dihydrofolate ($F_2$) to tetrahydrofolate ($F_4$, THF), the active form of folic acid. In this way the sulfonamides and trimethoprim block successive stages in folic acid synthesis, producing antibacterial synergism.

**PHARMACOLOGIC EFFECTS.** The sulfonamides are bacteriostatic and affect a number of bacteria both gram-positive and gram-negative. Unfortunately bacterial resistance is a major problem with the sulfonamides.

**TOXIC EFFECTS.** The adverse effects associated with the sulfonamides are 1) allergy, 2) crystalline aggregates in the urinary tract, 3) blood dyscrasias, 4) hepatitis, and 5) nausea and vomiting.

**THERAPEUTIC USES.** The sulfonamides and/or trimethoprim are agents of choice in the treatment of trachoma, commonly employed in urinary tract infections, and sometimes used in the treatment of menigococcal infections, nocardiosis, and the prophylactic prevention of rheumatic fever.

QUESTION

71. The mechanism of action of the sulfonamides is to prevent the bacterial formation of
    1. pyruvic acid
    2. DNA
    3. glycogen
    4. folic acid
    5. RNA polymerase

### Antibiotics

Antibiotics are chemicals produced by microorganisms that suppress the growth or actually kill other microorganisms.

**GENERAL THERAPEUTIC PRINCIPLES.** The vast majority of oral and facial infections are caused by gram-positive microorganisms, in particular *Streptococci* and *Staphylococci*. Therefore, the antibiotic agents of choice are those which possess a substantial gram-positive spectrum: the penicillins, the erythromycins, and the cephalosporins. The use of lincomycin and clindamycin has been severely restricted due to their propensity to produce severe diarrhea and pseudomembranous colitis. The tetracyclines are never considered as initial drugs of choice but may be considered for patients who are allergic to both penicillin and the cephalosporins and who experience severe gastrointestinal upset from erythromycin.

Intelligent use of antibiotics in dentistry dictates that they be employed only in the treatment of an established oral or facial infection as diagnosed by the presence of one or more of the following symptoms: purulence, fever, edema, cellulitis, and lymphadenopathy. The prophylactic use of antibiotics for patients with rheumatic or congenital heart disease and intracardiac prostheses is established clinical practice, but the prophylactic use of antibiotics in otherwise healthy patients prior to, during, and after such surgical procedures as impaction removal, endodontic therapy, and periodontal flap surgery is unnecessary and unwarranted. Clinical trials have not established the effectiveness of antibiotics in promoting wound healing nor their efficacy in the treatment of chronic periocornitis, maxillary sinus perforations, localized osteitis, or noncompounded facial fractures. Unnecessary antibiotic therapy only promotes the selection out and the dominance of resistant bacterial strains and increases the probability of antibiotic toxicity and allergy.

Antibiotic dosage is determined by the physical status of the patient and the anticipated course of the infection. Medicine must deal with "rebound" infections (urinary tract, upper respiratory), which tend to recur after the antibiotic therapy is discontinued, so prolonged antibiotic regimens are not uncommon. Dentistry is not faced with rebound infections since the vast majority of oral or facial infections are self-limiting, particularly if the source of the infection can be reached by therapeutic procedures (extraction, incision and drainage, endodontic therapy). Therefore, the duration of antibiotic therapy is determined solely by the need to produce clinical remission of the disease. If a 2-day therapy regimen will cure the patient, then so be it; if it takes 5 days, then a 5–day therapy is correct. Unnecessarily prolonged exposure to antibiotics only increases the likelihood of the emergence of resistant bacterial strains and the possibility of adverse reactions. Short-term, intensive antibiotic therapy is becoming the standard practice for routine oral and facial infections.

*Mechanism of Action.*   The antibiotics commonly employed in dentistry have as their mechanism of action either inhibition of the synthesis of the rigid bacterial cell wall or inhibition of bacterial protein synthesis. The former agents are bactericidal and the latter bacteriostatic. Penicillin and the cephalosporins prevent the formation of the bacterial cell wall by inhibiting enzyme reactions responsible for establishing the final three-dimensional structure of the rigid bacterial cell wall. The tetracyclines and lincomycin affect protein synthesis by preventing the attachment of transfer RNA (tRNA) to the ribosome. Erythromycin disrupts the bonding of the amino acid on the tRNA to the growing peptide chain. Nystatin acts on the bacterial cytoplasmic membrane within the cell wall to alter its permeability to vital intracellular substances.

*Drug-Resistant Bacteria.*   It is generally accepted that bacteria do not mutate to a resistant form in the presence of the antibiotic any more than in an antibiotic-free environment (27). Therefore, the presence of the drug has little to do with the emergence of new antibiotic-resistant strains of bacteria. Spontaneous mutations occur once in every ten million to one billion bacterial cell divisions (28). Most of the clinical problems with suprainfections from resistant bacterial strains are due to the selection out (by the antibiotic) of bacteria already resistant to the drug at the expense of those still susceptible to the antibiotic. This problem is most likely to occur with broad spectrum agents and prolonged antibiotic therapy.

Bacteria possess at least two mechanisms by which they exhibit antibiotic resistance: drug tolerance and drug destruction. Bacteria may become tolerant to the antibiotic because of an alteration in the permeability of the cell membrane which prevents antibiotic access to the ribosome, or bacteria may inactivate the antibiotic by producing enzymes (penicillinase, cephalosporinase) which alter the chemical structure of the antibiotic. Transferred (infectious) drug resistance, whereby resistant bacteria may transfer the genes for drug resistance via plasmids (transduction) or by resistance factors through actual mating to a nonresistant bacteria (conjugation) is becoming increasingly important clinically, particularly regarding gram-negative bacteria.

*Therapy.*   The use of antibiotics in combination requires a knowledge of whether the drugs are bactericidal or bacteriostatic. Bactericidal antibiotics affect only microorganisms in the process of cell division; therefore, the presence of an antibiotic which suppresses cell division (bacteriostatic) will be inhibitory to an antibiotic which acts upon the developing cell wall. For this reason the combination of penicillin and erythromycin is irrational and antagonistic. The combination of two bactericidal agents (penicillin and the cephalosporins) is synergistic.

The need for antibiotic prophylaxis for patients with rheumatic or congenital heart disease, intracardiac prostheses, and possibly metallic joint replacements, coronary bypass operations, and indwelling catheters (hemodialysis) is well known; however, the dosage regimen has been changed as of 1977 (29, 30). The standard oral adult therapy is 2 g penicillin V within 30–60 min prior to the dental procedure and then 500 mg every 6 hours thereafter for eight doses (a total of 12 500-mg tablets). Specialized drug and dosage regimens are required for patients with intracardiac valvular prostheses (29, 30). There is no present consensus for antibiotic prophylaxis in patients with metallic joint replacements, organ transplants, coronary bypasses and indwelling catheters. The patient's physician should be consulted and if prophylatic antibiotics are recommended, then the standard regimen as stated above should be employed. In adult patients allergic to penicillin, erythromycin is the drug of choice at a dosage of 1 g within 1–½ to 2 hours prior to the procedure and then 500 mg every 6 hours for eight doses (a total of ten tablets). For a thorough discussion of the newest concepts in the antibiotic chemoprophylaxis of these risk patients, the reader should consult the *Journal of the American Dental Association.* 95:600, 1977 (30) or *Circulation* 50:139A, 1977 (29). A copy of the publication *Prevention of Bacterial Endocarditis* can also be obtained by writing to the American Dental Association, 211 East Chicago Avenue, Chicago, Illinois 60611.

*Toxic Effects.*   There are three types of adverse reactions which may occur during antibiotic therapy: 1) direct toxicity, 2) allergy, and 3) the development of suprainfections. Fortunately most antibiotics employed in dentistry possess a very high therapeutic index (penicillin, erythromycin, the cephalosporins). However, large doses of the tetracyclines, which cumulate in patients with impaired renal function, may produce severe liver damage; clindamycin (Cleocin) may induce a potentially fatal pseudomembranous colitis. Penicillin is highly allergenic; the tetracyclines, moderately so; and erythromycin, rarely allergenic. Suprainfections, defined as the emergence of a new infection during the treatment of a primary one, occur most commonly, but not always, with broad spectrum antibiotics. They may take the form of gram-negative infections, staphylococcal enteritis or monilial infections.

SPECIFIC ANTIBIOTIC AGENTS. The antibiotics of importance in dentistry are the penicillins, the cephalosporins, the erythromycins, the tetracyclines, lincomycin and clindamycin, (the lincosamides), topical agents and the antifungal antibiotics.

*The Penicillins.* The penicillins can be classified into two broad categories: 1) benzylpenicillin (penicillin G) and 2) semisynthetic penicillins. The various penicillins differ as to their antibacterial spectrum and their degree of absorption when administered orally. Penicillin G has a predominantly gram-positive spectrum, is effective against aerobic and anaerobic organisms, and is poorly absorbed orally. The oral dose of penicillin G should be four to five times that of the parenteral dose of the drug to offset its degradation by gastric acid. All the penicillins are bactericidal and inhibit the final transpeptidation reaction required for the three-dimensional structure of the rigid bacterial cell wall.

Phenoxymethyl penicillin (penicillin V) possesses a bacterial spectrum essentially the same as penicillin G; roughly two-thirds to three-quarters of an oral dose is absorbed from the gastrointestinal tract. Ampicillin is effective against a number of gram-negative organisms and should be reserved for such infections. Sodium methicillin (Staphcillin) and dicloxacillin (Dynapen) are highly resistant to penicillinase. All the penicillins are cross-allergenic, and anaphylactic reactions have occurred by every route of administration. Penicillin V is still probably the initial drug of choice for the treatment of most oral and facial infections.

*The Cephalosporins.* Chemically related to the penicillins, the cephalosporin antibiotics are bactericidal and broad spectrum. They are also effective against penicillinase-producing staphylococci. Their mechanism of action is very similar, if not identical, to that of penicillin G. The cephalosporins must be used with caution in patients allergic to penicillin as there is some incidence (an average of 8%) of cross-allergenicity (31). The cephalosporins are superior antibiotics and should be reserved for severe oral or facial infections. The two oral preparations are cephalexin (Keflex) and cephradine (Anspor, Velosef).

*The Erythromycins.* The erythromycin antibiotics are bacteriostatic and possess a bacterial spectrum very similar to that of penicillins G and V. They are also drugs of choice in the initial therapy of dental infections and in penicillin-allergic patients. The erythromycins are essentially nontoxic, although they may produce severe gastrointestinal upset. They are all reasonably well absorbed orally. Some of the common preparations are erythromycin base (E-Mycin), erythromycin succinate (Erythrocin) and erythromycin estolate (Ilosone). Cholestatic hepatitis is an allergic reaction occurring only to the estolate salt form (Ilosone).

*The Tetracyclines.* The tetracycline antibiotics are broad spectrum and bacteriostatic. Bacterial resistance is common. They are not the initial drug of choice for oral or facial infections, but may be useful in patients who are allergic to penicillin and the cephalosporins and who develop severe gastrointestinal problems with erythromycin. Adverse effects are not uncommon with the tetracyclines, however; they include allergy, photosensitivity, liver damage (very high doses), suprainfections, gastrointestinal upset, tooth discoloration, and the Fanconilike syndrome if the drugs are taken after their expiration date. Tetracycline–staining of the dentition may occur from 6 months in utero to 8 years of age.

*Lincomycin and Clindamycin.* The severe adverse effects of pseudomembranous colitis with clindamycin (Cleocin) and severe diarrhea with lincomycin (Lincocin) have severely restricted their clinical usefulness. These drugs are now reserved only for some patients with staphylococcal infections who are allergic to pencillin and those with *Bacteroides fragilis* infections (32). The true incidence of the potentially fatal pseudomembranous colitis associated with clindamycin is not known, nor is it established whether allergy or toxicity is involved. The symptoms consist of diarrhea, abdominal pain, fever, and yellowish white plaque formation on the intestinal mucosa. Clindamycin should be employed for oral infection only when all other antibiotics have failed and when dictated by antimicrobial sensitivity tests. Oral vancomycin may be effective in the treatment of antibiotic–induced pseudomembranous colitis.

*Topical Antibiotics.* The three topical antibiotics in common usage are bacitracin, polymyxin B, and neomycin (Neosporin ointment). Bacitracin is grampositive in spectrum; polymyxin B, gram-negative; and neomycin, broad spectrum. The only firmly established uses for topical antibiotics are burns and eye infections (33).

*Antifungal Antibiotics.* The three antifungal antibiotics are nystatin, amphotericin B, and griseofulvin.

Nystatin (Mycostatin) is the drug of choice for the treatment of oral monilial infections.

## QUESTIONS

72. Pseudomembranous colitis is an adverse drug effect occurring with the use of
    1. erythromycin
    2. bacitracin
    3. clindamycin
    4. cephalexin
    5. None of the above

73. The initial oral dose of penicillin V in the prophylactic chemotherapy of adult patients with rheumatic or congenital heart disease prior to dental treatment is
    1. 250 mg
    2. 125 mg
    3. 500 mg
    4. 1 g
    5. 2 g

74. Which of the following statements are true regarding the cephalosporin antibiotics?
    a. They are potentially cross-allergenic with penicillin.
    b. They are ineffective against gram-negative microorganisms.
    c. They are bactericidal.
    d. They are resistant to penicillinase.
    e. They inhibit bacterial protein synthesis.

    1. a, b, and c
    2. b, c, and d
    3. c, d, and e
    4. a, c, and d
    5. a and e

75. The combination of bactericidal and bacteriostatic antibiotics is antagonistic because bacteriostatic antibiotics suppress protein synthesis and bacterial cell division.
    1. Both statement and reason are correct and related.
    2. Both statement and reason are correct but not related.
    3. The statement is correct, but the reason is not.
    4. The statement is not correct, but the reason is an accurate statement.
    5. Neither statement nor reason is correct.

76. Adverse effects associated with the tetracycline antibiotics are
    a. photosensitivity
    b. liver damage
    c. tooth discoloration
    d. renal damage
    e. psychotic behavior
    1. a, b, and c
    2. b, c, and d
    3. c, d, and e
    4. a and c
    5. d and e

77. Penicillin G is well absorbed from the gastrointestinal tract because penicillin G is inactivated by the enzyme penicillinase.
    1. Both statement and reason are correct and related.
    2. Both statement and reason are correct but not related.
    3. The statement is correct, but the reason is not.
    4. The statement is not correct, but the reason is an accurate statement.
    5. Neither statement nor reason is correct.

78. The penicillins are bactericidal because the penicillins suppress the formation of the rigid bacterial cell wall.
    1. Both statement and reason are correct and related.
    2. Both statement and reason are correct but not related.
    3. The statement is correct, but the reason is not.
    4. The statement is not correct, but the reason is an accurate statement.
    5. Neither statement nor reason is correct.

79. Which of the following antibiotics is a drug of choice in patients with a penicillin allergy?
    1. Lincomycin
    2. Erythromycin
    3. Tetracycline
    4. Neomycin
    5. Ampicillin

80. Which of the following antibiotics is effective against pathogenic fungi?
    1. Polymyxin B
    2. Cephalexin
    3. Tetracycline
    4. Nystatin
    5. Bacitracin

## Local Antiseptics

An antiseptic is a substance which inhibits bacterial growth when applied topically. A bactericide (germicide) and a fungicide kill bacteria or fungi, respectively. A disinfectant is lethal for pathogenic organisms.

TYPES OF TOPICAL ANTISEPTICS. Numerous chemicals are destructive to bacteria when applied topically. The most common of these are iodine, iodophors, alcohol, hexachlorophene, chlorhexidine and antibiotics. Agents of lesser importance are hypochlorite, mercurials (Merthiolate), phenols, and quaternary ammonium compounds (Zephiran).

MECHANISM OF ACTION. The alcohols denature protein. Iodine preparations are effective because they release free iodide. Phenols interfere with bacterial protoplasm. Quaternary ammonium compounds disrupt bacterial cell membranes, producing a loss of intracellular substances.

**PHARMACOLOGIC EFFECTS.** Iodine is among the most potent of all antiseptic agents, particularly when combined with alcohol (iodine tincture [USP]). The iodophors are aqueous solutions of iodine and are less effective than iodine tinctures. The alcohols (ethyl and isopropyl) are also highly effective, particularly in the presence of water; hence they are used as 70%–95% solutions. The alcohols are effective against both gram-positive and gram-negative organisms and should be rubbed on the skin or mucosa for 2 min for maximum effectiveness. Hexachlorophene, which is only effective against gram-positive organisms, is maximally effective when allowed to cumulate on the skin for several days. Chlorhexidine highly effective against gram-positive and gram-negative bacteria, is also maximally effective when it cumulates.

**TOXIC EFFECTS.** Iodine is irritating to the skin and allergenic. Alcohol is drying or irritating to skin and mucosa. Hexachlorophene is absorbed through the skin and may be toxic to the central nervous system, particularly in premature infants. The use of chlorhexidine (Hibiclens) as an antiplaque agent is associated with tooth discoloration and irritation of the oral mucosa.

**THERAPEUTIC AGENTS.** The most effective local antiseptics are iodine and chlorhexidine. The addition of alcohol potentiates both agents. Hypochlorite has a solvent action on pulpal tissue and organic intracanal debris. Local antiseptics can be used in dentistry as endodontic medications, as preparation for local anesthetic injections, and for minor mucosal infections.

### QUESTION

81. The most effective local antiseptics are
    a. iodine
    b. hexachlorophene
    c. chlorhexidine
    d. hypochlorite
    e. mercury
    1. a, b, and c
    2. b, c, and d
    3. c, d, and e
    4. a and c
    5. d and e

## ENDOCRINE SYSTEM

### Steroids

**ADRENAL STEROIDS.** Adrenocorticosteroids (adrenal steroids, corticosteroids) are endogenous hormonal substances released from the adrenal cortex or their synthetic derivatives. They effect 1) carbohydrate, protein, and fat metabolism; 2) electrolyte and water balance; 3) the functions of the cardiovascular and central nervous systems, the kidney, bone, and skeletal muscle; and 4) the inflammatory and immune processes. The prime organ of homeostasis, the adrenal cortex, is essential to life because it allows adaptation to a constantly changing environment. The drugs are classified as glucocorticoids or mineralocorticoids. The adrenal cortex also contains androgenic steroids.

*Mechanism of Action.* Like other hormones, the adrenocorticosteroids produce their effects by controlling the rate of physiologic occurrences. The prime biochemical action of the adrenal steroids is to affect RNA transcription within target cells. The adrenal steroids enter the cell, bind to a steroid receptor within the cytoplasm, producing conformational changes which allow the steroid–receptor complex to enter the nucleus, bind to chromatin, and control the transcription of RNA (34). This allows for the synthesis of specific proteins (anabolism). The corticosteroids are also catabolic in other tissues (skin, muscle, bone) because they inhibit RNA transcription and protein synthesis. Therefore, the principal effect of the adrenal steroids is on protein synthesis, either to inhibit or stimulate it. The prime biochemical actions of the adrenocorticosteroids are 1) stimulation of protein synthesis in the liver, 2) inhibition of peripheral tissue protein synthesis, and 3) stimulation of hepatic gluconeogenesis.

*Pharmacologic Effects.* The adrenocorticosteroids possess a wide variety of pharmacologic effects.

*Carbohydrate and Protein Metabolism.* The adrenal steroids are essentially antiinsulin in their effects. They promote liver and peripheral gluconeogenesis, increase liver glycogen storage, decrease peripheral glucose utilization, and decrease peripheral protein synthesis.

*Lipid Metabolism.* The adrenal steroids inhibit fatty acid synthesis, promote mobilization of fatty acids from adipose tissues, and redistribute fat to the neck and face (buffalo hump, moon face).

*Electrolyte and Water Balance.* The mineralocorticoids and some glucocorticoids increase sodium absorption in the renal tubules and decrease potassium reabsorption.

*Cardiovascular System.* The cardiovascular effects of the adrenal steroids are secondary to their effects on the kidney and sodium retention. A lack of adrenal steroids results in reduced blood volume and hypotension; hypertension is a cardinal finding in hyperadrenocorticism (Cushing's disease).

*Skeletal Muscle and Bone.* The adrenal steroids decrease protein incorporation into muscle and bone and also promote the breakdown of protein into glucose. The steroids also inhibit osteoblastic activity.

*Central Nervous System.* In both Addison's disease (hypoadrenocorticism) and Cushing's disease (hyperadrenocorticism) profound mental changes are apparent. Excess adrenal steroids result in mood elevation, euphoria, restlessness and psychosis. Addison's disease is associated with apathy, depression, and psychosis.

*Blood.* Addison's disease is associated with anemia, whereas the adrenal steroids produce a lymphocytopenia, reduced lymphoid tissue, and inhibition of phagocytosis.

*Antiinflammatory Effects.* The adrenal steroids suppress many of the signs and symptoms of inflammation (heat, erythema, edema, capillary dilation, fibroblastic proliferation, phagocytic activity, and collagen deposition), but they do not affect the cause of inflammation. These effects also substantially suppress wound healing. There is at present no unifying hypothesis to explain the antiinflammatory effects of the corticosteroids; however, it is agreed that the steroids act locally at the site of injury by effecting capillaries and cell mediators of inflammation. The steroids may prevent the release of lysosomal enzymes from damaged cells and inhibit the release of arachidonic acid by inhibiting phospholipase A activity thereby preventing the formation of the prostaglandins and thromboxane $A_2$ (see Prostaglandins).

*Immune Response.* The adrenal steroids do not prevent either the union of antibody and antigen in the immediate allergic response or the release of cell mediators (histamine, bradykinin) from affected tissue, nor do they suppress circulating antibodies (IgG or IgE). Their role in the acute allergic response is to reduce the signs and symptoms of cell disruption as they do in inflammation. In high doses the adrenal steroids suppress cell-mediated allergy (T cells), as in contact dermatitis and serum sickness (delayed allergy). The adrenal steroids may prevent graft rejection by reduction of inflammation, but they have no effect on the allergic component.

*Absorption, Distribution, Metabolism, and Excretion.* The adrenal steroids are well absorbed orally and may be administered parenterally, orally, or topically.

*Toxic Effects.* The adverse effects of the adrenocorticosteroids are myriad and are a direct extension of their pharmacologic effects. In addition, iatrogenic production of Addison's disease may result from suppression of adrenocorticotropic hormone (ACTH) secretion, atrophy of the adrenal cortex, and too rapid withdrawal of adrenal steroid therapy. The signs and symptoms of hyperadrenocorticism (Cushing's disease) are CNS disturbances, diabetes, hypertension, peptic ulceration, myopathy, osteoporosis, fat redistribution, skin atrophy, impaired wound healing, activation of latent infections, and suppression of the immune response. The signs and symptoms of hypoadrenocorticism (Addison's disease) are CNS disturbances, myocardial atrophy, hypotension, musculoskeletal weak-

ness, melanin deposition, hypoglycemia, reduced body fat, and marked inability to respond favorably to stress.

*Therapeutic Uses.* The adrenal steroids are curative for only one disease: Addison's disease. In other diseases they are essentially only palliative drugs. They may be effective in rheumatoid arthritis, rheumatic carditis, ulcerative colitis, asthma, hepatitis, blood dyscrasias, collagen diseases (systemic lupus erythematosus, polymyositis, polyarteritis nodosa, allergy, ocular diseases, lymphatic malignancies, and graft rejection. Topical corticosteroids have revolutionized the practice of dermatology.

*Representative Agents.* The various adrenocorticosteroids differ primarily in their potency, effects on carbohydrate metabolism, and degree of sodium retention. The principal endogenous mineralocorticoid is aldosterone. Endogenous glucocorticoids are cortisol (hydrocortisone), cortisone, and corticosterone. The synthetic corticosteroids in increasing order of potency are prednisolone, prednisone, methylprednisolone (Medrol), triamcinolone (Aristocort), paramethasone (Haldrone), betamethasone (Celestone), and dexamethasone (Decadron).

## QUESTIONS

82. The pharmacologic effects of the adrenocorticosteroids include the
    a. suppression of antibody formation
    b. prevention of histamine release in allergy
    c. inhibition of fibroblast proliferation
    d. suppression of lymphoid tissue
    e. suppression of signs of inflammation

    1. a, b, and c
    2. b, c, and d
    3. c, d, and e
    4. a and b
    5. d and e

83. The signs and symptoms of excess adrenocorticosteroids (hyperadrenocorticism) include
    a. hypertension
    b. hyperkeratosis of skin
    c. osteopetrosis
    d. myocardial atrophy
    e. peptic ulceration

    1. a, b, and c
    2. b, c, and d
    3. c, d, and e
    4. a and e
    5. All of the above

**FEMALE SEX HORMONES.** The female sex hormones are of two types: 1) estrogens and 2) progesterones (progestins). The estrogens and progesterones provide a negative feedback mechanism to reduce pituitary gonadotropin secretion.

*Estrogens.* The estrogens are secreted by the ovaries, which in turn are controlled by pituitary follicle-stimulating hormone (FISH). The psysiologic effects of the estrogens include 1) control of the growth of female reproductive organs, 2) keratinization of vaginal epithelium, 3) stimulation of cervical mucous secretions, 4) decrease in blood cholesterol, 5) increase in protein-bound iodine in the blood, 6) inhibition of pituitary FSH secretion and stimulation of luteinizing hormone (LH) release, 7) epiphyseal closure, 8) sodium retention, 9) increase in bone calcium deposition, and 10) increase in skin elastic fibers. The estrogens are employed in the treatment of menopausal symptoms, amenorrhea, osteoporosis, atrophic vaginitis, and some forms of prostatic and mammary carcinoma. Maternal estrogen use may increase the risk of vaginal carcinoma in offspring.

*Progesterones.* The progestins are secreted by the corpus luteum and the placenta. Their physiologic effects include 1) control of the secretory phase of the endometrium, 2) reduction in uterine contraction, 3) differentiation of female reproductive organs, and 4) production of menstruation. Progesterones are used therapeutically in cases of threatened abortions, amenorrhea or dysmenorrhea, inhibition of lactation, and endometriosis. The use of androgenic progestins in pregnant women may induce fetal masculinization.

MALE SEX HORMONES. The principal male sex hormone is testosterone, which is secreted by testicular Leydig cells. The protein anabolic effect of testosterone has been exploited to produce the anabolic steroids used by athletes and in certain metabolic disturbances.

*Testosterone.* The physiologic effects of the androgens include: 1) development and maintenance of male secondary sex characteristics and male sex organs, 2) closure of the epiphysis, 3) increase in tissue protein (anabolism), 4) cellular hypertrophy of the prostate gland, 5) increase in striated muscle, 6) increase in osteoblastic activity, 7) increase in sebaceous gland secretions, and 8) decrease in scalp hair and increase in body hair. The prime therapeutic use of the androgens is in the treatment of impaired or absent testicular secretion of testosterone. In addition, testosterone may be employed in the palliative treatment of premenopausal metastatic breast cancer in females.

*Anabolic Steroids.* These agents produce greater metabolic nitrogen retention than testosterone and have been used to treat certain growth disturbances and osteoporosis; they have also been used by athletes to increase muscle mass. Their side-effects include sodium retention, fetal masculinization, cholestatic jaundice, and aggravation of prostate cancer.

ORAL CONTRACEPTIVES. First used in 1955 to prevent pregnancy, the oral contraceptives are presently the most reliable agents (virtually 100% reliable if used properly) for this purpose.

*Types.* There are three forms of oral contraceptives: 1) estrogen–progestogen combinations, 2) sequential agents, and 3) low-dose progestogens. The estrogen–progestogen preparations contain both drugs; the sequential agents use estrogen alone for the first 14–15 days, and then a progestin is added for the last 4–5 days; the low-dose progestogens employ only a progestin. The sequential contraceptives were withdrawn from the market in the United States in 1976.

*Mechanism of Action.* The primary effect of the estrogen component is to inhibit ovulation by preventing the secretion of pituitary FSH and luteinizing hormone. The progesterone is synergistic in suppressing LH secretion and promotes endometrial maturation, allowing for proper menstruation. Other ancillary contraceptive effects include an alteration in the endometrium which produces an antinidation effect, changes in cervical mucous secretions which are spermicidal and restrict sperm mobility, and alterations in fallopian tube mobility.

*Toxic Effects.* The entire range of psychologic changes seen with the human psyche has been attributed to the "pill," most unjustifiably. Objective side-effects associated with the oral contraceptives probably include vascular headache, visual disturbances, acne, cholestatic jaundice, vaginal monilial infections, increased blood pressure, and breakthrough bleeding. Since the oral contraceptives produce endometrial changes resembling pregnancy, weight gain and breast enlargement are to be expected. Recent research indicates that the use of the oral contraceptives may be associated with increased risk of thromboembolic disease, cardiovascular disease, gallstones, and hepatic adenoma, but a decreased risk of malignant breast cancer. A woman taking the oral contraceptives undergoes much less physical risk than that associated with pregnancy, childbirth, and abortion. Absolute contraindications to the oral contraceptives include a current or past history of thromboembolic disease, undiagnosed genital bleeding, markedly impaired liver function, and known or suspected estrogen-dependent cancers.

## Nonsteroids

INSULIN AND THE ORAL ANTIDIABETIC AGENTS. Insulin is a hormone consisting of two amino acid chains joined by disulfide linkages and secreted by the $\beta$ cells of the pancreas after conversion from proinsulin. Insulin deficiency results in diabetes mellitus. The oral antidiabetic agents produce hypoglycemia via either an action on the $\beta$ cells or peripheral glucose utilization. There are two types: the sulfonylureas and phenformin hydrochloride (DBI).

*Diabetes Mellitus.* There are two types of diabetes mellitus: 1) juvenile onset (insulin-dependent, ketosis-prone) and 2) maturity onset (nonketotic). Juvenile onset diabetes is characterized by a deficiency in $\beta$-cell synthesis and secretion of insulin. Functional $\beta$ cells are present in maturity onset diabetes, but there is a time delay in insulin secretion in response to stimuli and also a reduction in the amount of insulin secreted.

Diabetes mellitus is characterized by hyperglycemia, hyperlipemia, ketonemia, and azoturia. Diabetes mellitus is also associated with thickening of capillary basement membranes resulting in atherosclerosis, diabetic retinopathy, renal glomerulosclerosis, neuropathy, and gangrene of the extremities. The hyperglycemia results from an overproduction and underutilization of glucose produced by an increased conversion of protein to glucose, a markedly reduced rate of glucose transport across cell membranes, and a reduction in the amount of glucose converted to glycogen. The hyperlipemia and ketonemia result from increased mobilization of free fatty acids from peripheral lipid sources and their liver metabolism to ketone bodies. Insulin deficiency encourages gluconeogenesis and increased production of urea and ammonia (azotemia).

*Regulation of Insulin Secretion.* Proinsulin is synthesized in the endoplasmic reticulum of the pancreatic $\beta$ cells and converted to insulin within the Golgi apparatus. Insulin secretion is regulated by a number of mechanisms: 1) food (glucose, amino and fatty acids) increases insulin secretion; 2) gastrointestinal hormones (secretin, gastrin, pancreozymin) increase insulin secretion; 3) a $\beta$-adrenergic response increases blood glucose and thereby insulin secretion, while $\alpha$-adrenergic stimulation reduces insulin secretion; 4) cholinergic drugs and vagus nerve stimulation increase insulin secretion; 5) the prostaglandins increase insulin secretion, and stomatostatin decreases insulin secretion. Glucose stimulates both insulin secretion and synthesis.

*Mechanism of Action.* The initial site of action of insulin is the cell membrane, but its precise biochemical mechanism of action is unknown. Insulin may reduce intracellular cyclic adenosine monophosphate (cAMP) by either inhibition of adenylate cyclase or stimulation of phosphodiesterase. A decrease in cAMP reduces the activity of a protein kinase responsible for the breakdown of glycogen; insulin reduces the sensitivity of the protein kinase to cAMP and also activates glycogen synthetase. Insulin also increases the active form of pyruvate dehydrogenase, which is responsible for the oxidation of pyruvate or its conversion to fat, thereby making it unavailable for glucose formation. Insulin also increases protein synthesis. The sulfonylureas stimulate the $\beta$ cells to secrete insulin. Phenformin acts peripherally to increase glucose utilization and decrease gluconeogenesis. Glucagon is a stimulant of cAMP synthesis and an insulin antagonist.

*Absorption, Distribution, Metabolism, and Excretion.* The various insulin preparations must be administered parenterally and differ only in their onset and duration of action. The various sulfonylurea preparations, which are intended for oral use, also differ only in onset and duration of action.

*Toxic Effects.* Hyperinsulinism frequently occurs in labile forms of the disease due to unpredictable changes in insulin requirements, failure to eat, unusual exercise, or insulin overdosage. The symptomatology is essentially due to a reduction in brain glucose. The initial signs and symptoms are those of epinephrine release from the adrenal medulla: sweating, hunger, weakness, and tachycardia. The later symptoms of brain glucose deprivation include headache, diplopia, mental confusion, speech impairment, and finally coma and convulsions. It is imperative to remember that it is very difficult to make a clinical differentiation between insulin shock and diabetic acidosis.

Patients treated with the sulfonylureas may have a greater incidence of cardiovascular disease than those treated with dietary control or insulin. Other adverse effects of the sulfonylureas include blood dyscrasias, skin lesions, hepatic dysfunction, gastrointestinal bleeding, and hypoglycemia. The Food and Drug Administration has removed phenformin from clinical use, since it produces lactic acidosis.

*Therapeutic Uses.* Insulin is the mainstay of therapy in juvenile onset diabetes. There is increasing emphasis on the management of adult onset diabetes with diet control and weight reduction alone, with the sulfonylureas being reserved for refractory patients.

*Representative Agents.* The insulin preparations include regular insulin (reserved for diabetic acidosis), isophane insulin (NPH) and protamine zinc insulin. The sulfonylureas include tolbutamide (Orinase), acetoheximide (Dymelor), tolazamide (Tolinase), and chlorpropamide (Diabinese).

## PITUITARY HORMONES

*Anterior Pituitary Hormones.* The anterior portion of the pituitary gland secretes seven hormones which control the hormonal secretions and metabolic functions in other organs and tissues:

1. thyroid-stimulating hormone (TSH)
2. adrenocorticotropic hormone (ACTH)
3. follicle-stimulating hormone (FSH)
4. luteinizing hormone (LH)
5. growth hormone (GH, somatotropin)
6. melanocyte-stimulating hormone (MSH)
7. prolactin (PL)

The secretion of these hormones is in turn inhibited by hormones secreted by their target organs (negative feedback mechanisms) and stimulated by hypothalamic releasing factors. TSH-releasing hormones (TRH), ACTH-releasing factor (CRF), LH-releasing factor (LRH), FSH-releasing factor (FRF), growth-hormone releasing and inhibiting factors (GRF and GIF), MSH-releasing and inhibiting factors (MRF and MIF) and prolactin-releasing and inhibiting factors (PRF and PIF). The hormone that inhibits the growth hormone (somatropin) releasing factor is somatostatin, which also inhibits glucagon and insulin secretion by pancreatic cells.

*Posterior Pituitary Hormones.* The two posterior pituitary hormones are vasopressin (Pitressin) and oxytocin (Pitocin). Vasopressin (antidiuretic hormone) acts on the kidney to increase water reabsorption by enlarging pores in the membranes of the distal tubule and collecting ducts. Oxytocin increases uterine muscle tone and is used for the induction of labor in gravid females.

**THYROID HORMONES.** Thyroid hormone is synthesized in the thyroid gland by the enzymatic oxidation of the iodide ion to active iodide; the active iodide then reacts with tyrosine groups on the thyroglobulin molecule, resulting in the formation of thyroxine and triiodothyronine. These hormones have physiologic effects on growth and development, metabolism, thermoregulation, skeletal muscle, water and electrolyte balance, and the cardiovascular and nervous systems. The metabolic effects of thyroid hormone include increased gastrointestinal absorption of glucose and galactose, potentiation of the metabolic effects of epinephrine, potentiation of insulin-induced glycogen synthesis and glucose utilization, increased glucose uptake by fat, increased mobilization of free fatty acids, and reduction in serum cholesterol levels.

Hypothyroidism as manifested in cretinism and myxedema is treated by thyroglobulin (Proloid), sodium levothyroxine (Synthroid), or sodium liothyronine (Cytomel). Hyperthyroidism as manifested by weight loss, anxiety, perspiration, heat production, increased appetite, tachycardia, and muscle weakness is treated by "antithyroid" drugs such as propylthiouracil (Propacil), and methimazole (Tapazole). Thyrotoxicosis is exacerbated by epinephrine.

**PARATHYROID HORMONE AND THYROCALCITONIN**
*Parathyroid Hormone.* The secretion of parathyroid hormone from the parathyroid glands is controlled by blood calcium levels. The major function of parathyroid hormone is to insure adequate tissue calcium levels, particularly for neuromuscular function. The sites of parathyroid hormone action are bone, the kidney, and the intestines. Parathyroid hormone increases the resorption of bone, probably through the action of cAMP and adenylate cyclase, and inhibits inorganic phosphate resorption in the renal tubules. It also stimulates gastrointestinal calcium absorption, although vitamin D is the most important hormone regulating dietary calcium absorption.

*Thyrocalcitonin.* Thyrocalcitonin (calcitonin) is secreted by the thyroid gland in response to elevated blood calcium levels. It inhibits bone resorption and increases urinary calcium and phosphate excretion. It is employed in the treatment of Paget's disease and osteoporosis.

QUESTIONS

84. The metabolic effects of insulin include
    a. regulation of cellular transport of glucose
    b. increased protein synthesis
    c. increased glycogen formation
    d. stimulation of ketone body formation
    e. increased gluconeogenesis

    1. a, b, and c
    2. b, c, and d
    3. c, d, and e
    4. a and b
    5. All of the above

85. The symptoms of hyperthyroidism (thyrotoxicosis) are exacerbated by an excess of
    1. acetylcholine
    2. histamine
    3. epinephrine
    4. lactic acid
    5. None of the above

86. The hormones primarily responsible for the maintenance of blood calcium levels is
    1. calcitonin
    2. thyroid hormone
    3. adrenal steroids
    4. parathyroid hormone
    5. testosterone

## NEUROMUSCULAR AGENTS

Neuromuscular blocking drugs are agents which interrupt nerve transmission at the skeletal neuromuscular junction.

### Classification

Neuromuscular blocking drugs are classified according to their mechanism of action: 1) competitive (stabilizing) and 2) depolarizing. D–tubocurarine (curare) is the prototype for the competitive agents; succinylcholine (Anectine), for the depolarizing agents.

### Mechanism of Action

Because D–tubocurarine is a competitive antagonist of acetylcholine at the postjunctional membrane of the neuromuscular junction, it prevents the nerve action potential from depolarizing the membrane. Succinylcholine depolarizes the postjunctional membrane in much the same manner as acetylcholine, preventing membrane repolarization. The end result of both mechanisms is neuromuscular paralysis. Anticholinesterase agents antagonize the competitive effects of d-tubocurarine but are synergistic with succinylcholine. Diethyl ether, the halogenated hydrocarbon general anesthetics, and the aminoglycoside antibiotics are synergistic with d-tubocurarine.

### Pharmacologic Effects

Both types of neuromuscular blocking drugs produce generalized muscle weakness. The smaller muscles of the fingers, toes, and eyes are affected first, followed by the muscles of swallowing and speech, the larger muscles of the limbs, and finally the intercostal muscles and diaphragm. These drugs do not produce any central nervous system depression; therefore, there is no analgesia, memory impairment, loss of consciousness, or impairment of special senses. Curare releases histamine from the mast cells.

### Toxic Effects

The prime adverse effect is prolonged apnea due to the neuromuscular blockade of the intercostal muscles and the diaphragm. Patients genetically deficient in serum (pseudo) cholinesterase are acutely sensitive to succinylcholine because of impaired metabolism. Histamine release by curare results in hypotension. Apnea resulting from succinylcholine is treated by mechanical ventilation with positive pressure oxygen; if it results from curare, it is treated by mechanical ventilation and anticholinesterase drugs.

### Therapeutic Uses

Neuromuscular blocking drugs are used 1) as adjuncts to general anesthesia, 2) in convulsive states, 3) for orthopedic manipulation, 4) for endotracheal intubation, and 5) for the treatment of laryngospasm.

### Representative Agents

The competitive drugs include d-tubocurarine (curare), gallamine (Flaxedil), and pancuronium (Pavulon). The depolarizing drugs are represented by decamethonium (Syncurine) and succinylcholine (Anectine).

#### QUESTIONS

87. Which of the following statements are true regarding d-tubocurarine (curare)?
    a. It produces significant central nervous system depression.
    b. It is a competitive antagonist of acetylcholine.
    c. It releases histamine from the mast cells.
    d. Its effects are potentiated by anticholinesterase drugs.

    e. It produces persistent motor endplate depolarization.
    1. a, b, and c
    2. b, c, and d
    3. c, d, and e
    4. b, c, and e
    5. All of the above

88. Succinylcholine (Anectine) produces a depolarizing blockade of the neuromuscular junction because succinylcholine possesses pharmacologic effects at the neuromuscular junction similar to acetylcholine.
    1. Both statement and reason are correct and related.
    2. Both statement and reason are correct but not related.
    3. The statement is correct, but the reason is not.
    4. The statement is not correct, but the reason is an accurate statement.
    5. Neither statement nor reason is correct.

89. Patients genetically deficient in serum (pseudo) cholinesterase may experience prolonged apnea when administered succinylcholine because serum cholinesterase inhibits the metabolism of succinylcholine.
    1. Both statement and reason are correct and related.
    2. Both statement and reason are correct but not related.
    3. The statement is correct, but the reason is not.
    4. The statement is not correct, but the reason is an accurate statement.
    5. Neither statement nor reason is correct.

## INORGANIC ION: FLOURIDE

Fluorine is a highly reactive chemical element which in nature is almost never found alone, but rather in combination with other elements. It is virtually impossible to avoid the fluoride ion, as it is present in almost all foods, air, water, and even some drugs.

### Absorption, Distribution, Metabolism, and Excretion

In its highly soluble sodium fluoride form, fluoride is very well absorbed from the gastrointestinal tract by passive diffusion. The presence of divalent metals (calcium, magnesium, and aluminum) retards fluoride absorption; calcium fluoride and crystalite are insoluble. Fluoride may also be absorbed through the skin and lungs.

The fluoride ion is distributed to all tissues of the body, but it is essentially concentrated in only calcified tissue (teeth and bone). The concentration of fluoride in soft tissue is the same as that in plasma; the mean plasma level is 0.14–0.19 PPM and remains stable even at doses of 2.5 PPM/day. The highest calcified tissue concentration of fluoride is in the cementum, followed in decreasing order by bone, dentin, and enamel. Skeletal uptake of fluoride increases with intake and age.

The vast majority of ingested fluoride ions is excreted

via the kidney. Certain important feedback mechanisms protect soft tissue from excessive fluoride exposure: reduced renal excretion of fluoride ions results in greater skeletal sequestration and reduced gastrointestinal absorption; increased oral intake results in greater skeletal uptake and greater renal excretion.

## Toxic Effects

Fluoride dosages at the level of 1 PPM/day are nontoxic to the human being. The low end of the dose–response curve for mottling of dental enamel has been established at 2 PPM/day during active tooth calcification. Chronic ingestion of 4–8 PPM/day may result in osteosclerosis. Crippling fluorosis is seen at doses of 20–80 mg/day for 10–20 years. The symptoms of endemic fluorosis are 1) stiffness of the limbs and decreased mobility of the spinal cord, 2) myopathy, 3) peripheral neuritis, 4) calcification of fibrocartilage and ligaments, 5) increased bone density, 6) exostosis formation, 7) bone resorption cavities, and 8) rapid osteoblastic and osteoclastic activity.

Acute fluoride intoxication is extremely rare, and the lethal acute dose range is approximately 5–10 g in the human adult. The signs and symptoms are 1) severe gastrointestinal irritation, 2) hemorrhagic gastroenteritis, 3) salivation and lacrimation, 4) muscular fibrillation, 5) convulsions, 6) cardiovascular and respiratory depression, and 7) coma and death. The Council on Dental Therapeutics has restricted the prescribing of fluoride tablets to only 264 tablets at one time, as an acute dose of 0.5 g may be fatal in children (35).

## Dosage

The optimum dose of fluoride in water is 1 PPM and must be adjusted according to climate (greater water ingestion in hotter climates). The optimum fluoride concentration in water in areas where the average daily temperature is 50° F is 1.2 PPM, whereas it is 0.7 PPM in climates averaging 85° F. The dosage of sodium fluoride (NaF) tablets must also be adjusted according to the natural fluoride content of the water: at 0.0 PPM, 2.2 mg NaF; at 0.2 PPM, 1.8 mg NaF; at 0.4 PPM, 1.3 mg NaF; and at 0.6 PPM, 0.9 mg NaF (36). Sodium fluoride should not be prescribed where the natural fluoride water concentration is 0.6 PPM or greater (37). A standard 2.2-mg tablet of sodium fluoride contains 1 mg available fluoride.

## Mechanism of Action

The precise mechanism by which the fluoride ion prevents dental caries is unknown but may involve any or all the following: 1) reduction of enamel solubility in the presence of acid, 2) inhibition of acid-producing

bacterial enzymes (plaque), 3) alteration in tooth protein matrix, and 4) alteration in tooth shape. The most likely mechanism by far is the reduction in enamel solubility to acid. This may be accomplished by the production of fluorohydroxyapatite (the replacement of the hydroxyl ion by the fluoride ion), which is less soluble and possesses lower chemical reactivity. Fluorohydroxyapatite also has larger crystals so that there is less surface area and thereby less susceptibility to resorption. Enamel solubility to acid may also be reduced by the precipitation of calcium phosphate on the enamel surface, resulting in enamel remineralization. The fluoride ion concentrates in bacterial plaque and may inhibit acid-producing enzymes. The proposed alteration of tooth shape or the protein matrix is probably of little if any importance.

## Therapeutic Uses

The fluoride ion is of unquestioned efficacy in the reduction of dental caries (50%–60%) in communities with fluoridated water, and the best source is water fluoridation. The maximum benefit is attained when the teeth are developing, and the maximum total benefit is attained with continued fluoride ingestion after the eruption of the permanent dentition. Maternally ingested fluoride reaches the fetal blood, but there is no consensus regarding the benefit of prenatal fluoride.

Sodium fluoride tablets are effective and should be chewed and dissolved in the mouth. Topical application of sodium (2% aqueous solution) fluoride or stannous (8% aqueous solution) fluoride may reduce caries incidence by 30%–40%. The maximum effect of topical sodium fluoride is attained by four treatments several days apart at ages 3, 7, 11, and 13 (35). Stannous fluoride is commonly applied in single applications 6–12 months apart. Acidulated phosphate (sodium fluoride and orthophosphoric acid) fluoride preparations are also effective. Dentifrices containing stannous fluoride or sodium monofluorophosphate have been judged effective in the prevention of dental caries.

Oral ingestion of large doses of fluoride in patients with osteoporosis, Paget's disease, and multiple myeloma promotes calcium retention. It is probable that chronic low-dose fluoride ingestion during the adult years may prevent the onset or reduce the severity of crippling osteoporosis (38).

QUESTIONS

90. The most probable mechanism by which the fluoride ion prevents dental caries is

    1. stimulation of dentinal protein formation
    2. alteration of tooth morphology
    3. reduction in enamel acid solubility
    4. chemical neutralization of bacterial acid
    5. destruction of plaque matrix

# MISCELLANEOUS

## Prostaglandins

The prostaglandins are acidic lipodinal substances present in most tissues of the body; they are released in response to various mechanical, nervous, and chemical stimuli. Discovered in the 1930s, the prostaglandins (PGs) derived their name from the fact that they were first isolated from seminal fluid.

CLASSIFICATION. The prostaglandins contain 20 carbon atoms and are classified according to the characteristics of their cyclopentanone ring as E, F, A, B, C, and D with a numerical subscript denoting the number of double bonds in their side chains ($E_1$, $E_2$, $F_2$).

MECHANISM OF ACTION. Since the prostaglandins possess such widespread and diverse activity, it is probable that they affect basic physiologic control mechanisms. The PGs affect adenylate cyclase and subsequent cAMP concentrations in many tissues, often producing antagonistic effects on various organs and physiologic functions. The prostaglandins are synthesized from essential fatty acids, primarily arachidonic acid, within cells by a complex of microsomal enzymes termed prostaglandin synthetase. The key precursors to the PGs are the endoperoxides which may be converted to either the prostaglandins or the thromboxanes; all three substances produce physiologic effects. Their duration of action is extremely short, lasting from a few seconds to a maximum of a few minutes.

PHARMACOLOGIC EFFECTS. The major loci of action of the endoperoxides, prostaglandins, and thromboxanes are the uterus, cardiovascular system, platelets, bronchi, gastrointestinal tract, nervous system, and inflammatory mechanisms. PGE and $PGF_{2\alpha}$ are potent stimulators of uterine contraction and are present in the ovary, fallopian tubes, endometrium, placenta, and amniotic fluid at the onset of labor or spontaneous abortion. Most of the PGs are vasodilators (except in the nasal mucosa) and increase the force of myocardial contraction. PGE decreases platelet adhesiveness, and $PGF_{2\alpha}$ increases platelet aggregation. A thromboxane ($TXA_2$) is a potent platelet aggregator and also a coronary vasoconstrictor. $PGI_2$ is formed by the action of an enzyme (prostacyclin synthetase) located in blood vessel walls and inhibits platelet clumping. The implications for the role of the PGs, endoperoxides, and thromboxanes in cardiovascular disease, particularly arterial clotting disorders (atherosclerosis), are obvious. PGF contracts bronchial smooth muscle (asthmatics are very sensitive to this effect), and $PGE_1$ and $PGE_2$ dilate bronchial smooth muscle. PGE and PGF contract longitudinal intestinal smooth muscle; PGE re-laxes and PGF stimulates circular intestinal smooth muscle. PGE decreases gastric secretions. Present throughout the peripheral and central nervous sytems, the PGs may play a role in nerve transmission. They are important in thermoregulation ($PGE_1$ is a potent pyretic), and $PGF_2$ induces convulsions. $PGE_1$ and $PGE_2$ play a role in inflammation and pain, as they increase capilary permeability which results in erythema and edema.

PROSTAGLANDIN ANTAGONISTS. The nonsteroidal antiinflammatory agents such as aspirin and indomethacin are potent inhibitors of prostaglandin synthetase (see Nonnarcotic Analgesics). The tricyclic antidepressants are competitive inhibitors of the prostaglandin receptor. The adrenal steroids inhibit the release of the prostaglandin precursor, arachidonic acid, by phospholipase A.

THERAPEUTIC USES. The PGs and related substances possess therapeutic potential in the treatment of cardiovascular disease (stroke, myocardial infarction, hypertension), asthma, peptic ulcer, and reproductive disorders. A prostaglandin, dinoprost tromethamine (Prostine $F_2$ Alpha) is approved for use as an abortifacient in the second trimester of pregnancy. Its side-effects include fever, hypertension or hypotension, cramps, syncope, pain, and thrombophlebitis at the injection site, paresthesia, cardiac arrhythmias, hemorrhage, cervical or uterine laceration, and placental retention.

QUESTION

91. Which of the following statements concerning the prostaglandins are true?
    a. They are oxytocic.
    b. They are pyretics.
    c. They inhibit platelet agglutination.
    d. They are vasodilators.
    e. They reduce gastric secretions.
    1. a, b, and c
    2. b, c, and d
    3. c, d, and e
    4. a and b
    5. All of the above

## Antihistamines

Antihistamines are drugs which selectively antagonize some of the pharmacologic actions of histamine. To varying degrees antihistamines also possess sedative, local anesthetic, anticholinergic, and antispasmodic effects.

PHARMACOLOGIC ACTIONS OF HISTAMINE. Although the enodgenous chemical histamine is found in many tissues, it is particularly abundant in the skin and gastrointestinal tract. It is bound to heparin in the mast cell and basophil. The pharmacologic effects of histamine include 1) vasodilation (edema and hypotension); 2) bronchial, uterine, and gastrointestinal smooth muscle contraction; 3) stimulation of secretions from the salivary, lacrimal, bronchial, and gastric exocrine glands, and 4) release of catecholamines from the adrenal medulla. Histamine is also a chemical mediator of pain and itch and, most importantly, the principal chemical mediator of systemic anaphylaxis. Histamine receptors are classified as $H_1$ and $H_2$. Activation of $H_1$ receptor, results in itch, pain, epinephrine secretion from the adrenal medulla, bronchoconstriction and gastrointestinal contraction. $H_2$ receptors are located in the brain, heart and stomach.

**MECHANISM OF ACTION.** Antihistamines are competitive antagonists of selected histamine receptors. The drugs are effective against edema and itching but poorly, if at all, effective against the bronchial, gastric, and vascular (hypotensive) actions of histamine. A specific $H_2$ receptor antagonist, cimetidine (Tagamet) is now used to reduce gastric secretions in peptic ulcer patients.

**PHARMACOLOGIC EFFECTS.** Many antihistamines possess sedative effects and are used for this purpose in over-the-counter sleeping preparations. Antihistamines may also produce central nervous system stimulation and xerostomia. Some agents possess antiemetic, antimotion sickness, and local anesthetic actions. Diphenhydramine (Benadryl) has been successfully used as a local anesthetic in dentistry (39). Antihistamines do not prevent the release of histamine from mast cells and basophils in a sensitization (allergic) reaction, but they do reduce some of the signs and symptoms of histamine release, particularly edema and itching.

**TOXIC EFFECTS.** The antihistamines generally possess a very high therapeutic index. Side-effects include sedation, gastric upset, constipation, headache, visual disturbances, allergic reactions, and hypotension. In adults acute toxicity usually results in central nervous system depression; in children, central nervous system stimulation followed by depression.

**THERAPEUTIC USES.** Antihistamines are used in the treatment of acute allergy, emesis, motion sickness, parkinson's disease, and as a local anestetic and expectorant.

**REPRESENTATIVE AGENTS.** Diphenhydramine (Benadryl) and chlorpheniramine (Chlor-Trimeton) are primarily employed in the treatment of allergic symptoms. Dimenhydrinate (Dramamine), cyclizine (Mare-zine), and meclizine (Bonine) are used in the therapy of emesis and motion sickness; and promethazine (Phenergan) is used as an expectorant and preoperative sedative.

QUESTION

92. Which of the following statements are true regarding the antihistamines?
   a. Sedation is a common side-effect.
   b. They effectively antagonize itching produced by histamine.
   c. Diphenhydramine is useful as a local anesthetic agent.
   d. They possess a relatively low therapeutic index.
   e. They prevent histamine release from mast cels and basophils.

1. a, b, and c
2. b, c, and d
3. c, d, and e
4. a and e
5. b and d

## Drug Abuse

The World Health Organization (WHO) (40) has defined **drug dependence** as a state of psychic or physical dependence, or both, on a drug, arising in a person following administration of that drug on a periodic or continuous basis, the characteristics of which state are designated by the particular type of drug dependence such as the morphine type, the barbiturate type, or the amphetamine type. WHO defined **drug abuse** as the use, usually by self-administration, of any drug in a manner that deviates from the approved medical or social patterns within a given culture. Serious drug abuse is present when the drug use produces mental or physical harm to the individual and/or seriously impairs function in society (work, family, school). The term drug addiction and habituation are no longer commonly used except by the lay public.

**TYPES OF DRUG DEPENDENCE AND ABUSE.** There are presently nine types of drug dependence: 1) narcotic (opioid), 2) alcohol, 3) barbiturate, 4) amphetamine, 5) cocaine, 6) hallucinogen (LSD and phencyclidine), 7) cannabis (marijuana), 8) nicotine, and 9) hydrocarbon ("glue sniffing"). These various types differ in the degree of physical dependence, psychic dependence, tolerance, and physical or mental injury to the individual associated with their acute or chronic use.

Drug abuse can be classified according to the pattern of use of the drug: 1) experimental—drug use on only one or a few occasions fostered by curiosity or peer group pressure; 2) casual or recreational—drug use in moderate amounts for pleasurable effects; 3) circumstantial—drug use to improve performance or relieve anxiety in certain circumstances; 4) intensive—drug use with increasing frequency; and 5) compulsive drug use to maintain personal well-being, causing a compulsive preoccupation with procuring adequate supplies of the drug (41).

**THEORIES OF DRUG DEPENDENCE.** There are presently five theories (42) that are exposed to explain the development of dependence upon a chemical:

1. Acquired Drive Theory: the repeated use of a drug produces pleasurable feelings and an acquired drive for repeated stimulation.
2. Avoidance Paradigm Theory: drug use must be repeated to prevent physical withdrawal symptoms.
3. Metabolic Disease Theory: there is a metabolic genetic defect in persons who become drug-dependent.
4. Conditioning Theory: drug dependence occurs due to learned behavior sustained by conditioning stimuli such as friends and environment.
5. Automedication Theory: the drug-dependent person is psychologically impaired and requires the drug to alleviate psychoneurotic symptoms (anxiety, depression).

All drugs of abuse alter the mood or mental attitude of the individual either by central nervous system stimulation or depression. The Automedication Theory is currently the most widely held, since seriously drug-dependent individuals appear to have certain neurotic symptoms in common: anxiety, depression, guilt, hostility, and an inability to accept or perceive pleasure. The drugs alleviate these distressing symptoms.

**PSYCHIC DEPENDENCE, PHYSICAL DEPENDENCE, AND TOLERANCE.** In order to appreciate more fully the vast complexities of drug dependence and abuse, it is imperative to understand the three underlying components of this epidemic disease: psychic dependence, physical dependence, and tolerance.

*Psychic Dependence.* All drugs of abuse can produce psychic dependence, defined as a feeling of satisfaction or as a psychic drive which requires periodic or continuous drug administration to produce pleasure (euphoria) or to avoid pain (anxiety, depression). Psychic dependence fits neatly into the Automedication Theory. The degree of psychic dependence associated with the various types of drug dependence may vary greatly. Strong psychic dependence is associated with the opioids, alcohol, barbiturates, nicotine, cocaine, and the amphetamines, but dependence is low to moderate with marijuana, LSD, and the hydrocarbons.

*Physical Dependence.* An altered physical state which requires repeated drug administration to prevent the onset of an intense physical disturbance indicates physical dependence. The only drugs associated with severe physical dependence are the CNS depressants: opioids, barbiturates, and alcohol. Physical dependence is a constant reinforcement (Avoidance Paradigm Theory) to psychic dependence, as the individual must continue to take the drug to prevent the abstinence, or withdrawal, syndrome (anxiety, pain, tremors, convulsions, hallucinations). Many efforts have been made to explain the development of physical dependence, but the most likely is the production of a condition which allows for rebound hyperexcitability of the CNS. The depressant drug may substitute for inhibitory neurons or their neurotransmitters, allowing for disuse atrophy of the neurons or reduction in the amount of the inhibitory neurotransmitters. As long as the drug is present, it functions as an inhibitory substance to maintain the balance between excitatory and inhibitory neurons. Once the drug is removed, the excitatory neurons act unopposed; the withdrawal syndrome ensues and remains until the inhibitory neurons regain their function.

*Tolerance.* An adaptive state of the individual, characterized by increasingly diminished responses to the drug over a period of time, is termed tolerance. Greater and greater doses must be used to attain the desired effect, requiring increasingly greater effort on the part of the individual to acquire increasingly greater doses of the drug. The tremendous tolerance associated with opioid (heroin) use leads to increasing illegal efforts (robbery, burglary, prostitution) to pay for the drug. Tolerance development is very high with the opioids and LSD; moderate with alcohol, barbiturates, amphetamines, and nicotine; and low with marijuana, cocaine, and the hydrocarbons.

**MENTAL AND PHYSICAL PATHOLOGY.** Psychotic reactions, including paranoid and aggressive behavior are very common with intravenous amphetamine use. There is no question that "speed kills," often through crimes of violence or renal aneurysms. Hydrocarbon inhalation (glue sniffing) induces cardiac arrhythmias. Chronic heavy alcohol ingestion results in alcoholic deterioration (dilated facial capillaries, bloated appearance, flabby muscles, tremors, memory impairment, and emotional instability), psychosis (delirium tremens), fatty liver, cirrhosis, and very importantly the fetal alcohol syndrome (a group of congenital abnormalities noted in infants born to women who imbibed moderate to large doses of ethyl alcohol during pregnancy) (43). There is no question that ethyl alcohol is preeminent as the most serious drug of abuse. The tissue pathology associated with cigarettes needs no repetition. Marijuana and LSD and its cogener phencyclidine hydrochloride ("angel dust," PCP) may induce impaired judgment, abnormal behavior, and psychotic reactions. Chronic opioid use does not produce any tissue pathology except that associated with unsterile needles.

QUESTIONS

93. A strong physical dependence is associated with drug dependence on

    a. phencyclidine
    b. diacetylmorphine (heroin)
    c. ethyl alcohol
    d. LSD
    e. marijuana

    1. a, b, and c
    2. b, c, and d
    3. c, d, and e
    4. a and e
    5. b and c

94. Psychic dependence is common to all forms of drug dependence because drugs of abuse affect the central nervous system and the mood of the individual.

    1. Both statement and reason are correct and related.
    2. Both statement and reason are correct but not related.
    3. The statement is correct, but the reason is not.
    4. The statement is not correct, but the reason is an accurate statement.
    5. Neither statement nor reason is correct.

## EMERGENCY TREATMENT

An emergency can be defined as a sudden, unexpected change in a person's health status which calls for immediate action.

### Types of Emergencies

Three types of emergencies can occur in the dental situation: 1) those of medical origin, 2) those due to a toxic drug overdosage, and 3) acute allergy. Medical emergencies may range from simple syncope to acute myocardial infarction; they may include epileptic seizures, acute asthma, angina pectoris, and insulin shock. The two most common acute adverse drug reactions are CNS depressant overdosage (narcotics, barbiturates) and local anesthetic toxicity. Acute allergic symptoms include skin lesions (erythema and urticaria), angioedema, exfoliative dermatitis, and systemic anaphylactic shock.

### Signs and Symptoms

Acute myocardial infarction is characterized by crushing substernal pain; angina pectoris, by substernal pain radiating to the arms and face; epilepsy, by tonic–clonic seizures; acute asthma, by chest distention and characteristic asthmatic wheezing; and insulin shock, by hunger, sweating, disorientation, and loss of consciousness. Overdosage with CNS depressants results in respiratory depression. Local anesthetic overdosage is characterized by early CNS stimulation (nervousness, muscle twitching, and tonic–clonic convulsions) followed by postseizure CNS depression (loss of consciousness, cardiovascular and respiratory depression). The symptoms of the acute fear reaction are identical to those of local anesthetic overdosage. If massive doses of a local anesthetic are administered, cardiac arrest may occur without any signs of CNS stimulation. The vast majority of allergic reactions are confined to the skin; erythema, itching, and vesicle formation (urticaria) are characteristic. Swelling localized to the eyes, lips, hands, or feet (angioedema) may occur with or without skin lesions. Exfoliative dermatitis is the loss of the skin barrier and constitutes a major medical emergency. Acute systemic anaphylaxis, the most serious of medical emergencies, is characterized by acute anxiety (fear of impending death), flushing, itching, urticaria, bronchoconstriction (asthmatic wheezing), and severe hypotension.

### The Emergency Kit

The list of drugs with potential and/or practical use in the treatment of emergency health situations is exceedingly long, highly complex, and, at best, intimidating. Close scrutiny of this list reveals that the majority of these agents should be reserved for hospital use by highly trained individuals. Drugs are two-edged swords; they may help, but they also may harm. However, a basic minimum of drugs and equipment must be available in the dental office to treat acute and potentially life-threatening emergencies.

The emergency kit has two components: physical equipment and drugs. The mechanical devices include intramuscular and/or intravenous syringes, a cricothyreotomy needle, and a mechanism by which to administer positive pressure oxygen (Robertshaw valve). The lack of a positive pressure oxygen system in a dental office is indefensible from a medicolegal standpoint. Plastic oropharyngeal airways are no longer recommended since the majority of patients vomit during their insertion, which in turn may result in airway obstruction and/or lung aspiration and subsequent abscess formation.

The essential drugs to be included in the emergency kit are epinephrine (Adrenalin), an antihistamine (diphenhydramine or chlorpheniramine), sugar, nitroglycerin, a Medihaler-Epi aerosol, aromatic ammonia ampules, and naloxone (Narcan). Drugs with potential usefulness are an analgesic (meperidine or pentazocine) and diazepam (Valium).

### Emergency Treatment

Before initiating therapy in any emergency situation, the diagnosis of whether the situation is one of acute allergy or something else must be made instantly.

There are only three emergency situations in which a drug is administered prior to proper patient oxygenation: acute allergy, narcotic overdosage, and insulin shock. The vast majority of emergency situations are treated in accordance with the ABCs of cardiopulmonary resuscitation (CPR): airway, breathing, and circulation. It is mandatory that all dental personnel be trained in this technique and take refresher courses periodically. It is also imperative to understand that serious emergencies cannot be handled by the dentist alone; trained medical personnel such as paramedics or their equivalents must be close at hand. The telephone number of the nearest paramedic or ambulance unit must be placed on each office phone.

Simple syncope is treated by aromatic ammonia inhalation and oxygenation; angina pectoris, by sublingual nitroglycerin; and insulin shock, by sugar. The only CNS depressants for which specific antidotal therapy is available are the narcotics; naloxone (Narcan) may be given in 0.4-mg (1 ml.) doses. Barbiturate overdosage can be treated only by oxygenation until the drug is metabolized. Local anesthetic and epileptic seizures are self-limiting, and the only treatment ordinarily necessary is prevention of physical harm to the patient during the clonic seizures. Intravenous diazepam terminates the seizures, but it is poorly absorbed by the intramuscular route. The life-threatening aspect of convulsions is the postseizure CNS depression, particularly the respiratory depression which inevitably occurs. Proper oxygenation is mandatory until full patient recovery. The bronchoconstriction seen in systemic anaphylaxis and the acute asthmatic attack are both treated with epinephrine (a β–adrenergic effect) either by intramuscular injection (0.5 ml of a 1:1000 solution) or by topical applicaiton (inhalation) from a Medihaler-Epi aerosol. Antihistamines are effective only in the treatment of allergic skin manifestations. It is wise to remember that a mild allergic skin reaction may be the forerunner of systemic anaphylaxis, however, and epinephrine must be available.

Two excellent texts—one by Malamed (44) and another by McCarthy (45)—are available which comprehensively discuss allergic, medical and drug emergencies in dental practice.

### QUESTIONS

95. Epinephrine (Adrenalin) is the drug of choice in the treatment of anaphylactic shock because β adrenergic drugs relax bronchial smooth muscle.
    1. Both statement and reason are correct and related.
    2. Both statement and reason are correct but not related.
    3. The statement is correct, but the reason is not.
    4. The statement is not correct, but the reason is.
    5. Neither statement nor reason is correct.

96. The agent of choice for the symptomatic treatment of a mild allergic skin reaction is
    1. adrenal steroids
    2. epinephrine
    3. isoproterenol
    4. antihistamine
    5. norepinephrine

97. The agent of choice to antagonize narcotic overdosage is
    1. isoproterenol
    2. nalorphine (Nalline)
    3. diphenhydramine (Benadryl)
    4. diazepam (Valium)
    5. naloxone (Narcan)

## CLINICAL PHARMACOLOGY

Clinical pharmacology is that branch of pharmacology that is directly involved with the efficacy and safety of drugs in humans. It deals with the examination and detection of drug actions, the elucidation of drug effects in man, and the correlation of these effects in man with pharmacologic observations in lower animals.

### The Clinical Trail

The purposes of the study of drugs in humans is to 1) find effective drug therapy for a particular disease state, 2) determine the adverse effects of drugs, and 3) find any clinical area of usefulness for a given drug. Human drug studies begin with the filing of an Investigational Exemption for a New Drug (IND) with the Food and Drug Administration (FDA). The IND must contain information about the chemical and biologic activity of the drug, specific dosage forms, manufacturing controls, names and qualifications of the clinical investigators, a description of the physical facilities where the drug study is to be performed, signed statements from the investigators that the rights of the human subjects will be protected, and statements as to the laboratory tests to be performed and any predictable toxicity.

After the FDA has approved the IND, the clinical trial is begun. It is divided into three clinical phases. Phase I trials are limited to only a few volunteers, and their aim is to determine the pharmacologic properties of the drug (absorption, distribution, metabolism, and excretion), its therapeutic effects, and therapeutic and toxic dose levels. Phase II studies are done (after FDA approval of Phase I data) on a larger number of volunteers, and the aim is to prove definite efficacy in the treatment of a specific disease state within reasonable bounds of adverse effects. Phase III trials, which take 1–3 years, are done in a number of clinical centers on a large number of patients to prove efficacy and delineate adverse effects in large, varied populations. If the FDA is satisfied with the data on efficacy and toxicity of the new drug, it issues a new drug application and the drug may be marketed. Since 1963 only 5% of investigational new drugs have reached the market place.

If the clinical evaluation of a new drug requires the investigator or the patient to make a judgment as to efficacy and toxicity, the study must be "blinded" to prevent bias. This is particularly critical for drugs which affect disease processes with a substantial subjective component (pain, anxiety, angina pectoris). In a single blind study the investigator, but not the patient, knows which is the drug under study (the new drug versus an established one, or the new drug versus a placebo). In a double blind study neither the patient nor the investigator knows which is the new drug.

## Ethics of Human Experimentation

It is imperative that the rights of the human subject be protected at all times during the clinical trial. Statements to this effect have been issued after the Nuremberg War Crimes trials (the Nuremberg Code), by the Judiciary Council of the American Medical Association, and by the World Medical Association (Helsinki Declaration). All these declarations have in essence the following conditions for human experimentation:

1. The subject must give voluntary, informed consent (free choice; no deceit or duress; legal capacity to make the choice as a subject; knowledge of all potential hazards, as well as the nature, purpose, and duration of the experiment).
2. All alternative modes of treatment must be explained to subject.
3. The subject is free to withdraw from the experiment at any time.
4. There must be a minimum number of volunteers.
5. The experiment should be of such a nature as to benefit society.
6. The experimental data must be unobtainable by any other means.
7. The experiment must be justified by animal studies.
8. All unnecessary physical and mental injury must be avoided.
9. No clinical experiment can be performed when there is any reason to believe that disabling injury or death may result.

THE PLACEBO. A placebo effect can be defined as any psychologic or physiologic effect attributable to a drug or physical procedure, but not to the pharmacodynamic properties of the drug or the procedure. The placebo effect may be due to the patient's confidence in

the practitioner or the treatment, expectation of relief from the drug or procedure, previous conditioning due to the purported fame and effectiveness of the drug or treatment, and previous experience with the drug or procedure. Most patients inherently desire to become well and benefit from the drug or treatment. The wise practitioner appreciates this fact and does nothing to destroy the placebo response. Since the placebo effect is very important in the treatment of pain and anxiety, a calm, controlled, empathetic attitude on the part of the dentist towards the patient and his or her problem, as well as the dentist's expressed confidence in the drug or therapeutic procedure, can greatly increase the success rate in the prevention and treatment of pain and anxiety.

BIOAVAILABILITY AND EQUIVALENCE. Bioavailability is the amount of the drug administered to the patient which is actually available in the tissues to interact with the drug receptor and produce a therapeutic response. Bioavailability is determined by many factors: the pharmaceutic preparation of the drug in a form which is adequately absorbed from the gastrointestinal tract or intramuscularly, the water and lipid solubility of the drug, its ability to transverse membranes, its rate of liver metabolism, and its rate of renal excretion. Combining a drug with other chemicals which render it insoluble in the intestine may retard or prevent its absorption. The strong binding of a drug to plasma proteins prevents its access to its receptor site. Very rapid liver metabolism or renal excretion greatly reduces the drug concentration in the blood and subsequent drug–receptor interaction.

Bioavailability is closely allied to equivalence. Chemically equivalent drugs meet certain chemical and physical standards established by agencies which regulate pharmaceuticals. Biologically equivalent drugs are capable of achieving the same concentrations of drug in the blood and tissues. Therapeutically equivalent drugs produce comparable efficacious effects in disease states. Therefore, for one drug to compare favorably with another in therapeutic effect, it must possess chemical, biological, and therapeutic equivalence; if two drugs are not equivalent, then they differ in their bioavailability, which may greatly affect their therapeutic efficacy.

QUESTIONS

98. Placebo drugs are incapable of producing therapeutic effects in patients because placebo drugs do not possess any demonstrable pharmacologic activity.
    1. Both statement and reason are correct and related.
    2. Both statement and reason are correct but not related.
    3. The statement is correct, but the reason is not.

(Continued)

4. The statement is not correct, but the reason is an accurate statement.
5. Neither statement nor reason is correct.

99. Which of the following statements is true regarding the Phase III clinical trial of a drug?
    1. It is performed only on primates such as monkeys.
    2. It is primarily intended to determine the $LD_{50}$ of a drug.
    3. It is intended to determine drug efficacy and toxicity on a large number of patients.
    4. It is primarily intended to determine the liver biotransformation rate of the drug.
    5. It is performed with only a few volunteer subjects.

# REFERENCES

1. STEPHENSON RP: A modification of receptor theory. Br J Pharmacol 11:379, 1956
2. ARIENS EJ, VAN ROSSUM JM, SIMONIS AM: Affinity, intrinsic activity and drug interactions. Pharmacol Rev 9:218, 1957
3. PATON WDM: A theory of drug action based on the rate of drug–receptor combination. Proc Roy Soc Biol 154:21, 1961
4. PATON WDM, WAUD DR: A quantitative investigation of the relationship between rate of access of a drug to receptor and the rate of onset or offset action. Arch Exp Path Pharmakol 248:124, 1964
5. TAUSSIG HB: A study of the German outbreak of phocomelia—The thalidomide syndrome. J Am Med Assoc 180:1106, 1962
6. CONNEY AH, COUTINHO C, KOECHLIN B, SWARM R, CHERIPHRO JA, IMPELLIZZERI C, BARUTH H: From animals to man: Metabolic consideration.Clin Pharmacol Therap 16:176, 1974
7. SINGER SJ, NICOLSON GL: The fluid mosaic model of the structure of cell membranes. Science 175:720, 1972
8. Drugs in Breast Milk. The Medical Letter of Drugs and Therapeutics. 16:25, 1974
9. KOCH–WESER J, GREENBLATT DJ: Drug interactions in clinical perspective. Europ J Clin Pharmacol 11:405, 1977
10. HARVEY SC: Hypnotics and sedatives: The barbiturates. In Goodman LS, Gilman A (eds.), The Pharmacological Basis of Therapeutics, 5th ed, New York, Macmillan, 1975
11. JORGENSEN NB: Local anesthesia and intravenous premedication. Anes Prog 13:168, 1966
12. WOODBURY DM, FINGL E: Drugs effective in the therapy of the epilepsies. In Goodman LS, Gilman A (eds). The Pharmacological Basis of Therapeutics, 5th ed. New York, Macmillan, 1975
13. GASTAUT H: Clinical and electroencephalographical classification of epileptic seizures. Epilepsia 11:102, 1970
14. PERT CB, SNYDER SH: Opiate receptor: Demonstration in nervous tissue. Science 179:1011, 1973
15. SNYDER SH, SIMANTOV R: The opiate receptor and opioid peptides. J. Neurochem. 28:13, 1977
16. MELZACK R, WALL PD: Pain mechanisms: A new theory. Science 150:971, 1965
17. MELZACK R: The Puzzle of Pain. New York, Basic Books, 1973
18. SIMON EJ, MILLER JM: The opiate receptors. Ann. Rev. Pharmacol. Toxicol. 18:371, 1978
19. HUGHES J, SMITH TW, KOSTERLITZ HW, FOTHERGILL LA, MORGAN BA, MORRIS HR: Identification of Two Related Pentapeptides from the brain with potent opiate agonist activity. Nature 258:577, 1975
20. MEHTA J, MEHTA P: Status of antiplatelet drugs in coronary heart disease. J Am Med Assoc 241:2649, 1979
21. HOLLISTER LE: Effective use of analgesic drugs. Ann Rev Med 27:431, 1976
22. COSTA E, GUIDOTTI A: Molecular mechanisms in the receptor action of benzodiazepines. Ann Rev Pharmacol Toxicol 19:531, 1979
23. GREENBLATT DJ, SHADER RI: Benzodiazepines. N Engl J Med 291:1011–1239, 1974
24. SUTTIE JW: Oral anticoagulant therapy: The Biosynthetic basis. Seminars Hematol 14:365, 1977
25. DEJONG RE: Neural blockade by local anesthetics. Life Sci 29:915, 1977
26. LINDORF HH, GANSSEN A, MAYER P: Thermographic repesentation of the vascular effects of local anesthetics. Electromedica 4:106, 1974
27. WEINSTEIN L: Chemotherapy of microbial disease: General considerations. In: Goodman LS, Gilman A (eds), The Pharmacological Basis of Therapeutics, 5th ed. New York, Macmillan, 1975
28. WATANABE T: Infectious drug resistance. Sci Am 217:19, 1967
29. American Heart Association: Prevention of Bacterial Endocarditis. Circulation 56:139A, 1977
30. Prevention of Bacterial Endocarditis: A Committee Report of the American Heart Association. J Am Dent Assoc 95:600, 1977
31. MANDELL GL: Cephaloridine. Ann Int Med 79:561, 1973
32. Colitis Associated with Clindamycin. The Medical Letter on Drugs and Therapeutics. 16:73, 1974
33. Topical Neomycin. The Medical Letter on Drugs and Therapeutics. 15:101, 1973.
34. O'MALLEY BW, SHADER WT: The receptors of steroid hormones. Sci Am 234:32, 1976
35. Fluoride Compounds. *Accepted Dental Therapeutics.* 37th Ed., American Dental Association, Chicago, 1977.
36. U. S. Department of Health, Education and Welfare, Public Health Service: Public Health Service Drinking Water Standards, 1962, PHS Pub. No. 956, Washington, D.C., 1962, U.S. Government Printing Office.
37. DRISCOLL WS, HOROWITZ HS: A discussion of optimal dosage for dietary fluoride supplementation. J Am Dent Assoc 96:1050, 1978
38. BERNSTEIN DS, SADOWSKY N, HEGSTEAD DM, GURI CD, STARE FJ: Prevalance of osteoporosis in high- and low-fluoride areas in North Dakota. J Am Dent Assoc 198:499, 1966
39. MALAMED SF: Diphenhydramine hydrochloride—Its use as a local anesthetic in dentistry. Anes prog 17:76, 1973
40. EDDY NG, HALBACK H, ISBELL H, SEEVERS MH: Drug dependence: Its significance and characteristics. Bull WHO 32:721, 1965
41. JAFFE JH: Drug Addiction and Drug Abuse. In: Goodman LS, Gilman A, (eds), The Pharmacological Basis of Therapeutics, 5th ed. New York, Macmillan, 1975
42. GREAVES G: Toward an existential theory of drug dependence. J Nerv Ment Dis 159:263, 1974
43. Fetal Alcohol Syndrome. FDA Drug Bulletin. Sept–Oct., 1977.
44. MALAMED SF: Handbook of Medical Emergencies in the Dental Office, St. Louis, CV Mosby, 1978
45. MCCARTHY FM: Emergencies in Dental Practice: Prevention and Treatment, 3rd ed. Philadelphia, WB Saunders, 1979

# SUGGESTED READING

PALLASCH TJ: Pharmacology for Dental Students and Practitioners. Philadelphia, Lea & Febiger, 1980

**MONTHLY PHARMACOLOGY UPDATES**

Dental Drug Service Newsletter. P.O. Box 1912, Glendale, California 91209

Facts and Comparisons, 111 West Port Plaza Drive, St. Louis, Missouri, 63141

## ANSWER KEY

| | | | | | | | |
|---|---|---|---|---|---|---|---|
| 1. 4 | 9. 1 | 17. 1 | 25. 5 | 33. 3 | 50. 5 | 67. 1 | 84. 1 |
| 2. 5 | 10. 4 | 18. 4 | 26. 2 | 34. 3 | 51. 1 | 68. 3 | 85. 3 |
| 3. 5 | 11. 4 | 19. 5 | 27. 5 | 35. 2 | 52. 4 | 69. 4 | 86. 4 |
| 4. 2 | 12. 3 | 20. 5 | 28. 4 | 36. 1 | 53. 3 | 70. 4 | 87. 4 |
| 5. 5 | 13. 3 | 21. 4 | 29. 3 | 37. 1 | 54. 3 | 71. 4 | 88. 1 |
| 6. 5 | 14. 3 | 22. 5 | 30. 4 | 38. 4 | 55. 4 | 72. 3 | 89. 3 |
| 7. 4 | 15. 3 | 23. 3 | 31. 1 | 39. 2 | 56. 1 | 73. 5 | 90. 3 |
| 8. 5 | 16. 1 | 24. 4 | 32. 3 | 40. 1 | 57. 1 | 74. 4 | 91. 5 |
| | | | | 41. 5 | 58. 5 | 75. 1 | 92. 1 |
| | | | | 42. 1 | 59. 4 | 76. 1 | 93. 5 |
| | | | | 43. 3 | 60. 3 | 77. 4 | 94. 1 |
| | | | | 44. 4 | 61. 2 | 78. 1 | 95. 1 |
| | | | | 45. 2 | 62. 1 | 79. 2 | 96. 4 |
| | | | | 46. 1 | 63. 5 | 80. 4 | 97. 5 |
| | | | | 47. 1 | 64. 3 | 81. 4 | 98. 4 |
| | | | | 48. 4 | 65. 4 | 82. 3 | 99. 3 |
| | | | | 49. 2 | 66. 3 | 83. 4 | |

# 16

# DENTAL BEHAVIORAL SCIENCES

## Joseph K. Wittemann / James E. Hardigan

Although specific questions on the behavioral sciences may not appear on the National Board Examinations, the principles of these disciplines, particularly those of psychology and sociology, are taught in the clinical/dental sciences. Topics related to these disciplines can be found in the literature and teaching of pedodontics, prosthodontics, oral surgery, occlusion, and general operative/restorative dentistry. The behavioral sciences are applied to the clinical sciences via discussions on patient fears and the related management of those fears, pain and pain control, child–parent–doctor interaction, and temporomandibular joint (TMJ) management. These topics are presented through behavioral principles related to motivation, perception, communication, and emotions. The management of patients is approached through learning theory, classical/operant conditioning, desensitization, modeling, and hypnosis.

## DENTAL FEAR AND ANXIETY

Fear and anxiety are emotions which are widespread and influential in the behaviors of all children and adults; both conditions are motivating forces in human behavior.

Fear typically refers to the anticipation of threat elicited by an external object that is perceived to be harmful (3). A fear is a very real thing which moves a person to action. The fear of being run over by an automobile keeps people from running indiscriminately into traffic. The fear of fire (or being burned) keeps people from reaching into a fire. The fear of being hurt keeps people away from the dentist's office. In each of the preceding, the object or the event which is potentially harmful can be easily identified—speeding cars, flames, dental needles, and drills. It must be emphasized that a fear is related to a threatening object or event in reality.

There are times when a patient uses the expression, "I am afraid of . . ." or "I fear . . ." without being able to identify clearly the source of the fear. In that case, the patient's aversive behavior would be more appropriately described as highly anxious. Anxiety is a fearful and apprehensive emotional state, usually in response to unreal or imagined dangers, that interferes with favorable and effective solutions to real problems. It is a coping mechanism accompanied by somatic symptoms which result in a continuous, physically exhausting state of tension and alertness. Grave apprehensions, insecurity, and gloominess are the behavior symptoms; gastrointestinal disturbances, insomnia, and fatigue are the physical symptoms.

A highly anxious person usually responds to an anxiety-producing situation by avoiding it or, once in it, attempting to flee it, but the dental patient does not act on the emotion because of social and situational constraints. Thereby the patient becomes more anxious. The dentist can usually diagnose anxiety by feeling the palm of the patient's hand. An anxious person perspires profusely; a fearful person's palms are dry. In addition to these changes, the inspiration–expiration ratio falls during anger and fear and rises during pleasant states. Pupils tend to dilate in moments of anger and pain.

### Acquisition of Fear and Anxiety

The fear response can be conditioned in two ways: through actual experience or through verbalization. A child or adult who experiences intense pain, annoyance, or any other unpleasant feeling—sharp pain, sudden or loud noise, rapid punishment—will experience it again each time the original stimulus occurs. A child develops a fear of fire by sticking a finger into a flame; a fear of dogs by being jumped on or knocked down by one, a fear of closed places by being locked in a closet, and a fear of dentists by being hurt.

Expressive language accompanied by some physical (nonverbal) act can be a powerful adjunct of fear and anxiety development. A significant person in the child's life—parent, sibling, teacher, or peer—can relate personal experiences in such a way that the aversive reaction is fostered and nurtured in the listener. A mother may shout, while leaping toward the child, "Don't touch that . . ." or "Drop that, it's dirty."

When anxieties and fears become exaggerated and their causes cannot be recalled, the individual enters into a phobic state. A phobia is a morbid fear or dread. While a fear is a result of a natural experience, a phobia is a prolonged and exaggerated dread of the experience. A child may be fearful of a bear encountered in the woods. As an adult, he or she may be able to recall the reason for this fear and laugh at it. If, however, this person avoids all zoos, furry animals, and woods without knowing why, then it could be said that he or she has developed a phobia. Phobias do occur in the dental setting, the most common being the dread of pain. This phobia is called algophobia. In addition, phobias related to entrapment (claustrophobia), suffering (pathophobia), sight of blood (hematophobia), and even needles have been identified in the dental situation.

### Stress, The Common Denominator

Aversive behavior or intensive expression of aversive feelings are indicators of stress. Situational stress generates multiple reactions: reactions of the nervous system (stress) and overt expressions that attempt to relieve inward emotions (psychologic stress). The most classic description of the "stress syndrome" was developed by Selye (8, 9). Stress, according to Selye, is "the nonspecific response of the body to any demand made upon it." The patients he saw as a student and the animals in his early experiments were suffering from stress (according to this definition) or responding to demands made by infectious or toxic substances. All living beings, Selye explains, are constantly under stress, and anything (pleasant or unpleasant, physical or emotional) that speeds up the intensity of life causes a temporary increase in stress. A painful blow and a passionate kiss, for instance, can be equally stressful. Indeed, he says, complete freedom from stress is death.

Stress itself can lead to disease and death. Selye, through what he calls the "general adaptation syndrome" (GAS), has explained how stress might be related to disease. The syndrome has three stages: an alarm reaction, resistance, and exhaustion. During the first stage, the body recognizes the stressor and the pituitary–adrenal–cortical system responds by producing the arousal hormones necessary for either flight or fight. Increased heart and lung operation, elevated blood sugar levels, increased perspiration, dilated pupils, and slowed digestion are among the physiologic responses to this initial GAS stage.

During the resistance (or adaptive) stage, the body begins to repair the damage caused by arousal, and most of the initial stress symptoms diminish or vanish.

But if stress continues, the acquired adaptation is lost because the body eventually runs out of energy with which to maintain its defenses and exhaustion sets in. During this final stage, body functions are slowed down abnormally or stopped altogether.

Continued exposure to stress during the exhaustion stage can lead to what Selye calls the "diseases of adaptation." Various emotional disturbances, such as schizophrenia, migraine headaches, certain types of asthma, as well as cardiovascular and renal disease, are among the conditions that have been linked to stress. Apparently, says Selye, conditioning (particularly hereditary predisposition, diet, and environmental factors) determines which organ or system is weakest and breaks down most readily under the influence of stress.

Levine (5) discusses Selye's work in regard to the endocrine system, specifically the pituitary and adrenal glands. He describes the response as follows:

The essentials of the system's operation in response to stress are as follows. Information concerning the stress (coming either from external sources through the sensory system or from internal sources such as a change in body temperature or in the blood's composition) is received and integrated by the central nervous system and is presumably delivered to the hypothalamus, the basal area of the brain. The hypothalamus secretes a substance called the corticotropin-releasing factor (CRF), which stimulates the pituitary to secrete the hormone ACTH [adrenocorticotropic hormone]. This in turn stimulates the cortex of the adrenal gland to step up its synthesis and secretion of hormones, particularly those known as glucocorticoids. In man the glucocorticoid is predominantly hydrocortisone; in many lower animals such as the rat it is corticosterone.

The entire mechanism is exquisitely controlled by a feedback system. When the glucocorticoid level in the circulating blood is elevated, the central nervous system, receiving the message, shuts off the process that leads to secretion of the stimulating hormone ACTH. Two experimental demonstrations have most clearly verified the existence of this feedback process. If the adrenal gland is removed from an animal, the pituitary puts out abnormal amounts of ACTH, presumably because the absence of the adrenal hormone frees it from restriction of this secretion. On the other hand, if crystals of glucocorticoid are implanted in the hypothalamus, the animal's secretion of ACTH stops almost completely, just as if the adrenal cortex were releasing large quantities of the glucocorticoid.

Now, it is well known that a high level of either of these hormones (ACTH or glucocorticoid) in the circulating blood can have dramatic effects on the brain. Patients who have received glucocorticoids for treatment of an illness have on occasion suffered severe mental changes, sometimes leading to psychosis. Also, patients with a diseased condition of the adrenal gland that caused it to secrete an abnormal amount of cortical hormone have also shown effects on the brain, including changes in the pattern of electrical activity and convulsions.

In addition to the affective and physiologic changes which result from stress, Dworkin (3) and his colleagues indicate that motor behaviors also indicate stress conditions. Increased muscle tension (rigidity), disturbance of speech, accentuated facial expressions, directionality of behavior (to or away from), and intensity of behavior are typically evident in an individual under stress. Furthermore, thinking, listening, memory recall, problem solving, and perceptual acuity are likewise affected by stress.

It must be noted that although the terms stress and psychologic stress are related, they are not synonymous. Psychologic stress includes the intervening variable of threat, and the identification of that threat provides the single most important clue to managing the anxious patient successfully.

## The Management of Stress

STRESS IN THE CHILD.   While there are many suggested approaches to reducing any stress connected with the dental experience, the most pervasive is that of preventive therapy during childhood. Simply stated, preventive management involves carefully introducing the child to the dental situation without negative, abrasive, or emotionally charged language. Smeltzer (10), in his text *Psychology for Student Nurses*, makes several suggestions for the health care deliverer:

1. Take extra precautions to avoid causing pain.
2. Never surprise a child by saying it will not hurt when you know very well that it will. When you are going to do something that will cause pain, tell the child beforehand.
3. Tolerate a reasonable amount of resistance, encourage and persuade to some extent, but never give the impression that you will back away. Your tone of voice and your gestures will be the cues for the child. After you have exhausted your repertoire of preliminary persuaders, go ahead and do what you intended in the first place.
4. Do not use promises and bribes to get a child to do what you want. Bright children will develop into regular horse traders, and you eventually will have to give more than the annoyance is worth.
5. Never hesitate to commend good behavior. If you had quite a problem of noncooperation, reduce the intensity of your commendations accordingly. However, do not shame the child afterwards. It is better to play an aloof or indifferent role instead.

Currier (2) suggests a series of behaviors which should be adopted and followed by the dentist and his or her entire staff at all dental visits for children and adolescents.

**Do**

Use a positive, firm, consistent approach.
Have a smooth, confident, relaxed manner.
Be truthful; do not lie.
Educate both the child and the parents; parents must become active in management.
Work from a comprehensive treatment plan, and have everything ready before the child arrives.
Make the first visit as pleasant as possible so that subsequent appointments are not spent counterconditioning disrup' ive behaviors.
Be time-oriented with the child, since a child has a short attention span and becomes restless within an hour if required to sit for that length of time.
Get an adequate history. Listen.
Direct your attention to the whole patient.
Introduce yourself to the child and offer your hand to the younger child, but do not insist on shaking hands.
Allow the child to get into the dental chair unassisted and adjust the chair for comfort.
Pin the napkin directly to the shirt or dress from around the front of the patient, not the neck side; do not let the napkin flow free.
Explain the sights and sounds of the dental equipment.
Tell, show, and do.
Keep the instruments, including the syringe and larger bur blocks, out of sight.
Use short, to the point statements with understandable words.
Assume the child who says it hurts is telling the truth; a child usually is not trying to be difficult. Give the child the benefit of the doubt the first time and reanesthetize.
Give the child a preview of what will occur at the next appointment.

**Don't**

Talk down to the child or adolescent.
Greet the patient in a loud voice.
Use baby talk
Shake the child's hand forcefully.
Ignore the child or adolescent.
Adjust the chair without first advising the child.
Ridicule the child.
Be oversympathetic.
Use fear-provoking words.
Use undesirable mannerisms or facial expressions.
Deceive the child.
Permit extraneous noises or interferences by the office staff or others in the office area.
Use words such as bite, drill, needle, pull, sharp, shot, stick.
Think that these rules apply to children and adolescents only; adults need the same thoughtful approach.

While these practices do not eliminate all apprehensions, they help the child develop the ability to cope with the dental situation as an adult.

STRESS IN THE ADULT. For the adult who has learned or otherwise acquired aversive reactions to the dental situation the problem of management is more complex. In part the complexity is due to conflict.

*Conflict.* By definition conflict is a struggle or controversy; disagreement of one idea, emotion, action, etc., with another. Mental conflict results when mutually exclusive or imposing impulses, drives, wishes, etc., operate at the same time. Research indicates that a person encountering two equally attractive but contradictory and mutually exclusive alternatives shows extreme agitation and disruption of normal functioning. Although there are various ways to escape from the conflict, the precise way in which the individual tries to cope with the conflict is determined in part by the type of conflict involved.

There are three distinct kinds of conflict situations: 1) the approach–approach conflict, in which two equally desirable but mutually exclusive alternatives are presented; 2) the avoidance–avoidance conflict, in which two equally aversive alternatives are presented in such a way that one but not both can be avoided; and 3) the *approach–avoidance* conflict, in which a positive alternative is inseparably paired with an equally aversive one. The dental experience is by and large an approach–avoidance conflict. The patient knows that dental treatment is necessary, but the treatment may involve some discomfort—real or imagined. The patient is in conflict.

The aversiveness or the attractiveness of one alternative over another changes with the temporal or spatial distance of the alternative from the individual. Conflict related to the dental situation, remains intense unless there is dramatic change in either the patient or the dentist. For example, if the pain of the tooth becomes great(er), it may override the anxiety or fear and move the individual to action. On the other hand, if the dentist announces (or the patient hears from a trusted friend) that he or she has developed "pain-free drilling," the patient's perception of the dentist can change; this favorable perception overrides the avoidance.

Some patients continue to have conflicting feelings toward dental care and repeatedly move between approach and avoidance. The professional must learn to recognize these feelings and be able to deal with them.

*Potential Approaches for Adults.* It is not the intent of dental schools to train psychotherapists, but the dentist as a professional has a personal, human quality which mediates his or her skills and permits him or her to render care. This quality is at times overshadowed by demands on the dentist's time, service, and skill, however. Because of these sometimes conflicting demands, the dentist may increase the anxiety of a highly anxious or fearful patient by being nonattentive, rushed, curt, demanding, or otherwise noncaring.

The management of the stressed adult depends upon 1) the dentist and his or her interpersonal skills, 2) the receptivity of the patient, and 3) the environmental factors surrounding both. Dworkin (3) suggests a series of factors a dentist can use in the stress response to an emergency dental situation:

1. How the dentist acts and talks may at least in part be determined by the type of situation, that is, whether it is highly perilous or devoid of any danger.
2. Only the dentist who understands and accepts atypical behaviors precipitated by the emergency can be of help to the stressed patient. Atypical behaviors at times of stress include irrational attitudes, disordered emotions, and negative or hostile responses.
3. The intensity of the patient's anxiety over the dental emergency is likely to be exaggerated in relation to the objective seriousness of the clinical emergency.
4. Body damage or its perceived threat often brings a fear of abandonment, feelings of helplessness, and the need for reassurance, affection, and protection.
5. Stress induces cognitive blocks and perceptual confusions, yielding misconceptions about the nature and implications of the emergency. These cognitive blocks and misperceptions are generally the result of denial, repression, and suppression. They may render the patient resistant to rational explanation and prone to forget postoperative instructions.
6. The typical dental crisis is self-limiting in time. Usually it is over quickly, for both dentist and patient.

It is essential that the dentist attend primarily to the person's chief complaint and the behaviors which accompany the description in an active manner. In the psychologic/human relations literature, this is called counseling.

### Counseling: The Primary Management Tool

An examination of the numerous definitions of counseling reveals certain recurring characteristics:

Counseling normally involves two willing participants who meet to consider a problem, question, or situation posed by one of the individuals.

Counseling is a face-to-face situation.

Counseling takes place in privacy.

Counseling demands a friendly, free atmosphere.

Counseling requires that the counselor have special skills and abilities acquired through prescribed professional training.

Counseling occurs as the result of either self-referral or referral by another individual.

To clarify the nature of counseling a bit further, it is helpful to consider what counseling is not:

Counseling is not advice-giving.
Counseling is not census-taking.
Counseling is not controlling.
Counseling is not simply an aimless exchange of pleasantries.

These statements indicate that practitioners who have not had specific training for counseling should not conduct counseling interviews, although this is not to say that practitioners cannot or should not confer with patients. They can and should. But, it must be recognized that such meetings are conferences, not counseling interviews.

Many of the conditions of counseling apply to conferences in the dentist–patient relationship. It is typically a face-to-face encounter which occurs in the privacy of the dentist's office, consultation room, or treatment room. The patient usually presents the problem to the practitioner, who is skilled in managing the clinical case. At this point, the practitioner should employ the techniques of counseling. Unfortunately, the process often breaks down in the dialogue stage. Rather than permitting the patient to give information, the dentist assumes control and gives advice. The act of obtaining information is hampered by excessive probing. The process of counseling is doomed to failure by these noncounseling activities.

The initial interview is typically the most difficult. It is during this time that the practitioner must establish a relationship with the patient and set the stage for its growth. By actions, words, gestures, and facial expressions the practitioner must communicate a feeling of acceptance, understanding, and sincerity to the patient. All the knowledge in the world is of no use if one of these qualities is absent.

ACCEPTANCE.   The dentist must keep in mind the patient's perception of the situation. It is imperative that the patient feel accepted by the dentist. Only in an air of acceptance can good rapport develop. Both verbal and nonverbal messages can transmit acceptance. Eye contact, facial expressions, hand and arm gestures, body position, and voice and questioning behaviors are some of the techniques which the practitioner can use to communicate acceptance.

A patient who senses, through verbal or nonverbal clues, that his or her honesty, sincerity, or good judgment is doubted will feel rejected. Rejection can also be inferred by the incorrect use of assurance. For example, the response, "It's okay if you eat candy, just brush your teeth when you can," to an overweight teenager exposes the dentist's insensitivity to the patient's needs. The patient will also feel rejected if the dentist insists on following his or her own line of thought rather than attending to what is on the patient's mind. Such behavior on the part of the dentist typically results from a lack of active listening and perception.

UNDERSTANDING.   In order to be helpful to a patient a practitioner must respond to what a patient is saying. Yet practitioners occasionally fail to realize the importance of the patient's information. Should a practitioner misread or completely ignore some information, the responses may be erroneous. Unfortunately the practitioner may continue to speak, lecture, or cajole and the patient may respond by becoming angry, apathetic, or noncompliant. The patient may ultimately respond by leaving the dentist's care.

Much of the patient's comfort is based on the dentist's verbal responses to information volunteered. Phrases such as "I see," "I understand," and "Could you explain?" are indicative of active listening. These expressions also provide an opportunity to obtain additional information: "I see, could you tell me more?", "How do you feel about_____?", and "You appear to feel strongly about _____." Such verbal expressions are only useful if accompanied by sincere expressions of intent, however. Therefore facial expressions and body gestures must coincide with verbal expression.

SINCERITY.   Sincerity in dealing with patients is imperative. The practitioner cannot do or say one thing and then do or say the opposite. Rogers (7) uses the word incongruence to describe this behavior. In addition, a practitioner who is interested in a patient's case does not permit him- or herself to be interrupted by telephone calls, auxiliaries, and so forth. Likewise, the patient's privacy is not being respected if an interview is conducted in the presence of others. Nevertheless group counseling, particularly for young patients with similar dentally related stress problems, may be an effective format for counseling, since it may promote congruence in the peer group and make better patients (11).

## Adjuncts to Adult Patient Management

There are several alternative psychologic management systems or processes available to a dentist who cares.

DENTIST AVAILABILITY.   A dentist or one of the staff may be called upon to help a patient over an immediate anxiety response. This is a common occurrence when dental surgery is necessary, for example. It should be made clear to the patient that the dentist understands he or she may be frightened, anxious, and in need of some reassurance and that the dentist will be available if needed. An able, skilled person with a willingness to listen and a prior knowledge of the patient should handle such a situation.

Few dentists use a formal crisis interview. Yet it is one of the most pervasive processes available to health professionals. It is often used as a postoperative procedure, but it could reduce fear, anxiety, and stress if its use were also extended to routine care.

**TOKEN REWARDS.** One major technique of behavior therapy which has been used with hospital patients is to substitute tokens for specific rewards such as food. A token stands for a reinforcer; it could be practically anything—a poker chip, a check mark, a green stamp. The most obvious token in real life is money. Tokens are easy to supply, and patients do not become satiated with them, as they do with food.

A token economy program was set up by Krasner and Ullmann (4) in a Veterans' Administration hospital in California. Most of the patients in the hospital had been diagnosed as chronic schizophrenics or as victims of organic brain damage. As a group they were apathetic, indifferent, dependent, and socially isolated. When these patients performed socially desirable behaviors such as attending an occupational therapy session Ullmann and Krasner reinforced their behavior with tokens that they could cash in for rewards, like candy, or for privileges, like time out of the ward. Before this token economy program, most of the patients had refused to participate in any of the hospital activities available to them. In fact their behavior represented the endpoint of years of compliance and apathy shaped by life in an institution. Token reinforcement sharply reduced the patients' apathy and made them more responsive, active, and productive. Staff morale also improved enormously because the staff felt that they were actually affecting the patients' lives.

While not directly related to the dental situation, the token reward system can influence the behavior of the dental patient. A token which can be used in the scheduling of appointments, discounts on services rendered, or even free prophylaxis can benefit the patient anticipating a dental visit. In effect, a token system serves to alter the environmental factors of the visit and thereby diminishes its aversive nature.

**SYSTEMATIC DESENSITIZATION.** The first step in systematic desensitization is to construct an anxiety hierarchy. The patient makes a list of experiences that make him or her anxious and arranges them in descending order of intensity. For example, a man who cannot stand the sight of blood might go to a behavior therapist for systematic desensitization because his fear reaction is so strong that he faints whenever he sees

anyone bleeding. At the bottom of his list he perhaps puts listening to a lecture on first-aid techniques; somewhere near the middle, watching a black and white newsreel of a medic dressing a soldier's wounds; and at the top, suddenly finding himself kneeling over a child with an open stomach wound.

After the list is complete, the therapist teaches the patient to relax, and while relaxing, to imagine the least disturbing scene or experience. The therapist makes the person repeat the imagined experience of this scene until it fails to generate anxiety. The same procedure is followed step by step up the list with the other anxiety-arousing events. The person is finally able to imagine the situations that are most threatening. At that point the therapist actually exposes the patient to one of the threatening situations in real life. For example, a therapist might take the man who faints at the sight of blood to a hospital operating room.

Systematic desensitization can be employed by dentists in the dental setting. It must begin with the "discovery" of what in this setting causes the fear, anxiety, or phobia. This can be partially identified during the initial interview. Once identified, a hierarchy of anxieties can be set, and a list of successive experiences can be established. The key to the effectiveness of this approach lies in the professional's ability to diagnose the aversive stimuli correctly and his or her willingness to spend the necessary time with the patient. Systematic desensitization has worked very effectively in the cure of many phobias or irrational fears, and the average cure usually takes only about six sessions.

**MODELING.** The idea behind modeling is quite simple. People tend to imitate other people—especially people they respect. At Stanford University Bandura (1) initiated a program using the principles of modeling to cure fear of snakes. He contacted people whose fear of snakes interfered seriously with their everyday lives. Some were anticipating Peace Corps assignments in foreign countries; others were afraid to go hunting, hiking, or camping; and others were in occupations that brought them in contact with snakes. Bandura and his colleagues put people who were afraid of snakes into one of four groups. The first group underwent systematic desensitization. The second watched films of children and adults playing with snakes. The third group watched a therapist through a one-way mirror as he played with a snake; these subjects then entered the room and slowly but surely approached the snake, touched it, and finally held it. The fourth group was a control group, which received no treatment. Each of the three experimental groups received ten treatment sessions.

The results of the experiment were unequivocal: people in the group who watched the model through the mirror and learned to touch the snake improved more than people in the group who watched the film or the group who engaged in the desensitization procedure but never actually observed a live model handling a snake. All of the people who had observed a live model were able to sit in a chair with their hands at their side and allow a snake to crawl on them for 30 sec.

After the experiment was over, the experimenters had all the people who had not done so earlier observe a live model and engage in guided participation with snakes. They succeeded in generating cures in 100% of the subjects.

Modeling has proven to be effective when working with young children in the dental office. Children who were able to observe the positive behaviors of other children, either via film or in person, acted more sure, controlled, and generally more relaxed. The same effect should occur in adults given positive stimuli prior to the dental treatment. This can be accomplished on film (vicariously) or in person. The former tends to be the preferred way, because it is more comfortable for the model patient.

AUTONOMIC CONDITIONING. Recently learning experiments have found that heart rate, sweating, blood pressure, and other responses controlled by the autonomic nervous system can be conditioned in much the same way as other behavioral responses. For example, if rewarded every time his or her heart rate spontaneously decreases, a patient will learn to make it go down. The techniques of autonomic conditioning—or operant conditioning of autonomic behavior—hold promise for curing psychosomatic disorders such as a chronically high heart rate, high blood pressure, gastrointestinal disorders, and other conditions caused by too little or too much activity in the autonomic nervous system.

Although autonomic conditioning has the potential to revolutionize psychosomatic medicine, the procedures do not always work effectively. For the human being rewarding reinforcers which can be administered quickly enough to reinforce only the desired responses are difficult to find. In addition, the reinforcer itself must not cause troublesome unconditioned responses. For example, a reinforcer that raises heart rate should not be used in attempts to achieve a lower heart rate.

The nontechnical application of the autonomic conditioning process is transcendental meditation (TM) or relaxation therapy, which can help to relieve stress in the situation. It follows logically that a person who can learn to relax in a natural setting should be able to employ these techniques to reduce stress. The dentist can serve as the guide in this process for the anxious patient by, for example, recounting a tranquil scene, having the patient concentrate on breathing or focus on a pleasant memory, etc. Through modulation of the voice, the dentist can induce relaxation.

GROUP INTERVENTION. A dentist who has a number of highly anxious patients may meet with them as a group to discuss their perceptions, fears, and stresses. It demands a willingness to give patients a different kind of time than a dentist customarily does, but its success has been demonstrated by Marbach and Dworkin (6). Given the appropriate skills, a dentist could help the participants to feel better about their dental visits in relatively few meetings. Clarity of intent and surety of skill are required for this modality, however.

### Recommended Modality

The most powerful strategy for anxiety, fear, and stress control and management is the dentist. Through attentiveness to the patient's "psychologic crisis," the dentist has the opportunity to motivate the patient positively. To do so demands an ability to listen with the eyes as well as the ears, to ask questions in a way which elicits understanding, and to speak positively, as well as a staff which mirrors these actions.

Webman (12) suggests five activities which the dentist should use in managing the patient. Although anxiety begins before the patient walks through the office door, the dentist can influence that anxiety by procedures undertaken in the office.

First, each patient should be attended to as an individual. Each patient has a unique dental history, and a great deal can be learned by asking about prior experiences with dentistry and dental pain during an initial conference. Patients who describe themselves as nonreactive should still be handled with care, and those who describe themselves as reactive should be made to feel during treatment that their message has been received.

Second, patients should be given an accurate description of what will be experienced during a procedure. Charged words such as pain, sharp, or hurt should be avoided, but in instances where pain is unavoidable accurate descriptions should be used. The brevity of the experience and the dentist's concern should be stressed.

Third, patients should be given a feeling of some control. A prearranged signal by which patients can "turn off the procedure" can be established. Perceived control is what is important, and even if a patient uses the panic button frequently at first, this behavior will likely taper off when a patient feels assured of some influence.

Fourth, the environment should be relaxed. Patients will be paying attention to the dentist's actions. Soothing music is useless if patients are paying no attention. Patients are more likely to be aware of the people present, so the behavior of the professional staff should be low key and soothing.

Finally, the dentist must pay attention to the patient.

Patients and dentists communicate both verbally or nonverbally, and dentists must be receptive to the messages of patients, especially new patients. The dentist should try to hear what is behind ostensibly simple statements or questions, and where possible, try to avoid pain games by attending to the needs that underlie them.

### QUESTIONS

1. The primary difference between fear and anxiety is that
   1. fear makes the hands perspire
   2. anxieties are real
   3. fears are related to real events
   4. anxiety is less severe than fear

2. Fears can be
   1. learned
   2. acquired
   3. conditioned
   4. All of the above

3. A child's negative response to a dental drill is a
   1. phobia
   2. fear
   3. anxiety
   4. Any of the above

4. The common denominator to fear and anxiety is (are)
   1. stress
   2. avoidance
   3. frustration
   4. anger

5. Selye described a syndrome which has three stages; the syndrome is called the
   1. Selye syndrome
   2. specific alienation syndrome
   3. general adaptation syndrome
   4. antistress syndrome

6. The correct order of the stages of the syndrome described by Selye is
   1. resistance, alarm, exhaustion
   2. exhaustion, resistance, alarm
   3. alarm, resistance, exhaustion
   4. alarm, exhaustion, resistance

7. The system within the endocrine system which is involved in the general adaptation syndrome is
   1. gastrointestinal
   2. adrenal–cortical (pituitary)
   3. cardiovascular
   4. lymphatic

8. The ultimate consequence of continued resistance in the GAS syndrome is
   1. chaos
   2. stress
   3. death
   4. alarm

9. In the stress situation the hypothalamus secretes a substance called

1. hydrocortisone
2. corticotesterone
3. corticotropin-releasing factor
4. adrenocorticotropin hormone

10. Stress and psychologic stress are
    1. synonomous
    2. identical
    3. related but not synonomous
    4. not related

11. The most pervasive approach to managing dental stress is
    1. preventive therapy
    2. psychomedication
    3. premedication
    4. hypnosis and feedback

12. The development of a positive dental attitude should begin
    1. on the child's first visit
    2. with the parents' feelings
    3. after the first visit by the child
    4. through education programs in public schools

13. The form of conflict which most adults experience in the dental situation is
    1. approach–approach
    2. approach–avoidance
    3. avoidance–avoidance
    4. double approach–avoidance

14. Conflicts can be resolved by
    1. changes in the person
    2. changes in the situation
    3. 1 and 2
    4. taking flight

15. The primary tool in patient management is the
    1. counseling interview
    2. dentist's rapport with the patient
    3. staff's attitude toward the patient
    4. All of the above

16. Teaching the person to relax and, while relaxed, to experience a series of increasingly threatening events is called
    1. modeling
    2. reinforcing
    3. desensitizing
    4. dreaming

17. In modeling, the patient
    1. learns to deal with increasingly threatening tasks
    2. learns to identify positively with other persons
    3. shows the dentist how brave he or she is
    4. identifies with the dentist

## STRESS RELATED OROFACIAL PAIN

In 1934 Costen (14) first described a complex syndrome of ear, sinus, and face pain; the syndrome included impaired hearing and tinnitus. Referred to as the "Costen syndrome," it was attributed to disturbed function of the temporomandibular joints and face. The term temporomandibular joint pain dysfunction was introduced in 1955. Schwartz presented data on 2500 patients showing the dysfunction was a syndrome of the muscles of mastication and not of the temporomandibular joints. Although Schwartz (24) found no single cause for the syndrome, he stated that "reacting to stress seems to be more important than any malocclusion the patient has." This work focused on the interaction of emotive states and somatic symptoms.

Laskin (18), building on prior research, introduced the term myofacial pain dysfunction syndrome. His work emphasized the role of the muscle in this syndrome. In order to understand this dysfunction, it is helpful to review Laskin's 1969 work.

## Diagnosis: The Four Symptoms

The most common finding in the pain dysfunction syndrome is pain of nonspecific origin. It is described as a dull ache felt in the ear or the preauricular area which may radiate to the mandible, the temporal area, or the lateral cervical region. The pain is reported as either more severe in the morning upon arising or as mild in the morning and increasing in intensity during the day. Accompanying pain is muscle tenderness which is readily determined upon examination. Tenderness extends "over the neck of the mandible and in the region distal and superior to the maxillary tuberosity" (15). In order to be diagnosed as the pain dysfunction syndrome (according to Laskin), the condition must involve pain or tenderness, or both. In addition, there occurs a clicking or popping noise in the temporomandibular joint. Limitation of jaw function is the fourth symptom.

Two negative characteristics must also be present: 1) absence of clinical, radiographic, or biochemical evidence of organic changes in the temporomandibular joint; and 2) lack of tenderness in the temporomandibular joint when palpated via the external meatus. These two negative conditions serve to distinguish the pain dysfunction syndrome from problems related to organic joint problems.

## The Psychophysiologic Theory of Causation

Tooth theories dominated the literature on the etiology of the temporomandibular joint syndrome. The proposition was that

when teeth are brought together during chewing or swallowing the discrepancies in occlusion produce a displacement of the mandible, usually in a posterior direction, with resultant compression of the highly vascular, densely innervated, loose retrocondylar connective tissue (18).

Continued compression of tissue would certainly cause pain (specificity theory) and ultimately degeneration of the tissues. Researchers found these theories to be inadequate, however.

The tooth theories were replaced by tooth–muscle theories which were less mechanically oriented but were still based on the belief that "incoordination spasms of some of the muscles of mastication" were organically caused by occlusal discrepancy and interference (18). In 1955 Schwartz reported that functional disturbances in the masticatory musculature could play a role in the etiology of temporomandibular joint dysfunction (24).

Laskin and his colleagues at the Temporomandibular Joint Research Center at the University of Illinois during the 1960s proposed a new concept of etiology—the psychophysiologic theory.

THE THEORY. The theory purports that the masticatory muscle spasm is the primary factor responsible for the signs and symptoms of the pain dysfunction syndrome. Extending both the pain dysfunction syndrome and temporomandibular joint dysfunction, it terms the condition myofacial pain dysfunction syndrome because pathologic involvement of the joint occurs, but in the latter states (Fig. 16–1).

The theory is psychophysiologic. While dental irritations such as overextension of masticatory muscles and loss of lateral teeth do occur, the most common cause of pain is seen to be muscle fatigue or muscle tension produced by chronic oral habits such as grinding or clinching. Certainly these habits can be caused by disturbances in function of teeth, but Laskin and his group believe these irritations to be involuntary tension-relieving behaviors rather than mechanical interferences—hence the term psychophysiologic.

If the theory is correct, then the syndrome self-perpetuates; that is, tension increases and adds to dental irritations which result in muscle fatigue which result in spasms. Ultimately the syndrome evolves into alterations in occlusion and mastication, and it can result in organic damage. The prime cause is tension.

THE TENSION COMPONENT. In early psychologic studies Lupton (19, 20) reported that about 75% of the patients in the Temporomandibular Joint Research Center displayed dominant personality characteristics described as "hypernormal." Hypernormal is defined as responsible, generous, managerial. In distinguishing this group from several other groups, Lupton assumes that these individuals work exceedingly hard to maintain their perception of normality.

When patients who suffer from the myofacial pain dysfunction syndrome were treated, it was found that the symptom could be alleviated or markedly reduced

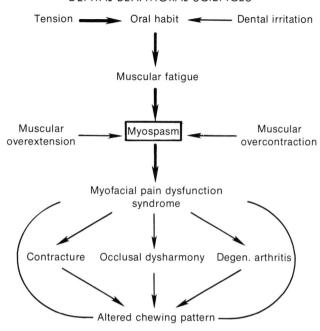

**FIG. 16-1.** Pain dysfunction syndrome. (Laskin DM: J Am Dent Assoc 79:147–153, 1969)

through psychologic counseling. Marbach and Dworkin (21), in their study of chronic myofacial pain dysfunction, found that patients consistently demonstrated a psychodynamic constellation comprised of depression, isolation, denial, and passive aggressive conflict. Their findings complement the early work of Moulton (22) in which he described most of his patients as having "life long problems requiring strict self-control to avoid conflict with people on whom they were dependent."

By repeated testing, i.e., using standardized psychologic tests, a profile of the myofacial pain dysfunction patient evolves:

1. The patient (20) typically has other psychologic related ailments—migraine headaches, ulcers, or dermatitis—which are psychoneurotic in etiology.
2. The patient typically demonstrates chronic oral habits—a habit being a behavior which is acquired and becomes fixed over a period of time.
3. The patient exhibits a wide range of behaviors associated with anxiety. The behaviors may be overt aggression, directed at others, or covert aggression, directed inward. The patient may appear to be restless or nervous or seem overly controlled, even rigid.

In most instances, tension is chronic and has been present for at least six months. It may be situational,

that is, caused by an "unhealthy" family, work, or peer group situation. It may be nonspecific—tension which is present but the person does not know why. When the reason is known, the person might be in an avoidance–avoidance or approach–avoidance conflict. These conflicts are difficult to resolve, since there is a perceived negative or harm component in them.

The effort to prevent bodily or psychic harm may result in aversive behaviors with which the dentist must deal. Typically the patient 1) is depressed about a situation, 2) feels isolated in the world, 3) denies that there is anything wrong, 4) wants to be dependent on someone else, 5) desires sympathy, and 6) may not want to be cured. With reference to the desirability of being cured, Marbach and Dworkin write (21), "the patient's persistent search for alternative mechanosurgical treatments may be a maneuver to give the illusion of seeking a cure." To the extent that these maneuvers are successful, the patient is not compelled to deal with the underlying psychodynamic conflicts.

The psychophysiologic theory is a powerful one. It involves an individual's emotional state in the etiology of the myofacial pain dysfunction syndrome. While it helps to explain possible relationships, it does not answer all the questions where somatic disturbance has been eliminated as a causative factor. It is difficult to assess the degree to which psychologic factors affect the somata or to understand the strength of the behavior's resistance to change or extinction once it develops.

## Treatment

If the theory holds, and it seems to be holding, then the emotional factors which help to initiate the syndrome must be sought. The dentist is the key to such discovery. Perhaps the single most powerful tool which a dentist has in identifying causality is diagnostic skill. Asking questions in a consistent nonthreatening manner can be most effective. There are a number of content–behavior areas which should be explored:

1. History of the pain. When did it start? How has it progressed? What is its continuity? Is there a pattern related to it?
2. Severity of the pain. How much pain is experienced? When? What is its duration?
3. Personal Factors. What was happening in the person's life when the pain began—death of a relative, injury, retirement, marriage, job loss, or relocation?
4. Continuing factors in the situation which cause stress. What is happening to you now? Last week?

It is particularly important to assess the stress component of the patient's life. Holmes and Masuda have expanded on the nonspecific pain theory of Selye and have developed a life stress checklist which can provide a stress score at any point in time (Table 16–1). The theory states that stress is definitely related to ill health and that the more stress one is under, the greater the propensity for illness. Holmes and Masuda (16) state,

the magnitude of life change is observed to be highly significant of life crisis. There is a strong positive correlation between magnitude of life change (life crisis) and seriousness of the *chronic* illness experienced.

It is interesting to note that Holmes and Masuda have assessed the impact of their stress scale across cultures and that the ranking of valued events is fairly consistent.

While the dentist is not expected to cure the patient of a stressful condition, the dentist's awareness of its cause can aid in the development of treatment modalities for the patient with the myofacial pain dysfunction syndrome. These modalities might involve operative or surgical procedures, and they should involve psychologic support as a precursor to other action. Psychologic support is rendered through 1) active listening, 2) empathetic understanding, 3) respectful questioning, and 4) nonverbalization of warmth. It states to the myofacial pain dysfunction patient that "I understand that you are in pain. I am willinng and capable to help you assess the cause of it. If possible, I will help you to obtain relief from it."

Relief may be obtained surgically or psychologically through various modalities. Among the more common

**Table 16-1. The Stress of Adjusting to Change**

| EVENTS | SCALE OF IMPACT |
| --- | --- |
| Death of spouse | 100 |
| Divorce | 73 |
| Marital separation | 65 |
| Jail term | 63 |
| Death of close family member | 63 |
| Personal injury or illness | 53 |
| Marriage | 50 |
| Fired at work | 47 |
| Marital reconciliation | 45 |
| Retirement | 45 |
| Change in health of family member | 44 |
| Pregnancy | 40 |
| Sex difficulties | 39 |
| Gain of new family member | 39 |
| Business readjustment | 39 |
| Change in financial state | 38 |
| Death of close friend | 37 |
| Change to different line of work | 36 |
| Change in number of arguments with spouse | 35 |
| Mortgage over $10,000 | 31 |
| Foreclosure of mortgage or loan | 30 |
| Change in responsibilities at work | 29 |
| Son or daughter leaving home | 29 |
| Trouble with in-laws | 29 |
| Outstanding personal achievement | 28 |
| Wife begins or stops work | 26 |
| Begin or end school | 26 |
| Change in living conditions | 25 |
| Revision of personal habits | 24 |
| Trouble with boss | 23 |
| Change in work hours or conditions | 20 |
| Change in residence | 20 |
| Change in schools | 20 |
| Change in recreation | 19 |
| Change in church activities | 19 |
| Change in social activities | 18 |
| Mortgage or loan less than $10,000 | 17 |
| Change in sleeping habits | 16 |
| Change in number of family get-togethers | 15 |
| Change in eating habits | 15 |
| Vacation | 13 |
| Christmas | 12 |
| Minor violations of the law | 11 |

(Holmes T, Masuda M: Life change and illness susceptibility. Separation and Depression. AAAS, 161–186, 1973)

modalities are hypnosis, acupuncture, biofeedback, behavior modification, and/or brief individual or group psychotherapy.

**HYPNOSIS.** In its broadest form hypnosis—general relaxation—is useful in redirecting a patient's awareness, altering the patient's mental set, and offering an opportunity for refocusing a patient's expectations and attitudes. In its extreme form, according to Joy and Barber (17), it is an altered state of consciousness characterized by a narrowed, heightened level of attention and the enhanced ability to accept suggestions uncrit-

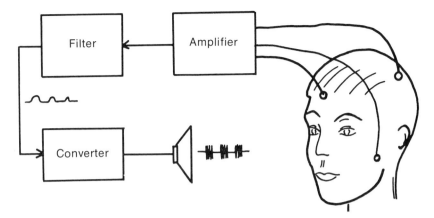

**FIG. 16-2** Schematic rendition of the feedback loop.

ically, including suggestions to relieve pain. Hypnosis has been used in the dental office for pain control, but it has been called other things, namely, successive relaxation, deep suggestion, image making, and the like. With an increased awareness of the psychologic overtones to dental fear, anxiety, and pain, hypnosis is gaining increased acceptance.

Hypnosis can be used for analgesia in the dental office and subsequently for reduction of pain associated with the myofacial pain dysfunction syndrome if the syndrome is not of an organic nature. Reducing or eliminating the pain if there is organic interference or tissue destruction can compound the problem. Barber (13), in the *American Journal of Clinical Hypnosis*, reported the development of a rapid analgesia induction system which is highly effective in the dental office. Whether or not hypnosis can lead to long-term positive effects for the myofacial pain dysfunction patient is questionable, especially since the psychologic overtones of the syndrome are so strong.

**BIOFEEDBACK.** Patients may learn to use biofeedback to control anxiety, frustration, despair, and other emotional reactions which can influence the normal functioning of the body. By definition biofeedback is an instrumented learning process for relaxation of the facial muscles; it is useful for treatment of bruxism, temporomandibular joint dysfunction, and pain control.

The basic concept is described by Rugh, Perles, and Desraeli (23): "A patient is provided continuous, detailed information about his bodily functions of which he is normally not aware. Given such information, the patient can learn to control specific body functions." The more accurate and consistent the information is, the better able the individual will be to do something

about it. The "doing something about it" closes the feedback loop (Fig. 16-2).

Rugh and his colleagues (23) utilized the biofeedback device in their efforts to identify stressors in the environment of patients with oral irritations. Of their 15 patients, 10 showed significant clinical improvement. All of the patients became more aware of their stressors (interaction with employer, children coming home from school, pending divorce, etc.)

The advantage of biofeedback in managing the patient with myofacial pain dysfunction syndrome is that it helps to break a habit which will result in destroyed tissue. By alerting the patient at the time destructive behavior is occurring, the person can stop and redirect energy.

**INDIVIDUAL OR GROUP PSYCHOTHERAPY—COUNSELING.** It could be effective to couple the treatment modality selected for the myofacial pain dysfunction with one-on-one counseling or even with group counseling. In this situation, the hypnotic and biofeedback modes would become primarily diagnostic aides for the skilled clinician to identify causes (problems) of the stressors which are believed to be triggering the MPD syndrome. Secondarily, they can be used to control the pain or to change damaging habits while attempts are made to improve the patient's ability to cope with the stressors.

Group and individual psychotherapy should be carried out only by competent therapists. The dentist can aid the patient by being an active–attentive listener, but the patient with chronic myofacial pain dysfunction may be better served if referred to such a therapist while dental treatment is planned. The dentist must ultimately make the decision regarding mode of treatment, and a referral is an acceptable mode.

18. The theory which supports behavioral interaction with somatic reactions is termed
    1. specific pain theory
    2. tooth muscle theory
    3. psychosomatic theory
    4. psychophysiologic theory

19. The psychophysiologic theory is based on the belief that pain occurs because of
    1. muscular fatigue
    2. dental irritation
    3. tension
    4. All of the above

20. The primary cause of myospasm is believed to be
    1. muscular over- or underextension
    2. tension
    3. headaches
    4. faulty diet

21. The myofacial pain dysfunction patient tends to be profiled as
    1. hyperkinetic
    2. hyperactive
    3. hypoactive
    4. anxious

22. The tension which is present in a myofacial pain dysfunction patient is typically
    1. acute and readily defined
    2. chronic and readily defined
    3. chronic and not readily defined
    4. Both 1 and 2

23. The single most significant contributor to adult stress is
    1. divorce
    2. change in a job
    3. death of spouse
    4. marriage

24. The life stress theory was developed by
    1. Selye
    2. Dworkin and Marbach
    3. Coury and Wittemann
    4. Holmes and Masuda

25. The life stress theory states that the greater the magnitude of change, the
    1. less the chance of ill health
    2. more severe the ill health will be
    3. greater the probability that disease will occur
    4. less the stress after health has been restored

26. The best modality for managing myofacial pain dysfunction patients is
    1. hypnosis
    2. biofeedback
    3. group counseling
    4. individual counseling

## CHILD–FAMILY–DENTIST INTERACTION

In managing children, the dental team should seek to provide positive experiences to the uninitiate. Bakwin and Bakwin (28) and Wright (51) have written two of the better texts on children's dental behavior, the role of the family in children's attitudes, and the interactions between children and the dental team. Both texts view the child as a positive force in the setting. They tend to take a humanistic–developmental approach to the management of the child and play down the psychoanalytic and behavioristic persuasions.

### Psychologic Theories

The model used by the psychoanalytic group, which stems from the work of Freud, is termed the medical model. It is a disease-oriented framework through which behavior could be explained. Erratic, anxious, "bad" behavior is treated either as a symptom of underlying psychologic dysfunction or as a manifestation of libidinal, instinctual energy which must be sublimated into socially acceptable channels or suppressed. In the dental office the untoward behavior of a child—whining, kicking, crying, yelling, flailing of arms—is seen as behavior to be suppressed or otherwise eliminated.

The behavioral school of psychology, greatly influenced by Skinner, is an empirical model. Its laws are based on observation, and in turn the behaviors are classifiable, hence definable. Behaviorists assume that it is possible to describe all behaviors in terms of objective observable events. Where the behavior is not describable through observation, a hypothetical construct is established to summarize the behavior pattern. Anxiety as a construct would include behaviors such as restlessness, sullenness, tenseness, jumpiness, etc., which are measurable (observable). The behaviorists then devise strategies to manage each of the component behaviors, and as each component is eliminated, the larger behavior pattern disappears. Unfortunately, the development of constructs, the decision strategies, and the implementation of them are difficult to do in practical dentistry—there simply is not enough time.

The humanistic approach to child management is perhaps the most effective one for the dental practitioner. It tends to view behavior as a part of the living complex developed through interaction with others, events in the environment, personal history, and genetic potentials. It recognizes behavior as a part of the child's reaction to a larger world. It rejects the medical disease model of the psychoanalyst and the fragmented, value-free approach characteristic of the behavioral model. It incorporates society in its framework. The humanists, study the healthy person, concentrating on those behaviors, qualities, and values which make him or her unique. Rather than studying specific behaviors, they study the individual's behavior as related to communication, motivations, perceptions, emotions, and beliefs. From these studies have emerged constructs which describe the self-actualized person (39), the fully functioning person (43), and the loving person (40).

Instead of perceiving anxiety as a negative value, or at best a neutral value, humanists see it as a positive force. Anxiety is viewed as a part of life, a legitimate coping response to threat of punishment, physical harm, or the unknown. In this sense the stimulus serves to energize the being to action, and the action is termed anxiety. It is both a warning system and a motivator. As a warning system, it is essential for well-being; as a motivator, it can save lives.

## Enter the Child

Before the child's behavior in the dental situation can be understood, the dentist must have some knowledge about the child's developmental stage and developmental tasks.

### CHILD DEVELOPMENT
#### Stages
#### Birth to 18 Months

The child has a strong tendency to become attached to another person, usually the mother.

The child's essential motives (drives) are physiologically oriented.

The child seeks "significant other" for relief from pain, food, and protection.

The child becomes more self-sufficient and begins to explore the larger world which is enhanced due to contact with mother.

Stranger anxiety develops at 7–8 months because of the child's uncertainty in which is perceived as being familiar.

Separation anxieties develop at 10–11 months due to unexpected absence of the mother.

If nurtured, the child develops attitudes of trust and affection and displays decreasing anxieties in mother's absence.

#### 18 Months to 3 Years

The child first encounters the demands of society.

The child discovers or learns about dangers.

Rules are discovered and tested.

The child encounters discipline.

The child learns to conform to rules of society and becomes toilet trained.

Through rewards and punishments the child learns *not* to do some things (inhibits forms of behavior).

The child becomes anxious over the prospect of punishment or losing affection from mother.

Through anxieties, the child becomes a social being.

The child identifies very closely with mother.

Separation anxiety persists if the child feels sufficiently insecure in his or her relationship to mother or if the child is overprotected.

The child plays alone to age 24 months.

#### Preschool Years: 4 and 5

The child uses language concepts.

The child begins to roam outside and play more regularly *with* other children.

The child develops first feelings of guilt, which represents the working of the conscience mechanism.

The child discovers boys and girls.

The child tries on specific sex-related roles.

The child needs and thrives on praise and other rewards.

The child molds behavior to avoid disapproval, punishment, or possible anxiety.

The child identifies with parents and tries to imitate them.

#### The Child and Peers: 6–10

The child's world expands significantly.

The child can accept extended separation from the familiar (mother, siblings, neighboring peers).

The child experiences formal systems of control.

The child experiences conflict with parent surrogate, especially boys who have a female teacher but identify with father.

The child experiences fear or failure.

Peers influence the child via comparisons of assigned roles and a sharing of mutual attitudes.

The child acquires patterns of dominance or submissiveness.

The child responds to self-set standards such as being valued by parents and peers, mastery of physical and mental skills, behavior appropriate to sex typing, and cognitive consonance between thought, word, and behavior.

The child continues to be anxious, relative to these self-set standards and develops preferences for various defenses against those anxieties. The most prominent coping mechanisms are withdrawal, denial, and compensation.

The child who does not cope well begins developing symptoms of neurosis found in later life—ticks, compulsive behaviors, obsessions, psychosomatic ailments.

The child is capable of performing a wide range of motor skills, has mastered language, is knowledgeable, and has developed a personality.

***Developmental tasks.*** Gilmore (47) has organized many of the developmental behaviors around tasks which a child needs to accomplish.

| Work | Explore and manipulate immediate environment. Acquire language and concepts. |
| --- | --- |
| Interpersonal relations | Approach others. Allow others to approach. Differentiate family, friends, and strangers. |
| Aloneness | Allow mothering person out of sight. Stand and walk alone. Separate sense of "me-ness." Play alone. |

***Developmental Tasks and Learning.*** Erikson (30) has developed a model which incorporates behaviors and learning, and relates learning to developmental tasks. He has established his model around eight dichotomies which must be reconciled as the child grows: 1) basic trust versus basic mistrust, 2) autonomy versus shame and doubt, 3) initiative versus guilt, 4) industry versus inferiority, 5) identity versus role confusion, 6) intimacy versus isolation, 7) generativity versus stagnation, and 8) ego integrity versus despair.

Psychosocial development proceeds through critical steps. Ages are critical in the sense that they are characteristic of turning points between progress and regression, integration and retardation. Each age can be represented in a ratio format; that is, a favorable ratio of basic trust over basic mistrust is the first step in psychosocial adaptation, a favorable ratio of autonomous will over shame and doubt, the second step, etc.

Each being comes to the stage, meets the crisis in it, finds the solution, and progresses to the next stage. All ages must be ascended to: The child must move through the first three on the way to adolescence. The degree of ascendance should be in the positive direction with the ratios favoring the positive aspects in development.

***Individual Development.*** Peters (42), in reviewing the development of the individual, identifies nine processes of personal development which tend to be basic to an individual's behavior pattern. The way these processes are used tends to differentiate the individual.

*Looking.* The infant learns to recognize those things which give pleasure or cause distress and to differentiate between familiar faces and places and those which are strange. Subsequently the infant learns the meaning of gestures—the frown and the smile—and interprets movements to and away. Inferences drawn from what the infant is watching may give the scene frightening importance.

*Listening.* Listening is certainly one of the basic experiences. It is in the privacy of listening that meaning is given to what is heard. By looking and listening children see the importance or lack of importance of doing what they are told. When children listen to an adult saying one thing and doing something else, they learn that "talk is cheap."

*Thinking.* Perhaps one of the most crucial processes, thought can mediate, make real, or dismiss that which is seen or heard. The fundamental cognitive skills of children become the backbone of complex operations, such as applying one kind of information to something else, putting two bits of information to derive a third, or evaluating the quality or integrity of the information given.

*Feeling.* Feelings are facts. A process of feeling develops in the same way that other processes develop. An individual who understands his or her own feelings learns to respond more effectively and more appropriately.

*Searching for Meaning.* The search for one's reason for being is critical at all ages of man. A child seeks to find his or her place in relation to parents, siblings, and peers, through a variety of trial and error activities. The number and types of successes (or failures) in these activities provide evidence for "who I am" and "where I am going." Although transitory, each encounter with the meaning of oneself contributes to the next; the child becomes a synergistic expression of all encounters—the good and the bad.

*Valuing.* Establishing a set of values involves the process of looking, listening, thinking, and feeling. To a great extent, parents are responsible for inculcating values. Children tend to value what their parents value—good health, money, attractiveness, religion, education, etc. As a child grows to adolescence, early values are questioned, redefined, and in some cases discarded. Values pertinent to good health (oral hygiene) are formed early in life, as early as age 5. Habits emanating from these values take a bit longer to establish, however.

*Focusing.* Children and adolescents (even adults) focus, attend directly, on events or people that are important to them. A child will focus on one parent, a toy, or a new situation to find relative meaning in it—relative to him or her. As the child grows older, focusing is extended to peers, school, churches, teachers, and significant others in the child's life. Focusing on events, such as a first dental visit, a shot from a physician, or a trip in a plane, can have significant impact on subsequent behavior.

*Choosing.* Choosing is the result of all the other processes. The child, adolescent, and adult must make decisions. Failure to choose leaves the decisions in the hands of someone else (autonomy versus dependency). Not all choices are pleasant, but they must be made. It is particularly difficult for a child to make choices about routine health matters, or for that matter, about what to eat, where to live, what to wear, and the like. Yet by being involved in discussions relating to such choices the child learns (models) the processes involved in making the choice.

*Becoming.* All the previous processes interact in the individual's total development as he or she is becoming the best person possible. This process does not ignore the past nor does it deny the present. It relies on the influences drawn from each experience—encounters with significant people or significant events.

**IMPACT ON DENTAL SITUATION.** Since the ages and stages do impact on the dental situation, Dworkin (29) suggests some guidelines for the dentist:

Age 0–2: The dentist should use secure and consistent physical support with slow, careful movements.

Age 2–4: Simple explanations can be given to the 4-year-old. This child also responds to appeals and to fantasy.

Age 4–6: The 4- to 6-year-old child can be treated as an adult—both through verbal and nonverbal communications.

Age 7–9: Long-range behavior change can be reinforced by schedules and checkpoints. The child approaching age 9 is willing to repeat tasks and perfect skills.

Age 10–12: Frequent praise still goes a long way, but realistic feedback can be given when the child does not perform well.

Age 12–18: A viable interpersonal relationship is the best lever for reaching the adolescent with persuasive communications.

### Enter the Parent

Adult behaviors influence child behaviors (34, 33, 49, 48, 31). In fact, Shoben and Barland (45) have stated that the single most important inculcator of attitudes relative to dental health or dental fear is the family. Moreover, Johnson and Baldwin (33) have reported that there is a significant relationship between a mother's anxiety and her child's cooperative behavior in a dental office. In other words; if Mom is nervous, the greater the chance that the child will be nervous (26, 35). This transference of anxiety is more pronounced with children 3–4 years old (48, 49), although there is some negative behavior in older children who are accompanied by nervous, anxious mothers (26).

**MANAGING THE ANXIOUS PARENT.** Most dentists are not overly concerned about a child's anxiety per se; what is of concern is the destructive and dysfunctional behavior which can be caused by anxiety. If the paren-

tal anxiety proposition holds, then the dentist or a member of the staff must prepare the parent for her child's visit to the dentist. Some approaches that have been tried with varying degrees of success include a preappointment consultation, a preappointment letter, or simply additional consideration at the time of the visit.

Much of the mother's anxiety revolves around her own personal experiences, her fears, and her concern for her child. Many of the anxious behaviors are due to the unknown—not knowing what might happen, anticipating problems, and not knowing how to prepare herself or her child for the experience (44). The dentist, or even a secretary or receptionist, can put the parent at ease by calmly discussing the procedures, expectations, and protocols for the dental visit. Attending to questions parents have in a straightforward way is very helpful in preparing them for their child's visit.

The preappointment letter (46, 48, 26, 42) can help a mother relax and prepare her child for a dental visit. Parents typically acknowledge such thoughtfulness by being more attentive to the requests of the dentist, which permits the dentist to be in better control. An appropriate letter should contain the dentist's appreciation for the mother's attention to the child's oral health needs and for being selected as the child's first dentist, a brief description of what will be done at the first visit, expected behavior, a general statement relating oral health to health in general, and an invitation to call if she has any questions.

A highly anxious mother finds it difficult to get the child to the office. Some times such a mother finds it difficult to stay, and if this is the case, the child's needs may be better served if the mother is elsewhere. It is imperative that a parent be recognized as highly anxious so that he or she can be greeted in person and made to feel relaxed, if possible. The child of this parent should receive immediate attention so that the child's attention is diverted from the anxious parent to some other object or event.

At the time of entry to the office, the focus must change from the mother to the child. This can be accomplished by 1) conducting an oral health history with the mother in a private section of a waiting room or preferably in the dentist's consultation room, 2) conducting a preliminary oral examination in the consultation room with the mother present, and 3) continuing the examination with the mother out of the treatment area.

**MANAGING SEPARATION.** As stated earlier, separaiton anxiety appears when the child is about 10–11 months old and may persist through age 5. Many children have resolved their dilemma by age 3, however. This depends upon the development of basic trust, autonomy, and initiative. It is the dentist's responsibility to recognize the varying perceptions of the child and parent. Helpful nonverbal clues include observations relative to 1) closeness to parent (on lap, clinging to legs and arms), 2) huddled or closed body position, and 3) the child being quiet and intense or staring as opposed to playing with available toys, exploring the office, smiling and generally being active. It must be emphasized, however, that not all quiet children are anxious children, nor are all active children nonanxious. Some children and adults do a lot of pacing to reduce their anxiety.

If the dentist perceives that a child is anxious and the mother is in control, she can become an ally in the treatment room. On the other hand, if she is the cause of much of the anxiety, she can help create chaos. In this case it is better to deal with the separation anxiety than the panic of two individuals.

The control factor is unique in managing the 3- and 4-year-old. Since the child is in the process of identifying (36) with like sex roles—boys with fathers (other males) and girls with mothers (other females)—the dentist should use this to advantage. If the child patient is a boy, a male dentist will have an advantage if he asserts himself and if in fact the boy has a father model at home. Similarly, if the child patient is a girl, a female dentist will have an advantage in dealing with the child. The dentist's knowledge about the child prior to the visit can also help in making management decisions. The dentist should be aware of

1. prior surgical procedures the child has had. Children with a history of prior surgery have a greater incidence of fear and anxiety.
2. prior health problems. Children who have had chronic ailments or repetitive acute ailments for which they were treated by a physician tend to be more anxious.
3. family relationship and parental concerns as discussed earlier.
4. socioeconomic or ethnic background. Differences in religion, ethnic origin, and family size can have an impact on the child's self-concept and parental responses.

### Enter the Dentist

There has been considerable research undertaken on the personality, values, interests, attitudes, and the like of the aspiring dental professional. (For a rather complete review see Hollinshead BS: *Survey of Dentistry*. Washington, DC: American Council on Education, 1962.) Little, however, is written about the interaction of the dentist with the anxious mother and anxious child patient. Yet the literature admonishes the dentist and the dental team to communicate with the parent and child, be a good model for the child, maintain

control in the situation, and try to make the experience comfortable for both the child and the parent. Ideally the dentist should also be relaxed and comfortable. There are some principles which may be followed to meet all these demands in treating the child.

**COMMUNICATION WITH THE CHILD.** Effective communication with the child is the precursor to all other techniques in managing the child. For the anxious child patient the nonverbal dimension of communication takes on great importance. Communication goes beyond conversation when touch, eye contact, and appropriate body posture is used. Touch can satisfy warmth; eye contact, sincerity or strength; and body posture, a willingness to meet the child at his or her level. Certainly the voice—choice of words, tonality, intensity, and the other verbal dimensions—are crucial to effective rapport with the child. Transmission should be constant, phrases short and precise, and the speech slow.

The terminology or jargon of dentistry is lost on a young child. Emotionally charged words such as air blast, x-ray film, and anesthetic can be replaced by words like wind, tooth picture, sleep juice. Because words such as hurt, pain, scratch, and pick have different meanings for different children, it is helpful to get the child's interpretation of the energized words in advance.

At times short and rapid commands followed by a physical act such as shaking one's hand or rapping a counter top can have a positive effect. The startle response can interfere with aversive behavior. The dentist must be ready, however, to capitalize on that second by once again becoming the controlled but kind dentist.

**BEHAVIOR MODIFICATION—SHAPING THE CHILD'S BEHAVIOR.** Behavior modification is a slow and deliberate process designed to alter the behavior of the child. It is a technique which attempts to teach the child what behavior is expected in the dental setting. At the same time it is an attempt to alleviate aversive reactions and apprehensions. The most widely used method is the tell–show–do technique developed by Addelston (25). (This method is equally effective for adults.) The procedure encourages the utilization of language appropriate to the child's age, ability, health knowledge, background, etc. delivered in a precise and slow manner as many times as necesary. It is nonpunitive in the sense that the child is given the freedom to err during the learning process. The showing aspect depicts the activity to be undertaken. Again, this is done in a quiet, matter-of-fact manner; any movement should be undertaken slowly. The gradual and ordered demonstration of what is to come is a desensitizing technique. By the time the patient has been talked to, shown, and has vicariously experienced the procedure through the voice of the dentist, the child should be ready for the actual performance of the procedure.

It is important to note that the verbal and nonverbal messages that accompany this technique should be reinforcing. Words and phrases like great, that's good, right, and the like, accompanied by a gentle touch or smile, are helpful in shaping the response. These positive reinforcers should occur as frequently as possible and must be coincident with the child's desirable behavior. To observe a positive action and then delay the gratification for 5–10 min is like not giving the reinforcer at all.

Every dental visit should be perceived as an opportunity for shaping behaviors, altering old, undesirable behaviors or helping to reinforce those desirable behaviors which have been forgotten.

**RETRAINING.** Sometimes a very anxious or frightened child has developed aversive behaviors at earlier visits to another dentist. The "new" dentist must shift his or her training (skill or behavioral development) emphasis. Since retraining is difficult, the dentist is not expected to change or modify the behavior at one sitting. Retraining demands the identification of the causes for the child's fears, avoiding the causes which trigger those fears, and displacing the aversive behaviors through reinforcement. Avoidance of the triggers is difficult, however, since some procedures must be accomplished. Preparation of the child requires a careful choice of words, phrases, and sequences of action.

**AVERSIVE METHODS OF RESTRAINT.** It is inevitable that a time will come when the dentist must physically restrain the child. Restraint is carried out by physically preventing aversive (interfering) behavior. The most common form of aversive restraint is the Hand Over Mouth Exercise (HOME):

1. It is used to gain control over the child.
2. It is used to reduce wild aversive behaviors.
3. It is not a scientifically proven method.
4. It does work.
5. There is no scientific evidence that it causes trauma.
6. It is a technique and as a technique it must be done correctly.

Levitas (38) describes it well:

I place my hand over the child's mouth to muffle the noise. I bring my face close to his and talk directly into his ear. "If you want me to take my hand away, you must stop screaming and listen to me. I only want to talk to you and look at your teeth." After a few seconds, this is repeated, and I add, "Are you ready for me to remove my hand?" Almost invariably there is a nodding of the head. With a final word of caution to be quiet, the hand is removed.

As it leaves the face, there may be another wail with the garbled request, "I want my mommy." Immediately the hand is replaced. The admonition to stop screaming is repeated, and I add, "You want your mommy?" Once again the head bobs. And then I say, "All right, but you must be quiet, and I will bring her in as soon as I am finished. O.K.?" Again, the nod—and the hand is slowly lowered. My assistant is always present during HOME to help restrain flailing arms and legs so that no one is physically injured. By restraining the child he can be made aware of the fact that his undesirable coping strategies are not necessary or useful.

While the child is composing himself, I begin to talk—about his clothes, about his freckles, about his pets, about almost anything, and no reference is made to what has gone before. As far as I am concerned, that is done and over. If there is an attempt on the part of the child to start again, a gentle but firm reminder that the hand will be replaced is usually enough to make him reconsider. It is sometimes difficult to convey HOME with the written word, for voice control and modulation are essential for HOME to be most effective.

The HOME method is a conditioning technique. Maladaptive behaviors (kicking, thrashing, hitting) are coupled with an unpleasant experience (HOME with modification; i.e., nose pinch, towel). It is hoped the action will reduce the probability of maladaptive behavior in the future. In order for it to work, since it involves punishment, it should be 1) precise, 2) physically relevant, and 3) constantly in contact with the child. Certainly, anyone giving punishment to change a behavior takes a risk. It can evoke additional fear, reinforce previously held fears, and result in continued avoidance of the dental situation. In essence, this technique has the potential to reaffirm the child's belief that dentists are not nice people and that dental offices are no place to go.

The best approach is one based on an honest communication between child, mother, and doctor. Positive attention during the child's early dental experiences will develop a healthy adult patient. It also aids in establishing health oral hygiene patterns out of the dentist's office. A summation of a total communication model is presented by Moss (41). In "On Communicating" Moss states:

I think of communication with parents and children as having three essential parts:
THE TRANSMITTER–The Dentist
THE AIRWAY–The Office Environment
THE RECEIVER–The Parent or Child
Each of these parts can be modified to help persuade for prevention.
*Transmitter*
—Send the message over a short distance by getting close to the parent or child.
—Send the message in a calm steady voice.
—Don't stand over the parent or child while talking with her.
—Keep the messages short.
—Keep your body in a relaxed position; it is talking for you.

### Airway

—Use soft background music, nothing too upbeat. There is already enough excitement in treating children.
—Maintain an environment that does not have too much "static" or distraction.
—Use chairs that are uncomplicated, and do not have too many cords and instruments around.
—Ask assistants not to move around while you are talking—parents' and children's attention wander toward movement.

### Receiver

—Use repetition. It helps keep the child–patient tuned in. By rephrasing an idea you can repeat it without seeming to be repetitious.
—Have child hold a mirror. It helps keep them tuned in and turned on.
—Let them be in a comfortable position without a light in their eyes.
—Use the rubber dam. It helps the parent and child see and understand what is being done.

The key elements are:
—Relay your message at eye level with the parent and child.
—Keep the message short and send it in a calm, steady voice.
—By rephrasing your ideas on good oral hygiene, you can repeat them and make a greater impact on the child patient.
—You can create an environment that will make the child more responsive to suggestions. It should be as calm and free from distractions as possible.
—Get the child involved by using a mirror, so that he can see what is going on.

## The Child at Home

As Herzberg (32) has stated, a person cannot be motivated; a person must motivate him- or herself. Yet people can be *moved* to act. The question which must be resolved regarding the oral health behaviors of children outside the dental office is whether the child should become intrinsically motivated or whether they should perform the behaviors which adults see as being in the children's best interest. Obviously they should do both. The first is far more difficult than the latter because it is so difficult for a child to control extraneous variables which interfere with the development of self-motivation.

Moving a child to action is far easier. Herzberg claims that "hygiene factors" in the environment reinforce desirable behaviors. Such factors as having toothbrushes and toothpaste available, understanding the reasons for oral hygiene, and having parents committed to a preventive philosophy moves the child to action. Such a model reflects the steps of habit formation:

1. Knowledge, that is, understanding the etiology of disease and the consequences of nonattentiveness to disease prevention.
2. Interest. In order to act, an individual must have some excitement about the process of the behavior being learned.
3. Belief in the value of the behavior. An individual not only must be excited about the behavior but also must see and feel that doing it is in his or her best interest. There should be repeated, concrete, and empirical verification.
4. Commitment. Belief is usually not enough to support action until it becomes a part of the individual's life and philosophy.
5. Action. Learning is manifested in overt behavior. Permanent learning requires commitment, and commitment is best demonstrated through action.
6. Habit. An action repeated successfully over time results in a habit, the ultimate step.

A child tends to become interested in that which is new or different. Since a child's attention span is limited, the interest waxes and wanes with different situations or stimuli. It becoms the parents' responsibility (with support of the dental staff) to help the child maintain interest in dental care, realize its goodness, and ultimately commit him- or herself to it. Without action this will not happen.

Baldwin (27) presents a series of behavioral targets for the 3- to 8-year-old child. The targets relate to responsibilities of the child, parent, and dentist regarding home care, dental treatment, and eating habits (Table 16–2).

### QUESTIONS

27. The psychoanalytic model of child development is the
    1. dental model
    2. medical model
    3. health model
    4. preventive model

28. The arch supporter and exponent of the behavioral school of psychology was (is)
    1. Freud
    2. Maslow
    3. Rogers
    4. Skinner

29. The behavioral model stresses the
    1. humanistic approach to child rearing
    2. classification and objectivication of behavior
    3. libidinal energy derived from anger
    4. the freedom of man to choose behavior

30. The humanists study the person who is
    1. sick
    2. pathologic
    3. healthy
    4. young

## Table 16-2. Behavioral Targets

| | THE CHILD WILL | THE PARENTS WILL | THE DENTAL STAFF WILL |
|---|---|---|---|
| For home care | Brush his or her teeth for a specified period of time and frequency, using a method appropriate for his or her age level | Provide the items required for the child's toothbrushing procedures<br><br>Oversee and periodically evaluate the child's toothbrushing practices as to method, duration, and frequency; adjust supervision in accord with performance<br><br>Brush the child's teeth and clean between his or her teeth with dental floss at least once daily until the child can accomplish these procedures effectively | Assess the homecare practices and determine the extent to which the child's practices are supervised<br><br>Correct any deficiencies in the home care practices of the child and parent<br><br>Stimulate parents to select a proper toothbrush and guide them toward having the child use an ADA-recognized dentifrice |
| For dental treatment | Accept dental treatment as a part of growing up by cooperating with the dentist and staff during the dental appointment by doing what is requested, i.e., sitting still, listening to the dentist, keeping his or her hands down, opening his or her mouth as needed | Utilize dental care services available for their family<br><br>Obtain appointments for the child's first and succeeding dental appointments and periodic examinations<br><br>Make arrangements for and see that the child keeps scheduled appointments<br><br>Help prepare the child for all dental visits in a positive manner<br><br>Accept the child management procedures of the dental facility<br><br>Accept the child's treatment proposed by the dental staff | Orient the parents and child to the dental office environment and to the general office treatment procedures<br><br>Explain to the parents the child's dental needs and the proposed treatment plan<br><br>Explain to the child all treatment procedures before they are initiated (tell–show–do)<br><br>Praise the child for good behavior |
| For eating habits | Restrict sweets and other decay-producing foods to mealtimes or special occasions or both<br>Restrict between-meal snacks to low-decay-producing items | Buy food items that provide the family with a low-decay-producing diet<br><br>Offer only low-decay-producing food items for between meal snacks<br><br>Restrict sweets and other decay-producing snacks to mealtimes or special occasions | Assess, on a routine basis the child's progress toward restricting sweets and between-meal snacks<br><br>Make a dietary analysis for children with complex dietary or decay problems<br><br>Make recommendations for improvement in eating practices |

(Baldwin DC Jr: The young child. In Dworkin S (ed): Persuasive Prevention. New York, MEDCOM, 1975)

31. The humanists perceive anxiety as
1. at least neutral
2. having positive value
3. debilitating
4. Both 1 and 2

32. During development a child moves through some specific
1. stages
2. tasks
3. events
4. All of the above

33. Most values are pretty well established by age
1. 3
2. 5
3. 10
4. 15

34. At what age is it safe to assume that a child has resolved the mother absence crisis, unless the child is insecure in the relationship with the mother?
1. 2
2. 5
3. 3
4. 4

35. Stranger anxiety develops between age
    1. 5–6 months
    2. 7–8 months
    3. 9–10 months
    4. 10–11 months

36. Separation anxiety develops at about age
    1. 5–6 months
    2. 7–8 months
    3. 9–10 months
    4. 10–11 months

37. Separation and stranger anxiety is represented in which age of man?
    1. First
    2. Second
    3. Third
    4. Fourth

38. The key to effective child control is
    1. imparting threats and fear
    2. developing rapport with the parent
    3. attending to the child
    4. Both 1 and 2

## THE HANDICAPPED CHILD

The Developmental Disabilities Services and Facilities Construction Act defines developmental disability as a disability attributed to mental retardation, cerebral palsy, epilepsy, or other substantially chronic neurologic condition either closely related to mental retardation or requiring similar treatment. The flexibility of this definition encompasses learning disabilities such as dyslexia, deafness, or impaired vision, and gross motor functioning and motor coordination. In general, disabilities are found in combination, that is, two-thirds of handicapped children have two or more handicaps.

### Mental Retardation

Mental retardation is not a classification of an individual's ability to function. It is a diagnostic term representing a combination of signs and symptoms. The intelligence quotient (IQ), which is found by dividing the child's mental age (figured via testing) by his or her chronological age (year and month) and multiplying the result by 100, is but one of the diagnostic signs. The three other signs or criteria are 1) significant impairment in adaptive behavior: language usage and development, school achievement, social adjustment–emotional control, and sensory motor skills; 2) combination of an IQ of less than 70 with impaired adaptive behavior; 3) presence of an IQ less than 70 prior to 18 years of age (54).

The IQ involves a score taken on one of several standardized developmental tests. The most frequently used tests for children in the first 3 years of life are the Cattell, Gesell, and Bayley Tests. They indicate normal and below normal functioning. The Stanford–Binet Test can be used for children and adolescents (ages 2–16), and the Wechsler Intelligence Scale for children can be used for nearly the same group (ages 5–16).

Although an intelligence test can give an indication of differing intellectual functioning, it is important to note that it is but one of the predictors. Even within a single test variations which can alter the diagnosis can occur. For example, the Stanford–Binet and Wechsler scales include a number of subtests to measure different aspects of mental functioning. If the child tests uniformly at a level within the normal range on all the subtests, then it can be assumed that the child is able to perform adequate school work. If the score is depressed—at below normal score—then it is imperative to examine each subtest in order to discern if one or all of the functions are subnormal. Such tests should be administered and analyzed by a professional.

Grossman (56) defines an individual with deficits in adaptive behavior as one who does not possess the personal independence and social responsibility expected of his or her age and cultural group. Independence and social responsibility may be measured by developmental tasks (milestones) such as talking, walking, eye movement, recognizing and approaching specific objects, transferring objects by using overhand movement, cooperating in getting dressed, developing table manners, and reading aloud. In adulthood these tasks are more complex and include gaining economic independence, earning a living wage, and the like.

The developmental period is relegated to the first 18 years of life. It is the time frame when most developmental tasks must be achieved so that the individual can function as an adult.

CLASSIFICATION. The mentally retarded are classified into four categories by the American Association of Mental Deficiency (56). The categories are based on scores obtained via standardized intelligence measures. They are 1) the educable mentally retarded, 2) the trainable mentally retarded, 3) the severely mentally retarded, and 4) the profoundly mentally retarded.

*Educable Mentally Retarded.* Typically the educable mentally retarded (EMR) are culturally deprived individuals. The deprivation (social, educational, nutritional, familial) results in an inability to manage the academic demands made of them. These children are readily recognized as early as first grade when they are confronted by examinations and IQ measures. Education with special attention to skill development should include the child's parents so that they can reinforce the messages and provide support. The goal in working with the EMRs is social and economic independence.

*Trainable Mentally Retarded.* The trainable mentally retarded (TMR) develop 40%–60% of normal intelligence and reach a mental age (via testing) of 4–8 years of age by adulthood (chronological age equals 21 years of age). TMRs are readily identified during infancy and early childhood because of a severe developmental lag, especially in language skills. They rarely use two-word sentences until they are beyond 4 years of age. Yet they can develop functional reading and writing skills. The goals for this group are to enhance their self-help skills and to increase their social skills so that they can live and work in a sheltered environment.

Often accompanying low intelligence are a number of undesirable and antisocial behaviors due to organic brain damage. Many of the children have short attention spans, can tolerate a minimum of frustration, and are easily distracted. In addition, they may display behaviors which resemble psychiatric disorders, i.e., head banging, rolling and rocking, finger display before eyes, kicking and biting, and mumbling and screaming.

The TMR can be trained to perform basic functions at a rudimentary level. The most effective tool currently available is behavior modification through the use of rewards and token economies.

*Severely/Profoundly Mentally Retarded.* The severely and profoundly mentally retarded are more seriously impaired than the TMRs. The primary goal for these children is to maximize their communication and social skills. Since only limited training is possible, these children require constant attention and care.

ACCOMPANYING SIGNS. Capute (54) reports that many of the trainable, severely, and profoundly mentally retarded children have certain physical characteristics in common. Among the features are

1. Hirsutism—excessive amounts of hair over body parts
2. Ossification disorders—delayed bone age, microcephaly, malformed or dysplastic teeth
3. Clinodactyly—medial or lateral curvature of the finger or toe
4. Brachydactyly—stubbiness of fingers or toes
5. Carotenemia—jaundiced look of skin

Language development is a key indication of a child's developmental progress. The Language Milestone Test (Table 16–3) is used at the J. F. Kennedy Institute.

## Other Disabilities

CEREBRAL PALSY. Cerebral palsy "is disorder of movement and posture resulting from a permanent nonprogressive defect or lesion of the immature brain" (52). In other words, it is descriptive of brain pathology produced during the developmental years (including the results of trauma) which involves those areas in the brain which regulate movement, posture, and function.

*Incidence.* Variance is significant; at birth it varies from 0.6 to 5.9 per 1000 (depends on source); among children aged 5–15 years it varies from 0.6 to 2.4 per 1000.

*Classification.* The Academy for Cerebral Palsy (57) established seven classifications of cerebral palsy. In brief they are

1. Physiologic—spasticity (the most common), athetosis (slow, ceaseless, sinuous, writhing movement), rigidity, ataxia (failure of muscle coordination), tremor, atonia (deficient muscle tone), and mixed types
2. Topographic—monoplegia, paraplegia, hemiplegia, triplegia, quadriplegia, diplegia, and double hemiplegia
3. Etiologic
4. Supplemental
5. Neuroanatomic
6. Functional
7. Therapeutic

The two most common classifications are the physiologic and topographical ones, and occupational and physical therapists provide treatment to the extremities affected. The topographical classification, if known by the dentist, can be helpful in the dental management of the child. For example, the hemiplegics have a higher risk of associated neurologic deficits such as visual field blindness and hearing loss. The quadriplegics are usually more mentally involved and have a lower incidence of convulsion. The paraplegics or diplegics usually have an even lower incidence of convulsions and better mentation than the quadriplegics (54).

MINIMAL CEREBRAL DYSFUNCTION. Minimal cerebral dysfunction, which includes learning disabilities and dyslexia (54), is also referred to as minimal brain damage, hyperkinetic syndrome, Strauss–Lehtin syndrome, minimal cerebral palsy, choreiform syndrome, or the brain damage syndrome. A syndrome is a set of symptoms which occur together or the sum of signs of any morbid state. Among the signs that occur in a child with minimal cerebral dysfunction are 1) behavioral aberrations such as inattention, emotional lability, impulsiveness; 2) "soft" neurologic findings such as asymmetric reflexes, left–right disorientation, wide variety of rapid, highly complex jerky movement; 3) slow wave (EEG) activity in posterior hemisphere of brain (53); 4) wide scattering of mental functioning with large dis-

**Table 16–3.  Developmental Language Milestone**

| AGE | DEVELOPMENTAL MILESTONE | QUESTIONS ASKED OF PARENTS |
|---|---|---|
| 1 mo | Alerting response to sound | At what month did your infant recognize the presence of sound by either blinking, startling, moving any part of the body, etc.? |
| 4–6 wks | Social smile | At what age did your infant look at you when you were talking to him or her or stroking his or her cheek or chin? |
| 4 mos | Orienting response to sound (voice) | At what age did your infant turn toward sound? |
| 6–7 mos | Babbling ("mama" and "dada" inappropriately) | At what age did your infant vocalize "mama" and "dada" but was not using it appropriately? |
| 7–8 mos | Gesture language | At what age did your infant wave "bye–bye" or play "pat-a-cake"? |
| 9–11 mos | "Mama" or "dada" appropriately | At what age did your infant use "mama" and "dada" appropriately? |
| 11 mos | First word | At what age did your infant say his first word other than "mama" and "dada"? |
| 12 mos | Two-word vocabulary | At what age did your infant say two words? |
| 14 mos | Three-word vocabulary | At what age did your infant say three words? |
| 15 mos | Two to six words; immature jargon | At 15 months what was your infant's vocabulary? or At what age did your infant have a two- to six-word vocabulary? At what age did your infant run unintelligible words together in an attempt to make a sentence? (Imitate for parents) |
| 18 mos | 2 to 20 words; mature jargon | At what age did your infant have a 2- to 20-word vocabulary? or How many words did your infant use at 18 months of age? At what age did your infant run many unintelligible words together in an attempt to say a sentence, but you did note several intelligible words said? (Imitate for parents) |
| 21 mos | Two words together | At what age did your infant put two words together? |
| 24 mos | 50 or more words; two word sentences using pronoun or noun (appropriately) and verb | How many words did your child use appropriately at 2 years of age? What is your estimate of your child's vocabulary at 2 years of age? At what age did your infant use a noun or pronoun (inappropriately) along with a verb, such as "me go" or "me like"? |
| 30 mos | Pronouns used appropriately | At what age did your infant use pronouns appropriately? |
| 36 mos | 200-word vocabulary; three-word sentences; plurals formed | What was your child's vocabulary at 36 months? When did your child use three-word sentences? When did your child use plurals? |
| 48 mos | Ability to tell stories and describe experience; interest in the meaning of words, particularly, abstract ones | At what age did your child tell stories? At what age did your child start asking the meaning of words? |

(Capute AJ: Developmental disabilities: an overview. In Fox L (ed): Dentistry for the Handicapped Child, D.C.N.A., Philadelphia, WB Saunders, 1974, p 1515)

crepancy between verbal and performance scores, combined with auditory and visual perceptual disabilities.

Approximately one-half to two-thirds of the children with minimal cerebral dysfunction have perceptual–cognitive impairments which result in a learning disability. A child with a learning disability is not globally retarded, but rather has a specific perceptual–cognitive disability which results in a specific retardation or disorder in one or more of the speech or language processes. Specific dyslexia is a disability in a child who is unable to learn to read with normal facility despite normal intelligence, intact senses, proper instruction, and normal motivation.

Approximately 10% of school children have minimal cerebral dysfunction. The majority of these become learning disabilities. The primary dyslexics comprise 0.5%–3% of this group. Dyslexia is more common in males than females.

## Implications for Dentistry

It is estimated that approximately 4 million American families are affected by a child who is either mentally or perceptually disabled or both. Of this group, only a small percentage is institutionalized (58); the rest are found within the community. Although they are all entitled to regular, routine, and high quality dental care, two powerful constraints continue to operate against the fulfillment of it. They are 1) the lack of dentists who possess the skills and knowledge necessary to manage the handicapped and 2) the community–family resources necessary to get the children to the office (60).

The number of dentists who are treating noninstitutionalized disabled children must be increasing. (Although this is difficult to document, the dental literature on this topic has increased since 1970). Some management strategies have shown promise in dealing with the educable and trainable mentally retarded. The key to all of the techniques—behavior modification, shaping, retraining, and the like—is the dentist's relationship with the child's family (59). Among the factors which must be considered are

1. Parental attitude regarding the child's disabilities
2. The child's behavioral history—aberrations
3. The child's health history
4. The parent's fear
5. The presence or absence of siblings and their attitudes
6. The parent's own health, dental, emotional history
7. The parent's understanding of child–parent–dental team capabilities and responsibilities

### Treatment Protocol for Behavior

A child who is seriously mentally retarded and is also hyperactive should be restrained. Troutman (59) indicates that the Pedi wrap is among the best restraints available. Should wraps not be available, the parent or hygienist or other team member should help control the child. A second form of restraint is premedication. Drugs used to control (quiet or stabilize) behavior can be helpful when dealing with a potentially active child, but a caution in the type and dosage of drug is essential because of possible untoward reactions.

**TECHNIQUES FOR BEHAVIOR MODIFICATION.** Among the strategies that can be used with the educable trainable mentally retarded children are shaping, prompting, fading, and chaining. These strategies are designed to effect long-term change and must be accomplished over a longer period of time. They are essential for developing new behaviors.

*Shaping.* Shaping is a technique whereby desired behavior is specified in objective terms and analyzed into its components. After accomplishing the component part, the child is reinforced.

*Prompting.* If the child makes no voluntary response to the desired behavior, some form of physical prompting may be used.

*Fading.* Fading involves shifting the physical prompting to the verbal command. That is, if the dentist wants the child to be still and says "lie still," while holding the child's shoulders, it will be necessary to "fade" out the tactile stimulus of the shoulders, while accentuating the verbal message.

*Chaining.* A series of relatively discrete behaviors which have been individually shaped are linked together to make a complex behavioral chain. A series of

behaviors may be 1) being on time for the appointment, 2) walking to the treatment room, 3) climbing into the chair, 4) sitting in the chair, 5) opening the mouth.

**BEHAVIOR MODIFICATION PROGRAM.** It is quite possible to incorporate these techniques into a more formal behavior modification program. Drash (55) suggests a procedure for designing such a program:

*Identification of the Desired Target Behavior or Terminal Response Repertoire.* In the dental setting, the overall behavior goal is usually the same for most children, that is, to have the child walk quietly and voluntarily into the dental office, get into the treatment chair, and sit quietly and cooperatively during treatment.

*Identification of Specific Behaviors To Be Produced or Conditioned.* Using the desired terminal behavioral repertoire as a guide, the initial behavior of the child is evaluated in order to determine what new behaviors must be produced. For example, a child may be generally pleasant and cooperative, but may totally refuse to get into the treatment chair. This then becomes the immediate target behavior to be shaped.

*Identification of Undesirable Behaviors To Be Weakened or Eliminated.* Many children who are considered behavior management problems exhibit a relatively large number of undesirable behaviors. While many of these behaviors, such as screaming, may be incompatible with the acquisition of good dental behavior, others, such as a generally negative attitude, may not be. The task of the dentist is to identify in precise operational terms those behaviors which must be decreased in frequency before dental work can proceed.

*Determination of Effective Reinforcers.* Since the success of a behavior modification program rests heavily upon the availability of appropriate reinforcing stimuli, it is essential to identify at the outset those reinforcers which will control the behavior of the child. This can be accomplished relatively quickly and efficiently through the procedure termed **reinforcement sampling.** The child is given an opportunity to look at, hold, taste, or listen to a variety of potential reinforcers which the dentist has available. Such a display is termed a **reinforcement lieu.** Those items in which the child displays high interest will in most cases serve as reinforcers.

*Determination of Procedures for Recording, Timing, and Tabulation of Data.* Although formal tabulation of behavioral data may not be necessary in all cases, behavior modification programs are based upon the premise that the reinforcement procedures used will, in fact, produce a measurable change in the frequency of the target behavior. An effective data recording system will give immediate feedback regarding effectiveness of the program. If no measurable change in the target behavior occurs, the procedures must be modified. While major changes in behavior, such as a rapid and dramatic decrease in the rate of crying, can be observed without benefit of measuring devices, other changes in behavior, such as a slight increase in the length of time that a child keeps his mouth open, may be impossible to assess without benefit of mechanical recording devices. It is therefore desirable to have available as minimum equipment a stopwatch, a counter, and a data sheet on which to record behavior frequency on a time base.

***Outlining the Reinforcement Program or the Shaping Sequence.*** After the basic details of identifying target behaviors, reinforcers, and recording procedures have been completed, the next step is to outline, either formally or informally, a tentative sequential program for moving the child from the baseline performance level to the desired target behavior. This is the heart of the behavior modification program and must be individually tailored to each child. This usually involves an identification of the various behaviors required to reach the final target performance and a sequencing of the behaviors in a logical step-by-step fashion so that at each stage of the reinforcement program, the child has mastered all of the previous steps. The initial program serves as a guide to action, but it should be considered tentative in the sense that if during programming it becomes obvious that the sequence should be changed or that additional behaviors are needed, appropriate revisions are made in the program (11).

### QUESTIONS

39. A mother brings her son to your office. Upon casual observation, you note some behavior which is in your estimation not normal. He is very erratic, displays jerky movements, and tends to mumble to himself. Your initial reaction is to
   1. classify him as being mentally retarded
   2. reserve judgment until you are able to interview the child and parent
   3. move him to the treatment room immediately so as to avoid other patients' negative reactions
   4. ignore him

40. Mental retardation is a disability which involves
   1. deficiency in intelligence
   2. impaired adaptive behaviors
   3. a chronic condition prior to age 18
   4. All of the above

41. The most common class of mental retardation is the
   1. trainable mentally retarded
   2. educable mentally retarded
   3. severely/profoundly mentally retarded
   4. chronic mentally retarded

42. Among the most common symptoms which the mentally retarded have in common are
   1. excessive amounts of hair over body parts
   2. delayed bone age
   3. delayed language development
   4. medial or lateral curvature of the fingers

43. If language milestones are not met on time, it means that the
   1. child is definitely retarded
   2. child needs tutoring
   3. child will become retarded
   4. child did not meet milestones on schedule

44. The language milestone test
   1. specifies absolute dates at which the language should develop
   2. provides a sequence of general linguistic development
   3. is a guide for observing linguistic development
   4. Both 1 and 3

45. The two most common classifications for cerebral palsy are
   1. etiologic and therapeutic
   2. etiologic and physiologic
   3. physiologic and topographic
   4. topographic and therapeutic

46. A learning disability is
   1. a specific retardation in one or more processes of language development
   2. an inability to think
   3. another term for global retardation
   4. All of the above

47. The key to the dentist's ability to work with a mentally retarded child is
   1. knowledge of the child's health history
   2. the dentist's relationship with the child's family
   3. the parents' attitude toward the child
   4. knowledge of the child's behavioral history

48. A child who kicks, flails, or exhibits other gross body movements should be
   1. allowed to wear him- or herself out
   2. premedicated
   3. restrained
   4. Both 2 and 3

49. A technique in managing a child whereby the desired behavior is specified, objectivized, analyzed, and reinforced is
   1. prompting
   2. fading
   3. chaining
   4. shaping

## REFERENCES

### DENTAL FEAR AND ANXIETY

1. BANDURA A: Principles of Behavior Modification. New York, Holt, Rinehart & Winston, 1969
2. CURRIER F: The child and adolescent: new rights for an old minority. In Wittemann JK (ed): Practical Behavioral Considerations, DCNA. Philadelphia, Saunders, 1977

3. DWORKIN SF, FERRENCE TP, GIDDON DB: Behavioral Science and Dental Practice. St. Louis, CV Mosby, 1978
4. KRASNER L, ULLMANN LP: Research in Behavior Modification: New Developments and Implications. New York, Holt, Rinehart, & Winston, 1965
5. LEVINE S: Stress and behavior. Sci Am 224:26–31, 1971
6. MARBACH JJ, DWORKIN SF: Chronic MPD, group therapy and psychodynamics. J Am Dent Assoc 90:827–832, 1975
7. ROGERS C: On Becoming a Person. Boston, Houghton Mifflin, 1961
8. SELYE H: The stress syndrome. Am Jr News 65:97–99, 1965
9. SMELTZER CH: Psychology for Student Nurses. New York, Macmillan, 1962
10. TROTTER, R: Stress, Sci News 107:356–359, 1975
11. WITTEMANN JK: Behavioral implications in successful dietary counseling. In Nutrition D.C.N.A. Philadelphia, WB Saunders, 1976
12. WEBMAN B: Psychological component of pain perception. In Pain D.C.N.A. Philadelphia, WB Saunders, 1978

## STRESS RELATED OROFACIAL PAIN

13. BARBER J: Rapid induction analgesia: a clinical report. Am J Clin Hypn 19:138, 1977
14. COSTEN JB: Syndrome of ear and sinus symptoms dependent upon disturbed function of temporomandibular joint. Ann Otol Rhinol Laryngol 43:1, 1934
15. GREEN CS, LERMAN M, SUTCHER H, LASKIN D, et al: The TMJ pain dysfunction syndrome: heterogeneity of the patient population. J Am Dent Assoc 79:1168, 1969
16. HOLMES T, MASUDA M: Life change and illness susceptibility. Separation and Depression. AAAS, 161–186, 1973
17. JOY ED, BARBER J: Psychological, physiological, and pharmacological management of pain. In Wittemann JK (ed): Practical Behavioral Considerations, D.C.N.A. Philadelphia, WB Saunders, 1977
18. LASKIN DM: Etiology of the pain-dysfunction syndrome. J Am Dent Assoc 79:147–153, 1969
19. LUPTON DE: A preliminary investigation of the personality of female temporomandibular joint dysfunction patients. Psychother Psychosom 14:149, 1966
20. LUPTON DE: Psychological aspects of temporomandibular joint dysfunction. J Am Dent Assoc 79:131, 1969
21. MARBACH JJ, DWORKIN SF: Chronic MPD, group therapy and psychodynamics. J Am Dent Assoc 90:827–833, 1975
22. MOULTON RE: Psychiatric considerations in maxillofacial pain. J Am Dent Assoc 51:408, 1955
23. RUGH JD, PERLES DB, DESRAELI RI: Biofeedback in Dentistry: Research and Clinical Application. Phoenix, Semantodondics, 1977
24. SCHWARTZ LL: Pain associated with the temporomandibular joint. J Am Dent Assoc 51:394, 1955

## CHILD-FAMILY-DENTAL INTERACTION

25. ADDELSTON HK: Child patient training. Fortnight Review, Chicago Dental Society, 38:7–8, 27–29, 1959
26. BAILEY PM, TALBOT A, TAYLOR PP: A comparison of maternal anxiety levels with anxiety levels manifested in the child dental patient. J Dent Child 40:277–84, 1973
27. BALDWIN DC JR: The young child. In Dworkin S (ed): Persuasive Prevention. New York, Medcom, 1975
28. BAKWIN H, BAKWIN R: Clinical Management of Behavior Disorders in Children. Philadelphia, WB Saunders, 1967
29. DWORKIN S (ed): Persuasive Prevention. New York, Medcom, 1975
30. ERIKSON E: Eight ages of man. In Lavatelli CS, Stendler F (eds): Readings in Child Behavior and Development. New York, Harcourt Brace Jovanovich, 1972, pp 19–30

31. HAWLEY B, MCCORKLE AD, WITTEMANN JK, et al: The first dental visit for children from two socioeconomic families. J Dent Child 41:376–381, 1974
32. HERZBERG F, MAUSNER B, SNYDERMAN B: The Motivation to Work. New York, John Wiley & Sons, 1959
33. JOHNSON R, BALDWIN D: Maternal anxiety and child behavior. J Dent Child 36:87, 1969
34. JOHNSON R, BALDWIN DC: Relationship of maternal anxiety to the behavior of young children undergoing dental extraction. J Dent Res 47:801–805, 1968
35. JOHNSON R, MACHEN JB: Behavior modification techniques and maternal anxiety. J Dent Child 40:20–24, 1973
36. KAGAN J: The concept of identification. In Musen P, Conger JJ, Kagan J (eds): Readings in Child Development and Personality. New York, Harper & Row, 1970
37. KAGAN J, HAVEMANN E: Psychology: An Introduction. New York, Harcourt Brace Jovanovich, 1972
38. LEVITAS TC: HOME—Hand over mouth exercise. J Dent Child 41:178, 1974
39. MASLOW A: Toward a Psychology of Being, 2nd ed. Princeton, Van Nestrand, 1968
40. MAY R (ed): Existential Psychology. New York, Random House, 1961
41. MOSS SJ: In Dworkin S (ed): Contemporary Dentistry: Persuasive Prevention. New York, Medcom, 1975
42. PETERS HJ: Processes of personal developing in adolescence. In Peters HJ, Bathory MJ: School Counseling: Perspectives and Procedures. Itasca, FE Peacock, 1968
43. ROGERS CR: On Becoming a Person. Boston, Houghton Mifflin, 1961
44. SALK L: What Every Child Would Like His Parents to Know. New York, Warner Paperback Library, 1973
45. SHOBEN E JR, BARLAND L: An empirical study of the etiology of dental fears. J Clin Psychol 10(4):171, 1954
46. TUMA CF: How to help your child be a good dental patient: an open letter to parents. J Dent Child 21:81–84, 1954
47. TYLER LE: The Work of the Counselor. New York, Appleton-Century-Crofts, 1969
48. WRIGHT GZ, ALPERN GD, LEAKE JL: Modifiability of maternal anxiety as it relates to children's cooperative behavior. J Dent Child 40:265–271, 1973
49. WRIGHT GZ, ALPERN GD: Variables influencing children's cooperative behavior at the first dental visit. J Dent Child 38:126–128, 1976
50. WRIGHT GZ: Children's behavior in the dental office. In Wright GZ: Behavior Management in Dentistry for Children. Philadelphia, WB Saunders, 1975
51. WRIGHT GZ: Behavior Management in Dentistry for Children. Philadelphia, WB Saunders, 1975

## THE HANDICAPPED CHILD

52. BAX MCO: Terminology and classification of cerebral palsy. Dev Med Child Neurol 6:295, 1964
53. CAPUTE AJ, NEIDEIMYER CFL, RICHARDSON F: The electroencephalogram in children with minimal cerebral dysfunction. Pediatrics 41:1104, 1968
54. CAPUTE AJ: Developmental disabilities: an overview. In Fox L (ed): Dentistry for the Handicapped Child, DCNA Philadelphia, WB Saunders, 1974, p 1515
55. DRASH PW: Behavior modification: new tools for use in pediatric dentistry with the handicapped child. In Fox L (ed): Dentistry for the Handicapped Child, DCNA. Philadelphia, WB Saunders, 1974, p 617–632
56. GROSSMAN HJ (ed): Manual on Terminology and Classification in Mental Retardation. Baltimore, Garamound/Pridemark Press, 1973
57. MINEAR WL: A classification of cerebral palsy. Pediatrics 18:841, 1956

58. Mental Retardation Source Book. Washington DC, Department of Health, Education and Welfare, US Printing Office, 1973
59. TROUTMAN K: Behavioral management of the mentally retarded. In Wittemann JK (ed): Practical Behavioral Consideration, DCNA. Philadelphia, WB Saunders, 1977
60. YOUNG WO, SHANNON JH: Providing dental treatment for handicapped children. J Dent Child 35:225–240, 1968

# SUGGESTED READING

## DENTAL FEAR AND ANXIETY

FOX L (ed): Dentistry for the Handicapped Child, DCNA. Philadelphia, WB Saunders, 1974

GORDON T: P.E.T.: Parent Effectiveness Training. New York, PW Wyden, 1970

HOLLINSHED BS: Survey of Dentistry. Washington DC, Am Council on Education, 1962

KAGAN J, HAVEMAN E: Psychology and Introduction. New York, Harcourt Brace Jovanovich, 1972

LAVATELLI CS, STENDLER F: Readings in Child Behavior and Development. New York, Harcourt Brace Jovanovich, 1972

MUSSEN PH, CONGER JJ, KAGAN J: Readings in Child Development and Personality. New York, Harper & Row, 1970

WRIGHT GZ: Behavior Management in Dentistry for Children. Philadelphia, WB Saunders, 1975

## CHILD-FAMILY-DENTIST INTERACTION

ADELSON R, GOLDFREED MR: Modeling and the fearful child patients. J Dent Child 37(6): 34, 1970

AYER WA: Use of imagery in needle phobic children. J Dent Child 39:34, 1972

CHAMBERS DW: Managing the anxieties of young dental patients. J Dent Child 37:5, 1970

CRAIG W: Hand over mouth technique. J Dent Child 38:387, 1971

GORDON T: Parent Effectiveness Training. New York, Wyden, 1970

GIFT H: Group persuasion. In Dworkin S (ed): Persuasive Prevention. New York, Medcom, 1975

HILL FJ, O'MULLANE DM: A preventive program for the dental management of frightened children. J Dent Child 43:30–36, 1976

JENKS L: How the dentist's behavior can influence the child's behavior. J Dent Child 31:358, (4th Quarterly), 1964

KOENGSBERG SR, JOHNSON R: Child behavior during three dental visits. J Dent Child 42:33–36, 1975

LEVITAS CC, STENDLER F: Readings in Child Psychology. New York, Harcourt Brace Jovanovich, 1972

LAZARUS PS: Four Stress and Coping Processes. New York, McGraw-Hill, 1966

LENCHNER V: The influence of the family. In Wright GZ (ed): Behavior Management in Dentistry for Children. Philadelphia, WB Saunders Co, 1975

MARTIN RB, SHAW MA, TAYLOR P: The influence of prior surgical experience on the child's behavior at the initial dental visit. J Dent Child 44:35, 1977

OPPENHEIM MN, FANKEL SN: A behavioral analysis of the preschool child when introduced to dentistry by a dentist or hygienist. J Dent Child 38:17, 1971

SHAUMA PS, SHAUMA A: Psychological management of anxiety in young adults. J Dent Child 43:25–29, 1976

Techniques for behavior management—A survey. J Dent Child 39:34, 1972

WILLIAMS QE, CLARK CM: Securing cooperation from the child dental patient. J Dent Child 43:36, 1976

## THE HANDICAPPED CHILD

DICKS JL: Effects of different communication techniques on the cooperation of the mentally retarded child during dental procedures. J Dent Child 41:35–40, 1974

KOHLENBERG R, GREENBERG D, REYMORE L, et al: Behavior modification and the management of mentally retarded dental patients. J Dent Child 39:61–68, 1972

NOWAK AJ: The role of dentistry in the normalization of the mentally retarded person. J Dent Child 41:34–38, 1974

NUSSBAUM B, CARREL R: The behavior modification of a mentally disabled child. J Dent Child 43:39–45, 1976

## BEHAVIORAL SCIENCES/GENERAL

ANOTTI WR, GREIDER A: Applied Psychology in Dentistry, 2nd ed. St. Louis, CV Mosby, 1972

BONICA JJ (ed): Advances in Neurology: International Symposium on Pain 1, Vol 4. New York, Raven Press, 1974

CURRO FA (ed): Pain Dental Clinics of North America. Philadelphia, WB Saunders, 1978

DWORKIN SF, FERENCE TP, GIDDEN DB: Behavioral Science and Dental Practice. St. Louis, CV Mosby, 1975

MELZAK R: The Puzzle of Pain: Revolution in Theory & Treatment. New York, Basic Books, 1973

PROTELL MR, KRASNER JD, FABIKANT B: Psychodynamics of Dental Practice. Springfield, IL, CC Thomas, 1975

WITTEMANN JK (ed): Practical Behavioral Considerations, DCNA. Philadelphia, WB Saunders, 1977

## ANSWER KEY

| | | | |
|---|---|---|---|
| 1. 3 | 14. 3 | 26. 4 | 38. 2 |
| 2. 4 | 15. 4 | 27. 2 | 39. 2 |
| 3. 4 | 16. 3 | 28. 4 | 40. 4 |
| 4. 1 | 17. 2 | 29. 2 | 41. 2 |
| 5. 3 | 18. 4 | 30. 3 | 42. 3 |
| 6. 3 | 19. 4 | 31. 4 | 43. 4 |
| 7. 2 | 20. 2 | 32. 1 | 44. 3 |
| 8. 3 | 21. 4 | 33. 2 | 45. 3 |
| 9. 3 | 22. 3 | 34. 4 | 46. 1 |
| 10. 3 | 23. 3 | 35. 2 | 47. 2 |
| 11. 1 | 24. 4 | 36. 4 | 48. 4 |
| 12. 1 | 25. 3 | 37. 1 | 49. 4 |
| 13. 2 | | | |

ISBN 0-06-142658-X

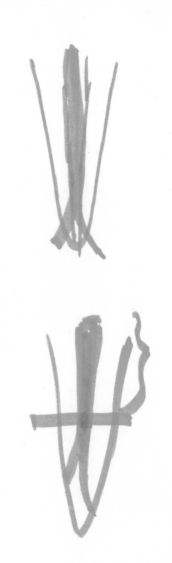